ULTRASOUND

The Core Curriculum

ULTRASOUND

WILLIAM E. BRANT, M.D.

Professor of Radiology
Chief of Thoracoabdominal Division
Department of Radiology
University of Virginia Health System
Charlottesville, Virginia

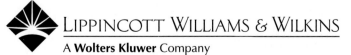
LIPPINCOTT WILLIAMS & WILKINS
A **Wolters Kluwer** Company
Philadelphia • Baltimore • New York • London
Buenos Aires • Hong Kong • Sydney • Tokyo

Acquisitions Editor: Joyce-Rachel John
Developmental Editor: Denise Martin
Production Editor: Sophia Elaine Battaglia, Silverchair Science + Communications
Manufacturing Manager: Benjamin Rivera
Cover Designer: QT Design
Compositor: Silverchair Science + Communications
Printer: Maple Press

Library of Congress Cataloging-in-Publication Data

Brant, William E.
    The core curriculum, ultrasound / William E. Brant.
      p. cm.
    Includes index.
    ISBN 0-683-30733-9
    1. Diagnosis, Ultrasonic. I. Title.

RC78.7.U4 B73 2001
616.07'543--dc21

               2001037732

Care has been taken to confirm the accuracy of the information presented and to describe generally accepted practices. However, the authors, editors, and publisher are not responsible for errors or omissions or for any consequences from application of the information in this book and make no warranty, expressed or implied, with respect to the currency, completeness, or accuracy of the contents of the publication. Application of this information in a particular situation remains the professional responsibility of the practitioner.

    The authors, editors, and publisher have exerted every effort to ensure that drug selection and dosage set forth in this text are in accordance with current recommendations and practice at the time of publication. However, in view of ongoing research, changes in government regulations, and the constant flow of information relating to drug therapy and drug reactions, the reader is urged to check the package insert for each drug for any change in indications and dosage and for added warnings and precautions. This is particularly important when the recommended agent is a new or infrequently employed drug.

    Some drugs and medical devices presented in this publication have Food and Drug Administration (FDA) clearance for limited use in restricted research settings. It is the responsibility of health care providers to ascertain the FDA status of each drug or device planned for use in their clinical practice.

10 9 8 7 6 5 4 3 2 1

I dedicate this book to my wife, Barbara, whose great love, titanic patience, and quiet vigilant support I treasure beyond words. She tolerated my "absence" without complaint during the uncountable hours it took to create this text. She served as my critic, copyeditor, and cheerleader and contributed immensely to its completion.

CONTENTS

PREFACE

Why should I write another ultrasound book when so many excellent ultrasound texts are already available? One niche that seemed underemphasized is a succinct, yet detailed and heavily illustrated, reference for the busy resident alone in the radiology department in the middle of the night. I submit this text with that goal in mind. I hope to follow the example set by my treasured friend, Clyde Helms, in his self-proclaimed "comic book," *Fundamentals of Skeletal Radiology*. This text is loaded with images to provide ready comparison and recognition. It expands the coverage of ultrasound begun in our *Fundamentals of Diagnostic Radiology* text.

Normal anatomy is emphasized because it is the foundation on which the abnormal is recognized. We must recognize what it is that we are looking at and the subtle and dramatic anatomic variations from normal before we can identify and interpret the abnormal. Ultrasound requires a systematic and detailed inspection of anatomy using a small field-of-view. The mind must be connected to the hand and the hand to the eye to keep pace with the changing image as we position the transducer and visualize moving structures within the living patient.

Important and diagnostic sonographic findings for pathological conditions are listed in bullet format with the intent of stating the findings clearly and succinctly while making them memorable. Descriptions of pathology are intentionally limited because full-length renditions are easily found in other texts.

It is my hope that radiologists, sonographers, and, most important, radiology residents find this text useful in learning sonography and comforting as a middle-of-the-night reference.

A great joy of performing ultrasound imaging is associating with dedicated, highly motivated, and greatly talented sonographers. I have had the extreme pleasure of working with exceedingly gifted sonographers at a number of institutions. These sonographers are responsible for the majority of images included in this text. I wish to thank them for their talent and extraordinary efforts and express my appreciation for the privilege of working with them.

At David Grant United States Air Force Medical Center, Travis Air Force Base, California, I would like to thank Diane Green, Tammy (McMahon) Paliari, Christine (Mangabay) Winston, and LaVerne (Martin) Jones.

At the University of California Davis Medical Center, Sacramento, I would like to thank Michael Cronan, Lorelei Maslen, Anna MacKenzie, Robin Stading, Marvin Courtright, Elizabeth Taylor, Sylvia Crane, Mark Johnson, Moonju Choi, Kim Heiser, Katie Hogan, Wendy McGrew, Joanne Mazzone, and Evelyn Byrne.

At Harborview Medical Center, University of Washington, Seattle, I would like to thank David Green and Colleen Elerick.

At the University of Utah Hospital, Salt Lake City, I would like to thank Johanna Semon, Ida Williams, Naomi Cummings, Kathleen Donner, Deanna Hecker, Catherine Townsend, Jodee Winter, Ruth Zollinger, and Becky Weintraub.

My physician colleagues in ultrasound have provided much inspiration, insight, and consultation over the years. I wish to especially thank Drs. Terry Collins, John McGahan, Kirin Jain, Eugenio Gerscovich, Ted Dubinsky, Karen Lindfors, Ray Dougherty, Darryl Jones, Cathy Babcook, Mark Anderson, and Terry Coates for their encouragement and support.

I also wish to thank my friend and former fellow, Joel Gross, M.D., for his review and helpful suggestions for many of these chapters during their formative stages.

ULTRASOUND

ULTRASOUND BASICS— GETTING STARTED

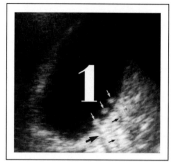

This chapter is *not* a grueling review of the sometimes tedious physics of US but is a discussion of "how to": turn on the machine, understand the US image, perform an examination, recognize and use US artifacts, and problem-solve when nothing seems to work. It is written to help the novice radiology resident deal with the sometimes terrifying nights on call alone in the hospital with surgeons hovering and the friendly sonographers at home in bed. The use and interpretation of Doppler US are covered in Chapter 11.

GETTING STARTED

Surely the most basic, but commonly ignored, aspect of learning to perform an US examination is how to turn on the machine. A wide variety of US units made by many different manufacturers are in everyday use. For reasons forever unknown, the power-on switch is often wickedly hard to find. The beginning student of sonography should spend 30 minutes of initial training with an experienced sonographer reviewing machine start-up, patient data entry, image storage, the procedure for changing transducers, and basic "knobology" for all the US units you are likely to use. Your expertise is immediately suspect, by both patient and referring physician, if you need to spend 10 embarrassing minutes finding the "on" switch.

US examinations are routinely performed by placing the transducer on the patient's skin. Because resistance to sound penetration is high at the skin surface, a sonolucent gel is used on the skin surface to promote sound transmission from the transducer into the patient through the skin. For patient comfort, the US gel should be kept warm in specially designed gel-warmers. For intracavitary US (transvaginal, transrectal), gel is placed on the transducer face. Then the transducer is covered with a sterile condom. The condom is in turn covered with additional sterile gel to promote sound transmission within the vagina or rectum. For intraoperative US, the exposed surgical bed is filled with sterile saline and the sterile condom-covered US probe can be placed directly on the structure of interest.

UNDERSTANDING THE US IMAGE

The design of the transducer determines the shape and field of view of the US image. Basic transducer formats are sector, linear array, and curved array (Fig. 1.1) [1]. **Sector** transducers produce slice-of-pie-shaped images that are narrow in the near-field but have a wide view in the *far-field*. These transducers are optimal for examining larger organs from between the ribs. Vector transducers are basically sector transducers with the tip of the pie-slice-image cut off. Vector transducers provide slightly wider near field of view than do sector transducers. **Linear array** transducers produce rectangular images with width of the image determined by the physical width of the transducer face. Linear array transducers often offer the best overall image quality and are preferred for examining anatomy in the *near-field*, just beneath the skin surface. **Curved array** transducers are a cross between linear and sector transducers providing a broader view in the near-field while retaining a broad view in the far-field. The transducer face is wide and gently curved.

All US images are obtained by using a pulse-echo technique (Fig. 1.2). All US transducers are sound transmitters and receivers. A brief (microsecond) pencil-beam-shaped pulse of US energy is directed into the patient. The transducer then becomes a receiver for echoes reflected back to the transducer from along the directed path of the US beam. All sound reflections detected are assumed to originate from the original "line-of-sight" of the

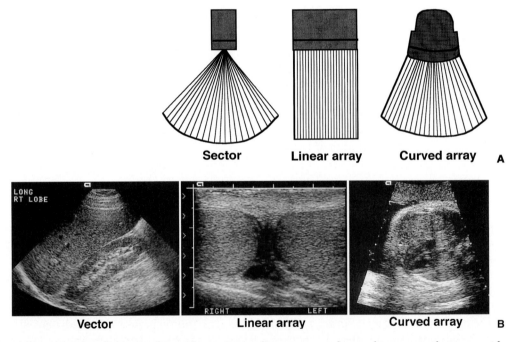

Figure 1.1 *Types of Ultrasound Transducers.* Sector, linear array, and curved array transducers provide differing shapes in the ultrasound field-of-view. *A.* Note that the US beams from sector and curved array transducers diverge as they penetrate deeper into tissue. This divergence decreases lateral (perpendicular to the US beam) resolution compared to the linear array transducer. *B.* **Sector** transducers are optimal for imaging large structures deep in tissue, such as the kidney. The small face of the transducer allows imaging through the narrow sonographic window of the intercostal spaces. The diverging field of view allows visualization of the entire kidney. True sector transducers produce a "piece-of-pie" shaped image originating from a point source on the transducer face as shown in *A.* **Vector** transducers are sector transducers with the origin of the image on the transducer face widened slightly as in *B.* **Linear** array transducers are optimal for visualizing smaller structures, like the testes, breast, and thyroid, that are just beneath the skin. The wider field-of-view in the near field improves visualization of these superficial structures. **Curved array** transducers combine advantages of the sector and linear formats. These transducers are optimally used when the sonographic window is broad, such as in the second and third trimester of pregnancy.

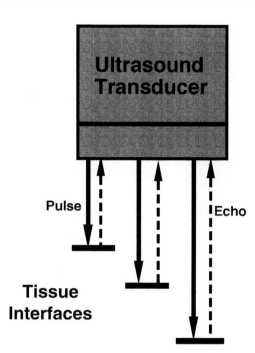

Figure 1.2 *Pulse-Echo Ultrasound.* The US transducer sends a series of US beams into patient tissue. The US image is produced by the pattern of reflected beams (echoes) detected. All echoes are assumed to originate along the "line-of-sight" of the originally transmitted beam. The depth of an echo is determined by measuring the round trip time-of-flight from beam transmission to echo reception. Assuming that the speed of sound in human tissue is a constant 1540 m/sec, the depth of an echo can be accurately plotted on the resulting US image.

transmitted beam. Sound reflections from directions other than the "line-of-sight" are either not detected or produce artifacts that impair image quality (Fig. 1.3). Dots (pixels) in the US image are placed along the "line-of-sight" according to the strength of each echo (brightness = sound intensity) and the time at which the echo is received. Depth is directly proportional to time of echo receipt. The US computer assumes that the speed of sound in tissue is a constant (**1540 m/sec**). Thus the depth of a sound reflector is determined by the time from pulse transmission to echo reception divided by two (allowing for the beam to go out and the echo to return).

US transducers are designed to operate at a specified sound frequency. Medical *ultrasound* is performed using very high sound frequencies in the range of 1–20 MHz. The best image resolution is obtained by using the highest frequency possible. However, the higher frequencies are more limited in ability to penetrate tissue. Thus, lower frequencies are often used, accepting lower resolution as a trade-off for better penetration.

Images are displayed on a computer monitor. During the infancy of diagnostic US there was some controversy whether images should be displayed as "white on black" or "black on white." White on black won. So virtually all gray-scale US images are displayed as tiny white dots on a black background (Fig. 1.4). Transverse images are routinely displayed with the

Higher frequency provides better image resolution. Lower frequency provides better tissue penetration. Therefore always use the highest frequency possible for the depth of the structure examined.

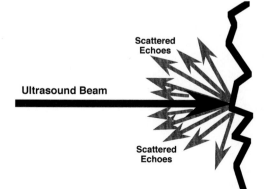

Figure 1.3 *Ultrasound Scatter.* As the US beam passes through tissue, it encounters irregular reflecting surfaces that scatter echoes in many directions. Only the echoes that return to the transducer at the site of origin of the US beam are displayed on the image. Progressive scattering of the echoes attenuates the sound beam as it passes deeper into tissues. Scattering of the echoes also degrades the US image and produces artifacts by multipath reflection.

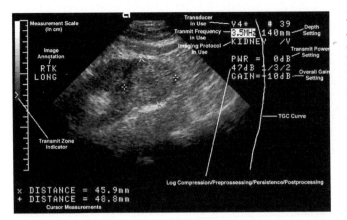

Figure 1.4 *Ultrasound Image Annotation.* This image is produced on an Acuson (Acuson Medical Ultrasound Company, Mountain View, CA) US unit and also shows the typical image annotation of technical settings used to produce the image. The nature of each annotation is indicated in small print. Other manufacturers have similar technical annotations. The image shows a renal cell carcinoma (*between cursors, +, x*) arising from the right kidney.

US images are displayed with the patient's right side or the patient's head toward the left side of the image.

patient's right side on the left side of the image as if we are examining the patient's cross-section anatomy from below looking upward toward the patient's head. This image display matches the convention for display of CT and MR images. Longitudinal images are displayed with the cranial aspect of the patient's anatomy at the left side of the image.

HOW TO SCAN

When first encountering a modern computerized US unit, any novice will be impressed with the number of knobs, switches, track balls, display screens, and gadgets to be used and mastered. To simplify the process and diminish the intimidation factor, I suggest the beginner concentrate on finding and using only the following, much reduced, list of controls. Concentrate on your scanning technique and optimize the use of these controls. Depend upon experienced sonographers to help you with the fine-tuning that produces the dramatic images in the "sonogenic" patient or saves the study in the nearly impossible-to-image patient.

THE KNOBS

Depth
The depth knob controls the deep portion of the field of view of the US image. As shown in Figure 1.4, the depth setting of 140 mm indicates the distance in the patient from the transducer face on the patient's skin to the curved bottom of the image. Depth should be adjusted to match the anatomy under inspection. Depth set too deep will minify the image, cramming the useful information into the top part of the image and wasting the bottom portion of the image. Depth set too superficial will fail to display the entirety of larger organs. You won't know where you are. Depth should be adjusted constantly to show the structure of interest and to optimize resolution (Fig. 1.5).

RES
RES (Resolution Expansion Selection) is another form of depth control. When the RES knob is pushed a RES box is displayed on the image (Fig. 1.6). Additional controls allow the operator to adjust the location and size of the RES box. When the RES knob is pressed a second time the image within the RES box is magnified to occupy the full image display. RES is useful for displaying and measuring small structures such as the common bile duct in the porta hepatis. RES is an Acuson (Acuson Medical Ultrasound Company, Mountain View, CA) trademark function. Other US manufacturers have similar functions identified by a variety of different names.

Gain
Gain is the US term for amplification. The intensity of returning echoes is amplified to produce a pleasing image. Gain is similar to the volume control on a stereo music system. Turn

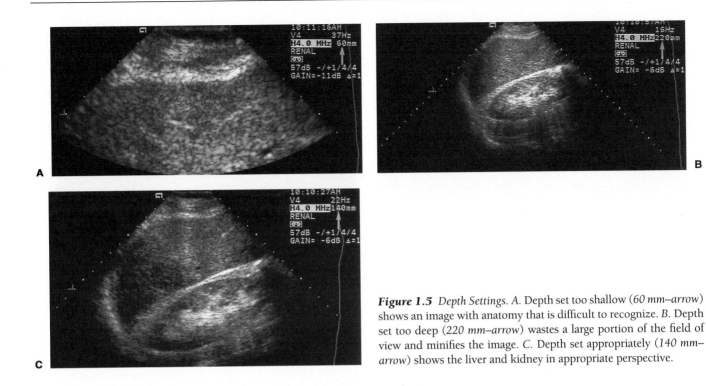

Figure 1.5 *Depth Settings. A. Depth set too shallow (60 mm–arrow)* shows an image with anatomy that is difficult to recognize. *B.* Depth set too deep (*220 mm–arrow*) wastes a large portion of the field of view and minifies the image. *C.* Depth set appropriately (*140 mm–arrow*) shows the liver and kidney in appropriate perspective.

gain up to produce an overall brighter image. Turn gain down to produce a darker image. Too much gain will display false echoes in cystic structures and make them appear complex or solid. Too little gain may make solid lesions appear cystic. One knob controls overall gain of the entire image. An array of time-gain-compensation (TGC) knobs controls gain at various depths in the image.

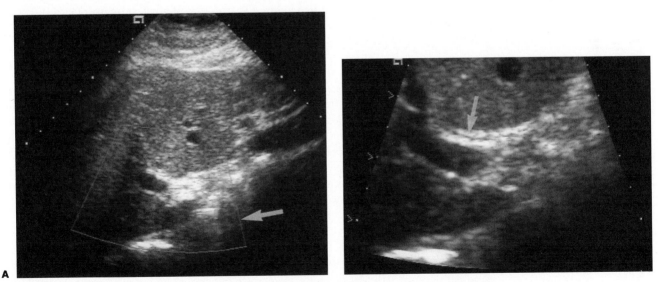

Figure 1.6 *Resolution Expansion Selection (RES) Function. A.* Image of the liver shows the porta hepatis. The portal vein and common bile duct are small structures, and their visualization is limited. The operator has placed a RES box (*arrow*) around the portion of the image to be magnified with improved resolution. *B.* By pressing the RES button a second time, the RES function is activated, and the anatomy of interest fills the image. Larger image size allows more accurate measurement of this normal common bile duct (*arrow*).

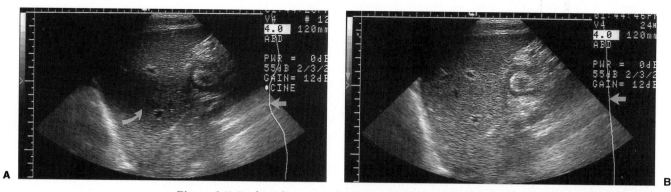

Figure 1.7 *Faulty Adjustment of Time-Gain-Compensation (TGC) Curve. A.* Image through the liver shows a central band of dark echoes (*curved arrow*) caused by faulty adjustment of the TGC curve (*short arrow*). *B.* Proper adjustment of the TGC curve (*short arrow*) produces a uniform appearance to the liver. Note that image resolution is the best at the level of the transmit zone (*long arrow*).

Time-Gain-Compensation

As the US beam travels deeper in tissue, its intensity is progressively attenuated by tissue absorption of sound energy and by scattering of the beam in different directions by tissue interaction. To compensate for this loss of sound energy, the returning echoes are progressively amplified proportional to the time of their return to the transducer. Echoes from deeper in the tissue return later to the transducer and are amplified to a greater degree. This method of amplification is called *time-gain-compensation.*

The controls for TGC are a series of sliding knobs corresponding to depth in the image. Gain can be individually adjusted for multiple levels of depth. The resulting TGC curve is often displayed on the side of the US image. The knobs should be aligned in an even curve that produces a pleasing image (Fig. 1.7).

Transmit Zone

Transmit zone is an operator-adjustable, transmit-focus function that allows for additional image enhancement of the structures adjacent to the transmit zone marker. The transmit zone marker should be set at, or just below, the structure of greatest interest (Figs. 1.7, 1.8). When no moving structures are within the field of view, multiple transmit zones can be used to improve quality of the entire image (Fig. 1.1B).

Freeze and Store

US examination is a dynamic process that allows viewing of enough frames of information per second to be considered "real-time." Just as in a movie, the "real-time" image is actually made up of numerous individual frames or "snapshots." These are captured and displayed quickly enough to evaluate motion of the beating heart, the moving diaphragm, or the pulsating aorta. To view and record individual images, press the FREEZE button. To store the image for viewing later and to create a permanent image file of the examination, press the STORE button. A CINE function is usually available to review and store recent images, just in case your finger is too slow hitting the FREEZE button.

SCAN TECHNIQUE

The physician sonologist has the opportunity to combine clinical diagnosis with sonographic examination. Any pertinent previous imaging studies should be reviewed and correlated with the current clinical problem. The examining physician should query the patient regarding current symptoms and past medical history, especially noting any previous surgical procedures. Suspected masses can be evaluated by physical examination as well as by sonography. Focal areas of pain or tenderness can be examined dynamically and correlated with the US images.

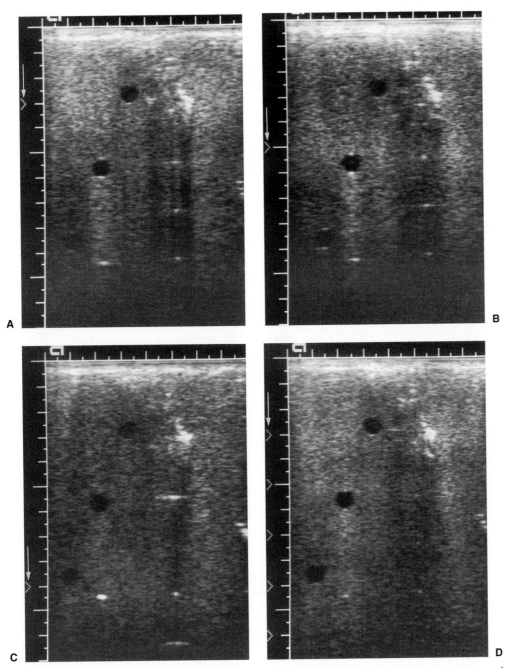

Figure 1.8 *Effect of Transmit Zone Focusing Shown on an Ultrasound Phantom.* US phantoms are used to quality control US equipment. This tissue-equivalent phantom simulates three cysts at different depths in tissue. In *A*, the transmit zone (*arrow*) is set at a superficial depth. The upper and middle cysts are well seen, but the deepest cyst is barely visible. In *B*, the transmit zone (*arrow*) is set at the level of the middle cyst. Now the deepest cyst is seen but not well characterized. In *C*, the transmit zone (*arrow*) is set at the level of the deepest cyst, providing a quality image of it, but a poor image of the most superficial cyst. In *D*, multiple transmit zones (*arrow*) are used to provide a quality image of all three cysts. Multiple transmit zones are effectively used whenever there is little or no motion of the imaged structures.

Table 1.1: Choosing a Transducer

Examination	Recommended Transducer
Abdomen	2.5–4.0-MHz sector or vector
Kidneys and bladder	Harmonics often provide the best images
Gastrointestinal tract	
Liver and renal transplants	
Pelvis	
Obstetric first trimester	
Transabdominal	2.5–4.0-MHz sector or vector
Transvaginal	4.0–8.0-MHz curved or sector intracavitary
Superficial parts	7.0–10.0-MHz linear array
Scrotum	
Thyroid	
Breast	
Extremity	
Chest	5.0–7.5-MHz linear array for superficial pleural space
	3.5–4.0-MHz sector or vector
Neonatal brain	5.0–7.0-MHz sector
Obstetric second/third trimester	3.5–5.0-MHz curved array or
	3.5–5.0-MHz wide linear array
Prostate	4.0–8.0-MHz curved or sector intracavitary

The first step in US examination is to select the transducer most appropriate for the examination at hand (Fig. 1.1). Experience makes this selection easy. Table 1.1 provides some suggestions for the novice. Make sure the patient's name and medical record number are entered into the US unit's database to properly identify the examination. Position the patient appropriately for the examination to be performed. Explain what you are doing and why. Make sure the US gel is warmed and use it to cover the area of examination.

Wear examination gloves for any intracavitary examination or examination around open wounds or with broken skin. Many sonographers wear gloves for all examinations. Hold the transducer firmly with your thumb against the ridge or groove that marks the orientation of the transducer. This marker should always be directed toward the patient's right side or toward the patient's head to properly orient the image. Place the edge of your hand against the patient's skin to stabilize the transducer and allow you to make fine gentle movements of the transducer. Begin scanning in an area where you think that recognizable anatomy should be. For example, start in the right upper quadrant of the abdomen to find the liver. Adjust the controls to fill the image with the anatomy of interest. Orient yourself to the three-dimensional anatomy of the patient. Move the transducer slowly to identify additional structures. The transducer can be moved freely in many directions to change the anatomy displayed. Don't bounce around but stay focused in one area and use small adjustments. You can slide the transducer right or left, craniad or caudad. You can angle the transducer up or down. You can turn the transducer into transverse, longitudinal, or oblique orientations [2].

Practice, practice, practice. You cannot fly an airplane, or perform a diagnostic US examination, without plenty of time spent behind the controls.

US TERMINOLOGY

Like so many other areas of medicine, US comes with its own unique terminology, both professional and slang. If you want to practice sonography you have to speak the language.

- **Sonographer.** An US technologist highly skilled in all aspects of US examination.
- **Sonologist.** A physician highly skilled in all aspects of US examination.
- **Anechoic—Echolucent.** These terms describe the complete absence of echoes. Usually applied to describe the contents of a cystic mass containing simple clear fluid. The inside of the cyst is black and contains no real echoes (see Fig. 1.15).

- **Hypoechoic** describes a structure that has fewer echoes (is darker) than the surrounding tissue. A hypoechoic lesion in the liver has fewer echoes than liver parenchyma.
- **Hyperechoic—Echogenic.** These terms describe structures that have more echoes (are whiter) than surrounding tissue. An echogenic liver mass has more echoes (is brighter) than surrounding liver parenchyma.
- **Transverse** means the image is oriented generally in the axial plane of the patient. The patient's right side is displayed on the left side of the image.
- **Longitudinal** means the image is oriented in the long axis of the patient and may be sagittal, coronal, or more often, in between. The patient's head is toward the left side of the image.

ARTIFACTS

US artifacts are errors in the presentation of anatomic structures (Fig. 1.9). Some artifacts, like acoustic shadowing and acoustic enhancement, are useful in diagnosis. Others are undesirable, obscure anatomy, and must be recognized to prevent errors in interpretation [3].

Several assumptions are made during the production of an US image. US beams are assumed to travel in straight lines in the direction that the beam is originally transmitted into tissue. Returning echoes are assumed to originate only from objects along the path of the transmitted beam. The intensity of a returning echo is proportional to the reflective strength of the tissue interface encountered. The speed of sound in tissue is presumed to be constant at 1540 m/sec. The depth of an echo source is proportional to the round-trip travel time of the US beam. When an imaging assumption is invalid an image artifact is produced [4]. Artifacts are common and an intrinsic part of US imaging (Fig. 1.9).

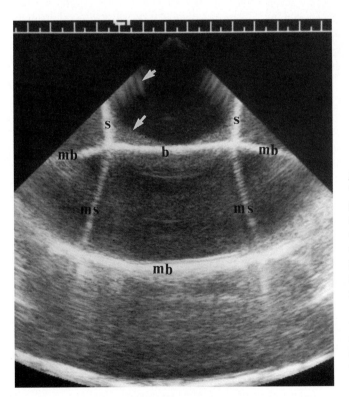

Figure 1.9 *A Glass of Water.* This image was produced by immersing the tip of a sector transducer into a plastic cup of water. The sides (s) and bottom (b) of the cup are indicated. Because the cup of water is surrounded by air, mirror image artifact reproduction of the sides (ms) and bottom (mb) of the container are prominent. Ghosting artifact (grating lobe or side lobe artifact) produces prominent artifactual echoes (*arrows*) within the water.

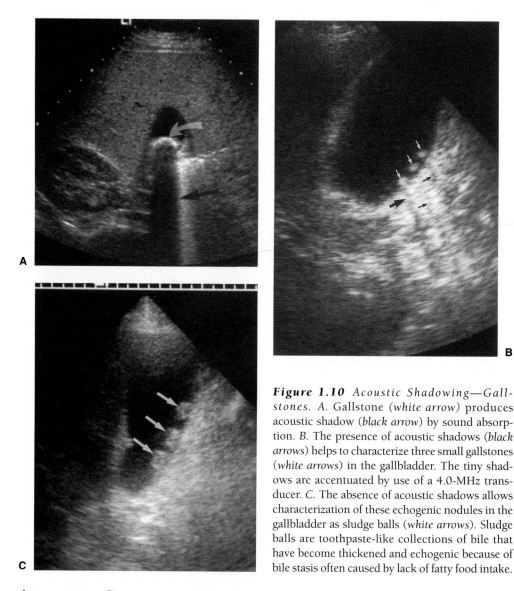

Figure 1.10 *Acoustic Shadowing—Gallstones. A.* Gallstone (*white arrow*) produces acoustic shadow (*black arrow*) by sound absorption. *B.* The presence of acoustic shadows (*black arrows*) helps to characterize three small gallstones (*white arrows*) in the gallbladder. The tiny shadows are accentuated by use of a 4.0-MHz transducer. *C.* The absence of acoustic shadows allows characterization of these echogenic nodules in the gallbladder as sludge balls (*white arrows*). Sludge balls are toothpaste-like collections of bile that have become thickened and echogenic because of bile stasis often caused by lack of fatty food intake.

ACOUSTIC SHADOWING

Acoustic shadowing is an artifactual reduction in the amplitude of echoes displayed on the US image. Sound absorption, sound reflection, or sound refraction may produce acoustic shadows. Shadowing is most commonly caused by sound absorption produced by intervening structures of high sound attenuation. Bone attenuates (absorbs) sound energy 20× greater than soft tissue. Reflective shadows, which commonly contain reverberation echoes, suggest the presence of gas [5]. Refractive shadows are produced by critical angle refraction at the edges of fluid-filled structures and aid in the recognition of cysts.

- **Sound Absorption.** Acoustic shadows caused by sound absorption aid in the recognition of gallstones, renal calculi, calcifications, foreign bodies, and bones (Figs. 1.10, 1.11) [6]. The shadows of sound absorption are "clean shadows," a uniform dark band of no anatomic information. The presence of a visible US shadow is related to imaging technique, the size of the object, the radius of curvature of the object, and the surface contour (smoothness or roughness) of the object. The chemical composition of gallstones or renal stones does not affect the presence or nature of stone shadowing.
- To produce or to improve the visualization of an acoustic shadow to identify a renal calculus or gallstone [7]:
    - Use a higher transducer frequency to produce a higher resolution image.

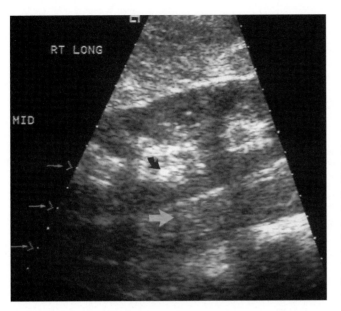

Figure 1.11 *Acoustic Shadowing—Renal Stone.* Harmonic imaging at 4.0 MHz allows demonstration of a tiny renal stone (*black arrow*) within the echogenic sinus of the kidney by visualization of a discrete acoustic shadow (*large white arrow*). This image was obtained using multiple transmit zones (*small white arrows*).

   — Adjust the focal zone or transmit zone to improve resolution at the level of the suspected stone.
   — Center the suspected stone in the US beam.
   — Optimize the gain and power settings to visualize the shadow.

■ **Sound Reflection.** A tissue-air interface causes near-complete (99%+) reflection of the US beam. This near-total blockage of sound penetration results in a blank band of absent anatomic information (an acoustic shadow) deep to the tissue-air interface. Because sound reflection is so intense, reverberation occurs, which results in bright echoes being displayed within the acoustic shadow. This is the "dirty shadow" characteristic of an US beam encountering air (see Fig. 1.19).

■ **Sound Refraction—Edge Shadow.** When the US beam encounters a curved interface at an oblique angle, such as the edge of a cyst within solid tissue, the beam transmission is diverted (refracted) to a new direction. Refraction results in few echoes returning to the transducer from the original "line-of-site" of the US beam causing an acoustic shadow (Fig. 1.12). This "edge shadow" is characteristic of a cyst and accen-

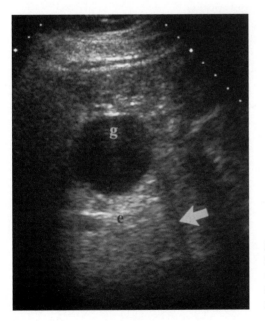

Figure 1.12 *Edge Shadow.* The gallbladder (g) in transverse section shows an edge shadow (*arrow*) produced by sound refraction adjacent to acoustic enhancement (e) produced by its fluid content.

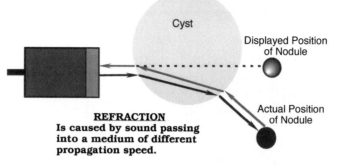

Figure 1.13 *Refraction Artifact.* The direction of the US wave is changed as it passes into a tissue of different speed of sound transmission. Although the US instrument assumes that the speed of sound in all tissue is constant, the speed of sound in soft tissue is 1540 m/sec while the speed of sound in simple fluid (water) is 1480 m/sec. A structure deep to the refracted sound wave is displayed in false position on the US image.

tuates the visualization of acoustic enhancement resulting from transmission of the US beam through the cyst. Refraction at boundaries between juxtaposed tissue types or the curved margins of anatomic structures is a cause of shadowing from solid tissue such as leiomyomas [8].

REFRACTION ARTIFACTS

Sound refraction may also displace the position of anatomic structures displayed on the image (spatial distortion artifacts) (Fig. 1.13). Sound refraction occurs most commonly at soft tissue-fluid and soft tissue-fat interfaces.

- Diaphragm discontinuity artifact occurs in patients with ascites (Fig. 1.14). Sound is refracted when entering or exiting the liver or spleen surrounded by ascites. A portion of the diaphragm is falsely positioned on the resulting US image [9].

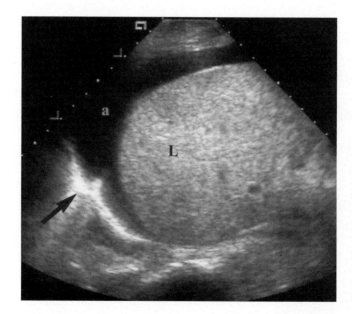

Figure 1.14 *Discontinuous Diaphragm Artifact.* Longitudinal image of the liver (L) taken through ascites (a) shows an apparent defect (*arrow*) in the diaphragm. This artifact is caused by refraction of the US beam as it passes through tissues, which transmit sound at slightly different speeds (the liver and ascites fluid).

■ Split image artifact duplicates structures imaged in the upper abdomen and pelvis [10,11]. Sound is refracted at the interface between anterior abdominal wall muscles and the layer of fat deep to the muscles. Split image artifact may falsely result in the display of two gestational sacs in the uterus when only one is present.

ACOUSTIC ENHANCEMENT

Acoustic enhancement, also called "accentuated through transmission," refers to echoes of increased amplitude that are seen deep to fluid-containing structures (Fig. 1.15). Fluid-filled structures, such as cysts, cause minimal sound attenuation as the US beam passes through them resulting in echoes of high intensity deep to the cysts. US beams that have passed through adjacent solid tissue have lower intensity at the same depth

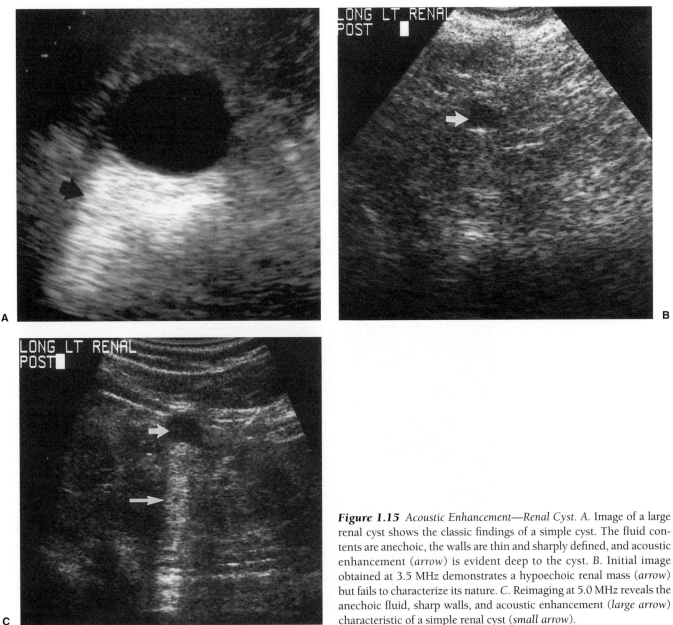

Figure 1.15 *Acoustic Enhancement—Renal Cyst. A.* Image of a large renal cyst shows the classic findings of a simple cyst. The fluid contents are anechoic, the walls are thin and sharply defined, and acoustic enhancement (*arrow*) is evident deep to the cyst. *B.* Initial image obtained at 3.5 MHz demonstrates a hypoechoic renal mass (*arrow*) but fails to characterize its nature. *C.* Reimaging at 5.0 MHz reveals the anechoic fluid, sharp walls, and acoustic enhancement (*large arrow*) characteristic of a simple renal cyst (*small arrow*).

because of greater sound attenuation in the solid tissue. TGC built in to all US displays to counter the effects of progressive sound absorption further accentuates acoustic enhancement.

- Acoustic enhancement, like acoustic shadowing, is technique dependent.
- To improve visualization of acoustic enhancement to confirm the nature of a small cyst, make the technique adjustments listed previously for demonstration of acoustic shadowing (Fig. 1.15).

REVERBERATION ARTIFACTS

Reverberation artifact is the improper display of echoes on the US image that is caused by multiple reflections between strongly reflective surfaces. Reverberation artifacts may obscure tissue anatomy or simulate soft tissue within cysts. A variety of artifacts are created by reverberation.

- **Reverberation bands** are produced by repeated reflection between an air interface and the transducer face (Fig. 1.16). The sound beam makes multiple round trips between the air interface (air bubble in bowel, air-filled lung, etc.) and the transducer face, producing a regularly spaced series of reverberation bands on the US image. Recognition of the presence of gas can be an important diagnostic finding indicating abscess, emphysematous cholecystitis or pyelonephritis, or anomalous communication of the biliary and intestinal tract [12].
- **Comet tail artifacts** are a form of reverberation artifact that appear as a dense tapering V-shaped trail of echoes beyond strong reflectors (Fig. 1.17). Short-range rapid reverberations, which can occur between the walls of a hollow structure or metallic object, produce comet tail artifacts. Comet tails are seen in association with and help to identify gas bubbles in fluid, catheters, surgical clips, metal-wrapped intrauterine devices, cholesterol crystals in bile, and inspissated colloid in thyroid cysts [13].
- **Ring-down artifacts** are reverberation echoes similar to comet tail artifacts except that the bright artifactual echoes are displayed in a much longer stream [14]. A line of bright continuous echoes is seen deep to a strong reflector, commonly a cluster of tiny

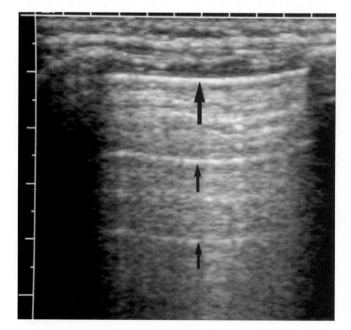

Figure 1.16 *Reverberation Bands.* Intercostal linear array image of the normal lung surface shows intense reflection at the soft tissue-air interface (*large arrow*) that reflects back and forth between the transducer surface and the interface to produce a series of reverberation bands (*small arrows*) deeper in the image.

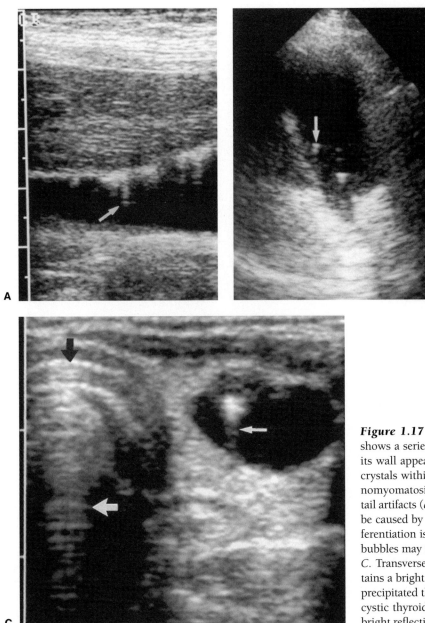

Figure 1.17 *Comet Tail Artifacts.* A. Image of the gallbladder shows a series of bright tapering echoes (*arrow*) extending from its wall appearing similar to stalactites. Precipitated cholesterol crystals within Rokitansky-Aschoff sinuses associated with adenomyomatosis produce these comet tail artifacts. *B.* Tiny comet tail artifacts (*arrow*) suspended in bile within the gallbladder may be caused by air bubbles or precipitated cholesterol crystals. Differentiation is made most confidently by CT. The presence of air bubbles may indicate highly lethal emphysematous cholecystitis. *C.* Transverse image of the thyroid gland shows a cyst that contains a bright comet tail artifact (*small white arrow*) produced by precipitated thyroid colloid. This finding is indicative of a benign cystic thyroid nodule. Air in the trachea (*black arrow*) causes a bright reflection and a ring-down artifact (*large white arrow*).

air bubbles in fluid. Ring-down echoes help to identify gas collections and commonly emanate from gas bubbles within intestine fluid (Fig. 1.18). Ring-down artifacts are also produced by metallic objects, like bullets or lead shot, suspended in liver or other solid tissue.

- **Near-field artifacts** are commonly displayed beyond the near wall of fluid-filled structures like cysts, the gallbladder, and urinary bladder (Fig. 1.19). The soft tissue-fluid interface produces strong reflection that bounces between the wall and the transducer producing artifactual bright echoes within anechoic fluid.

SLICE THICKNESS ARTIFACT

Slice thickness artifact, also called volume averaging, results from the finite thickness of the US beam. The two-dimensional US image displays information from three dimensions of

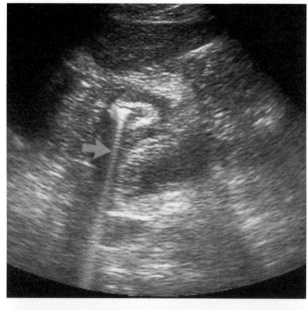

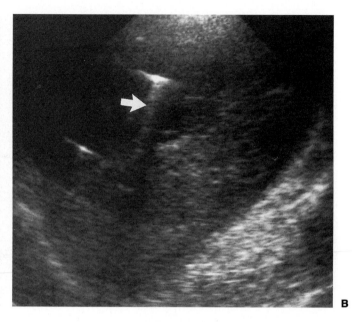

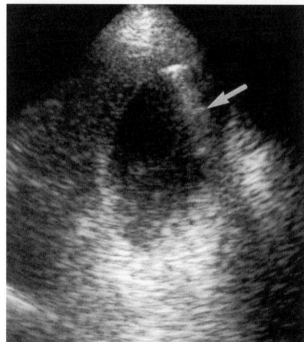

Figure 1.18 *Ring-Down Artifact—Air Bubbles. A.* Longitudinal image of the gastric antrum shows a prominent ring-down artifact (*arrow*) caused by air bubbles in the stomach. *B.* Similar ring-down artifact (*arrow*) identifies air bubbles that aid in the diagnosis of a splenic abscess. *C.* Ring-down artifact (*arrow*) emanates from the wall of the gallbladder in a patient with emphysematous cholecystitis. Recognition of air in the gallbladder wall is critical to diagnosing this condition with high mortality.

tissue interrogated by the US beam. This may result in echoes from the side wall being displayed within an otherwise anechoic cystic structure. Similar slice thickness effects are intrinsic to CT and MR imaging.

MIRROR IMAGE ARTIFACT

Mirror image artifact most often results from US reflection from a large air surface such as the lung or a gas-filled bowel. The interface between soft tissue and air acts like a mirror by reflecting sound of high intensity, which causes re-reflection within tissue and a delayed return of echoes to the transducer.

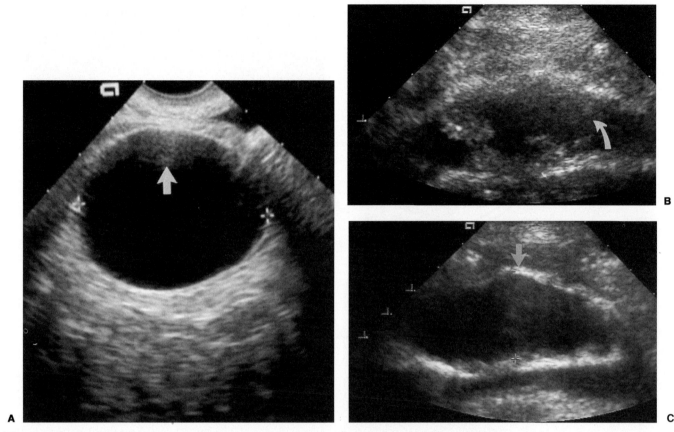

Figure 1.19 *Near-Field Reverberation Artifact. A.* Reverberation artifact causes echoes (*arrow*) to be displayed adjacent to the near wall of this ovarian cyst. This artifact must not be mistaken for solid tissue, which, if present, would characterize this benign cyst as an ovarian tumor. Imaging the cyst from different angles confirms that the artifact is always displayed on the wall nearest the transducer and is not fixed in location within the cyst. Color Doppler would show blood flow in solid tissue, but not in the artifact. *B.* Near-field reverberation (*arrow*) obscures the near wall of this small aneurysm of the abdominal aorta, making measurement of the aneurysm difficult. *C.* Repositioning the transducer and use of multiple transmit zones decrease the artifact and make confident identification of the near wall (*arrow*) possible.

Mirror image artifact is most apparent around the diaphragm, which reflects the US beam because of the presence of air-filled lung at the surface of the diaphragm (Fig. 1.20). High-intensity reflected sound is reflected several times within the liver or spleen prolonging the time of return of the resulting echoes to the transducer [15]. Prolonged time-of-flight is interpreted as being deeper in tissue. Thus images of the liver, or spleen, are displayed above, as well as below, the diaphragm. Mirror image artifact occurs only when air-filled lung is present above the diaphragm. Thus mirror image artifact of the liver and spleen above the diaphragm should be considered normal. When pleural effusion is present, or when the lower lobes of the lung are consolidated, sound penetrates the diaphragm and lung or fluid and the chest wall and ribs are displaced. Mirror image artifacts may be seen elsewhere as well (Fig. 1.21).

GHOSTING ARTIFACTS

Each sound-producing element in an US transducer produces a main lobe projected in the axis of the US beam and lesser-intensity side lobes projected at angles to the main lobe [16].

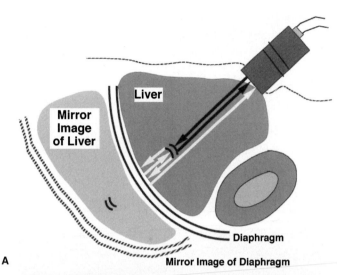

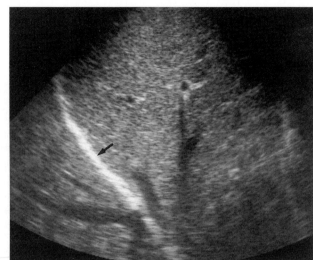

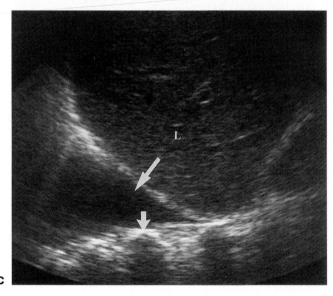

Figure 1.20 *Mirror Image Artifact. A.* Near-complete reflection of the US beam from the surface of the air-filled lung above the diaphragm causes reflection of the US beam back and forth within the liver before finally returning to the US transducer. The prolonged time-of-flight of these delayed echoes results in artifactual display of liver parenchyma above the diaphragm. *B.* Mirror image artifact duplicates the hepatic veins and liver above the diaphragm (*arrow*). The presence of mirror image artifact above the diaphragm confirms the presence of air at the lung base. *C.* A right pleural effusion prevents the mirror image duplication of liver (L) above the diaphragm. The effusion is seen as a triangular echolucency (*large arrow*) in the deep costophrenic angle. The chest wall with shadowing ribs (*small arrow*) is visualized through the effusion.

Grating lobes are higher-intensity side lobes produced by all multi-element electronic transducers in current use. Echoes produced by grating lobes may simulate septations, debris, or solid tissue within cystic masses (Fig. 1.22). These ghosting artifacts are particularly prominent with curved array transducers.

ANISOTROPIC EFFECT

Anisotropy in US refers to the difference in the echogenicity of a structure caused by its orientation relative to the US beam. Reflections from parallel structures are increased when they are perpendicular to the sound beam and are decreased when imaged obliquely (Fig. 1.23). Anisotropic effect must be recognized because increased or decreased echogenicity is commonly an US sign of pathologic change. Anisotropy is most commonly noted during US examination of tendons, which are made up of a series of parallel fibrous strands [17]. Tendons appear brightly echogenic when the US beam is perpendicular and they appear hypoechoic when imaged at angles other than 90 degrees. Anisotropy is the reported cause of the echogenic appearance of the fetal and neonatal brain when imaged in axial plane compared to the basal ganglia appearing isoechoic to the thalamus when imaged in the neonatal brain in coronal planes [18].

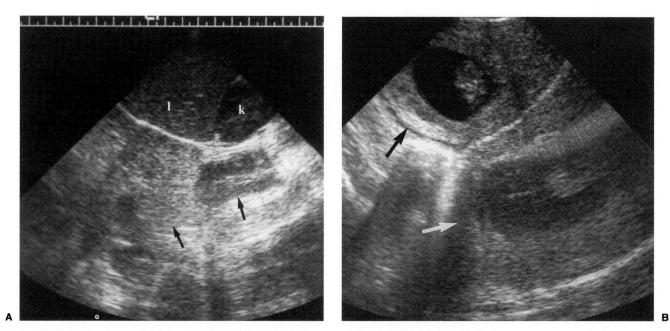

Figure 1.21 *Mirror Image Artifacts. A.* A faulty depth setting, way too deep, results in mirror image duplication (*arrows*) of the liver (l) and kidney (k) of an infant. Mirror image reflection in this case is caused by reflection at the posterior skin surface. *B.* An intrauterine gestational sac (*black arrow*) is duplicated (*white arrow*) on a transvaginal US examination by re-reflection from gas in the rectum.

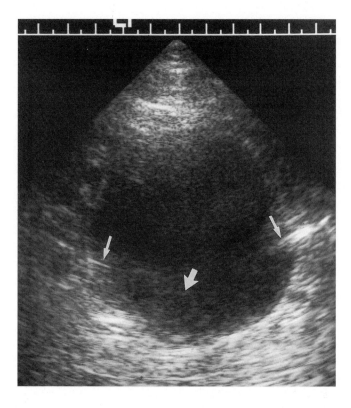

Figure 1.22 *Ghosting Artifact.* Artifactual internal echoes in this cyst are caused by reflection of low-intensity grating lobes from the wall of the cyst. These artifacts may simulate septations (*small arrows*) or echogenic debris (*large arrow*) within cyst fluid. These artifacts are identified during real-time US by moving the transducer to different orientations and observing that the "septations" and "debris" change location and appearance with the transducer movement.

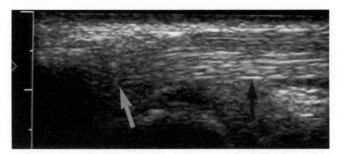

Figure 1.23 *Anisotropic Effect.* Longitudinal linear array image of a flexor tendon at the wrist demonstrates the anisotropic effect. The tendon appears as a group of very echogenic linear strands when the US beam is perpendicular to the tendon (*black arrow*). Where the tendon curves away and the US beam strikes the tendon at an angle, the tendon appears hypoechoic (*white arrow*). To properly examine a tendon, every effort must be made to keep the US beam perpendicular to the tendon strands. Hypoechoic zones produced by anisotropic effect may simulate tendon tears.

PRINCIPLES OF INTERPRETATION

The physician interpreting the US examination should check any questionable abnormalities by personally scanning the patient. Real-time scanning produces many thousands of images within a few minutes compared to the isolated images captured by the sonographer. Recorded images serve only to provide long-term documentation of the real-time examination. All questions of interpretation should be answered by dynamic real-time examination before the patient is allowed to leave the US suite.

FLUID-CONTAINING STRUCTURES

Structures that contain fluid (cyst, bladder, gallbladder, etc.) characteristically demonstrate accentuated through transmission. While the near wall of the fluid-filled structure may be obscured by reverberation artifact (Fig. 1.19), the far wall is sharply defined. Anechoic fluid is indicative of simple fluid (serous fluid, bile, and urine). Fluid that is echogenic is complicated by the presence of blood, pus, mucin, debris, or other materials in suspension.

- **Simple cysts** are well defined, are anechoic internally, have thin walls, and demonstrate accentuated through transmission (Figs. 1.15, 1.19). Simple cysts are common in the kidney, liver, and breast. Small simple cysts on the ovaries are properly called follicles.
- **Echogenic cysts** contain fluid with suspended particulate matter. Echogenic cysts may be hemorrhagic cysts, abscesses, or mucin-producing tumors. Echogenic cysts are easily mistaken for solid masses. Clues to the correct diagnosis include the following (Fig. 1.24):
  - The contents of echogenic cysts are commonly homogeneous.
  - Echoes within fluid will shift and swirl with compression of the cyst or with changes in patient position.
  - Doppler shows no internal blood vessels within an echogenic cyst.
  - Fluid layering may be seen with echogenic cysts. Fluid levels may be recognized only when imaging in a plane perpendicular to gravity.
  - Acoustic enhancement is usually but not universally present.
  - Echogenic cysts commonly have well-defined boundaries, uncommon with solid masses.

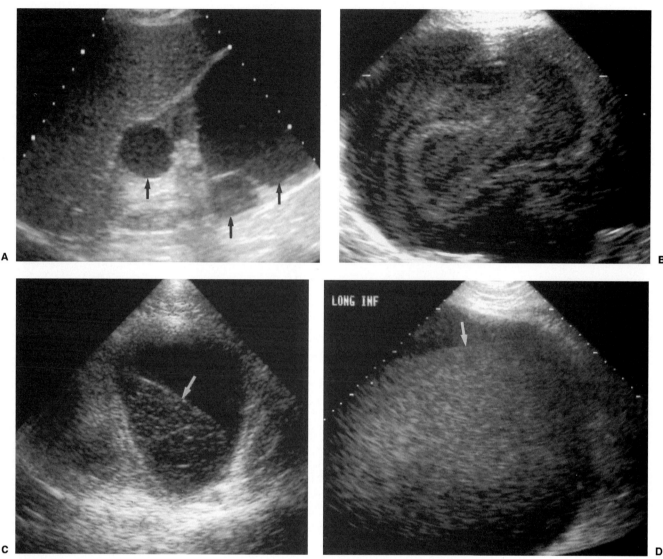

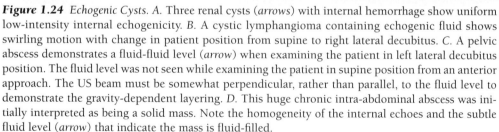

Figure 1.24 *Echogenic Cysts. A.* Three renal cysts (*arrows*) with internal hemorrhage show uniform low-intensity internal echogenicity. *B.* A cystic lymphangioma containing echogenic fluid shows swirling motion with change in patient position from supine to right lateral decubitus. *C.* A pelvic abscess demonstrates a fluid-fluid level (*arrow*) when examining the patient in left lateral decubitus position. The fluid level was not seen while examining the patient in supine position from an anterior approach. The US beam must be somewhat perpendicular, rather than parallel, to the fluid level to demonstrate the gravity-dependent layering. *D.* This huge chronic intra-abdominal abscess was initially interpreted as being a solid mass. Note the homogeneity of the internal echoes and the subtle fluid level (*arrow*) that indicate the mass is fluid-filled.

SOLID TISSUE

Solid tissue characteristically demonstrates a salt-and-pepper speckled pattern of tissue texture characteristic of each normal organ. Blood vessels are demonstrated coursing through normal organs in an organized pattern. Degree of echogenicity is relative and is routinely compared to adjacent organs. Normal liver and kidney parenchyma are very close in echogenicity. A notable difference in echogenicity of the parenchyma of the two organs is indicative of diffuse abnormality. The pancreas is significantly more echogenic than the liver, kidneys, or spleen. Normal testes are always exactly equal to each other in echogenicity and should always be compared on the same image.

■ Fat is routinely more echogenic than the organs it surrounds. However, in some circumstances, notably in the breast, fat may appear hypoechoic to surrounding tissue [19,20].
■ Masses within organs are recognized by the following characteristics:
  – Masses produce an alteration in tissue texture (the speckle pattern) or in echogenicity. Masses of lower echogenicity than surrounding parenchyma are termed hypoechoic. Masses of higher echogenicity are called hyperechoic or echogenic.
  – The surface contour of an organ is altered by the presence of a mass, which may cause a focal bulge or nodular appearance.
  – Blood vessels are commonly altered by masses. Color flow US shows an increased concentration of blood vessels with hypervascular masses and may show displacement or bowing of normal blood vessels around a hypovascular mass.
■ Masses arising within an organ will move with that organ during respiration or with palpation or changes in patient position. Masses arising adjacent to and only touching an organ will show a "sliding sign" of movement disparate from the organ.

GOODIES

TISSUE HARMONIC IMAGING

Conventional US images are obtained by transmitting an US beam at a primary or "fundamental" frequency designated by the transducer and frequency setting utilized. Echoes are detected by the transducer at the same fundamental frequency. **Harmonic** frequencies are produced as this primary beam passes through tissue. Harmonics occur at integer multiples of the fundamental frequency. For instance, an US beam with a fundamental frequency of 5 MHz will produce, in tissue, harmonic frequencies at 10, 15, and 20 MHz, etc. Conventional US utilizing the fundamental frequency is degraded by grating lobe and reverberation artifacts that arise primarily as the US beam passes through the body wall. The formation of harmonic frequencies is minimal at the body wall but progressively increases deeper in tissues. Most grating lobe and reverberation artifacts are eliminated and images appear cleaner and crisper. Image quality is improved and images provide more diagnostic information [21]. Images are of higher contrast and have a lower dynamic range (Fig. 1.25). Harmonic echoes are inherently much lower in amplitude than echoes at the fundamental frequency. Higher amplitude of the fundamental frequency will increase the amplitude of the harmonic frequencies. In practice, only the first harmonic, at twice the fundamental frequency, is used for tissue harmonic imaging. Typically, manufacturers lower the transmission frequency when "harmonics" is turned on. A 5-MHz probe set to harmonic imaging transmits at 2.5 MHz and receives the harmonic echoes at 5.0 MHz [22]. Harmonic imaging is most useful in obese patients, in the characterization of renal cysts, in the detection of urinary and biliary stones (Fig. 1.11), and in detecting tumors in the difficult-to-image liver. Harmonic imaging is now the default mode in many US imaging laboratories.

Tissue harmonic imaging decreases US artifacts and improves image quality in about 80% of patients.

US CONTRAST AGENTS

Contrast agents are currently being investigated for use in a number of US applications. Intestinal contrast agents may improve US diagnosis in the gastrointestinal tract or improve visualization of other abdominal organs by replacing the intestinal gas usually present. Vascular US may be improved by contrast agents that improve visualization of the vascular tree, improving detection of plaques and identifying areas of stenosis. Contrast agents may be used to provide enhancement of organ parenchyma to improve lesion detection. Partic-

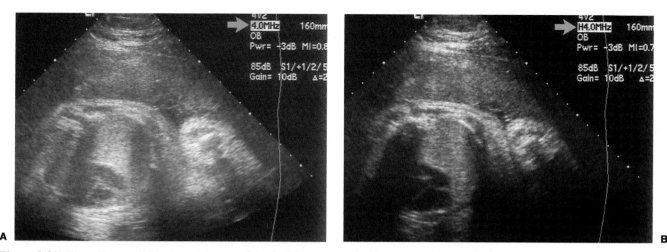

Figure 1.25 *Tissue Harmonic Imaging. A.* Image of the fetal heart is obtained using 4.0-MHz (*arrow*) fundamental frequency in a large pregnant woman. Details are obscured. *B.* The same image is obtained using tissue harmonics with transmission frequency of 2.0 MHz receiving harmonic echoes at 4.0 MHz (*arrow*). Note the increase in contrast and improved clarity of the image.

ulate agents taken up by Kupffer cells in the liver may improve detection of hepatic tumors. All sonographic contrast agents are investigational at this time.

THREE-DIMENSIONAL US

Three-dimensional US provides a novel display of US anatomy that may prove to be clinically useful [23]. Fetal anatomy is strikingly demonstrated making fetal anomalies easier to recognize and understand. Volume-rendered computer display techniques, such as shaded surface display and maximum intensity projection in common use in CT and MR, can also be applied to US to improve diagnosis and communication with patients, parents, and referring physicians. The prominence of US artifacts may, however, limit the usefulness of three-dimensional US.

REFERENCES

1. Kremkau F. Multiple-element transducers. RadioGraphics 1993;13:1163–1176.
2. American Institute of Ultrasound in Medicine. Technical Bulletin—Transducer manipulation. J Ultrasound Med 1999;18:169–175.
3. Scanlan KA. Sonographic artifacts and their origins. AJR Am J Roentgenol 1991;156:1267–1272.
4. Kremkau F, Taylor K. Artifacts in ultrasound imaging. J Ultrasound Med 1986;5:227–237.
5. Sommer F, Taylor K. Differentiation of acoustic shadowing due to calculi and gas collections. Radiology 1980;135:399–403.
6. Shiels WI, Babcock D, Wilson J, et al. Localization and guided removal of soft-tissue foreign bodies with sonography. AJR Am J Roentgenol 1990;155:1277–1281.
7. Kimme-Smith C, Perrella R, Kaveggia L, et al. Detection of renal stones with real-time sonography: effect of transducers and scanning parameters. AJR Am J Roentgenol 1991;157:975–980.
8. Kliewer M, Hertzberg B, George P, et al. Acoustic shadowing from uterine leiomyomas: sonographic-pathologic correlation. Radiology 1995;196:99–102.
9. Middleton W, Melson G. Diaphragmatic discontinuity associated with perihepatic ascites: a sonographic refractive artifact. AJR Am J Roentgenol 1988;151:709–711.
10. Sauerbrei E. The split image artifact in pelvic sonography: the anatomy and physics. J Ultrasound Med 1985;4:29–34.
11. Vandeman F, Meilstrup J, Nealey P. Acoustic prism causing sonographic duplication artifact in the upper abdomen. Invest Radiol 1990;25:658–663.

12. Horrow M, Kirby C, Enu B, et al. Sonography of gas in the abdomen: a help rather than a hindrance. Radiologist 1998;5:85–94.
13. Shapiro R, Winsberg R. Comet-tail artifacts from cholesterol crystals: observations in the postlithotripsy gallbladder and an in vitro model. Radiology 1990;177:153–156.
14. Avruch L, Cooperberg P. The ring-down artifact. J Ultrasound Med 1985;4:21–28.
15. Gardner F, Clark R, Kozlowski R. A model of a hepatic mirror-image artifact. Med Ultrasound 1980;4:19–21s.
16. Laing F, Kurtz A. The importance of ultrasonic side-lobe artifacts. Radiology 1982;145:763–768.
17. Fornage B. The hypoechoic normal tendon: a pitfall. J Ultrasound Med 1987;6:19–22.
18. Ashraf V, Feldstein V, Filly R. Variation in the echogenicity of the basal ganglia: anisotropic effect. J Ultrasound Med 1999;18:153–158.
19. Jain K. Hypoechoic fat on ultrasound: a diagnostic dilemma. Radiologist 1995;2:215–220.
20. Spencer G, Rubens D, Roach D. Hypoechoic fat: a sonographic pitfall. AJR Am J Roentgenol 1995;164:1277–1280.
21. Hann L, Bach A, Cramer L, et al. Hepatic sonography: comparison of tissue harmonic and standard sonography techniques. AJR Am J Roentgenol 1999;173:201–206.
22. Desser T, Jeffrey RJ, Lane M, et al. Tissue harmonic imaging: utility in abdominal and pelvic sonography. J Clin Ultrasound 1999;27:135–142.
23. Downey D, Fenster A, Williams J. Clinical utility of three-dimensional US. RadioGraphics 2000;20:559–571.

ABDOMEN ULTRASOUND

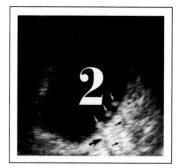

IMAGING TECHNIQUE

The abdomen is examined with sector or curved array transducers using frequencies of 5.0 to 2.25 MHz. The highest frequency that allows adequate penetration is used [1]. Routine examinations are conducted following a minimum fast of 4 hours to allow for filling of the gallbladder. Emergency examinations are conducted without patient preparation.

The **liver** is examined in transverse and longitudinal planes. The entire liver, porta hepatis, portal veins (PVs), hepatic veins, and intrahepatic inferior vena cava (IVC) are examined and documented on recorded images. Much of the liver is examined using an intercostal approach. Having the patient breathe in deeply will depress the liver for examination along the costal margin. An image that includes the liver and the right kidney should always be obtained to compare the relative echogenicity of the parenchyma of each organ. The right pleural space and right hemidiaphragm are included in the examination.

The intrahepatic **bile ducts** are examined along with the PVs and peripheral portal triads. Recorded images should include the right and left branches of the PVs and bile ducts. The common bile duct (CBD) is visualized in the porta hepatis and its diameter is measured (see Figs. 2.6, 2.7). Its course should be followed through the pancreatic head to its terminus in the descending duodenum.

The **gallbladder** (GB) is examined in its long and short axes with careful inspection for gallstones, luminal contents, wall thickness, and surrounding pathology. The examination is conducted with the patient in supine, left lateral decubitus, erect (sitting), and prone positions as needed to aid in the detection of gallstones and to document their mobility.

The **pancreas** is examined by transverse and sagittal imaging in the epigastrium. The left lobe of the liver serves as a sonographic window to the pancreas. Visualization of the pancreas is easy when the left lobe is large and is difficult when the left lobe is small. Air in the transverse colon and small bowel may obscure the pancreas and must be moved out of the way by graded transducer pressure. The patient is told that the examiner will "press hard" and is asked to tell the examiner if the maneuver becomes painful. In my experience other touted maneuvers, such as filling the stomach with water, seldom are worth the effort. Only graded compression works reliably to visualize the hidden pancreas. The splenic vein (SV) serves as the major sonographic landmark for the neck, body, and tail of the pancreas. The tail region is often obscured by gas in overlying small bowel. Masses in the tail region may be seen by using a left lateral approach to image the tail in the splenic hilum region through the spleen. The pancreatic head is identified by finding the PV commencement at the junction of the SV and superior mesenteric vein (SMV). The head envelops this confluence and extends caudally to wrap under the SMV as the uncinate process. This caudal extension of the head and the uncinate process is best shown in transverse plane. This area is particularly important to examine because it includes the terminus of the CBD and the pancreatic duct into the duodenum. Many disease processes (tumors, obstructing stones) involve this area.

The **spleen** is best imaged with the patient supine utilizing a posterior intercostal approach in the left upper quadrant [2,3]. Unless the spleen is enlarged, placing the patient in a right lateral decubitus position may be counterproductive because hyperexpansion of the left lung obliterates the narrow intercostal window to the spleen.

The **peritoneal cavity** is carefully inspected for the presence of ascites, blood, abscess, or tumor. Examination should include the major peritoneal recesses including the subdiaphragmatic spaces on both sides, the hepatorenal fossa (Morison's pouch), the paracolic gutters, and the pelvis and cul de sac.

US examination of the abdomen is commonly extended to include the retroperitoneum, kidneys, abdominal aorta, and IVC. These examinations are discussed in subsequent chapters.

ANATOMY

LIVER

Localization of tumors to segments of the liver is critical in the planning of surgical resection. The international Couinaud (pronounced "kwee-NO") system of hepatic nomenclature is currently utilized [4–6]. This system is based on the distribution of portal and hepatic veins. The right and left lobes are divided by the main hepatic fissure defined by the middle hepatic vein in the superior portion of the liver and by a line connecting the GB with the IVC in the inferior portion of the liver. Each segment has a branch PV at its center and a hepatic vein at its periphery. Segments are numbered clockwise starting with the caudate lobe (segment 1), left lobe (segments 2–4), and right lobe (segments 5–8) (Table 2.1, Fig. 2.1). The caudate lobe is anatomically distinct, extending between the IVC and the left lobe and separated from the left lobe by the fissure of the ligamentum venosum (Fig. 2.2).

Blood supply to the liver is provided by both the PV (~70%) and the hepatic artery (~30%). This dual blood supply makes infarction rare in the liver. Both enter the liver at the porta hepatis and divide into right and left lobe branches. Doppler documents blood flow direction in both vessels as into the liver (hepatopetal). Spectral Doppler shows a low-resistance, arterial flow pattern for the hepatic artery with forward flow throughout the car-

Table 2.1: Couinard's Liver Segments

Couinard Segment	American Name	International Name
1	Caudate lobe	Caudate lobe
2	Left lobe, lateral segment	Left lateral superior subsegment
3	Left lobe, lateral segment	Left lateral inferior subsegment
4	Left lobe, medial segment	Left medial subsegment
5	Right lobe, anterior segment	Right anterior inferior subsegment
6	Right lobe, anterior segment	Right anterior superior subsegment
7	Right lobe, posterior segment	Right posterior inferior subsegment
8	Right lobe, posterior segment	Right posterior superior subsegment

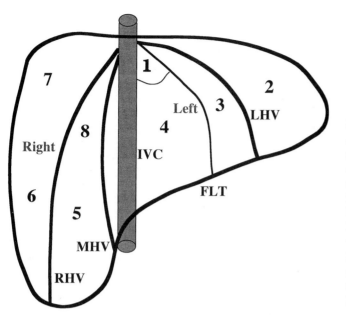

Figure 2.1 *Couinaud's Liver Segments.* Diagrammatic representation of Couinaud's numerical liver segments. FLT, fissure of the ligamentum teres; IVC, inferior vena cava; LHV, left hepatic vein; MHV, middle hepatic vein; RHV, right hepatic vein. *Adapted from Smith D, Downey D, Spouge A, et al. Sonographic demonstration of Couinard's liver segments. J Ultrasound Med 1998;17:375–381.*

diac cycle. Diastolic flow velocity increases and resistance index decreases after eating. The PV shows continuous antegrade venous flow with small pulsations that mirror the cardiac cycle. Mean velocity in the PV is 15–18 cm/sec.

Venous drainage of the liver is by three major hepatic veins that enter the IVC just below the diaphragm (Fig. 2.3). The right hepatic vein divides the anterior and posterior segments of the right lobe and enters the IVC separately. The middle and left hepatic veins may join just before entering the IVC. The middle hepatic vein separates the right and left lobe while the left hepatic vein divides the medial and lateral segments of the left lobe. Hepatic veins have no valves and their blood flow reflects the triphasic pulsatility of the IVC and right atrium. Spectral Doppler shows prominent antegrade flow toward the heart during systole reflecting movement of the tricuspid valve toward the cardiac apex. A second antegrade peak is produced in early diastole by opening of the tricuspid valve. In late diastole flow is reversed in the hepatic vein owing to atrial contraction. The caudate lobe drains directly into the IVC via small venous channels.

The liver parenchyma has homogeneous echogenicity equal to or slightly greater than the echogenicity of renal parenchyma (Fig. 2.4). Liver echogenicity is slightly less than that of the spleen. Portal triads are seen as echogenic foci well out into the periphery of the liver

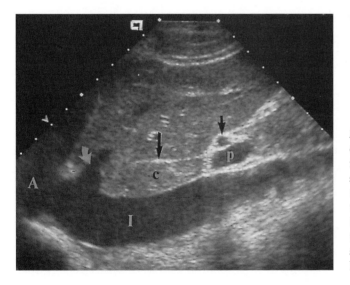

Figure 2.2 *Caudate Lobe.* The caudate lobe (c) is between the inferior vena cava (I) and the fissure of the ligamentum venosum (*long arrow*). The inferior vena terminates in the right atrium (A). The curved arrow indicates the right hepatic vein. Also seen are the portal vein (p) and the hepatic artery (*short arrow*).

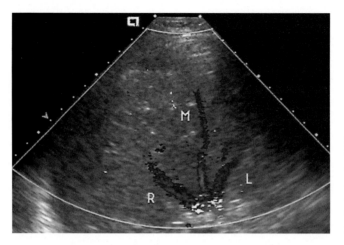

Figure 2.3 *Normal Hepatic Veins.* Transverse image through the liver obtained just below the diaphragm shows the right (R), middle (M), and left (L) hepatic veins converging to enter the inferior vena cava.

(Fig. 2.4). Fissures and ligaments are usually invested in fat and are highly echogenic (Fig. 2.2). The fissure of the ligamentum teres in the left lobe must not be mistaken for an echogenic mass (Fig. 2.5).

BILIARY TREE

Intrahepatic bile ducts (IHBD) course in the portal triads with the PVs and hepatic arteries. In the portal triads the relationship of the three structures to each other is not constant. The bile ducts may be anterior to, posterior to, or wrap around the PV [7]. Small bile ducts progressively anastomose to form the right and left lobe bile ducts that join in the porta hepatis to form the common hepatic duct. The common hepatic duct becomes the CBD approximately 3 cm distally at the junction of the cystic duct. The common hepatic duct and CBD are approximately 10 cm in length (Figs. 2.6, 2.7). Since they course outside of the liver parenchyma both are considered extrahepatic bile ducts (EHBD). The CBD joins with the main PV and the proper hepatic artery to cross the foramen of Winslow in the hepatoduodenal ligament. In this region the three structures maintain a constant relationship with the larger PV posterior and the smaller CBD and hepatic artery anterior. In cross section the three structures resemble Mickey Mouse with the vein being his face, the CBD his right ear, and the hepatic artery his left ear (Fig. 2.8). Dilatation of the CBD enlarges Mickey's right ear. The distal CBD passes behind the duodenum to run in a groove formed by the posterior pancreatic head and the medial aspect of the duodenum (see Fig. 2.14). The CBD enters the duodenum opposite the uncinate process of the pancreas.

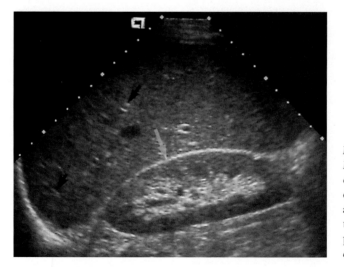

Figure 2.4 *Normal Liver and Kidney Echogenicity.* The parenchyma of the liver and kidney are equal in echogenicity. The white arrow indicates the location of the hepatorenal fossa (Morison's pouch). The portal triads (*black arrows*) are well visualized.

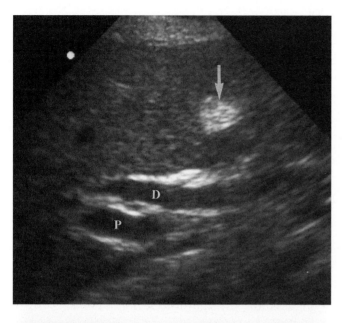

Figure 2.5 *Normal Fat in Fissure of Ligamentum Teres.* Transverse image through the left lobe of the liver demonstrates a focal echogenic area (*arrow*) that might be mistaken for an echogenic mass. This is the characteristic appearance and location of fat in the fissure of the ligamentum teres. Imaging in the longitudinal plane shows an elongated appearance to fat in the fissure. This patient also has a dilated bile duct (D) anterior to the portal vein (P).

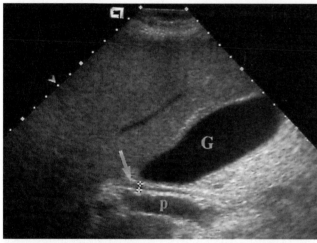

Figure 2.6 *Common Bile Duct.* The common bile duct (*arrow*) anterior to the portal vein (p) is measured with cursors (+). Compare to appearance of the dilated common bile duct in Figure 2.5. The gallbladder (G) is also seen.

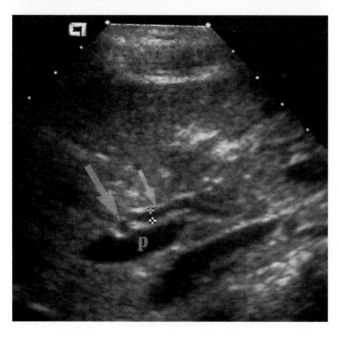

Figure 2.7 *Porta Hepatis.* The portal vein (p), common duct (*short arrow*), and hepatic artery (*large arrow*) course in the hilum of the liver, the porta hepatis. Note the oblique orientation of the hepatic artery as it courses between the common duct and the portal vein. Cursors (+) measure the diameter of the common bile duct.

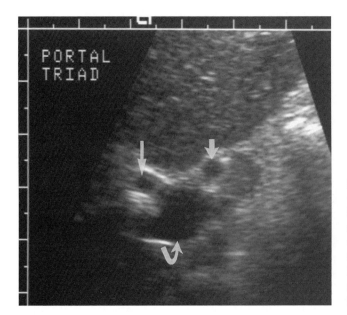

Figure 2.8 *Mickey Mouse.* Transverse image of the portal triad as it crosses the hepatoduodenal ligament resembles Mickey Mouse with the face being the portal vein (*curved arrow*), the hepatic artery being the left ear (*short arrow*), and the common bile duct being the right ear (*long arrow*).

GALLBLADDER

The GB is a pear-shaped, bile-filled sac nestled in a concave fossa on the visceral surface of the liver (Figs. 2.6, 2.9). The fundus usually projects beyond the edge of the liver while the body and neck extend dorsally toward the porta hepatis. The hepatic surface of the GB is attached to the liver by blood vessels and connective tissue whereas the inferior surface and fundus of the GB are covered by visceral peritoneum. Occasionally the GB is suspended on a mesentery and is not closely applied to the liver. The GB wall is made up of three layers of tissue. The inner mucosa is redundant and loosely connected to the fibromuscular layer. The mucosa is mucin-secreting columnar epithelium and is continuous with the epithelium of the cystic duct and biliary tree. The fibromuscular layer provides the framework of the sac with interlaced fibrous tissue and smooth muscle. The external coat is the covering peritoneum. The cystic duct is 4 cm long extending from the GB neck to the hepatic duct which it joins to form the CBD. The mucosal lining of the cystic duct forms 5–12 folds that constitute the spiral valve of Heister. These folds may cast acoustic shadows and mimic small stones lodged in the cystic dust. After a fast of 4 or more hours the normal GB is well distended and easily visualized by US as a gourd-shaped sac of fluid. Normal bile is echo-free. The normal GB does not exceed 5 cm in transverse diameter. In 4% of patients the fun-

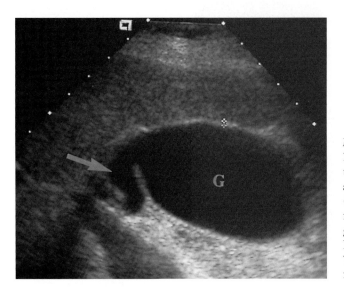

Figure 2.9 *Normal Gallbladder.* Image through the long axis of the gallbladder (G) demonstrates a tortuous gallbladder neck (*arrow*). Gallbladder wall thickness is measured between the gallbladder lumen and the hepatic parenchyma (*cursors*, +). This gallbladder wall measures a normal 2 mm.

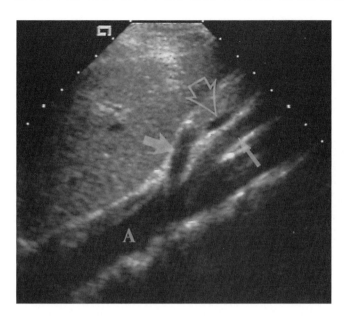

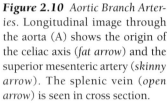

Figure 2.10 *Aortic Branch Arteries.* Longitudinal image through the aorta (A) shows the origin of the celiac axis (*fat arrow*) and the superior mesenteric artery (*skinny arrow*). The splenic vein (*open arrow*) is seen in cross section.

dus folds back on itself forming a "Phrygian cap." Additional normal folds may be seen near the neck of the GB. The GB wall is visualized as a thin echogenic line at the GB interface with the liver. Wall thickness is measured between the liver parenchyma and the GB lumen. This measurement, which includes the liver capsule, the entire GB wall, and intervening tissue, is normally less than 3 mm.

The normal GB does not exceed 5 cm in diameter. The normal GB wall does not exceed 3 mm in thickness.

PANCREAS

The pancreas is identified on US by recognition of the blood vessels within and around the pancreatic parenchyma (Figs. 2.10–2.14). The neck, body, and tail of the pancreas course anterior and parallel to the SV. The total length of the pancreas from head to tail is 12–15 cm. The neck of the pancreas is anterior to the confluence of the SV and the SMV that forms the PV. The SV is of uniform diameter (<10 mm) until its junction with the SMV where the combined veins form a teardrop-shaped dilatation (Figs. 2.12–2.14). The SMV courses in sagittal plane just to the right and usually slightly anterior to the superior mesenteric artery (SMA). The uncinate process of the pancreas extends leftward beneath the SMV to form a

The normal maximum diameter of the pancreas is 3.0 cm in head, 2.5 cm in the body, and 2.0 cm in the tail.

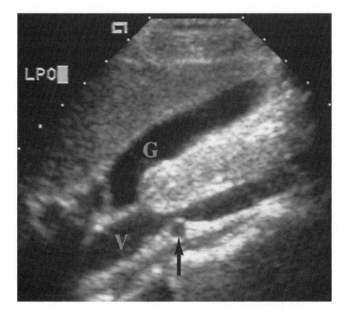

Figure 2.11 *Inferior Vena Cava.* Longitudinal image through the inferior vena cava (V) shows the right renal artery (*arrow*) crossing behind the cava. G, gallbladder.

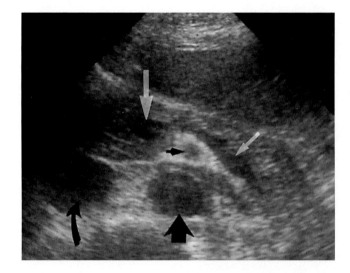

Figure 2.12 *Normal Pancreas—Transverse.* The pancreas is recognized by identifying its adjacent vasculature: the splenic vein (*small white arrow*), the superior mesenteric artery (*black arrowhead*), the inferior vena cava (*curved black arrow*), and the aorta (*fat black arrow*). The junction of the splenic vein with the superior mesenteric vein marks the commencement of the portal vein and is recognized by its teardrop shape (*large white arrow*) at the right end of the splenic vein.

tapered projection. Blunting of the normally tapered uncinate process is a sensitive sign of pancreatic enlargement or tumor. The SMA arises anteriorly from the aorta at or near the level of the crossing SV (Fig. 2.10). The SMA is surrounded by a collar of echogenic fat and appears, on transverse section, as the hole in a doughnut (Figs. 2.12, 2.14). The left renal vein and the transverse portion of the duodenum course underneath the SMV and SMA caudal to the level of the pancreas. The celiac axis arises from the aorta just cephalad to the pancreas (Fig. 2.10). In transverse plane the bifurcation into the hepatic and splenic arteries resembles a seagull in flight. The left gastric artery origin off the celiac axis may be seen in longitudinal plane.

The CBD extends caudally in the posterior aspect of the pancreatic head where it is commonly visualized as a tubular structure that ends at the major papilla entering the descending duodenum (Fig. 2.14). The pancreatic duct courses centrally within the pancreatic parenchyma from the tail to the head (Fig. 2.15). It joins the CBD to drain into the major papilla in 80% of individuals. In the remaining 20% the pancreatic duct enters the duodenum separately at the minor papilla. The hypoechoic muscular wall of the stomach should not be mistaken for the pancreatic duct (Fig. 2.16). The gastroduodenal artery courses anterior and parallel to the CBD. Doppler US confirms its identification.

The normal echogenicity of the pancreatic parenchyma depends upon the amount of fatty infiltration. The pancreas has no distinct capsule and, with aging, fat infiltrates between the lobules of parenchyma and increases the echogenicity. In children and younger adults the pancreas resembles a slab of meat and has well-defined margins with echogenic-

The pancreatic duct tapers from head to tail with normal maximum diameter of 3 mm.

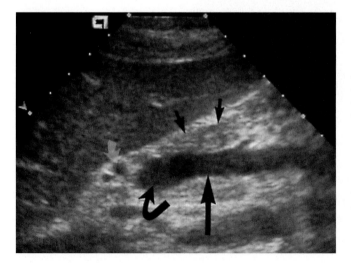

Figure 2.13 *Normal Pancreas—Sagittal.* Longitudinal image demonstrates the superior mesenteric vein (*long arrow*) extending cranially to its junction with the splenic vein to form the portal vein (*black curved arrow*). The hepatic artery (*white curved arrow*) is seen in cross section. A portion of the neck of the pancreas (*2 small arrows*) is seen anterior to the superior mesenteric vein.

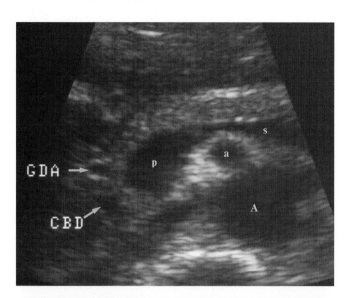

Figure 2.14 *Normal Head of the Pancreas.* Transverse view demonstrates the gastroduodenal artery (GDA) and the common bile duct (CBD) coursing adjacent to the head of the pancreas. The splenic vein (s) extends rightward to the commencement of the portal vein (p). Also seen are the superior mesenteric artery (a) and the aorta (A).

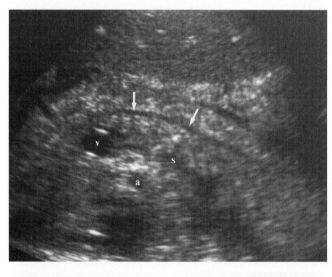

Figure 2.15 *Normal Pancreatic Duct.* A normal pancreatic duct (*2 white arrows*) courses in the substance of the pancreas anterior to a collapsed splenic vein (s). The portal vein origin (v) and superior mesenteric artery (a) are also seen on this transverse image.

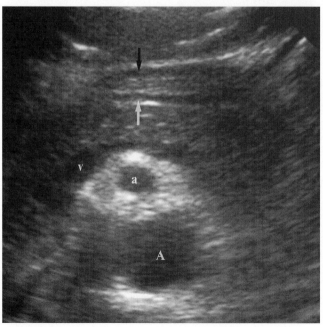

Figure 2.16 *Stomach Wall Mimics the Pancreatic Duct.* The hypoechoic posterior wall of the stomach (*white arrow*) may be mistaken for the pancreatic duct. This error is avoided by recognizing that the stomach wall is anterior to, rather than within, the pancreas and by identifying the anterior wall of the stomach (*black arrow*). Also seen on this transverse image are the superior mesenteric vein (v) and artery (a) and the aorta (A).

ity approximately equal to liver parenchyma. In older patients the pancreas resembles a dust mop and has poorly defined margins with echogenicity just slightly less than fat.

SPLEEN

The spleen is normally visualized in the left upper quadrant of the abdomen between the diaphragm and the fundus of the stomach (Fig. 2.17). The spleen is soft and pliable allowing it to conform to the shape of the structures around it. Its diaphragmatic surface is smooth and convex, matching the concavity of the diaphragm. Its visceral surface is rounded and smooth with concavities for the stomach, left kidney, and the splenic flexure of the colon. Usual dimensions in adults are 12 cm in length, 7 cm in breadth, and 3–4 cm in thickness.

> The normal spleen does not exceed 14 cm in any dimension.

The spleen parenchyma is a network of lymphatic follicles (the white pulp) surrounded by vascular lakes filled with blood (the red pulp). On US the splenic parenchyma is extremely homogeneous with mid-to-low-level echogenicity slightly greater than that of the liver. The SV runs a relatively straight course rightward from the splenic hilum to the commencement of the PV dorsal to the neck of the pancreas. The SV receives the small inferior mesenteric vein in the region of the distal body of the pancreas and joins with the larger SMV to form the PV. The splenic artery is tortuous as it courses from the celiac axis to the splenic hilum. As the splenic artery enters the hilum it divides into six or more branches which ramify throughout the parenchyma. The capsule of the spleen is covered by closely applied visceral peritoneum except at the hilum and a small "bare area" at the posterior dome of the diaphragm. The spleen is anchored by phrenicolienal, lienorenal, and gastrolienal ligaments that converge at the hilum.

PERITONEAL CAVITY

The peritoneal cavity is that portion of the abdominal cavity that is bounded by the parietal peritoneum. It consists of numerous recesses formed by organs, ligaments, and peritoneal reflections [8]. The lesser sac is the large potential space behind the stomach. It communicates with the remainder of the peritoneal cavity only by the small opening of the foramen of Winslow. Fluid in the lesser sac usually occurs only as a result of disease in structures bordering the lesser sac [9]. The major recesses of the greater peritoneal cavity are the right

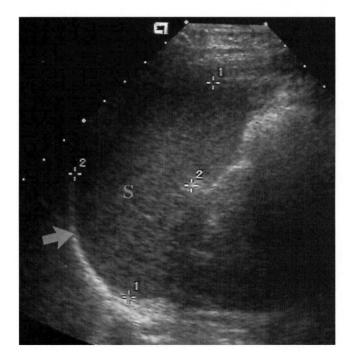

Figure 2.17 *Normal Spleen.* Longitudinal image shows a normal spleen (S; *between cursors, +, 1, 2*) conforming to the smooth curve of the diaphragm (*arrow*).

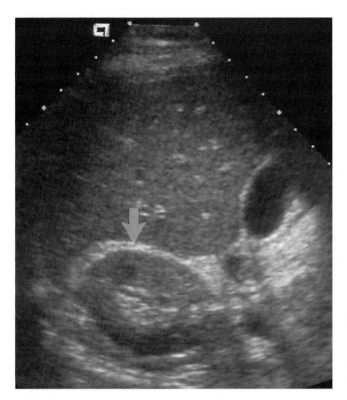

Figure 2.18 *Hepatorenal Recess.* Transverse image shows the location of the hepatorenal recess (Morison's pouch) (*arrow*) between the liver and the right kidney.

and left subdiaphragmatic spaces, the hepatorenal recess (Morison's pouch) (Fig. 2.18), the paracolic gutters, and the pelvic cul-de-sac. These recesses are most apparent when fluid is present in the peritoneal cavity.

LIVER

DIFFUSE HEPATIC DISEASE

Hepatomegaly

Hepatomegaly is a nonspecific finding in primary and systemic diseases of the liver. Causes include vascular congestion, infection, tumors and cysts, diffuse cellular infiltration (lymphoma, leukemia), storage diseases, and fatty infiltration.

- Length of the right lobe >15.5 cm is 87% accurate in the diagnosis of hepatomegaly (Fig. 2.19) [10].
- Extension of the right lobe beyond the lower pole of the right kidney suggests hepatomegaly (Fig. 2.19).
- Rounding of the inferior edge of the liver suggests pathologic enlargement (Fig. 2.20).
- Reidel's lobe is an elongation of the right lobe of the liver that may extend to the iliac crest. It is commonly found as a normal variation in thin women and may be mistaken for hepatomegaly. Reidel's lobe is recognized by noting an associated decreased volume of the left hepatic lobe.

Viral Hepatitis

Viral hepatitis is a common illness throughout the world. It is classified as hepatitis A (spread by fecal-oral contamination), hepatitis B (spread by blood products and sexual contact), and hepatitis C (spread by blood transfusion).

- **Acute hepatitis** causes diffuse interstitial edema and infiltration of inflammatory cells. US examination is commonly normal but may show hepatomegaly, GB wall edema, and

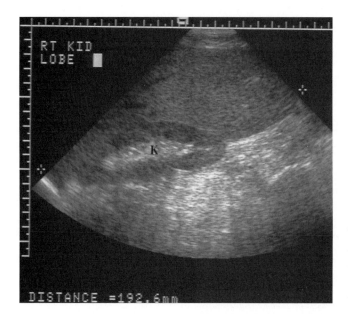

Figure 2.19 *Hepatomegaly.* The right lobe of the liver extends well below the lower pole of the right kidney (K) and measures 20 cm (*between cursors*, +), well exceeding the normal limit of 15.5 cm.

diffuse decrease in parenchymal echogenicity. The latter finding has been called the *starry sky liver* because the bright portal triads stand out as "stars" against a background of dark parenchyma (Fig. 2.21). Differential diagnosis of starry sky liver includes acute hepatitis, glycogen storage disease, leukemia, passive hepatic congestion, and toxic shock syndrome [11].

■ **Chronic hepatitis** implies continuing, usually low-grade, liver injury. US findings are usually normal until cirrhosis develops.

Fatty Liver

Infiltration of hepatocytes with lipid is a common and non-specific reaction to hepatocyte injury. This abnormality has a multitude of causes (Box 2.1).

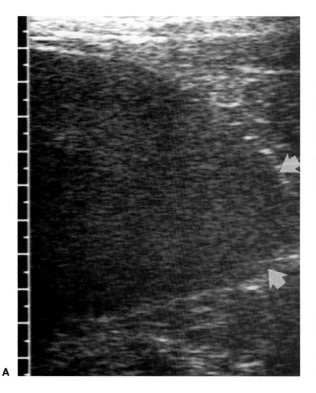

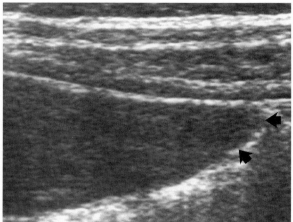

Figure 2.20 *Blunting of the Liver Edge. A.* A high frequency linear array transducer shows blunting of the edge of the liver (*arrows*). This finding is a sign of hepatomegaly or diffuse hepatic disease. *B.* A normal sharp liver edge (*arrows*) is shown for comparison.

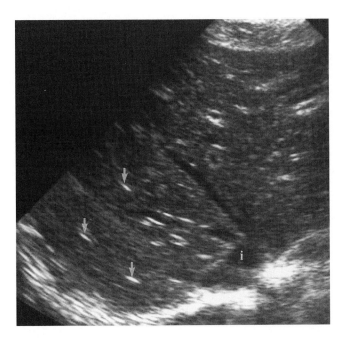

Figure 2.21 *Acute Hepatitis.* Transverse image at the level of the hepatic veins and inferior vena cava (i) shows the "starry sky" appearance of bright portal triads (*arrows*) on a background of edematous hypoechoic liver parenchyma.

■ Fatty infiltration increases the echogenicity of the liver parenchyma and causes increased attenuation of the US beam resulting in poor definition of the deep portions of the liver and the diaphragm (Fig. 2.22). The fatty liver significantly exceeds the echogenicity of normal renal parenchyma.

■ **Diffuse fatty liver** involves all of the liver parenchyma. Vessels course normally through the parenchyma without distortion, encasement, or mass effect.

■ **Focal fatty liver** usually occurs in a lobar or segmental distribution. Angulated geometric boundaries between involved and spared areas of liver parenchyma are characteristic.

■ Single or multiple nodular areas of focal fatty infiltration may occur and simulate tumors and metastatic disease [12]. A key finding is the absence of mass effect on vessels within and adjacent to the focal fatty nodules. Focal fatty nodules tend to occur in the same areas as focal fatty sparing [13].

■ An interdigitating pattern of fatty infiltrated and spared parenchyma is an uncommon but characteristic pattern of involvement.

■ **Focal sparing in diffuse fatty liver** simulates hypoechoic masses (Fig. 2.23). Recognizing that the liver parenchyma is diffusely echogenic and that the spared, more hypoechoic areas are in characteristic locations makes this diagnosis. Common areas for focal sparing (and for focal fat infiltration) are the medial segment of the left lobe (segment IV), anterior to the PV bifurcation, near the GB bed, and in subcapsular parenchyma.

Fatty livers are highly echogenic and difficult to penetrate with ultrasound.

Box 2.1: Causes of Fatty Liver

Common	Less common
Obesity	Steroid therapy
Alcohol abuse	Malnutrition
Chemotherapy	Parenteral nutrition
Diabetes mellitus	Glycogen storage disease
	Drugs

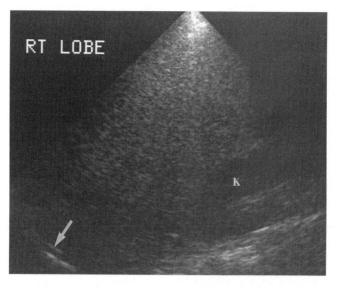

Figure 2.22 *Diffuse Fatty Liver.* The liver is markedly echogenic and difficult to penetrate with US despite the use of a 2.5-MHz transducer. The diaphragm (*arrow*) and right kidney (K) are barely visualized. The liver parenchyma is markedly more echogenic than the renal parenchyma.

- Correlation with CT of the liver that shows low attenuation in areas of fatty infiltration and normal attenuation in areas of fatty sparing is diagnostic in problem cases.
- The patterns of fatty infiltration are related to the relative blood flow distributions of the PV and hepatic artery either preferentially carrying toxins to, or preferentially sparing, portions of the liver [14].

Cirrhosis

Cirrhosis is the final common pathway of chronic injury to the liver from many causes (Box 2.2). Parenchymal necrosis is followed by extensive fibrosis and nodular regeneration of hepatocytes with progressive distortion of lobar and vascular architecture [15].

Cirrhosis alters hepatic echotexture and causes nodularity, whereas fatty infiltration alters hepatic echogenicity. Often the two conditions coexist.

- Cirrhosis alters hepatic echotexture resulting in liver parenchyma that appears heterogeneous, nodular, grainy, or coarse (Figs. 2.24, 2.25). Visualization of portal triads in the periphery of the liver is decreased. The echotexture of hepatic parenchyma does not correlate well with hepatic function or the severity of cirrhosis. In addition, this appearance is not specific and may be seen in other conditions such as diffuse metastatic disease (especially from breast cancer) or infiltrative hepatocellular carcinoma (HCC).
- Increased echogenicity of the liver indicates fatty infiltration, which is commonly present in cirrhosis.

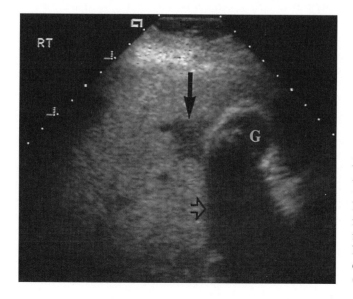

Figure 2.23 *Focal Sparring in Fatty Liver.* A hypoechoic area (*arrow*) with angulated margins located near the gallbladder (G) is characteristic of focal sparring in a markedly echogenic fatty liver. Gallstones in the gallbladder cast an acoustic shadow (*open arrow*).

Box 2.2: Causes of Cirrhosis

Common
Alcohol abuse (75% of cases)
Viral hepatitis (B, C) (10% of cases)
Idiopathic (10% of cases)

Less common
Primary biliary cirrhosis
Primary sclerosing cholangitis
Drug-induced hepatotoxicity
Parasitic diseases
Metabolic disorders
    Wilson's disease
      Hemochromatosis

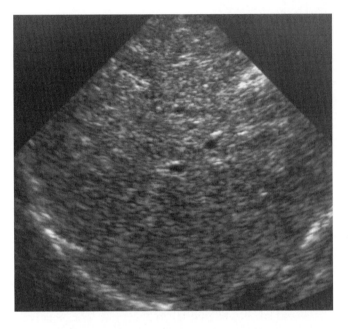

Figure 2.24 *Cirrhosis*. The fibrosis and altered architecture of cirrhosis cause a coarse appearance of the hepatic parenchyma with limited visualization of portal triads.

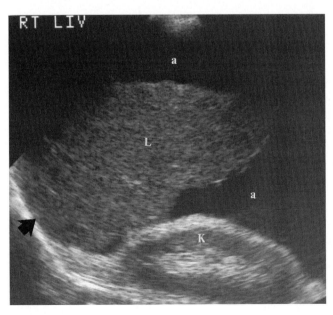

Figure 2.25 *Cirrhosis and Ascites*. The liver (L) appears shrunken and nodular as it is suspended in a sea of ascites (a). Note the echogenicity of the liver is nearly identical to the echogenicity of the right kidney (K) parenchyma. The "bare area" of the liver (*arrow*) is closely applied to the diaphragm and is not covered by ascites.

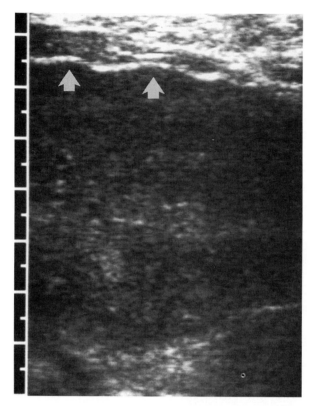

Figure 2.26 *Nodular Liver Surface in Cirrhosis.* Inspection of the liver surface with a high-frequency, linear array transducer demonstrates the surface nodularity (*arrows*) characteristic of cirrhosis.

- Scarring and nodular regeneration result in a nodular surface of the liver best seen with a linear array transducer (Fig. 2.26) or when ascites is present (Fig. 2.25) [16]. This finding is more specific for cirrhosis than is altered echotexture. The nodular contour varies from fine to coarse to grossly lobular [17].
- Asymmetric shrinkage of the right lobe with relative hypertrophy of the left lobe and caudate lobe are common findings in alcoholic cirrhosis. Portal venous flow from the stomach, where most alcohol is absorbed, is preferential to the right lobe, relatively sparing the left and caudate lobes.
- Nodules are a constant and problematic feature of cirrhosis.
- Portal hypertension is evidenced by splenomegaly, ascites, enlargement of the PV and mesenteric veins, and the presence of portosystemic collaterals.
- The hepatic artery is enlarged and tortuous in advanced cirrhosis.
- Patients with cirrhosis are prone to PV thrombosis.
- Cirrhosis decreases the compliance of the walls of hepatic veins resulting in spectral Doppler waveforms that are dampened and lack the normal pulsatility and flow reversal with atrial contraction that is characteristic of the hepatic veins [18]. This finding has been called *portalization of the hepatic veins.*
- HCC develops in 5–12% of patients with cirrhosis.

Nodules in Cirrhosis
Patients with cirrhosis are at high risk of developing HCC. Detection of this tumor is markedly impaired by the scarring and nodule formation that is characteristic of cirrhosis. A variety of nodular masses are seen in cirrhosis [19].

- **Regenerative nodules** are present in all cirrhotic livers; however, imaging studies demonstrate them in only 25–50% of patients. Each nodule consists of a group of regenerating hepatocytes surrounded by fibrous septa. Regenerating nodules are usually <10 mm in size. Most regenerating nodules are isoechoic and are poorly seen on US. When seen,

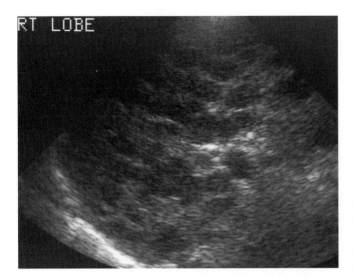

Figure 2.27 *Regenerative Nodules in Cirrhosis.* Innumerable small hypoechoic nodules are seen throughout the liver in this patient with cirrhosis.

the nodules are hypoechoic (Fig. 2.27). Nodularity is best appreciated by examining the surface of the liver with a high-frequency, linear array transducer (Fig. 2.26) [16].

- **Dysplastic regenerative nodules** (adenomatous hyperplasia) contain areas of cellular atypia without distinct malignancy. These nodules are a precursor of HCC. Most exceed 10 mm in size. These nodules are best recognized as a solid hypoechoic dominant nodule surrounded by a group of smaller nodules [20].
- **Small HCCs** (<3 cm) are difficult to differentiate from regenerative nodules. US detection rates of these small cancers are reported at 55–84%. Most small HCCs are hypoechoic solid tumors without necrosis. A thin peripheral hypoechoic halo, corresponding to a fibrous capsule, is a characteristic finding. Spectral Doppler shows high-velocity flow (70–90 cm/sec) in feeding arteries [21].
- **Focal confluent fibrosis** may be seen as a mass replacing hepatic parenchyma. Focal fibrosis may occur in any form of cirrhosis but is most common in primary sclerosing cholangitis [20]. Confluent fibrosis may be wedge-shaped, peripheral, segmental, or lobar [22]. Associated parenchymal atrophy is prominent.
- Hemangiomas and cysts are rare in cirrhotic livers, probably because they get obliterated by the cirrhotic process [20].
- Metastatic disease from primary cancers outside of the liver is uncommon in cirrhotic livers, probably because cirrhosis creates an unfavorable environment for metastatic tumor growth [23].

One of the unsolved problems of hepatic imaging is the detection of small HCCs in cirrhotic livers and the differentiation of small tumors from regenerating nodules and dysplastic nodules. All appear on US as small hypoechoic solid masses.

Portal Hypertension

US diagnosis of portal hypertension depends on indirect signs because non-invasive measurement of PV pressure is not currently possible.

- PV diameter >13 mm and SV or SMV diameter >10 mm suggests portal hypertension (approximately 80% sensitivity and specificity) (Fig. 2.28) [24].
- PV flow velocity < 21 cm/sec is 80% predictive [24].
- Splenomegaly and ascites are usually present with significant portal hypertension.
- Identification of porto-systemic collateral vessel enlargement (varices) is the most specific evidence of portal hypertension. A patent enlarged paraumbilical vein coursing through the fissure of the ligamentum teres (Fig. 2.29) and along the falciform ligament to the anterior abdominal wall and umbilicus is highly indicative. Additional enlarged collateral vessels may be seen along the lesser curve of the stomach (in the gastrohepatic ligament), in the hilum of the spleen (Fig. 2.30), and in the retroperitoneum especially near the renal hilum [25].

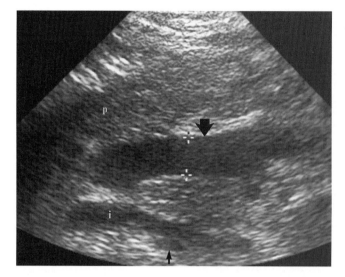

Figure 2.28 *Portal Hypertension—Dilated SMV.* Longitudinal image shows dilatation of the superior mesenteric vein (*large arrow*) to 12 mm (*between cursors, +*). This finding is highly indicative of portal hypertension. Seen posterior to the enlarged superior mesenteric vein is the inferior vena cava (i) and right renal artery (*small arrow*). p, neck of pancreas.

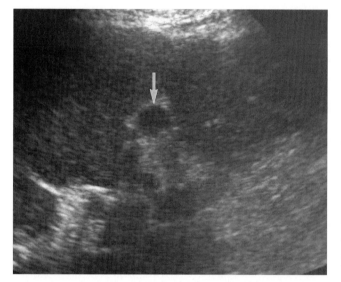

Figure 2.29 *Portal Hypertension—Enlarged Paraumbilical Vein.* Transverse image shows a dilated paraumbilical vein (*arrow*) seen as a "hole" in the normally echogenic fissure of the ligamentum teres. Enlarged paraumbilical vein collaterals are definitive evidence of portal hypertension.

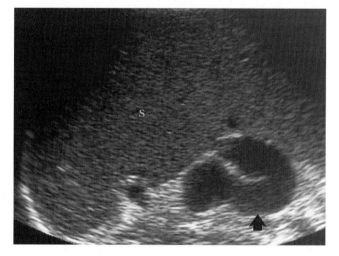

Figure 2.30 *Portal Hypertension—Collaterals.* The spleen (S) is massively enlarged, and a markedly dilated and tortuous portosystemic collateral vein (*arrow*) is seen in the splenic hilum.

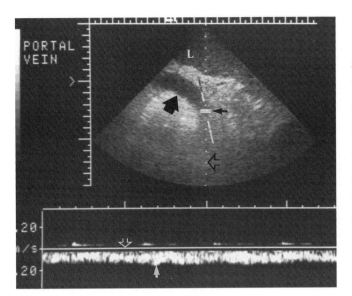

Figure 2.31 *Portal Hypertension—Reversed Flow in Portal Vein.* Spectral Doppler shows flow in the portal vein (*fat black arrow*) to be out of the liver (L). The spectral trace (*short white arrow*) is below the baseline (*open white arrow*), indicating flow away from the Doppler US pulse shown by the dotted line (*open black arrow*). When correlated with the anatomic position of the Doppler sample volume (*small black arrow*), this finding confirms reversed blood flow direction in the portal vein.

- Retrograde flow in the PV (hepatofugal flow—away from the liver) (Fig. 2.31) is indicative of advanced portal hypertension.
- Calcification may be seen in the wall of the portal, splenic, or mesenteric veins with long-standing portal hypertension [26].

Portal Vein Thrombosis
PV thrombosis occurs in association with cirrhosis, HCC, portal hypertension, hypercoagulable states, pancreatitis, and cholecystitis. Clinical presentation is non-specific.

- The PV is enlarged and filled with hypoechoic thrombus (Fig. 2.32) [27].
- Color flow US shows complete absence of blood flow or blood flow around an intraluminal thrombus (Fig. 2.32).

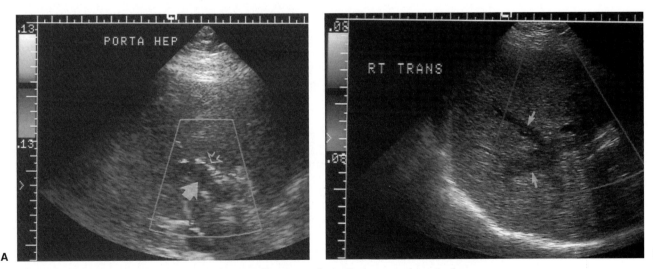

Figure 2.32 *Thrombosed Portal Vein.* A. Color Doppler image through the porta hepatis shows absence of blood flow in the dilated portal vein (*fat arrow*). High-velocity turbulent blood flow (mixed colors) is evident in the adjacent hepatic artery (*open arrow*). B. Transverse color Doppler image of the right lobe reveals extension of blood clot into intrahepatic branches (*arrows*) of the portal vein (see Color Figure 2.32A,B).

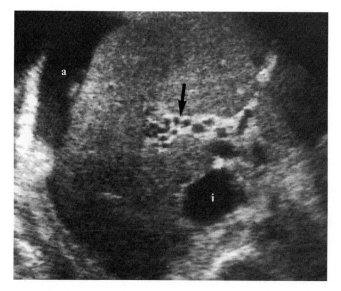

Figure 2.33 *Cavernous Transformation of the Portal Vein.* Transverse image through the porta hepatis shows multiple small collateral veins (*arrow*) in the bed of the occluded portal vein. Ascites (a) is present. The inferior vena cava (i) is dilated.

- **Cavernous transformation of the PV** refers to PV thrombosis with collateral flow in multiple tortuous collateral vessels that course in the bed of the PV (Fig. 2.33) [28].
- Hepatic artery resistance index (RI) is lowered (RI <0.50) by PV thrombosis [29].
- Normal color flow US examination excludes the diagnosis.

Passive Hepatic Congestion

Compromise of hepatic venous drainage by congestive heart failure or constrictive pericarditis causes stasis of blood in the liver parenchyma. Elevated central venous pressure is transmitted to the hepatic veins and the hepatic parenchyma. The liver becomes engorged and edematous [30].

- The IVC and hepatic veins dilate with increasing central venous pressure. The hepatic veins are considered dilated when their diameter exceeds 9–10 mm [31].
- The IVC and hepatic veins lose their normal triphasic pulsatility on spectral Doppler and show an abnormal pattern of continuous blood flow toward the heart [30].
- Portal venous blood flow becomes pulsatile as elevated pressure from the right heart is transmitted to the PV [32].
- Additional non-specific findings that are commonly present include cardiomegaly, pleural effusions, pericardial effusions, ascites, and hepatomegaly [30].

Budd-Chiari Syndrome

Budd-Chiari syndrome is characterized by obstruction or severe stenosis of hepatic venous outflow at the level of the hepatic veins or extrahepatic IVC. In Western countries Budd-Chiari syndrome is most often caused by thrombosis induced by systemic or malignant diseases. In Asian countries the cause is most often a membranous or segmental obstruction of the IVC. Patients present with abdominal pain, hepatomegaly, and ascites.

- Color Doppler shows no flow in one or more of the hepatic veins or the IVC. Retrograde flow away from the IVC into intrahepatic venous collaterals may be seen [33].
- Intrahepatic veno-venous collaterals are characteristic. These may appear as large tortuous intrahepatic veins or tiny "spider web" small vessel collaterals deep within the parenchyma or in the subcapsular area [34].
- Occlusion of the hepatic veins may result in portal hypertension with reversed flow in the PV and enlarged porto-systemic collateral veins. These changes may reverse after therapy.
- Webs appear as echogenic flap-like structures in the IVC near the junction with hepatic veins. IVC occlusion may be short segment (1 cm) or long segment (5 cm). The thrombosed IVC may be calcified [35].

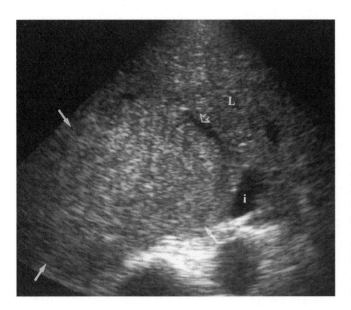

Figure 2.34 *Hepatocellular Carcinoma.* A large hepatocellular carcinoma (*small arrows*) replaces the right hepatic lobe and bows the right hepatic vein (*open arrow*). The margins of the hepatoma are poorly defined. The liver parenchyma (L) is heterogeneous because of cirrhosis. i, inferior vena cava.

- When the syndrome is chronic, the caudate lobe is classically hypertrophied whereas the involved lobes are atrophic. The involved parenchyma is heterogeneous in echogenicity. The caudate lobe drains directly into the IVC via small veins and is typically spared by hepatic vein thrombosis.

LIVER MASSES

Hepatocellular Carcinoma

HCC is the most common primary hepatic malignancy. It nearly always occurs in a setting of cirrhosis or chronic hepatitis. Serum alpha-fetoprotein is often elevated.

- US findings are usually non-specific in HCC. Tumors occur as a solitary mass (Fig. 2.34), as a dominant mass with small satellite lesions, as multiple nodules, or as diffuse parenchymal infiltration.
- Small HCCs (<3 cm) are usually homogeneous, solid, hypoechoic nodules that are difficult to differentiate from regenerative nodules in the cirrhotic liver. A thin peripheral hypoechoic halo corresponding to a fibrous capsule favors HCC [21]. Pulsatile blood flow shown by color Doppler or power Doppler US favors HCC [36].
- Larger HCCs are more variable in appearance with heterogeneous solid areas and areas of hemorrhage and necrosis.
- Intratumoral fat deposits cause diffuse or focal areas of increased echogenicity. Small HCCs with high fat content are echogenic masses that resemble hemangiomas. Because hemangiomas are uncommon in cirrhotic livers, HCC should always be considered the prime diagnosis.
- Many tumors are hypervascular with arteriovenous shunting. Doppler demonstrates high-velocity pulsatile flow most conspicuous in the periphery of the tumor. Color and power Doppler show a fine network of blood vessels around the periphery of the tumor or a branching network of internal vascularity [37].
- Tumor invasion of PVs (25–40%) and hepatic veins (16%) is characteristic of HCC. Tumor thrombus is visualized as a low-density plug within a dilated vein (Fig. 2.35). Doppler shows complete venous occlusion or flow around a partially obstructing thrombus. Extension of tumor into the IVC is a cause of Budd-Chiari syndrome.

HCC is associated with tumor invasion of portal veins, hepatic veins, and the IVC.

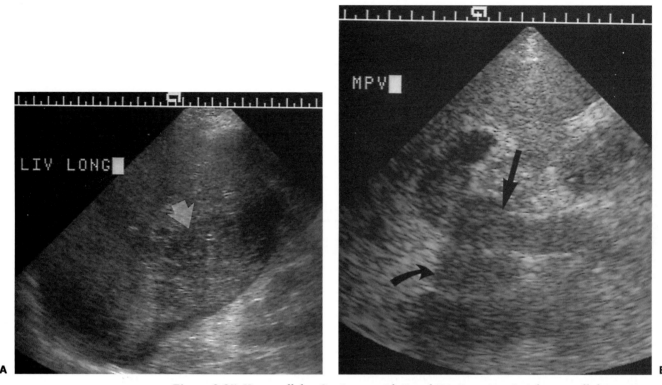

Figure 2.35 *Hepatocellular Carcinoma with Portal Vein Invasion. A. A hepatocellular carcinoma (*arrow*) is seen as an irregular heterogeneous hypodense mass in the inferior right lobe. B. The tumor (*curved arrow*) invades the portal vein, filling and expanding the vein with tumor thrombus (*straight arrow*).*

Fibrolamellar Carcinoma

Fibrolamellar carcinoma is a distinct variant of HCC in its clinical, pathologic, and imaging features. It is characteristically found in adolescents and young adults who lack the risk factors for HCC. Hemorrhage and necrosis are characteristically absent from the tumor [38].

- A large, lobulated, well-defined hepatic mass in a young person (mean age, 23) is characteristic (Fig. 2.36) [38].
- A central stellate fibrous scar is common. The scar may include calcification that is also stellate in appearance.
- Echotexture is variable and usually mixed with hyperechoic and isoechoic components [38].
- Hemorrhage, necrosis, vascular invasion, and multifocal disease are usually conspicuously absent.
- The major differential diagnosis is focal nodular hyperplasia (FNH).

Calcifications are much more common in fibrolamellar carcinoma (30–40%) than in HCC (<10%).

Hepatic Cavernous Hemangioma

Cavernous hemangioma is the most common primary neoplasm of the liver. Fortunately, all are benign with no malignant potential. Most cause no symptoms and are discovered incidentally by US or CT. Hemangiomas consist of a mass of blood-filled vascular channels lined by endothelial cells. Thrombosis in the vascular channels leads to fibrosis, scarring, and calcification.

- The characteristic US appearance is a well-defined, homogeneous, hyperechoic solid mass (Fig. 2.37). Accentuated through-transmission is often present. High echogenicity is produced by the numerous interfaces of the interlacing vascular spaces. Acoustic enhancement results from the fact that the lesion is mostly slow-flowing liquid blood.

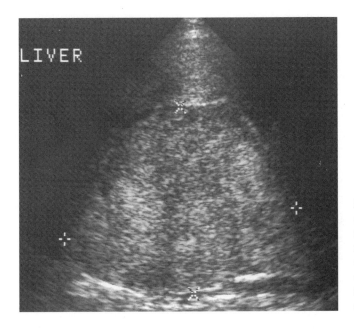

Figure 2.36 *Fibrolamellar Carcinoma.* A heterogeneous but rather well-defined solid mass is measured between the cursors (+, x). The patient is a 37-year-old male with no clinical or imaging evidence of hepatitis or cirrhosis.

The demonstration of a liver mass with these classic features is considered sufficient to make a definite diagnosis of hemangioma by many radiologists, particularly if the patient has no history of malignant disease and if liver chemistries are normal [39].

- When lesion size is >3 cm, thrombosis and scarring commonly result in an ill-defined central hypoechoic zone. Calcification may be present within the hypoechoic zone. Lesions with large hypoechoic areas have a characteristic thin hyperechoic border [40].

- In 10% of patients, multiple hemangiomas are present, often raising concern for metastatic disease.

- In a fatty-infiltrated liver, hemangiomas may appear hypoechoic compared to the abnormal liver parenchyma (Fig. 2.38).

- Most cavernous hemangiomas remain stable in size over time [41]. However, lesions that double or triple in diameter have been reported [42].

- Blood flow within hemangiomas is exceedingly slow. Typically, color and spectral Doppler will show no detectable signal within the lesion [43]. Power Doppler may show a diffuse color "blush" believed to be caused by the architecture of the lesion rather than

Hepatic cavernous hemangiomas are commonly discovered as an incidental finding on routine US examination of the abdomen.

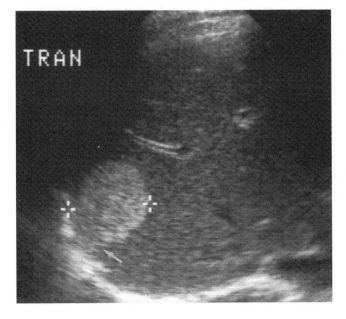

Figure 2.37 *Classic Appearance of Cavernous Hemangioma.* A solid, well-defined, uniformly echogenic mass is indicated by the cursors (+). Accentuated through-transmission (*arrow*) is seen distal to the mass. Color Doppler demonstrated no Doppler signal within the mass. Blood flow is usually too slow to be detected by Doppler.

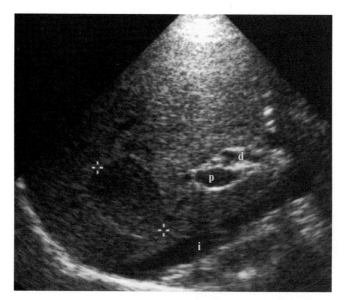

Figure 2.38 *Cavernous Hemangioma in Fatty Liver.* The cavernous hemangioma (*between cursors,* +) is well defined and uniformly low in echogenicity compared to the diffusely fatty infiltrated liver. d, common bile duct; i, inferior vena cava; p, portal vein.

by blood flow [44]. Doppler findings are not specific for hemangiomas, because metastatic lesions may also show the absence of internal vascularity [43].

■ A specific diagnosis of cavernous hemangioma can be made by radionuclide-labeled, red blood scintigraphy and by contrast-enhanced CT and MR [45].

■ Atypical appearance on imaging studies may lead to image-guided biopsy. Fine needle aspiration yields only blood and endothelial cells, results usually considered inadequate for a specific diagnosis. Core biopsy with an 18-gauge needle has been shown to be definitive and safe [46]. The needle path selected for biopsy should always pass through normal parenchyma before entering the lesion to prevent unimpaired bleeding into the peritoneal cavity.

Focal Nodular Hyperplasia

FNH is the second most common benign tumor of the liver. The lesion is a proliferation of nonneoplastic hepatocytes held together in abnormal arrangement by a network of fibrous tissue with a dominant scar [47]. Abundant, thick-walled arteries and sinusoids lined by endothelial and Kupffer cells are present within the mass. FNH is more common in women and is usually discovered as an incidental finding.

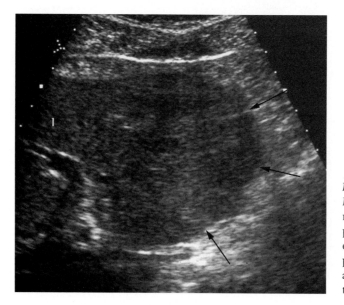

Figure 2.39 *Focal Nodular Hyperplasia.* The mass is recognized by the focal bulge (*arrows*) it produces in the liver contour. Its echogenicity is isoechoic to liver parenchyma (l). Note the slightly altered echotexture and lack of portal triads in the mass.

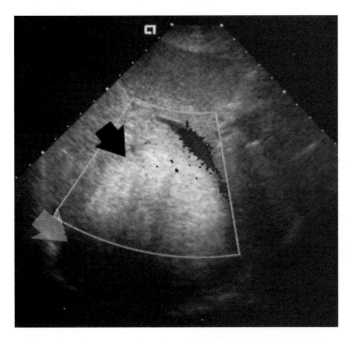

Figure 2.40 *Hepatic Adenoma.* This hepatic adenoma (*black arrow*) is strikingly echogenic and causes marked attenuation of the US beam (*white arrow*). These findings are caused by high fat content of the tumor confirmed by its low density on computed tomography and on pathologic examination following surgical resection.

- The lesion is typically solitary (80–95%) and homogeneous. Because of its excellent blood supply necrosis and hemorrhage are rare. Most lesions are smaller than 5-cm diameter [47].
- US shows a homogeneous solid mass that is isoechoic or slightly hypoechoic compared to normal liver parenchyma (Fig. 2.39) [47]. Only surface mass effect or displacement of vessels may identify the mass.
- A central scar with fibrous septations extending from it is a characteristic finding often not shown well by US. When seen, the scar is echogenic and hypervascular. The central hypervascular nidus may be shown by color flow US even when the scar is not evident [47].
- Radiocolloid scintigraphy is commonly diagnostic. Because of the presence of Kupffer cells in FNH, radionuclide activity within the lesion is equal to or greater than normal liver in 50–70% of lesions.
- On follow-up, the lesions may decrease in size or disappear [48].
- Calcifications are an atypical feature of FNH. When present the lesion is difficult to differentiate from fibrolamellar carcinoma [49].

Hepatocellular Adenoma

Hepatocellular adenoma (HA) is a rare benign neoplasm of hepatocytes proliferating in an abnormal pattern that lacks portal triads, central veins, and Kupffer cells [47]. The tumor is seen most often in women and may be related to use of oral contraceptives. Multiple HAs are seen in association with glycogen storage disease, type I (von Gierke's disease). Hemorrhage is common and malignant degeneration may occur. Surgical removal is recommended.

- Lesions are typically solitary, solid, and may be hypoechoic (20–40%), hyperechoic (30%), or mixed (50%). Fat is sometimes present with the tumor causing focal or diffuse areas of increased echogenicity (Fig. 2.40).
- HA tends to be larger than FNH at discovery with an average size of 10 cm [47]. HA lacks the central scar characteristic of FNH.
- Color Doppler shows intratumoral veins usually 1–5-mm diameter with characteristic continuous flat venous flow [50].
- Hemorrhage may occur into the tumor with rupture into the peritoneal cavity.

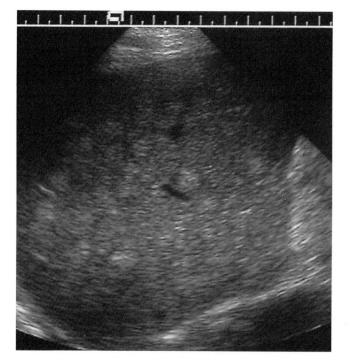

Figure 2.41 *Multiple Metastases from Breast Carcinoma.* The liver is riddled with numerous small echogenic nodules.

Metastases to the Liver

The liver is a common site of metastases from intestinal, pancreas, breast, and lung carcinoma.

Metastatic disease must be considered in the differential diagnosis of all solid hepatic lesions.

- Multiple lesions (Fig. 2.41) are a characteristic of metastatic disease, although solitary metastases are sometimes seen especially with colon carcinoma (Fig. 2.42).
- Metastases may resemble any other hepatic lesion and must always be considered in the differential diagnosis.
- A target or bull's eye appearance is common with lesions being hypoechoic with an echogenic center.
- A hypoechoic peripheral rim of parenchyma compressed by an expanding lesion is most often seen with a metastatic lesion [51].
- Calcified lesions are seen most often with mucinous adenocarcinoma and sarcomas.
- Cystic metastases usually occur with cystic primary lesions such as cystadenocarcinoma.
- Homogeneous solid hypoechoic lesions are seen with lymphoma.

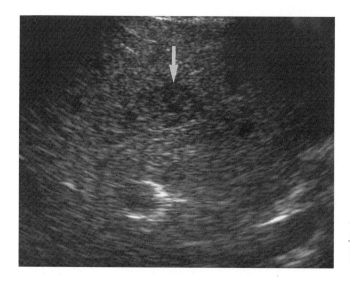

Figure 2.42 *Solitary Metastases from Colon Carcinoma.* A solitary metastasis is barely seen as a subtle hypoechoic solid mass (*arrow*).

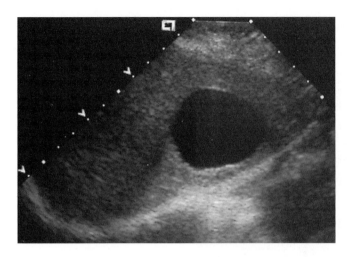

Figure 2.43 *Benign Hepatic Cyst.* This lesion is sharply defined, completely lacking in internal echoes, has a thin wall, and shows accentuated through-transmission seen as bright echoes deep to the lesion.

Benign Hepatic Cysts

Benign hepatic cysts are seen in 2–5% of the population. Rarely, cysts may develop internal hemorrhage or infection.

- Simple hepatic cysts are anechoic with thin walls and show posterior acoustic enhancement (Fig. 2.43). They are easily overlooked on US because of their similarity to blood vessels on initial inspection.
- Many benign hepatic cysts have septations that are thin and avascular and most have lobulated contours. Size varies from tiny to huge.
- Cysts are commonly multiple and occur in clusters of two or three.
- Doppler confirms that the cysts are avascular and that no flow is present in the cyst wall or septa.

Pyogenic Liver Abscess

Pyogenic liver abscesses develop as complications of biliary tract infection, sepsis, or trauma. Often no precipitating cause is evident. Patients present with fever, pain, and jaundice.

- Abscesses have a variable appearance. Most common is a cystic mass with irregular, thick, shaggy walls containing echogenic fluid with particulate matter (Fig. 2.44) and clumped debris that may layer [52].

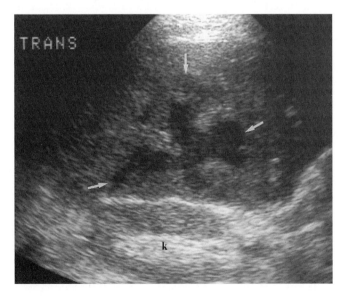

Figure 2.44 *Pyogenic Abscess.* The margins of this abscess (*arrows*) are ill defined. An irregular central fluid collection contains fluid with suspended particulate matter. k, right kidney.

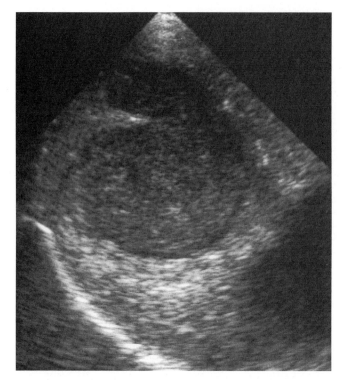

Figure 2.45 *Amebic Abscess.* This amebic abscess is much better defined than are most pyogenic abscesses. A hypoechoic wall surrounds the lesion. Internal contents show hypoechoic echoes but no internal vascularity was detected with Doppler.

- Internal septa are common. Air may be present within the abscess.
- Early, pre-abscess phlegmon may be seen as a subtle alteration of hepatic echotexture.
- US is commonly used to guide aspiration and catheter drainage.

Amebic Liver Abscess

Amebic abscess is the most common form of liver abscess worldwide. PVs carry amebic organisms to the liver from infestations in the colon. Patients present with pain and malaise and are usually much less acutely ill than patients with pyogenic abscess.

- The appearance of amebic abscess overlaps that of pyogenic abscess. Lesions are round or oval, hypoechoic or anechoic, and have echo-poor walls (Fig. 2.45) [52]. Lesions are multiple in 25% of cases and vary in size up to 20 cm.
- Characteristic features are a pattern of fine homogeneous granular internal echoes (Fig. 2.45) and location in the right lobe near the liver capsule.
- Complications include rupture of the abscess through the liver capsule and diaphragm into the right pleural space and free rupture into the peritoneal cavity.
- Diagnosis is made by serology and evidence of intestinal amebiasis. Guided fluid aspiration is needed only if pyogenic abscess is a strong consideration. Treatment is medical with amebicides.
- Lesions require 2 years or longer to resolve. Continued presence of cystic lesions does not imply that therapy has failed [53].

Hepatic Hydatid Cyst

Hydatid disease is caused by infestation with the parasite, *Echinococcus granulosus*. Hydatid cysts are most common in the liver, but may be seen in any organ. Patients present with low-grade fever and a tender liver [54].

- The appearance of the cyst is variable and dependent upon the stage of disease.
- Unilocular, anechoic cysts with walls of variable thickness characteristically contain **hydatid sand**, fine particulate parasitic debris that layers in the most dependent portion of the cyst. A second diagnostic finding is the visualization of two parallel echogenic

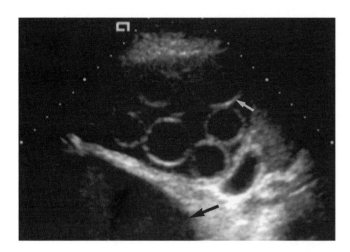

Figure 2.46 *Hydatid Cyst.* This cystic mass contains multiple daughter cysts (*white arrow*) characteristic of hydatid disease. Partially seen adjacent to this cyst is a large unilocular hydatid cyst (*black arrow*).

lines in the cyst wall. The outer line represents the **pericyst**, a dense fibrous capsule, and the inner line represents the **endocyst**, a thin membranous wall.

- The *water lily sign* refers to the presence of floating, undulating membranes within a cystic mass. The floating membrane is the detached endocyst that has ruptured.
- Small cystic masses with walls of variable thickness are "daughter cysts" within the "mother cyst." Visualization of daughter cysts is pathognomonic of hydatid disease (Fig. 2.46).
- Hydatid fluid may evolve from being thin and anechoic to becoming echogenic viscous gel. This results in the cyst appearing more like a solid mass. Recognition of the folds of collapsed membranes is diagnostic [55].
- Calcification in the walls and septa is common. Calcifications become thicker and denser with age.
- Diagnosis is made by serologic testing. Effective treatment is often difficult and may be medical, surgical resection, or catheter drainage.
- Complications include rupture into the peritoneal cavity reported to sometimes cause anaphylactic reaction, obstruction of the PV causing portal hypertension, obstruction of or rupture into the biliary tree causing jaundice or cholangitis, and rupture into the pleural space.

Microabscesses

Microabscesses are usually the result of opportunistic infection in immunocompromised patients. Causative organisms include *Candida* and other fungi, *Pneumocystis carinii*, cytomegalovirus, *Mycobacterium avium intracellulare*, and *M. tuberculosis*.

- Multiple small (<10 cm) target lesions with a central echogenic dot surrounded by a hypoechoic halo are typical of fungal infections. Lesions are found in both liver and spleen (see Fig. 2.97) [56].
- Innumerable tiny echogenic lesions seen diffusely throughout the liver and spleen are characteristic of *Pneumocystis*.
- Lesions may calcify with healing.

Biloma

Bilomas are collections of bile leaked from the biliary system as a complication of trauma, surgery, or instrumentation.

- Most bilomas are found within or adjacent to the liver, although they may be anywhere in the peritoneal cavity.
- Collections are anechoic and well defined with acoustic enhancement. Within the liver, bilomas are rounded cystic masses (Fig. 2.47). Outside of the liver the fluid assumes the shape of the space available to it.

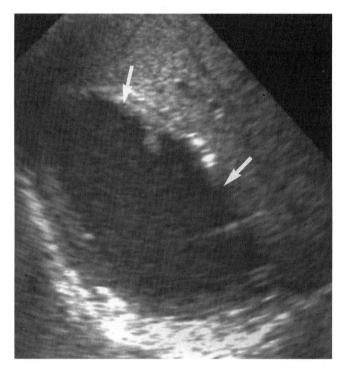

Figure 2.47 *Biloma.* This biloma (*arrows*) occurred as a complication of partial hepatic resection. Internal echoes indicate that some blood is present within the lesion.

- Internal septations, debris, and layering fluid within a biloma are caused by traumatic hemorrhage.
- Diagnosis of a bile leak is made most easily by hepatobiliary scintigraphy.

Hematoma
Hematomas also result from trauma or surgery. The appearance changes with time.

- Fresh clot within a hematoma appears echogenic compared to hepatic parenchyma.
- Within a few days the hematoma becomes progressively cystic and begins to shrink. Septations and internal debris are common (Fig. 2.48).

Hepatic Calcifications
Patterns of hepatic calcifications (Fig. 2.49) are listed in Table 2.2 [126].

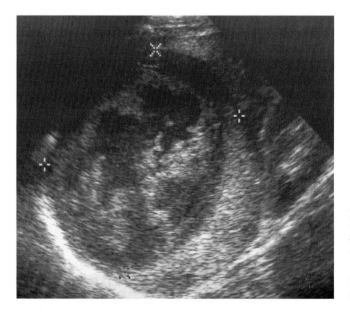

Figure 2.48 *Hematoma.* This hematoma (*between cursors, +, x*) was discovered a few days after laparoscopic cholecystectomy. The hematoma is becoming cystic but still contains echogenic clot and debris.

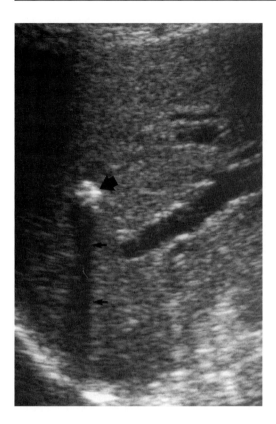

Figure 2.49 *Granuloma.* Calcification from previous granulomatous disease is seen as a bright echogenic focus (*fat arrow*) that casts a dense acoustic shadow (*small arrows*).

BILIARY TREE

BILIARY OBSTRUCTION

US is approximately 90% accurate in differentiating obstructive from non-obstructive jaundice by depicting the presence of biliary dilatation. The 10% inaccuracy arises from the fact that biliary obstruction is not always accompanied by biliary dilatation and that biliary dilatation does not always mean biliary obstruction (Box 2.3). US accurately determines the

US is commonly and effectively used as the imaging method of first choice in the diagnosis of obstructive jaundice. However, a number of pitfalls in the diagnosis of biliary obstruction must always be kept in mind.

Table 2.2: Patterns of Hepatic Calcifications

Lesion	Pattern of Calcification
Granulomas	Multiple, discrete calcifications with no associated mass.
Echinococcus cyst	Peripheral, rim calcifications in wall of main cyst or daughter cysts. Old healed lesions show coarse calcification.
Hepatic cavernous hemangiomas	Solitary, dense, coarse calcification in central hypoechoic zone within a solid echogenic mass.
Hepatocellular carcinoma	Dystrophic coarse calcification in necrotic heterogeneous mass. Fine granular or punctate calcification also occurs.
Fibrolamellar carcinoma	Calcification in central stellate fibrous scar with a well-defined solid mass without necrosis.
Metastatic disease	Stippled, granular, amorphous calcification is common in mets from mucinous cystadenocarcinomas. Sarcoma mets may have chondroid or osteoid calcification.

Adapted from: Stoupis C, Taylor H, Paley M, et al. The rocky liver: radiologic-pathologic correlation of calcified hepatic masses. RadioGraphics 1998;18:675–685.

Box 2.3: Pitfalls in Sonographic Diagnosis of Biliary Obstruction

. . . .

Biliary dilatation without biliary obstruction may occur as a result of aging, previous cholecystectomy, previous biliary surgery, spastic contraction of the sphincter of Oddi, intestinal hypomotility, or previous long-term obstruction with smooth muscle atony. *Biliary obstruction without biliary dilatation* occurs when obstruction is acute. Several days are required for the bile ducts to dilate even when obstruction is complete. In addition, partial or intermittent biliary obstruction, especially when caused by stones, commonly does not raise intrabiliary pressures enough to cause dilatation. Severe cirrhosis and periportal fibrosis may prevent the bile ducts from dilating.

---

level of obstruction in 92–95% of cases and the cause of obstruction in 71–88% of cases (Table 2.3) [57].

- Enlargement of the intrahepatic biliary tree distorts the normal anatomy of the portal triads as the IHBD become tortuous and more prominent than the PVs. IHBD are dilated when their diameter exceeds 2 mm or exceeds 40% of the diameter of the adjacent PV. Color Doppler is used to confirm the absence of blood flow in the enlarged tubes (Fig. 2.50). Enlargement of the bile duct to the size of the adjacent PV has been called the *parallel tube sign* or the *shotgun sign* (Fig. 2.5).
- As IHBD enlarge they become tortuous and irregular like the gnarly branches of an oak tree (Fig. 2.50). Confluence of enlarged IHBD creates a stellate appearance of merging tubes.
- Acoustic enhancement may be seen distal to dilated bile ducts but is not seen distal to intrahepatic veins or arteries (Fig. 2.51).
- Debris in the bile ducts caused by blood, pus, or sludge may make dilated bile ducts isoechoic to liver parenchyma and difficult to visualize.
- The common duct is considered dilated in adults when the internal diameter of the duct in porta hepatis exceeds 7 mm. The more distal common duct coursing adjacent to the pancreas is commonly larger especially in older adults. For patients older than 60 years of age, the distal common duct may be considered normal up to 10 mm in internal diameter.

Table 2.3: Causes of Biliary Obstruction

Level of Obstruction	Most Common Causes
Porta hepatis	Cholangiocarcinoma (Klatskin tumor)
	Enlarged metastatic lymph nodes in the hilum
Suprapancreatic	Cholangiocarcinoma
(between porta hepatis and pancreas)	Enlarged metastatic lymph nodes
	Impacted gallstone
	Benign stricture
Pancreatic	Gallstone impacted at ampulla
(most common level of obstruction)	Periampullary neoplasm
	Pancreatic carcinoma
	Cholangiocarcinoma
	Duodenal carcinoma
	Benign stricture
	Chronic pancreatitis
	Iatrogenic (biliary surgery)
	Cholangitis

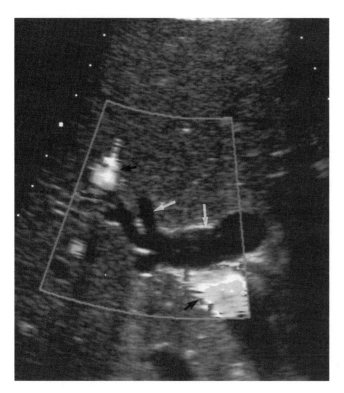

Figure 2.50 *Dilated Bile Ducts.* Dilated bile ducts (*white arrows*) are seen as tortuous tubular structures in the liver. Color Doppler (shown in black and white on this image) makes differentiation of bile ducts (*white arrows*) and blood vessels (*black arrows*) easy.

- In neonates and infants, 2 mm is the upper limit of normal size for the common duct. In children up to age 13, 3 mm is the upper limit of normal diameter [58].
- The normal size of the common duct after cholecystectomy remains controversial, with a number of studies indicating that mild post-operative dilatation of the common duct is common [59]. A reasonable approach is to consider 10 mm to be the upper limit of normal diameter for asymptomatic patients and 7 mm to be the upper limit of normal in symptomatic patients following cholecystectomy.

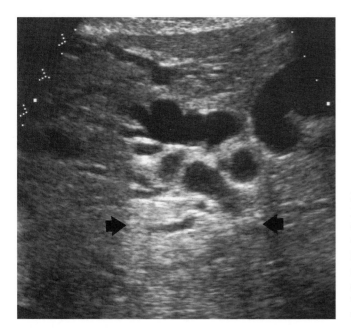

Figure 2.51 *Dilated Bile Ducts.* Dilated bile ducts are seen throughout the liver in this patient with long-standing jaundice. The larger bile duct shows accentuated through-transmission (*between arrows*). This finding may be seen with enlarged bile ducts but not with blood vessels.

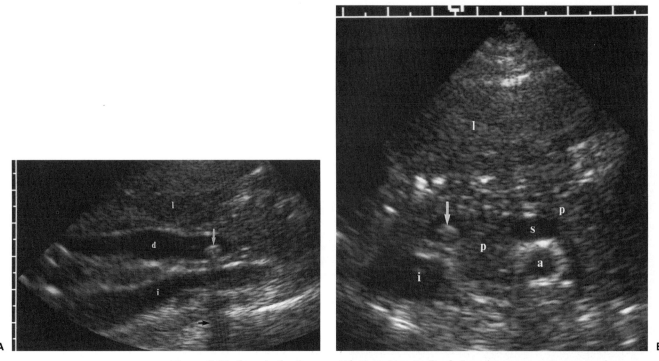

Figure 2.52 *Stone in the Common Bile Duct.* Longitudinal, *A*, and transverse, *B*, images show a stone as an echogenic focus (*white arrow*) in the dilated distal common bile duct (d). Acoustic shadowing (*black arrow*) is clearly seen in the longitudinal image but not on the transverse image. Stone shadowing was subsequently demonstrated on the transverse image by centering the stone in the US beam. a, superior mesenteric artery; i, inferior vena cava; l, liver; p, pancreas; s, splenic vein.

CHOLEDOCHOLITHIASIS

Common duct stones are the most common cause of obstructive jaundice (36–50% of cases). Stones are found in the bile ducts in 12% of patients undergoing cholecystectomy. The fact that 4% of patients in autopsy series have biliary stones is evidence that biliary stones may be relatively asymptomatic and pass spontaneously. Sensitivity of US in the diagnosis of stones in the CBD is only approximately 55–75%. Careful scanning technique is required.

- Biliary stones appear as shadowing echogenic foci within the duct (Fig. 2.52). The demonstration of shadowing is technique dependent.
- False-positive US diagnosis of biliary stones may result from surgical clips, air in the biliary tree, hepatic artery calcification, calcified lymph nodes, or tumor within the duct.
- The presence or absence of stones within the GB is not predictive of biliary stones as a cause of obstructive jaundice.

AIR IN THE BILIARY TREE

Pneumobilia is most often caused by sphincterotomy or surgical biliary-enteric anastomosis. Other causes include incompetence of the sphincter of Oddi or fistulas between the biliary tree and intestine. Air may be mistaken for stones in the biliary tree.

- Air is seen as linear or punctate foci of high echogenicity (Fig. 2.53) associated with acoustic shadowing and ring-down artifact. Air bubbles will commonly move with changes in patient position. Shimmering ring-down artifact seen with real-time scanning is characteristic.
- Air is preferentially seen in the non-dependent bile ducts.

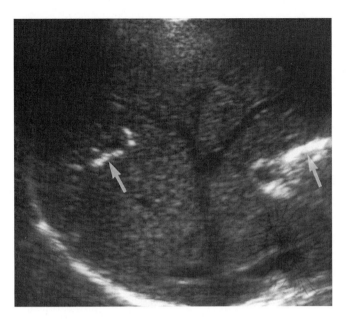

Figure 2.53 *Air in the Biliary Tree.* Air in the biliary tree appears as brightly echogenic branching structures (*arrows*). With patient movement, air will rise into non-dependent bile ducts. Reverberation artifact and acoustic shadowing are transiently visualized during real-time scanning. This patient's pneumobilia was caused by choledochojejunostomy.

- Extensive atherosclerotic calcification of intrahepatic arteries may mimic air or stones in the biliary tree [60].

ASCARIS IN THE BILIARY TREE

Ascariasis is the most common parasitic infection worldwide. The roundworm usually lives in the intestine but may migrate through the ampulla of Vater and gain access to the biliary tree and pancreatic duct resulting in cholangitis, acute cholecystitis, or, often fatal pancreatitis.

- The roundworm appears as an echogenic tubular structure within the bile duct (Fig. 2.54), the GB, or the pancreatic duct. Most striking is to observe a living worm moving within the bile duct. Adult worms are 15–50 cm in length and 3–6 mm thick. A central hypoechoic tube that extends the length of the worm is a characteristic finding. This tube is the worm's digestive tract [61].

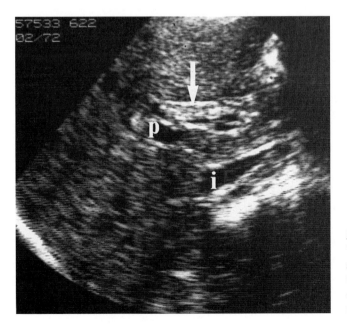

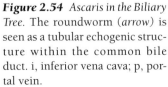

Figure 2.54 *Ascaris in the Biliary Tree.* The roundworm (*arrow*) is seen as a tubular echogenic structure within the common bile duct. i, inferior vena cava; p, portal vein.

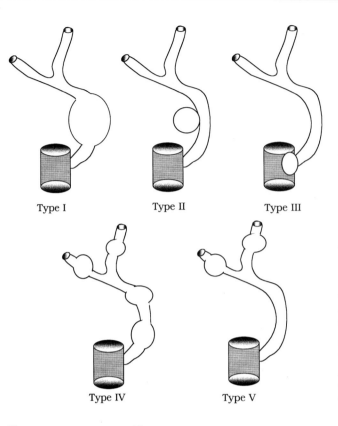

Type I   Type II   Type III

Type IV   Type V

Figure 2.55 *Classification of Congenital Biliary Cysts.* Type I choledochal cysts are focal, saccular or fusiform, dilatations of the common bile duct. Type II cysts are true diverticuli of the common bile duct. Type III, choledochoceles, are dilatations of the terminal intraduodenal portion of the common bile duct. Type IV cysts refers to multiple intrahepatic and extrahepatic bile duct cysts. Caroli's disease is classified Type V. *Reproduced with permission from Brant WE, Helms CA, Fundamentals of Diagnostic Radiology, Lippincott-Williams & Wilkins, Baltimore, 1999.*

CHOLEDOCHAL CYSTS

Choledochal cysts are uncommon congenital anomalies of the bile ducts characterized by cystic dilatation of portions of the intra- or extrahepatic biliary tree [62,63]. Choledochal cysts are usually discovered in infancy or childhood (60%). However, diagnosis may be delayed until adulthood. Patients are usually female (70–81%) and present with abdominal mass, jaundice, pain, or pancreatitis. Biliary stasis results in an increased incidence of gallstones and carcinoma of the bile ducts or GB. The Todani classification is commonly used (Fig. 2.55) [64].

- US demonstrates cystic dilatation of portions of the biliary tree.
- Type I choledochal cyst is most common (80–90%) and consists of dilatation of the CBD (Fig. 2.56). The dilatation may be focal or diffuse, saccular or fusiform. The GB commonly arises from the cyst. The IHBD are normal.
- Type II (2%) is a true diverticulum of the CBD. The connection to the CBD is usually small and may be occluded.
- Type III is a choledochocele (1.4–5.0%). Similar in appearance to a ureterocele, it involves dilatation of the distal CBD within the duodenum.
- Type IV (19%) refers to multiple cystic dilatations of both IHBD and EHBD.
- Type V is Caroli's disease.

CAROLI'S DISEASE

Caroli's disease is a rare congenital malformation of the IHBD characterized by non-obstructing saccular or fusiform dilatation of the IHBD. The condition presents in childhood and has an autosomal recessive inheritance pattern. Complications include biliary stones, recurrent bacterial cholangitis, hepatic fibrosis, portal hypertension, and hepatic failure [65].

- Segmental and saccular dilatation of the IHBD is characteristic. The EHBD are normal.
- Additional findings include biliary calculi, hepatic abscesses, and evidence of cirrhosis and portal hypertension.

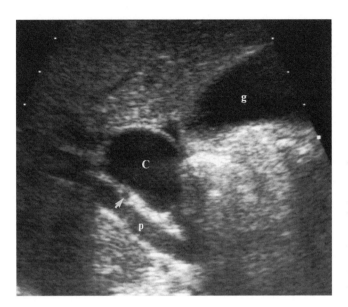

Figure 2.56 *Type I Choledochal Cyst.* Marked focal dilatation of the common bile duct (C) to 18 mm is evident. The intrahepatic bile ducts and the remainder of the common bile duct were normal in size and appearance. Also evident are the portal vein (p), hepatic artery (*arrow*), and gallbladder (g).

- Caroli's disease is found in association with autosomal recessive polycystic kidney disease and medullary sponge kidney.

SCLEROSING CHOLANGITIS

Sclerosing cholangitis is characterized by intra- and extrahepatic biliary fibrosis with progressive obliteration of the bile ducts. Primary sclerosing cholangitis is idiopathic but associated with ulcerative colitis, Crohn's disease, and retroperitoneal fibrosis. It eventually leads to biliary cirrhosis and hepatic failure [66].

- Bile ducts show focal areas of dilatation and focal areas of narrowing with wall thickening and irregularity. Both IHBD and EHBD may be affected. Bile duct dilatation that is focal and discontinuous is characteristic.
- Debris representing sludge, pus, or desquamated epithelium is commonly present within the bile ducts. Biliary calculi are seen in approximately 8% of patients. Stones create a linear cast of the bile duct with variable acoustic shadowing, or appear as a discrete echogenic focus within a dilated duct [67].
- The GB may show mild to marked wall thickening.
- Some cases have extensive fibrosis with minimal ductal dilatation. These cases are difficult to recognize with US. Cholangiography is the preferred method of making this diagnosis [66].

RECURRENT PYOGENIC CHOLANGITIS

Also called *Oriental cholangiohepatitis* in the literature, recurrent pyogenic cholangitis is related to infestation with *Clonorchis sinensis* and other parasites. Bacterial superinfection by *Escherichia coli* and other enteric pathogens is nearly always present. It is one of the most common diseases of the biliary tract in Southeast Asia and Hong Kong, and is seen in the United States primarily in Asian immigrants [68].

- The major US features are diffuse dilatation of the intra- and extrahepatic bile ducts associated with numerous biliary calculi.
- Fibrosis and inflammation thicken the walls of the bile ducts and cause increased echogenicity of the portal triads.
- Gallstones are usually present in the GB.

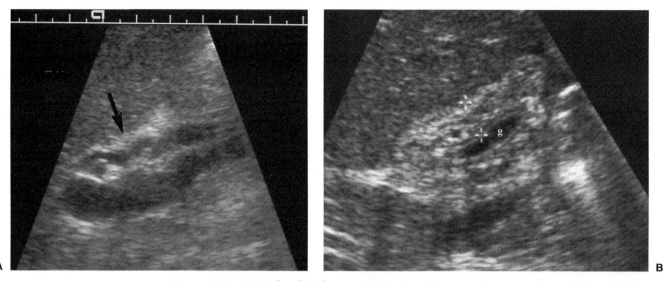

Figure 2.57 *AIDS-Related Cholangiopathy. A.* View of the porta hepatis reveals marked irregular thickening of the wall of the common bile duct (*arrow*). *B.* Image of the gallbladder shows marked thickening of the gallbladder wall (*between cursors*, +) with a small gallbladder lumen (g).

ACQUIRED IMMUNODEFICIENCY SYNDROME–RELATED CHOLANGIOPATHY

Acquired immunodeficiency syndrome (AIDS)–related cholangiopathy encompasses several types of biliary diseases encountered in patients with AIDS. Opportunistic infection plays a role in the illness with cytomegalovirus, *Cryptosporidium* species, and *Enterocytozoon bieneusi* organisms cultured from the bile. Patients present with abdominal pain and markedly elevated serum alkaline phosphatase [69].

- The walls of the bile ducts and GB are thickened, often markedly, because of mucosal inflammation and edema (Fig. 2.57) [69].
- IHBD and EHBD are usually dilated.
- Edema of the ampulla causes an echogenic nodule and tapered narrowing at the termination of the CBD [70].
- Findings may mimic sclerosing cholangitis with irregular narrowing of the IHBD and EHBD.

PERIPHERAL CHOLANGIOCARCINOMA

Cholangiocarcinoma may be peripheral presenting as a solid hepatic mass, hilar causing diffuse intrahepatic biliary dilatation, or distal presenting as a small obstructing mass in the CBD.

Cholangiocarcinoma arising in small bile ducts in the periphery of the liver is the second most common primary hepatic malignancy. Approximately 10% of cholangiocarcinomas are peripheral. Intrahepatic cholelithiasis, Caroli's disease, *Clonorchis* infestation, and Thorium exposure are predisposing factors. The tumor is an adenocarcinoma and is rare before age 40 [71,72].

- Peripheral cholangiocarcinoma presents as an intrahepatic mass similar to HCC and must be considered in the differential diagnosis of intrahepatic neoplasms. Peripheral cholangiocarcinoma often occurs in the absence of cirrhosis.
- The most common appearance is a solitary hyperechoic or hypoechoic mass (78%). Multiple nodules or a dominant mass with satellite nodules is less common (17%). A peripheral hypoechoic rim is frequently present (35%). Size ranges from 1–20 cm. Intrahepatic biliary dilatation may be seen peripheral to the mass [73].

- An infiltrative tumor is occasionally seen (5%) and is recognized by heterogeneous echogenicity of the involved parenchyma [73].
- Calcifications are occasionally present. Unlike HCC, peripheral cholangiocarcinoma rarely invades portal or hepatic veins.

HILAR CHOLANGIOCARCINOMA

Cholangiocarcinoma that arises in the hilum of the liver (the porta hepatis) is commonly called a *Klatskin tumor*. The tumor occurs at the confluence of the right and left bile ducts. Approximately 25% of cholangiocarcinomas are hilar [74].

- The IHBD are diffusely dilated whereas the EHBD remain normal size [72]. The GB is not obstructed provided the tumor has not extended to the cystic duct.
- The mass itself is usually small, scirrhous, echogenic, poorly defined, and difficult to visualize. The dilated ducts end abruptly at the hilum. The tumor mass itself is seen in 37–87% of cases [75,76].
- Lobar parenchymal atrophy occurs proximal to obstructed ducts. The dilated ducts are crowded together and unusually close to the liver surface [72].
- Metastases extend to regional lymph nodes, liver, and peritoneal cavity. The hilar tumor may invade the adjacent PV and hepatic artery [76].

DISTAL CHOLANGIOCARCINOMA

Distal cholangiocarcinoma occurs in the EHBD and presents early with biliary obstruction and jaundice. The prognosis is better than with peripheral or hilar cholangiocarcinoma because the tumors are small and more often resectable.

- A polypoid, echogenic, or hypoechoic mass is seen within the lumen at the abrupt termination of a dilated CBD (Fig. 2.58).
- If the mass is scirrhous, which is frequent, it is commonly not visible. The dilated common duct just ends abruptly. A similar appearance may be produced by benign strictures.
- Sludge in the distal duct may mimic tumor (Fig. 2.59).

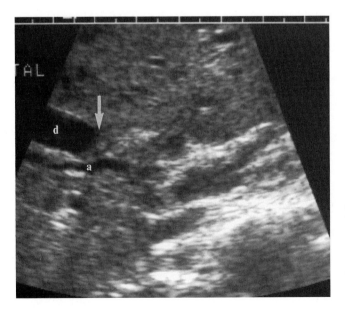

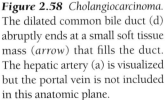

Figure 2.58 *Cholangiocarcinoma.* The dilated common bile duct (d) abruptly ends at a small soft tissue mass (*arrow*) that fills the duct. The hepatic artery (a) is visualized but the portal vein is not included in this anatomic plane.

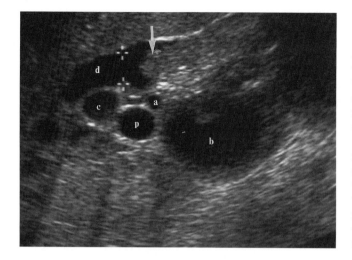

Figure 2.59 *Sludge in the Common Bile Duct.* Long-term impaction of a gallstone in the distal common bile duct resulted in the more proximal duct (d; *between cursors*, +) filling with sludge (*arrow*) mimicking a polypoid mass in the dilated duct. Also seen in this image are the portal vein (p), hepatic artery (a), a portion of the neck of the gallbladder near the cystic duct (c), and a transiently distended portion of the duodenum (b).

GALLBLADDER

THICKENING OF THE GALLBLADDER WALL

Thickening of the gallbladder wall is a common and non-specific finding.

Thickening of the GB wall is a non-specific finding caused by diseases of the GB as well as by extrinsic conditions (see Box 2.4 for differential diagnosis).

- The standard measurement of GB wall thickness is made from the GB lumen to the liver parenchyma (Fig. 2.60). This measurement includes the GB mucosa, smooth muscle of its wall, liver capsule, and any tissue between the liver and GB. The normal measurement is 3 mm or less. Greater than 5 mm is unequivocally thickened. Between 3 and 5 mm is equivocal.
- Thickening of the GB wall with striations and fluid pockets is evidence of acute gangrenous cholecystitis in the appropriate clinical setting [77].

SLUDGE

Sludge refers to bile that appears echogenic due to the presence of calcium bilirubinate granules and cholesterol crystals mixed with mucus. Sludge is commonly an incidental finding that is related to the lack of bile turnover in patients who are fasting for prolonged periods of time. Sludge is especially common in hospitalized patients. However, sludge may also be seen in patients with obstruction of the cystic duct or more distal bile ducts. Sludge

---

Box 2.4: Causes of Gallbladder Wall Thickening

Normal contracted gallbladder
Diseases of the gallbladder
    Acute cholecystitis
    Chronic cholecystitis
    Adenomyomatosis of the GB
    GB carcinoma

Extrinsic diseases
    Hypoalbuminemia
    Ascites
    Congestive heart failure
    Hepatitis
    Chronic renal failure
    Excessive fluid resuscitation
    AIDS-related cholangiopathy
    Varices in the GB wall

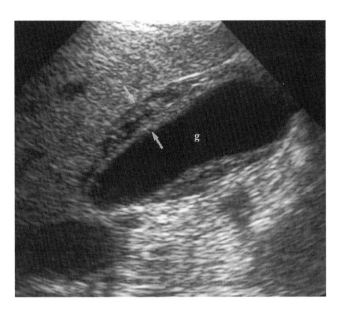

Figure 2.60 *Thickened Gallbladder Wall.* The standard measurement of the gallbladder (g) wall is made between the gallbladder lumen and the parenchyma of the liver (*between the arrows*). This gallbladder wall is thickened to 8 mm and appears edematous with echolucent striations within the wall. This patient has acute acalculous cholecystitis.

requires 5–7 days to form and is not caused by routine overnight fasting requested in preparation for GB US. Sludge may fill the entire GB, layer below anechoic bile, or form into balls or masses (tumefactive sludge). Sludge may become viscous and thicken to the consistency of toothpaste (see Fig. 2.62).

- Echogenic bile is commonly called *sludge* (Fig. 2.61) (see Table 2.4 for differential diagnosis).
- Sludge layers dependently and does not cause acoustic shadowing (Fig. 2.61).
- Tumefactive sludge is viscous and forms intraluminal masses that mimic GB carcinoma (Fig. 2.62).
- Mobile "sludge balls" move within the GB but do not cast acoustic shadows.

GALLSTONES

Gallstones affect 10–15% of the population and are a major cause of GB morbidity (Box 2.5). Most gallstones are mixtures of cholesterol, calcium bilirubinate, and calcium carbonate. Key US findings are

- Gallstones appear as rounded echodensities in the GB lumen that cast acoustic shadows and move with changes in patient position (Fig. 2.63). When all three features are

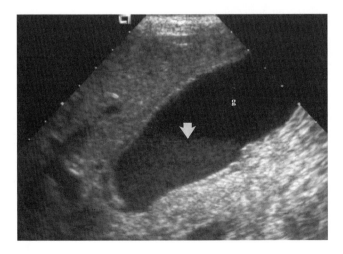

Figure 2.61 *Layering Sludge in the Gallbladder.* Sludge layers dependently within the gallbladder (g) to form a fluid-fluid layer (*arrow*) with echolucent bile.

Table 2.4: Echogenic Debris in Gallbladder Lumen

Diagnosis	US Findings
Sludge	Echogenic material layers but causes no shadowing. Found in patients with prolonged fasting or biliary obstruction.
Pus	Particulate matter disperses throughout the GB lumen or layers without shadowing. Findings of acute cholecystitis are present.
Blood	Particulate debris, no shadowing, in patient with hemobilia.
Pseudosludge	Caused by volume averaging of the GB wall and adjacent liver into the GB lumen. Seen in longitudinal but usually not in transverse views of the GB. Disappears when higher frequency (narrower beam) transducer is used.
Layering tiny gallstones	Echogenic layer causes acoustic shadow. Surface of the layer is often bumpy. Changing patient position may allow visualization of individual stones.
Sludge with gallstones	Layering nonshadowing echogenic bile contains discrete stones that shadow.
Milk of calcium bile	Echogenic bile with high calcium carbonate content layers and causes acoustic shadowing. May be indistinguishable from multiple tiny stones.
Cholesterol crystals	Tiny 1–2-mm floating particles produce comet tail artifacts.
Gas bubbles	Tiny echodensities cause comet tail or reverberation artifact and rise to the most nondependent portion of the GB.

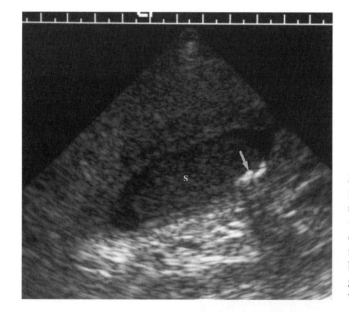

Figure 2.62 *Tumefactive Sludge in the Gallbladder.* Toothpaste-like sludge forms an echogenic mass (s) filling the gallbladder. Doppler examination showed no vascularity within the mass excluding gallbladder carcinoma. Several small gallstones (*arrow*) are trapped within the sludge.

Box 2.5: Complications of Cholelithiasis

Gallbladder colic
Acute cholecystitis
Chronic cholecystitis
Gallbladder perforation

Choledocholithiasis
Gallstone pancreatitis
Gallbladder carcinoma

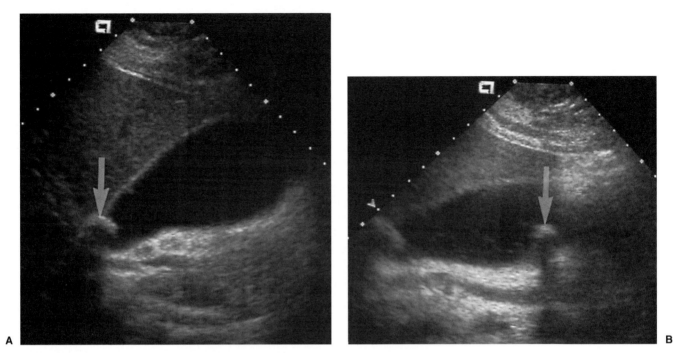

A   **B**

Figure 2.63 *Rolling Stone.* A. With the patient supine the gallstone (*arrow*) is in the neck of the gallbladder. B. With the patient in left lateral decubitus position the gallstone (*arrow*) rolls to the gallbladder fundus.

present, the accuracy of US diagnosis is nearly 100%. Most gallstones are round in shape, although some appear angulated or faceted.

■ The acoustic shadow is usually dark and clean (Fig. 2.64). Stones with a rough surface may cause reverberation artifact that produces a dirty shadow. Shadowing is produced by sound absorption. Depiction of shadowing depends upon stone size and US technique. Stones smaller than 3 mm may not cause shadows. To improve visualization of an acoustic shadow use a higher-frequency transducer, insure that the stone is centered in the beam, and adjust the transmit zone or focal zone to depth of the stone (Table 2.5).

Demonstration of acoustic shadowing from gallstones is dependent on US technique.

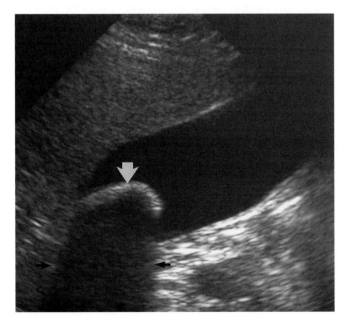

Figure 2.64 *Gallstone.* A large gallstone within the gallbladder produces a bright surface echo (*white arrow*) and causes a dark acoustic shadow (*between black arrows*).

Table 2.5: Differential Diagnosis of Gallstones in the Gallbladder

Diagnosis	US Findings
Gallstones	Echogenic balls in GB lumen
	Acoustic shadow
	Move within GB lumen
Sludge ball	Nodule of medium echogenicity in GB lumen
	No acoustic shadow
	Moves slowly
Blood clot	Hypoechoic nodule
	No acoustic shadow
	Moves
Polyp	Hypoechoic to echogenic nodule
	No acoustic shadow
	Fixed position
Gas bubbles	Bright echoes
	Comet tail/reverberation artifacts
	Move to nondependent lumen
Parasites	Elongated or oval shape
(Ascaris, Clonorchis)	May shadow
	May move spontaneously if still alive

- Movement of gallstones is called the *rolling stone sign* (Fig. 2.63). Move the patient into upright or lateral decubitus positions to demonstrate stone mobility. Stones typically layer dependently. However, stones may "float" following administration of contrast agents into the biliary system or when bile is highly concentrated.
- All gallstones show similar US features. US cannot be used to detect stone calcification or determine stone composition.
- Cholelithiasis is rare in infants and uncommon in children except for those with hemolytic anemia who are prone to develop calcium bilirubinate stones.

GALLBLADDER FILLED WITH GALLSTONES

A GB filled with gallstones may be difficult to differentiate from a gas-filled bowel loop. Characteristic findings have been described as the wall-echo-shadow sign (WES triad) or the double-arc-shadow sign [78].

- Two parallel echogenic lines represent the wall of the GB (proximal arc) and the surface of the packed gallstones (distal arc) separated by a thin anechoic space of residual bile (Fig. 2.65). A dense acoustic shadow emanates from the gallstones (see Table 2.6 for differential diagnosis) [79].
- A normal GB is not visualized.

ACUTE CHOLECYSTITIS

Acute cholecystitis is most commonly caused by impaction of a gallstone in the GB neck obstructing the GB and resulting in inflammation of the GB wall. Ischemia and bacterial infection are contributing and inciting factors. Patients present with pain, right upper quadrant tenderness, and leukocytosis. The differential diagnosis of patients with this set of symptoms is extensive and US is usually the first imaging study performed. No US finding is pathognomonic. The more findings that are present, the greater the likelihood of the diagnosis. The obstructing stone may spontaneously disimpact resulting in resolution of symptoms.

- Gallstones are present in 90–95% of cases. An immobile stone impacted in the GB neck is a key finding that is easily overlooked. Careful attention to the GB neck region is required for diagnosis.

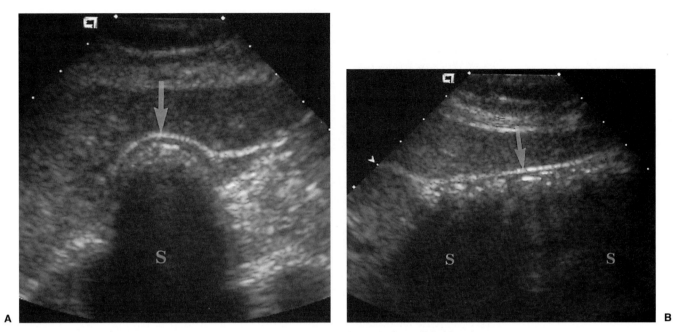

Figure 2.65 *Gallbladder Filled with Gallstones. A.* Transverse image through the gallbladder shows two arching echogenic lines (*arrow*) and a dense acoustic shadow (S), the WES sign or double-arc-shadow sign. *B.* In longitudinal plane the two echogenic lines (*arrow*) are more linear in configuration and the shadow (S) from the gallstones is elongated.

■ A positive sonographic Murphy's sign is strong evidence of acute cholecystitis. Transducer pressure is gently applied to multiple areas of the abdomen. When maximum tenderness is elicited directly over the visualized GB, the sonographic Murphy's sign is considered positive. The sonographic Murphy's sign is negative if no tenderness is present, if tenderness is diffuse, or if maximum tenderness is not clearly localized to the GB. An "equivocal" Murphy's sign is a negative Murphy's sign. Demonstration of Murphy's sign is usually not possible in obtunded patients.

Table 2.6: Differential Diagnosis of Double-Arc-Shadow Appearance or Non-Visualization of the Gallbladder

Diagnosis	US Findings
GB filled with gallstones	The proximal arc, representing the GB wall, is smooth and uniform in thickness. The second arc, representing the gallstones packed within the GB, is commonly bumpy because many stones are present. The acoustic shadow is dark and "clean."
Air in bowel loop	The soft tissue-air interface is seen as a single, curving, very bright echo. The shadow is "dirty" due to reverberation and ring-down artifacts produced by gas.
Porcelain GB	Calcification of the GB wall is often non-uniform in thickness and may be discontinuous. Acoustic shadowing is clean.
Air in the GB wall (emphysematous cholecystitis)	The soft tissue-air interface is bright. Bright ring-down artifact emanates from air bubbles in the wall. Confirm with plain radiography or CT. Patient is usually seriously ill.
Adenomyomatosis with cholesterol crystals in Rokitansky-Aschoff sinuses	GB wall is thickened and irregular. Cholesterol crystals in small intramural diverticuli (Rokitansky-Aschoff sinuses) produce echogenic foci with comet-tail artifacts. Patient is not seriously ill.
Agenesis of the GB	This is a rare condition (0.04% of the population). It is usually associated with other congenital anomalies.

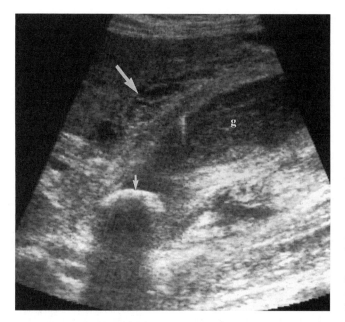

Figure 2.66 *Acute Cholecystitis.* The gallbladder (g) is filled with echogenic bile. A gallstone (*small arrow*) is impacted in the gallbladder neck. The gallbladder wall (*large arrow*) is markedly thickened with a striated appearance indicative of wall edema. Murphy's sign was strikingly positive.

- Thickening of the GB wall (>5 mm) with striated appearance of linear echolucencies is caused by edema and inflammation (Figs. 2.66, 2.67).
- Pericholecystic fluid is seen as discrete fluid collections between the GB and liver.
- Distended GB (GB hydrops) with diameter >5 cm is indicative of GB obstruction.
- Echogenic debris in GB lumen may be sludge, pus, blood, or necrotic tissue (Figs. 2.66, 2.68).
- Doppler findings are non-specific in acute cholecystitis with patients showing hypervascularity, normal flow, and no flow [80].

Atypical forms and complications of acute cholecystitis include the following:

Acalculous cholecystitis refers to acute cholecystitis developing in the absence of gallstones. In children, approximately one-half of the cases of acute cholecystitis are acalculous. Adults rarely develop acalculous cholecystitis unless they have a predisposing condition. Most cases occur in adult patients, who are hospitalized because of recent major surgery, trauma, burns, or debilitating diseases, are immunocompromised, or who are receiving intravenous hyperalimentation. Most cases are related to prolonged biliary stasis,

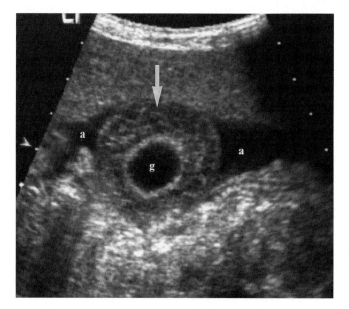

Figure 2.67 *Acalculous Cholecystitis.* Transverse image of the gallbladder (g) shows marked circumferential striated thickening of the gallbladder wall (*arrow*) in this post-operative patient with ascites (a).

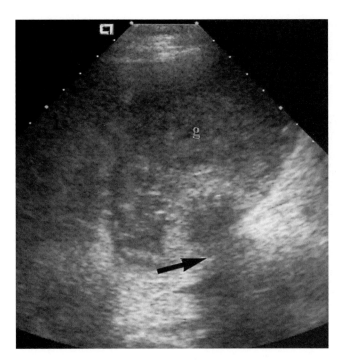

Figure 2.68 Gangrenous Cholecystitis. The gallbladder (g) is markedly distended and so filled with echogenic debris, pus, and blood that it is difficult to recognize as the gallbladder. A stone casts an acoustic shadow (*arrow*).

ischemia, and biliary infection. Outpatients who develop acalculous cholecystitis are usually elderly males with advanced arterial disease.

■ Findings are identical to acute calculous cholecystitis (Figs. 2.60, 2.67), except that gallstones are absent and the cystic duct is often patent on biliary scintigraphy.

Gangrenous cholecystitis refers to necrosis, hemorrhage, ulceration, and microabscess formation in the GB wall. Gangrenous changes complicate 20–30% of cases of acute cholecystitis. Patients are at high risk for perforation and mortality is in the 5–10% range. Findings that suggest gangrene in acute cholecystitis include:

■ Linear echogenic membranes within the lumen represent sloughed mucosa.
■ Coarse echogenic material within the bile represents necrotic debris (Fig. 2.68).
■ A striated appearance of GB wall thickening is more common in gangrenous cholecystitis.
■ Murphy's sign is absent in 70% of cases because the GB is denervated.
■ Perforation is a common sequela of gangrenous cholecystitis and occurs in approximately 10% of acute cholecystitis. Perforation occurs most commonly near the fundus and results in generalized peritonitis or a pericholecystic abscess.

Emphysematous cholecystitis is characterized by the presence of gas in the GB wall and lumen. It is associated with gangrene (75%), early GB perforation (20%), and high mortality (15%). Gas-producing bacteria are causative. Most patients are elderly and up to 50% have diabetes [81].

■ Intraluminal gas causes a dense band of bright echoes with prominent reverberation echoes [82].
■ Gas bubbles in bile appear similar to gas bubbles in a glass of champagne—the "effervescent GB sign"[81].
■ Intramural gas causes a string of bright, comet tail artifacts that emanate from the GB wall (Fig. 2.69) [82]. Similar echoes occur in association with adenomyomatosis of the GB, but patients with this condition are not acutely ill.
■ The presence of air in the GB wall is easily confirmed with CT and is often evident on plain radiographs.
■ Additional findings of acute cholecystitis are commonly present. Gallstones are absent in most cases.

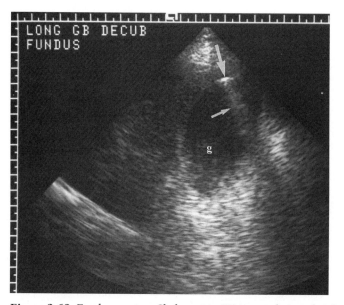

Figure 2.69 *Emphysematous Cholecystitis.* US image shows a bright echogenic focus (*large arrow*) in the gallbladder wall that produces a reverberation artifact (*small arrow*) and acoustic shadow in an acutely ill elderly man. The importance of this finding was not immediately recognized. The diagnosis of emphysematous cholecystitis was delayed for 8 hours and the patient died during emergency surgery. In the acute setting US signs of air in the gallbladder or its wall must be immediately recognized and confirmed with radiographs or computed tomography. The gallbladder (g) contains echogenic bile that proved to be blood, pus, and cellular debris.

CHRONIC CHOLECYSTITIS

Chronic cholecystitis occurs as a result of continued irritation by gallstones. Patients have recurring symptoms of biliary colic. The cystic duct is usually chronically obstructed.

- Gallstones are usually present.
- Thickening of the GB wall reflects chronic inflammation but is not always present. The GB wall may remain normal on US examination but show the pathologic changes of chronic inflammation [83].

PORCELAIN GALLBLADDER

Calcification of the GB wall in chronic cholecystitis is referred to as *porcelain GB.* Porcelain GB is associated with an increased risk of GB carcinoma (11–22%) [84].

- The calcified wall appears as a hyperechoic semilunar-shaped structure with posterior acoustic shadowing (Fig. 2.70). Calcifications may be thin and regular, clump-like, or discontinuous [84].
- Reverberation and comet tail artifacts seen with emphysematous cholecystitis are absent.

GALLBLADDER POLYPS

GB polyps are quite common being present in 4–6% of the population [85]. Most (90%) are cholesterol polyps, which are abnormal deposits of cholesterol in a polypoid mass. Cholesterol polyps have no neoplastic potential and are incidental findings. The remainder (10%) are adenomatous polyps that have potential for malignant transformation.

- Polyps appear as echogenic nodules attached to the GB wall (Fig. 2.71). They do not cause acoustic shadowing. They do not move from their attachment site with changes in patient position.

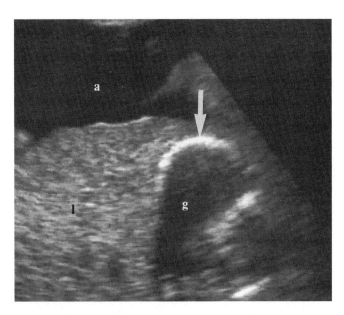

Figure 2.70 *Porcelain Gallbladder.* Calcification (*arrow*) in the wall of the gallbladder (g) produces a uniform arching echodense line with acoustic shadowing. The liver (l) is cirrhotic and ascites (a) is present.

■ Polyps <10 mm size are most likely incidental cholesterol polyps. Follow-up is not warranted because the incidence of malignant transformation is extremely low [85].
■ Polyps >10 mm are also most likely cholesterol polyps, but probably should be followed for evidence of growth because some are adenomas that could eventually becomes cancerous.
■ *Cholesterolosis* refers to the presence of deposits of cholesterol esters in the GB mucosa resulting in numerous tiny polypoid mucosal projections [86].

ADENOMYOMATOSIS OF THE GALLBLADDER

Adenomyomatosis is a benign hyperplasia of the epithelium and smooth muscle of the GB wall with herniations of mucosa forming tiny pockets in the wall called *Rokitansky-Aschoff sinuses* [86]. The condition is entirely benign with no malignant potential, although the findings may mimic GB carcinoma [87].

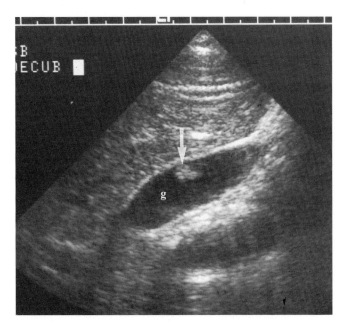

Figure 2.71 *Gallbladder Polyp.* A small lobulated echogenic mass (*arrow*) is suspended from the non-dependent wall of the gallbladder (g). No acoustic shadowing is present.

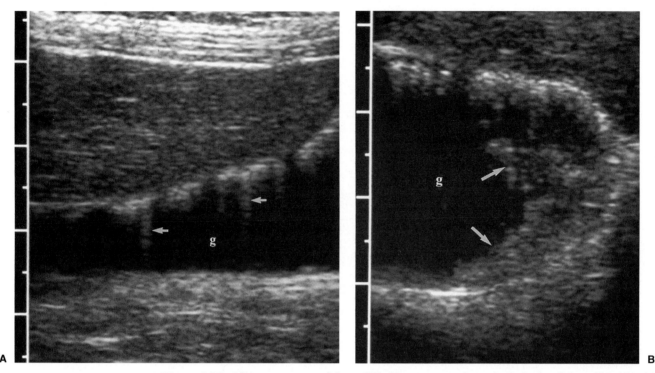

Figure 2.72 *Adenomyomatosis of the Gallbladder. A.* Image through the body of the gallbladder (g) shows the characteristic comet tail artifacts (*arrows*) produced by cholesterol crystals within Rokitansky-Aschoff sinuses in the gallbladder wall. *B.* Image through the fundus of the gallbladder (g) shows irregular thickening (*arrows*) of the fundal wall characteristic of adenomyomatosis.

- Adenomyomatosis may be diffuse, segmental, or focal. The GB fundus is nearly always involved (Fig. 2.72).
- The GB wall is thickened diffusely or focally.
- The most characteristic findings are comet tail artifacts that project from the thickened wall (Fig. 2.72). These are caused by the presence of cholesterol crystals that precipitate in the Rokitansky-Aschoff sinuses.
- Gallstones are commonly present but are not related to the disease process.

GALLBLADDER CARCINOMA

GB carcinoma affects primarily older individuals (>60 years). Pathologic types are adeno-carcinoma (90%) and squamous cell carcinoma (10%). GB carcinoma has a variety of appearances [88].

- An intraluminal polypoid soft tissue mass >2 cm size is likely carcinoma (Fig. 2.73). Polyps are often sessile and fungating. Color flow US shows vessels extending into the mass and differentiates tumor from tumefactive sludge.
- The GB may be partially or entirely replaced by a soft tissue mass that extends into the liver.
- Focal or diffuse, asymmetric, irregular thickening of the GB wall may be carcinoma.
- High-velocity, arterial blood flow (mean peak velocity, 34 cm/sec) is characteristic of tumor masses [89].
- Gallstones are present in 60–90% of cases. Gallstones may distort or obscure findings of GB carcinoma [90].
- Porcelain GB is present in 4–20% of cases.

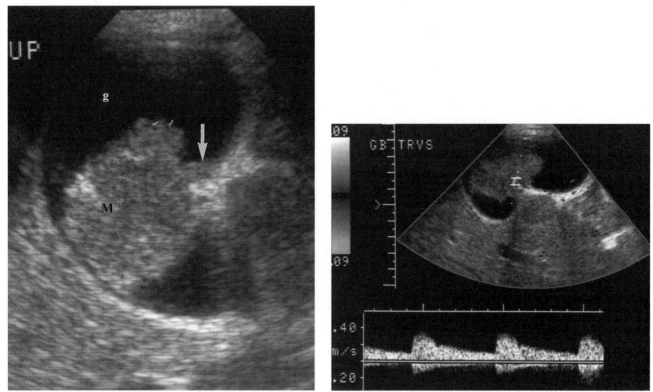

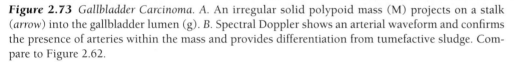

Figure 2.73 *Gallbladder Carcinoma. A.* An irregular solid polypoid mass (M) projects on a stalk (*arrow*) into the gallbladder lumen (g). *B.* Spectral Doppler shows an arterial waveform and confirms the presence of arteries within the mass and provides differentiation from tumefactive sludge. Compare to Figure 2.62.

- Tumor spread is commonly directed into the adjacent liver and may cause biliary obstruction.
- Hematogenous metastases nearly always involve the liver.
- Lymphatic spread involves nodes in the porta hepatitis, around the celiac axis or SMA, and in peripancreatic areas.
- Fine granular or punctate calcification occurs with mucinous adenocarcinoma.
- Metastases to the GB from other tumors have findings similar to GB carcinoma.

PANCREAS

ACUTE PANCREATITIS

Acute pancreatitis is most commonly caused by alcohol abuse or a gallstone impacted in the distal CBD. Additional causes include trauma, surgery, endoscopic pancreatography, and drugs. Inflammatory changes vary from mild interstitial edema to extensive necrosis with hemorrhage. Contrast-enhanced CT is used for initial evaluation to detect necrosis [91]. US is utilized for follow-up, to detect complications, and to guide intervention.

US examination in acute pancreatitis must be comprehensive to detect a wide array of possible complications.

- US may be normal in mild pancreatitis.
- Edema causes focal or diffuse enlargement of the pancreas with ill-defined margins and hypoechoic parenchyma in areas of fluid infiltration (Figs. 2.74, 2.75). Edematous peripancreatic fat is decreased in echogenicity with hypoechoic stranding densities.
- Hemorrhage may cause hyperechoic masses of clot blood in association with the other findings described.

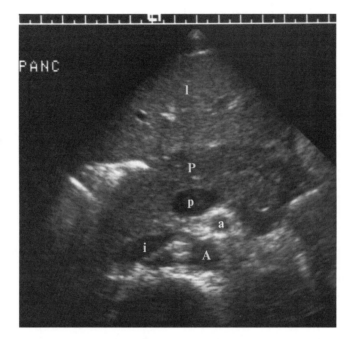

Figure 2.74 *Diffuse Acute Pancreatitis.* The pancreas (P) is diffusely enlarged and diffusely decreased in echogenicity because of edema. A, aorta; a, superior mesenteric artery; i, inferior vena cava; l, liver; p, commencement of portal vein.

- **Unencapsulated pancreatic fluid collections** containing high levels of amylase and lipase may be found anywhere, but are most common in the pancreatic bed (Fig. 2.76), lesser sac, perirenal areas, and small bowel mesentery. Fluid is usually anechoic unless complicated by hemorrhage or infection (Fig. 2.77). Thin fascial membranes limit the fluid collections. This fluid may resolve spontaneously or require drainage. US is commonly used to measure the fluid dimensions and follow changes in size and appearance. Fluid collections may extend into the mediastinum, groin, beneath the serosa of the intestinal tract, or beneath the capsule of the liver or spleen (see Fig. 2.94) [92].

- **Pancreatic pseudocysts** are encapsulated by a distinct wall of granulation tissue and fibrosis. Pseudocysts complicate 10–20% of cases of acute pancreatitis. They are well defined with distinctly visualized walls of measurable thickness (Fig. 2.78). Unencapsulated fluid collections develop into pseudocysts when the fluid collection has been present for approximately 6 weeks. Small pseudocysts usually resolve spontaneously but large pseudocysts commonly require surgical or catheter drainage.

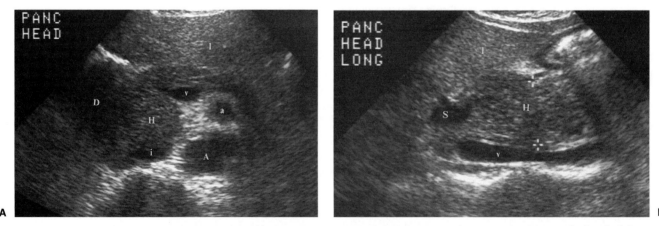

Figure 2.75 *Focal Acute Pancreatitis.* A. Transverse scan. B. Longitudinal scan. The head of the pancreas (H) is enlarged and decreased in echogenicity because of edema. Cursors (+) measure the enlarged pancreatic head. A, aorta; a, superior mesenteric artery; D, duodenum; i, inferior vena cava; l, liver; S, stomach; v, superior mesenteric vein.

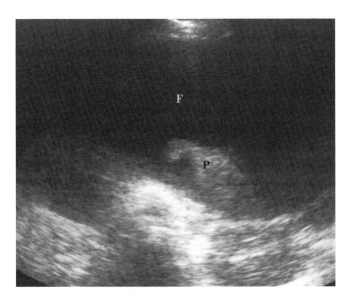

Figure 2.76 *Pancreatic Fluid Collection in Lesser Sac.* Transverse image shows a huge fluid collection (F) surrounding a portion of the pancreas (p) and extending anteriorly through the peritoneum into the lesser sac.

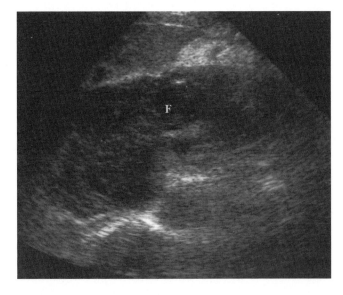

Figure 2.77 *Necrotizing Pancreatitis.* A complex echogenic fluid collection (F) replaces the pancreatic parenchyma. The fluid appears echogenic and septated because of tissue necrosis and hemorrhage.

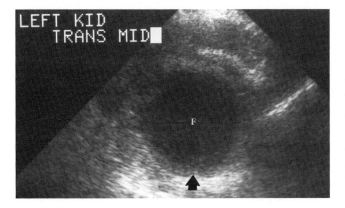

Figure 2.78 *Pancreatic Pseudocyst.* A well-defined fluid collection (F) in the pancreatic tail region has a measurably thick wall (*arrow*). It was proven to be a pancreatic pseudocyst by its high amylase content. The lesion was initially mistaken for a left renal cyst.

- **Pancreatic ascites** is found in approximately 7% of cases and is associated with increased morbidity and a high rate of recurrence. Debris and septations may be seen within the ascites.
- **Infection** may complicate an area of pancreatic necrosis, an unencapsulated fluid collection, or a pseudocyst. Progressive infection may evolve into a discrete **abscess**. Diagnosis commonly requires percutaneous aspiration with Gram's stain and culture of the fluid. The US appearance alone cannot accurately diagnose the presence or absence of infection. Infected fluid collections may remain anechoic, but infection is more likely if a fluid collection contains gas bubbles or if the fluid is echogenic with debris and floating particulate matter. Surgical or catheter drainage of abscesses is required [93]. Mortality of an untreated pancreatic abscess exceeds 50% [94].
- **Pancreatic-intestinal fistula** results in extraluminal gas collections with wall thickening or mass in the affected portion of the intestinal tract.
- **Biliary obstruction** may be caused by impacted stones, inflammation, or fibrosis.
- **Pseudoaneurysms** result from erosion of the pancreatic inflammation into an artery. Hemorrhage is contained by the adventitia and fibrosis. The splenic, gastroduodenal, left gastric, and pancreaticoduodenal arteries are commonly involved. The diagnosis is made by Doppler confirmation of pulsatile blood flow within a cystic mass. Prior to aspiration or catheter placement every pancreatic fluid collection should be examined with Doppler to diagnose the unrecognized pseudoaneurysm [95].
- **Venous thrombosis** may also result from the inflammatory process. The SV is commonly affected and results in development of enlarged collateral vessels around the spleen, stomach, and left kidney. Thrombosis may extend into the PV. Splenomegaly and splenic infarction may result. Doppler should be utilized to confirm patency of all visualized veins in the pancreatic area.

CHRONIC PANCREATITIS

Chronic pancreatitis is a chronic inflammatory disease of the pancreas characterized by progressive pancreatic damage with irreversible fibrosis. This process results in major structural abnormalities in varying combination including parenchymal atrophy, calcifications, stricture and dilatation of the pancreatic duct, fluid collections, pseudomass formation, and alteration of peripancreatic fat [94,96]. Although many patients with chronic pancreatitis have recurrent episodes of acute pancreatitis, chronic pancreatitis appears to be a separate entity. Patients with chronic pancreatitis average 13 years younger than those with acute pancreatitis. Acute pancreatitis seldom results in the development of chronic pancreatitis. Causes of chronic pancreatitis include alcoholism (70%), autoimmune disease, tropical pancreatitis [97], and non-alcoholic duct-destructive pancreatitis [98].

Acute pancreatitis and chronic pancreatitis are distinct and separate disease entities.

- Punctate echodensities, with or without acoustic shadowing, are commonly present (50%) and represent ductal calculi or parenchymal calcifications (Fig. 2.79) [99].
- The gland is focally or diffusely atrophic (54%) [99]. The parenchyma is heterogeneous, coarsened, and increased in echogenicity with irregular contours. Atrophy may result in exocrine insufficiency and diabetes.
- The pancreatic duct has focal strictures and dilated segments (68%) [99]. This "beaded" dilatation is characteristic.
- Focal areas of pancreatic enlargement (Fig. 2.80) caused by focal inflammation are common (30%) and must be distinguished from tumors [96]. The presence of calcifications within the mass strongly favors pancreatitis over tumor. Percutaneous biopsy, guided by US or CT, is commonly needed to make an accurate diagnosis.
- Bile ducts may be dilated because of inflammatory stricture of the CBD.
- Fluid collections are caused by superimposed acute pancreatitis (30%).
- Pancreatic pseudocysts are found in 25–40% of patients.

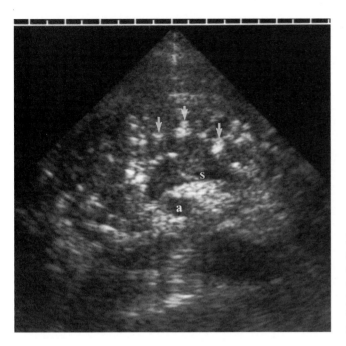

Figure 2.79 *Chronic Pancreatitis.* Transverse image of the pancreas demonstrates numerous calcifications in the pancreatic parenchyma seen as punctate echodensities (*arrows*). a, superior mesenteric artery; s, splenic vein.

■ Peripancreatic tissues show inflammatory change with fascial thickening and stranding densities in peripancreatic fat. These changes result in poor definition of the pancreatic margins.

ADENOCARCINOMA OF THE PANCREAS

Pancreatic carcinoma is an aggressive and usually fatal tumor. The only realistic hope for cure is early detection and aggressive surgery (Whipple procedure). US is highly accurate in the detection of the pancreatic carcinoma with reported sensitivity of 88–94% [100]. Color Doppler is used to assess vascular involvement by tumor [101]. Approximately 70% of tumors occur in the pancreatic head.

US examination in suspected adenocarcinoma of the pancreas should include Doppler US to detect vascular involvement and complete survey of the abdomen to detect distant metastases.

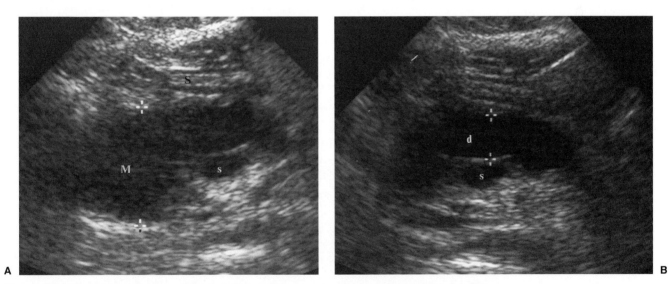

Figure 2.80 *Chronic Pancreatitis.* Chronic inflammation was the biopsy-proven cause of enlargement of the pancreatic head (M; *between cursors*, +) seen in *A* and the massive dilatation of the pancreatic duct (d; *between cursors*, +) to 21 mm seen in *B*. This mass is indistinguishable from pancreatic carcinoma and must be biopsied for diagnosis. Both *A* and *B* are transverse images through portions of the pancreas. s, splenic vein; S, stomach.

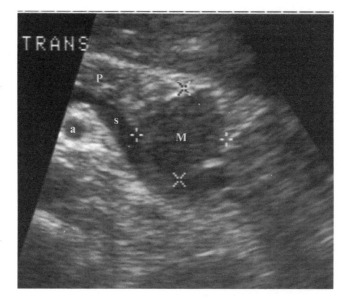

Figure 2.81 *Adenocarcinoma of Pancreas.* A mass (M; *between cursors, +, x*) in the pancreatic tail region is homogeneous, solid, and hypoechoic. This tumor proved to be resectable. P, pancreas; a, superior mesenteric artery; s, splenic vein.

- Small pancreatic carcinomas (2–3 cm) are homogeneous, solid, hypoechoic, and ill defined (Fig. 2.81) [100].
- Larger tumors (>3–4 cm) are more heterogeneous with well-defined, irregular, or lobulated margins (Fig. 2.82) [100].
- Dilatation of the bile ducts and/or pancreatic ducts is commonly caused by the tumor, but is rarely the only sign of tumor.
- Calcifications are not a feature of pancreatic adenocarcinoma.
- Tumors may cause proximal acute pancreatitis or pancreatic atrophy due to obstruction.
- Tumor invasion of the PV, SMA, SMV, hepatic artery, or celiac trunk makes the tumor non-resectable. Involvement of the SV or artery does not preclude surgical resection. Absence of vessel involvement is indicated by clear visualization of the hyperechoic vessel wall or demonstration of unaffected pancreatic parenchyma between the hypoechoic tumor and the vessel wall [101]. Vascular encasement is considered to be present when hypoechoic tumor surrounds 50% or more of the vessel wall. Reduction in size or change in shape of the vessel lumen indicates vascular compression. Thrombosis is visualized as soft tissue density in the vessel lumen with diversion of blood flow around the intraluminal mass or absence of blood flow with the vessel.
- The tumor metastasizes to the liver, regional nodes, and peritoneal cavity. These areas should always be carefully inspected for metastatic disease.

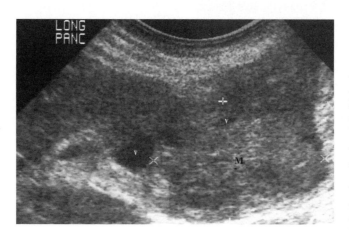

Figure 2.82 *Adenocarcinoma of Pancreas.* This large mass (M; *between cursors, +, x*) in the pancreatic head was initially missed because of failure to examine in detail the pancreatic head. Although the superior mesenteric vein (v) is compressed, the bile and pancreatic ducts were not yet affected. This is a sagittal plane image.

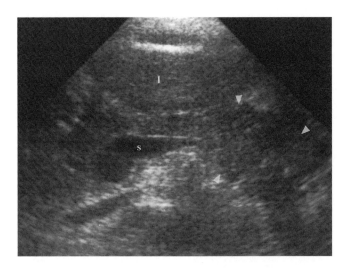

Figure 2.83 *Insulinoma.* A small functioning islet cell tumor (*between arrowheads*) is poorly visualized in the pancreatic tail. Careful examination is required to detect these small, often iso-echoic, tumors. l, liver; s, splenic vein.

ISLET CELL TUMORS

Islet cell tumors may function and secrete hormones (insulin, gastrin, glucagon), or be non-functional and grow to large size prior to detection. Tumors may be benign or malignant but are characteristically slow growing.

■ Small functioning tumors are often not detected by transabdominal US (Fig. 2.83). Intraoperative US is commonly used to improve detection and limit surgery even when the tumor location has been previously shown by other imaging methods. Tumor localization by palpation and intraoperative US approaches 100%.

■ Small tumors are solid, homogeneous, and may be isoechoic or hypoechoic and relatively well defined (Fig. 2.84). Functioning tumors are hypervascular.

■ Larger tumors are heterogeneous with areas of necrosis and hemorrhage commonly present. Calcifications are found in 20% of large lesions.

■ Tumors may invade adjacent organs or metastasize to lymph nodes and liver.

MUCINOUS CYSTIC NEOPLASM OF THE PANCREAS

Mucinous cystic neoplasm (macrocystic tumor) occurs as a malignant tumor (mucinous cystadenocarcinoma) or as a benign tumor with malignant potential (mucinous cystade-

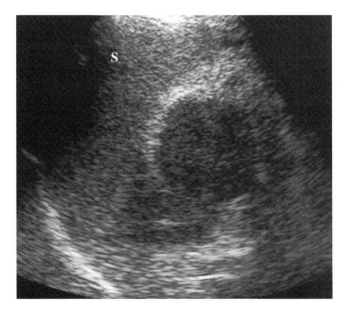

Figure 2.84 *Malignant Islet Cell Neoplasm.* A round homogeneous solid mass occupies the pancreatic tail in the hilum of the spleen (S). Although the mass appears well defined, surgery demonstrated invasion of the spleen, left kidney, and stomach.

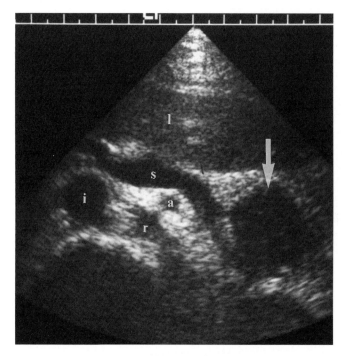

Figure 2.85 *Mucinous Cystadenocarcinoma of the Pancreas.* A well-defined multiloculated cystic mass (*arrow*) is seen in the tail of the pancreas. a, superior mesenteric artery; i, inferior vena cava; l, liver; r, left renal vein; s, splenic vein.

noma). Tumors are characterized by copious mucin production that may result in multicystic masses, striking dilatation of the pancreatic duct, or diffuse multicystic enlargement of the pancreas [102–104]. Tumors that arise in peripheral pancreatic ducts are mucinous cystadenomas/carcinomas. Tumors that arise in the main pancreatic duct are called *intraductal papillary mucinous tumors* [103].

- Multilocular cystic mass with six or fewer cysts of 2-cm diameter or larger is highly characteristic of mucinous cystic neoplasm (93% of cases) (Fig. 2.85) [104]. Mucin within the cysts is commonly echogenic. Mural nodules and solid components may be present.
- Calcifications may be seen in the cyst walls or septa.
- Intraductal papillary tumors dilate the main pancreatic duct by massive mucin secretion. Because the mucin is echogenic, the dilated duct may be difficult to visualize [102,103]. Ductal dilatation may be segmental or diffuse. Filling defects within the dilated duct may represent papillary tumor or globs of mucin. Ectasia of branch pancreatic ducts results in multicystic change throughout the pancreas. Endoscopic pancreatography confirms the diagnostic findings.
- Metastases to the liver are usually cystic.

SEROUS CYSTADENOMA OF THE PANCREAS

Serous cystadenoma (microcystic tumor) is a benign cystic neoplasm without malignant potential. The tumor grows slowly and is commonly large at presentation.

- Cysts are commonly so small that the mass appears solid and highly echogenic because of the numerous reflective surfaces. Occasionally cysts 5–10 mm in size are visible.
- A central stellate echogenic scar is sometimes present.

TRUE PANCREATIC CYSTS

Pancreatic lesions in von Hippel-Lindau syndrome include multiple cysts, islet cell tumors, and serous cystadenoma [105].

True pancreatic cysts are rare and are seen far less frequently than pancreatic pseudocysts. Congenital epithelial lined cysts are usually solitary. Multiple pancreatic cysts are seen with von Hippel-Lindau syndrome and autosomal dominant polycystic disease.

- Cysts are well-defined, spherical anechoic masses with thin walls (Fig. 2.86).

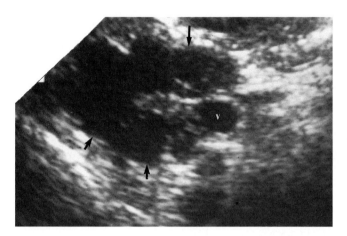

Figure 2.86 *Multiple Pancreatic Cysts in von Hippel-Lindau Syndrome.* Multiple, well-defined small cysts (*arrows*) occupy the pancreatic head as seen on this transverse image. v, superior mesenteric vein.

PANCREATIC LYMPHOMA

Pancreatic or peripancreatic lymphoma may be difficult to differentiate from primary pancreatic malignancy.

- Lymphoma appears as single or multiple homogeneous hypoechoic masses within or around the pancreas.
- Lymphadenopathy may be prominent elsewhere in the abdomen.

METASTASES TO THE PANCREAS

Metastases to the pancreas are uncommon; they are reported in autopsy series in only 3–11% of patients with known malignancy. Common primary tumors are melanoma, breast, lung, and renal carcinoma [106].

Hypoechoic pancreatic masses may be caused by adenocarcinoma, chronic pancreatitis, metastases, or lymphoma.

- Metastases appear as single or multiple hypoechoic masses (Fig. 2.87).
- Renal cell carcinoma metastases may be cystic and appear many years after the primary lesion [106].

CYSTIC FIBROSIS

Cystic fibrosis is a genetic disease characterized by increased volume of abnormally viscous mucous secretions from exocrine glands. The pancreas is a major site of involvement. Secretions precipitate within the pancreatic ducts and result in obstruction, dilatation, and creation of small cysts. Patients develop exocrine pancreatic insufficiency and malabsorption [107].

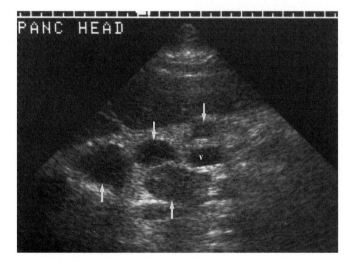

Figure 2.87 *Colon Carcinoma Metastases to Pancreas.* The metastases are seen as multiple hypoechoic nodules (*arrows*) in the pancreas. v, superior mesenteric vein.

- The affected pancreas is decreased in size and increased in echogenicity because of diffuse atrophy and fatty infiltration (70–100% of patients) [107].
- Cysts of varying size (1 mm to several cm) and calcifications are uncommonly seen throughout the pancreatic parenchyma.
- The GB is small and sclerotic and occasionally is not visualized. Sludge and gallstones are common.
- The bile ducts have thick walls and contain viscous echogenic bile.
- The liver may show the diffuse increased echogenicity of fatty infiltration and changes of cirrhosis.

SPLEEN

ACCESSORY SPLEENS (SPLENULES)

Isolated nodules of functioning splenic tissue are found separated from the spleen in 10% of the population. They vary in size from a few millimeters up to several centimeters. They must be recognized as normal splenic tissue to avoid mistaking them for pathological masses [108].

- Round or oval solid masses with echogenicity identical to parent spleen are characteristic (Fig. 2.88).
- Splenules are found most often near the splenic hilum.
- Blood supply is from the splenic artery and SV.
- Accessory spleens are multiple in 10% of patients.

SPLENOSIS

Splenosis refers to the implantation of ectopic splenic tissue on peritoneal surfaces resulting from trauma with fragmentation of the spleen. Severe traumatic injury to the spleen commonly results in splenectomy. The residual implanted splenic tissue then hypertrophies and assumes the function of the parent spleen. A clinical clue to this condition is the absence of Howell-Jolly bodies in the peripheral blood in a patient with a history of splenectomy. Howell-Jolly bodies are fragments of nuclear material within red blood cells. When functioning splenic tissue is present, these red blood cells are filtered from the blood.

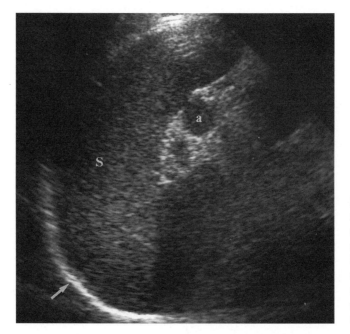

Figure 2.88 *Accessory Spleen.* A round nodule (a) identical in echogenicity to the parent spleen (S) is seen in the splenic hilum. This is the characteristic appearance and location of an accessory spleen. Note how the spleen conforms to the shape of the left hemidiaphragm (*arrow*).

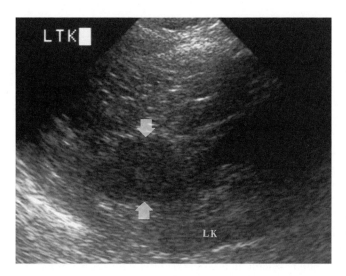

Figure 2.89 *Splenosis.* A round nodule (*between arrows*) of uniform echogenicity similar to spleen is seen in the left upper quadrant anterior to the left kidney (LK) in a patient with a history of previous splenectomy. Technetium-99m sulfur colloid radionuclide imaging confirmed functioning splenic tissue. *Reproduced with permission from Brant WE, Jain KA. Current imaging of the spleen. Radiologist 1996;3:185–192.*

- Rounded nodules of solid tissue of varying size are seen in the left upper quadrant. Nodules have the homogeneous echotexture of splenic tissue. Most are less than 5 cm in size (Fig. 2.89).
- Functioning splenic tissue may be confirmed with a radionuclide sulfur colloid scan.

Splenules and splenosis appear as nodules with echogenicity identical to parent spleen.

SPLENOMEGALY

US measurement of the maximum splenic dimension shows good correlation with the volume and weight of the spleen [109]. Splenomegaly may be the only sign of disease. The causes of splenomegaly are many. Unfortunately, US is unable to differentiate the various etiologies in the majority of cases because the echotexture of the spleen remains normal despite the presence of disease. Causes of splenomegaly include portal hypertension, lymphoproliferative disorders (lymphoma, leukemia, polycythemia vera, hereditary spherocytosis, etc.), infiltrative disorders (Gaucher's disease, amyloidosis), infections (malaria, infectious mononucleosis, AIDS), and vascular disorders (acute SV thrombosis) [110].

- Longest splenic dimension greater than 14 cm is diagnostic of splenomegaly (Fig. 2.90).
- The spleen tip commonly extends over the lower pole of the left kidney.
- The presence of focal defects, other pathological findings in the abdomen, and clinical history provide clues to the etiology of splenomegaly.

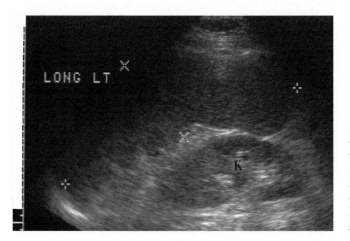

Figure 2.90 *Splenomegaly.* This enlarged spleen measures over 18 cm in length (*between cursors, +*). The tip of the spleen overlies the lower pole of the left kidney (K). These findings are signs of splenomegaly.

WANDERING SPLEEN

In rare cases the spleen lacks its normal attachments and has a long vascular pedicle that allows the spleen to move freely within the abdomen. The misplaced spleen may present as an abdominal mass or may cause abdominal pain because of torsion.

Wandering spleen is a cause of an abdominal mass.

- Solid abdominal mass has the characteristic homogeneous echotexture and shape of the spleen.
- The spleen is absent from the left upper quadrant of the abdomen.
- The wandering spleen is supplied by the splenic artery and SV.
- Findings of torsion include rapid enlargement of the spleen, splenic infarction, and dilatation of the SV near the spleen with no dilatation of the SV near the PV [111].

WRAPAROUND LIVER

In some individuals the left lobe of the liver is exceptionally elongated and partially envelops the spleen simulating a subcapsular splenic hematoma or fluid collection. This wraparound portion of the liver is often thin and not obviously part of the liver on initial inspection.

- The normal liver is slightly hypoechoic compared to the normal spleen. Envelopment of the spleen may suggest a pathological condition such as subcapsular hematoma (Fig. 2.91).
- Careful examination confirms that the tissue partially enveloping the spleen is contiguous with the parenchyma and vascularity of the liver. The liver is observed to move separately from the spleen during respiration.

FOCAL CALCIFICATIONS

Calcifications reflect previous granulomatous disease, most commonly histoplasmosis or tuberculosis. Splenic artery calcifications are a common manifestation of atherosclerotic disease. Splenic artery aneurysm is the most common visceral artery aneurysm.

- **Granulomatous calcifications** appear as focal bright echodensities with or without acoustic shadowing. No associated mass is evident (Fig. 2.92).

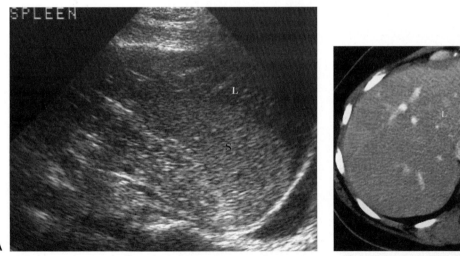

A **B**

Figure 2.91 *Wraparound Liver. A.* Transverse US image. *B.* Axial CT scan in the same anatomic plane. An elongated left lobe of the liver (L) wraps around the spleen (S) and simulates a subcapsular splenic fluid collection or mass. Demonstrating continuity of the elongated left lobe with the rest of the liver as clearly seen on the CT scan confirms this anatomic variant.

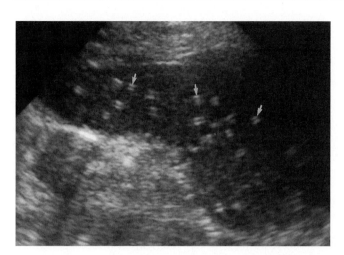

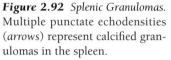

Figure 2.92 *Splenic Granulomas.* Multiple punctate echodensities (*arrows*) represent calcified granulomas in the spleen.

- **Splenic artery calcifications** are linear and within the wall of the tubular artery. Doppler confirms arterial flow.
- **Splenic artery aneurysms** commonly occur near the splenic hilum. Two-thirds are calcified. Aneurysms larger than 2 cm require treatment because of increased risk of rupture.

POSTTRAUMATIC SPLENIC CYST

Posttraumatic cysts are the most common cystic lesion of the spleen [112]. They occur as the end result of an intrasplenic hematoma.

- Cystic lesion has a thick fibrous wall.
- Calcification of the wall is very common (Fig. 2.93).
- Floating and layering internal echodensities are caused by hemorrhagic debris.

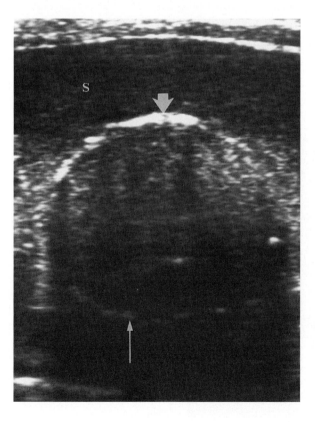

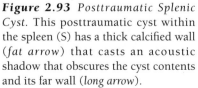

Figure 2.93 *Posttraumatic Splenic Cyst.* This posttraumatic cyst within the spleen (S) has a thick calcified wall (*fat arrow*) that casts an acoustic shadow that obscures the cyst contents and its far wall (*long arrow*).

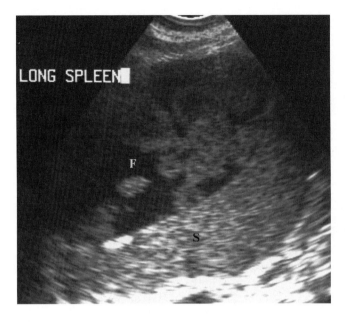

Figure 2.94 *Pancreatic Fluid Collection in the Spleen.* Pancreatic juices released during episodes of acute pancreatitis may gain access to the spleen by migrating along the splenic artery or vein as these vessels pass through pancreatic parenchyma. Digestive enzymes necrose splenic tissue (S) and result in complex fluid collections (F). *Reproduced with permission from Brant WE, Jain KA. Current imaging of the spleen. Radiologist 1996;3:185–192.*

PANCREATIC PSEUDOCYST IN THE SPLEEN

Fluid associated with acute pancreatitis may dissect along the splenic vessels to the splenic hilum and subcapsular locations in the spleen.

- Subcapsular fluid collection is found in association with pancreatitis (Fig. 2.94) [92].

TRUE SPLENIC CYST

True splenic cysts are congenital lesions that are lined by epithelium. These are often discovered *in utero* or in early childhood.

- The well-defined anechoic mass has smooth thin walls (Fig. 2.95).
- The cyst may have fine septations or low levels of internal echoes caused by floating cholesterol crystals.

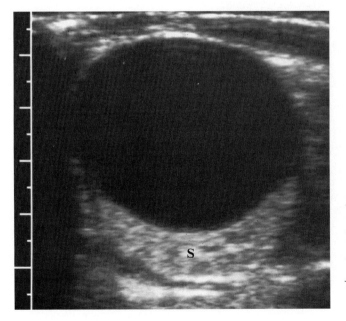

Figure 2.95 *Congenital Spleen Cyst.* A well-defined cyst in the spleen (S) of a young child contains anechoic fluid and has thin walls. *Reproduced with permission from Brant WE, Jain KA. Current imaging of the spleen. Radiologist 1996;3:185–192.*

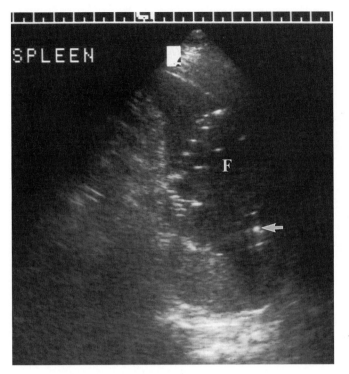

Figure 2.96 *Pyogenic Splenic Abscess.* A large portion of the spleen is replaced by a fluid collection (F) that contains numerous gas bubbles that are seen as floating echodensities (*arrow*). US-guided aspiration confirmed pyogenic abscess. *Reproduced with permission from Brant WE, Jain KA. Current imaging of the spleen. Radiologist 1996;3:185–192.*

PYOGENIC SPLENIC ABSCESS

Pyogenic splenic abscesses are caused by hematogenous infection (75%), penetrating trauma (15%), or as a complication of splenic infarction (10%) [112]. Fever, chills, and pain may be pronounced, or the patient may be relatively asymptomatic.

- Single or multiple, poorly defined hypoechoic or anechoic masses in a septic patient suggest splenic abscess.
- Gas within the abscess produces focal echodensities with shadowing and ring-down artifact (Fig. 2.96).
- Debris within the abscess layers and moves with changes in patient position.
- Aspiration and catheter drainage may be guided by US.

SPLENIC MICROABSCESSES

Microabscesses occur in the setting of an immunocompromised patient with an opportunistic infection [113]. Common causative organisms include *Mycobacterium tuberculosis* and *M. avium-intracellulare*, *Pneumocystis carinii*, candidiasis, and other fungal infections. Kaposi's sarcoma may produce similar lesions. Tiny lesions are best visualized with higher-frequency transducers (5 MHz).

- Multiple echolucencies 1–10 mm in size (Fig. 2.97).
- Multiple echodensities 1–10 mm in size.
- Both the liver and spleen are commonly affected.

HYDATID DISEASE OF THE SPLEEN

Involvement of the spleen is seen in only 2% of human infestations with *Echinococcus* [114].

- Cystic lesions are solitary and anechoic in most cases.
- Intracystic daughter cysts are highly characteristic when present. They have a cyst within a cyst appearance (Fig. 2.46).
- Layering debris within the cyst is hydatid sand, a mixture of parasite fragments and debris.

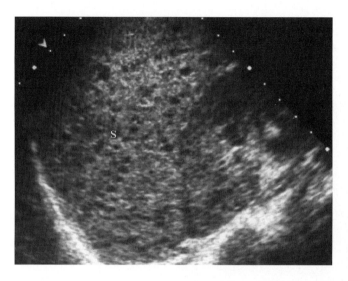

Figure 2.97 *Splenic Microabscesses.* Numerous small echolucencies throughout the splenic parenchyma (S) were caused by *Mycobacterium tuberculosis* in a patient with AIDS.

- Some lesions appear more solid with infolded membranes and hydatid sand filling the fluid spaces.
- The wall of the lesion calcifies in chronic cases.

LYMPHOMA/LEUKEMIA

As the major organ of the lymphatic system the spleen is commonly affected by lymphoma and leukemia [115]. Patterns of disease involvement include infiltrative without discrete masses, miliary with numerous tiny lesions (<2 cm), and massive with extensive replacement of spleen parenchyma [112].

- Splenic enlargement is a frequent finding when the spleen is diffusely infiltrated. A normal-sized spleen does not, however, exclude involvement.
- Focal lesions are hypoechoic. Lesions may be multiple and small, or large and confluent replacing most of the parenchyma. Most lesions are strikingly homogeneous.
- Occasionally, lesions are cystic because of massive necrosis.

METASTASES TO THE SPLEEN

Metastases to the spleen are usually a late manifestation of disseminated malignancy in terminal patients. The most common primary tumors are melanoma and breast, lung, or ovary carcinoma. Isolated metastases (without mets seen elsewhere) are rare but are reported with colon and renal carcinomas and gynecologic malignancies [116].

- Intrasplenic masses of variable and non-specific appearance. Lesions may be solitary or multiple and appear hypoechoic, hyperechoic, mixed, or partially cystic.

SPLENIC INFARCTION

Infarction occurs as a result of occlusion of branches of the splenic artery, or of thrombosis of venous sinusoids when the spleen is massively enlarged [112]. Arterial occlusion is associated with hemolytic anemias, endocarditis, arteritis, and pancreatic carcinoma. Most patients present with pain, but up to 40% are asymptomatic [117].

- In the first 24 hours, infarctions are well defined, wedge shaped, and hypoechoic (Fig. 2.98). Extension to the splenic capsule is characteristic. Some lesions are round or oval rather than classic wedge shaped.

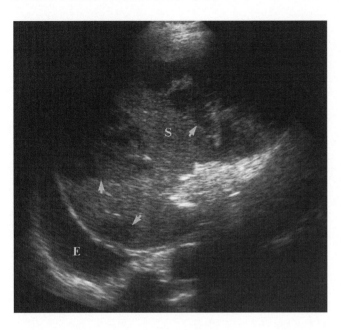

Figure 2.98 *Infarction of the Spleen.* Several areas of acute infarction are seen as irregular or wedge-shaped areas of mixed hypoechogenicity (*arrows*) in the spleen (S). A left pleural effusion (E) is also evident. *Reproduced with permission from Brant WE, Jain KA. Current imaging of the spleen. Radiologist 1996;3:185–192.*

- With time, echogenicity increases and the size of the lesion decreases. Liquefaction may occur. The parenchyma may eventually return to normal appearance or show a vague area of heterogeneous echogenicity.
- Complications include subcapsular hemorrhage and rupture with free bleeding into the peritoneal cavity.

SPLENIC HEMANGIOMA

Hemangiomas are found much less commonly in the spleen than in the liver. Although scarce, hemangiomas are the most common primary neoplasm of the spleen. Multiple splenic hemangiomas are seen with Klippel-Trenaunay-Weber syndrome [118].

Splenic hemangiomas are much less common than liver hemangiomas.

- Most appear as well-defined, homogeneous, echogenic masses, identical to the typical appearance of hemangioma in the liver.
- Some have cystic spaces of varying size.
- Lesions may contain areas of fibrosis and focal calcification.
- Doppler usually shows no signal because blood flow is very slow. High-sensitivity settings on high-grade modern equipment may demonstrate slow flow in some areas of the lesion.

SPLENIC LYMPHANGIOMA

Lymphangiomas are similar to hemangiomas except that the vascular spaces are filled with lymph rather than blood [112]. The lesions may be solitary or multiple.

- A well-defined cystic appearing mass is typical. Internal septations are common. Echogenic debris may be present within the locules.

ANGIOSARCOMA

Angiosarcomas of the spleen are rare lesions, accounting for less than 2% of all soft tissue sarcomas [119]. Exposure to thorium dioxide (Thorotrast), vinyl chloride, and arsenic are predisposing factors.

- Splenic parenchyma is nodular and heterogeneous.
- Prominent tortuous vessels with turbulent flow on Doppler are seen in and near the lesion.

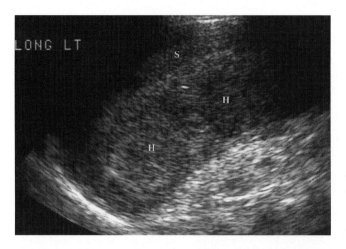

Figure 2.99 *Splenic Hematoma.* An intraparenchymal hematoma (H) is seen as a solid-appearing mass with variable echogenicity within the spleen (S).

- Pulsatile, high-velocity flow is present in the splenic and, occasionally, the portal veins.
- The splenic artery is enlarged with high-flow velocities.

SPLENIC PELIOSIS

Traumatic injury to the spleen may be reliably demonstrated by US.

Splenic peliosis is a rare cause of spontaneous splenic rupture [120]. *Peliosis* refers to the presence of multiple blood-filled cystic spaces (1–10-mm size) in the spleen or liver parenchyma. Both organs are usually affected. The etiology is unknown. Most patients are asymptomatic and the lesion is discovered incidentally.

- Multiple hypoechoic or hyperechoic lesions with ill-defined margins.
- Doppler characteristics have not been described. On CT enhancement is delayed and from the periphery similar to enhancement of hemangiomas.

SUBCAPSULAR/INTRAPARENCHYMAL SPLENIC HEMATOMA

The spleen parenchyma is injured and bleeding occurs, but the splenic capsule remains intact.

- The blood of a subcapsular hematoma appears hypoechoic and flattens or indents the spleen parenchyma. The splenic capsule is seen as a bright crescentic line providing the outer boundary of the hematoma.
- Intraparenchymal hematomas appear as intraparenchymal masses of varying echogenicity (Fig. 2.99).
- Beware the wraparound liver described previously.

SPLENIC RUPTURE

Injury lacerates the splenic parenchyma and the splenic capsule resulting in fragmentation of the spleen and blood in the peritoneal cavity.

- Fluid seen in the peritoneal cavity is indicative of hemoperitoneum. The fluid may be anechoic or contain particulate matter or clots.
- Immediately after injury, liquid blood defines splenic lacerations as irregular jagged lines (Fig. 2.100).
- With clotting of blood 24–48 hours after injury the laceration may not be identifiable because the blood is isoechoic with splenic parenchyma.
- When the clotted blood liquefies, lacerations are again easily seen.

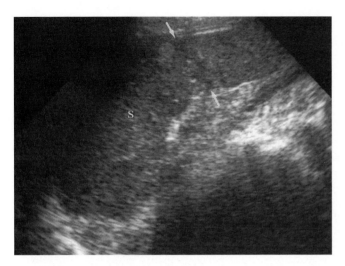

Figure 2.100 *Splenic Laceration.* A splenic laceration appears as a slightly hypoechoic jagged line (*arrows*) extending through the spleen (S). The patient had a hemoperitoneum.

PERITONEAL CAVITY

ASCITES

Ascites is an accumulation of fluid within the peritoneal cavity. Ascites may be a transudate or exudate, blood, pus, bile, urine, pancreatic juice, or lymphatic fluid. US is highly sensitive in detecting intraperitoneal fluid and demonstrates as little as a few mL of fluid.

Anechoic ascites may be a transudate or an exudate.

■ Gravity and peritoneal reflections determine the location of fluid in the peritoneal cavity (Fig. 2.101). Fluid in the subdiaphragmatic spaces separates the liver and spleen from the diaphragm. Fluid in the hepatorenal fossa (Morison's pouch) is seen as an echolucent band between the liver and right kidney. Fluid in the pelvis fills the cul-de-sac and outlines pelvic organs. Loops of bowel float freely within copious ascites.
■ Transudative ascites is always anechoic. Exudative ascites may also be anechoic; however, the presence of floating particulate matter or septations is definitive evidence of exudate (Fig. 2.102).

HEMOPERITONEUM

US is currently frequently used to detect the presence of hemoperitoneum in the setting of abdominal trauma [121]. Detection of even a tiny amount of fluid is used to triage patients urgently to CT or laparotomy. Fluid in the abdominal cavity in this setting is considered evidence of organ injury. US detection of solid organ injury is insensitive and clearly inferior to contrast-enhanced CT [122,123]. In addition, hemoperitoneum is absent in 17–34% of patients with abdominal visceral injuries, most commonly in patients with bowel and mesenteric injury [124,125].

■ Acute intraperitoneal hemorrhage is anechoic to hypoechoic. Floating particulate matter may be seen and may produce fluid-fluid levels.
■ Blood clots appear as echogenic masses within the intraperitoneal fluid. The clot evolves with time to become more hypoechoic.

PSEUDOMYXOMA PERITONEI

Implants of mucin-producing cells on peritoneal surfaces results in a gelatinous form of ascites that tends to loculate and produce cystic pseudomasses. Causes include mucinous cystadenomas and cystadenocarcinomas of the appendix, colon, and ovary.

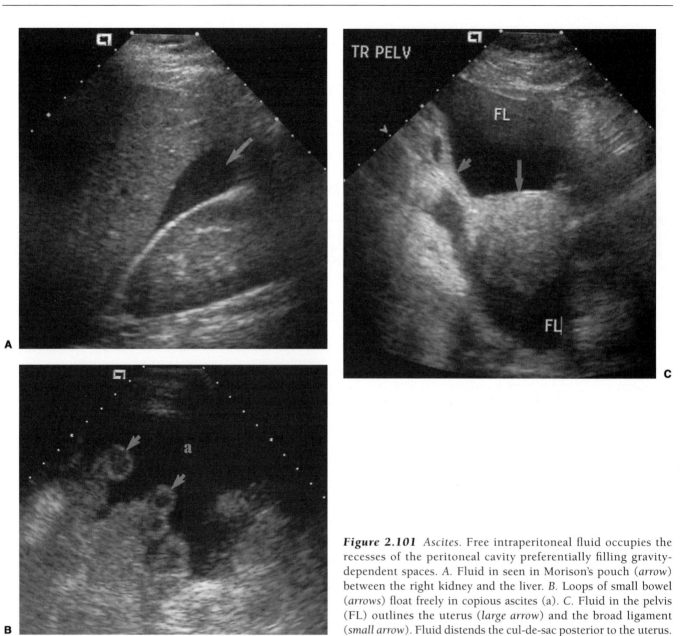

Figure 2.101 *Ascites.* Free intraperitoneal fluid occupies the recesses of the peritoneal cavity preferentially filling gravity-dependent spaces. *A.* Fluid in seen in Morison's pouch (*arrow*) between the right kidney and the liver. *B.* Loops of small bowel (*arrows*) float freely in copious ascites (a). *C.* Fluid in the pelvis (FL) outlines the uterus (*large arrow*) and the broad ligament (*small arrow*). Fluid distends the cul-de-sac posterior to the uterus.

- Fluid is loculated and usually multiseptated. Internal fluid shows low-level echogenicity caused by mucinous debris (Fig. 2.103).

PERITONEAL METASTASES

Peritoneal implantation of metastatic tumor nodules occurs most commonly with ovarian, gastric, colon, and pancreas carcinomas.

- Peritoneal implants are seen as soft tissue nodules that extend from peritoneal surfaces (Fig. 2.104). They are best visualized when ascites is present. Tiny tumor implants, most common with ovarian carcinoma, may not be visualized with US.
- The normal flow of peritoneal fluid determines the pattern of intraperitoneal seeding. Peritoneal tumor is commonly seen in the cul-de-sac and hepatorenal fossa. Tumor implants are most easily recognized on the peritoneal surface of the diaphragm and on the liver.

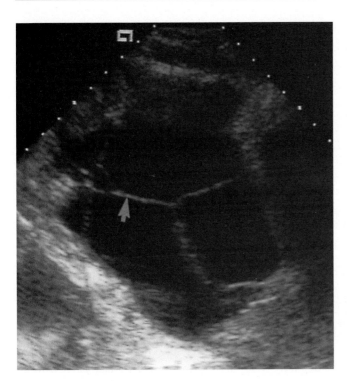

Figure 2.102 *Malignant Ascites.* Fluid pockets in the peritoneal cavity are spanned by fine septations (*arrow*) in this patient with widespread malignant melanoma.

■ Tumor implantation on the greater omentum causes irregular nodular thickening of the omentum seen between the bowel and the anterior abdominal wall. This flattened mass of tumor has been called *omental cake*.

INTRAPERITONEAL ABSCESS

US is an excellent screening method for the detection of intraperitoneal abscesses; however, abdominal wounds, surgical dressings, drainage tubes, and bowel gas limit its use to a small subset of patients. Interloop abscesses, between loops of small bowel, are better demonstrated by CT. Abscesses are caused by spillage of contaminated fluid into the peritoneal cavity as a result of trauma, surgery, pancreatitis, bowel perforation, or by infection elsewhere.

■ Any loculated fluid collection in the peritoneal cavity is suspicious for abscess in a high-risk patient. The presence of mass effect with the fluid collection making its own space and displacing adjacent structures is strong evidence of loculation.

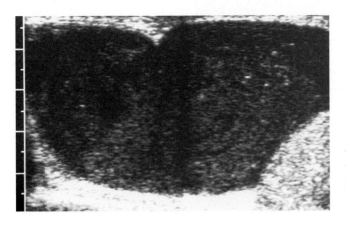

Figure 2.103 *Pseudomyxoma Peritonei.* Mucinous fluid is echogenic and gelatinous filling loculated recesses in the peritoneal cavity.

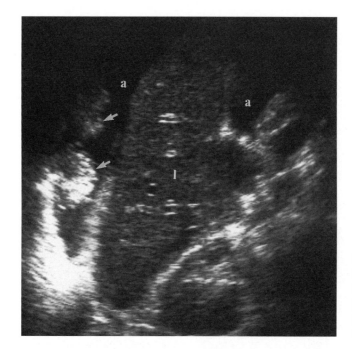

Figure 2.104 *Peritoneal Metastases.* Tumor implants (*arrows*) project from the diaphragm into ascites (a) in this patient with peritoneal spread of colon carcinoma. l, liver.

- Internal debris, fluid levels, and septations are commonly present (Fig. 2.105). A large amount of conglomerated internal debris may suggest a solid mass.
- Air within the fluid collection is strong evidence of abscess. Air bubbles within fluid are seen as bright floating foci with comet tail artifacts. Pockets of air are seen as bright interfaces with acoustic shadowing and reverberation artifacts. This appearance is difficult to differentiate from air within bowel. A fixed position and unusual shape are suggestive.

LYMPHOCELE

Lymphoceles are cystic collections of lymphatic fluid that occur as a result of surgical or traumatic disruption of lymphatic vessels. They are seen commonly after lymphadenectomy in the retroperitoneum or pelvis and following renal transplantation.

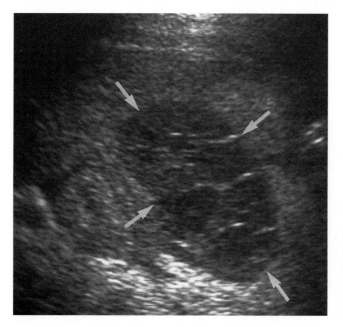

Figure 2.105 *Intraperitoneal Abscess.* An abscess appears as an echogenic fluid collection (*between arrows*) with septations in the gallbladder fossa complicating a cholecystectomy.

- Lymphoceles are typically anechoic loculated fluid collections located in or near an area of previous surgery. Size varies from a few cm to huge.
- Internal septations and debris occur with complicating hemorrhage or infection.
- Diagnosis is confirmed by image-guided percutaneous aspiration.

REFERENCES

1. American Institute of Ultrasound in Medicine. Guidelines for performance of the abdominal and retroperitoneal ultrasound examination. Rockville, MD: AIUM, 1991.
2. Brant WE, Jain KA. Current imaging of the spleen. Radiologist 1996;3:185–192.
3. Goerg C, Schwerk WB, Goerg K. Sonography of focal lesions of the spleen. AJR Am J Roentgenol 1991;156:949–953.
4. Smith D, Downey D, Spouge A, et al. Sonographic demonstration of Couinaud's liver segments. J Ultrasound Med 1998;17:375–381.
5. Lafortune M, Madore F, Patriquin H, et al. Segmental anatomy of the liver: a sonographic approach to the Couinard nomenclature. Radiology 1991;181:443–448.
6. Dodd GD. An American's guide to Couinaud's numbering system. AJR Am J Roentgenol 1993;161:574–575.
7. Lim J, Ryu K, Ko Y, et al. Anatomic relationship of intrahepatic bile ducts to portal veins. J Ultrasound Med 1990;9:137–143.
8. Meyers MA. Dynamic radiology of the abdomen: normal and pathological anatomy. (3rd ed.) New York: Springer Verlag, 1988.
9. Dodds WJ, Foley WD, Lawson TL, et al. Anatomy and imaging of the lesser peritoneal sac. AJR Am J Roentgenol 1985;141:567–575.
10. Gosink B, Leymaster C. Ultrasonic determination of hepatomegaly. J Clin Ultrasound 1981;9:37–42.
11. Cazier PR, Sponaugle DW. "Starry sky" liver with fasting: variations in glycogen stores? J Ultrasound Med 1996;15:405–407.
12. Wang S-S, Chiang J-H, Tsai Y-T, et al. Focal hepatic fatty infiltration as a cause of pseudotumors: ultrasonographic patterns and clinical differentiation. J Clin Ultrasound 1990;18:401–409.
13. Rubaltelli L, Savastano S, Cellini L, et al. Hyperechoic pseudotumors in segment IV of the liver. J Ultrasound Med 1997;16:569–572.
14. Itai Y, Matsui O. Blood flow and liver imaging. Radiology 1997;202:306–314.
15. Brown JJ, Naylor MJ, Yagan N. Imaging of hepatic cirrhosis. Radiology 1997;202:1–16.
16. Di Lelio A, Cestari C, Lomazzi A, et al. Cirrhosis: diagnosis with sonographic study of the liver surface. Radiology 1989;172:389–392.
17. Dodd GI, Baron R, Oliver JI, et al. Spectrum of imaging findings of the liver in end-stage cirrhosis: part I, gross morphology and diffuse abnormalities. AJR Am J Roentgenol 1999;173:1031–1036.
18. Colli A, Cocciolo M, Riva C, et al. Abnormalities of Doppler waveform of the hepatic veins in patients with chronic liver disease: correlation with histologic findings. AJR Am J Roentgenol 1994;162:833–837.
19. Taylor AJ, Carmody TJ, Quiroz FA, et al. Focal masses in cirrhotic liver: CT and MR imaging features. AJR Am J Roentgenol 1994;163:857–862.
20. Dodd GI, Baron R, Oliver JI, et al. Spectrum of imaging findings of the liver in end-stage cirrhosis: part II, focal abnormalities. AJR Am J Roentgenol 1999;173:1185–1192.
21. Choi BI, Takayasu K, Han MC. Small hepatocellular carcinomas and associated nodular lesions of the liver: pathology, pathogenesis, and imaging findings. AJR Am J Roentgenol 1993;160:1177–1187.
22. Ohtomo K, Baron RL, Dodd GD, III, et al. Confluent hepatic fibrosis in advanced cirrhosis: appearance at CT. Radiology 1993;188:31–35.
23. Mergo PJ, Ros PR, Buetow PC, et al. Diffuse disease of the liver: radiologic-pathologic correlation. Radiographics 1994;14:1291–1307.
24. Haag K, Rössle M, Ochs A. Correlation of duplex sonography findings and portal pressure in 375 patients with portal hypertension. AJR Am J Roentgenol 1999;172:631–635.
25. Subramanyam BR, Balthazar EJ, Madamba MR, et al. Sonography of portosystemic venous collaterals in portal hypertension. Radiology 1983;146:161–166.

26. Ayuso C, Luburich P, Vilana R, et al. Calcifications in the portal venous system: comparison of plain films, sonography, and CT. AJR Am J Roentgenol 1992;159:321–323.
27. Parvey HR, Raval B, Sandler CM. Portal vein thrombosis: imaging findings. AJR Am J Roentgenol 1994;162:77–81.
28. De Gaetano A, Lafortune M, Patriquin H, et al. Cavernous transformation of the portal vein: patterns of intrahepatic and splanchnic collateral circulation detected with Doppler sonography. AJR Am J Roentgenol 1995;165:1151–1155.
29. Platt J, Rubin J, Ellis J. Hepatic artery resistance changes in portal vein thrombosis. Radiology 1995;196:95–98.
30. Gore RM, Mathieu DG, White EM, et al. Passive hepatic congestion: cross-sectional imaging features. AJR Am J Roentgenol 1994;162:71–75.
31. Henriksson L, Hedman A, Johansson R, et al. Ultrasound assessment of liver veins in congestive heart failure. Acta Radiol 1982;23:361–363.
32. Hosoki T, Arisawa J, Marukawa T, et al. Portal blood flow in congestive heart failure: pulsed duplex sonographic findings. Radiology 1990;174:733–736.
33. Millener P, Grant E, Rose S, et al. Color Doppler imaging findings in patients with Budd-Chiari syndrome: correlation with venographic findings. AJR Am J Roentgenol 1993;161:307–312.
34. Kane R, Eustace S. Diagnosis of Budd-Chiari syndrome: comparison between sonography and MR angiography. Radiology 1995;195:117–121.
35. Chou Y-H, Tiu C-M, Hwang J-I, et al. Primary Budd-Chiari syndrome: duplex ultrasonic diagnosis. J Med Ultrasound (Taiwan) 1993;2:78–83.
36. Koito K, Namieno T, Morita K. Differential diagnosis of small hepatocellular carcinoma and adenomatous hyperplasia with power Doppler sonography. AJR Am J Roentgenol 1998;170:157–161.
37. Tanaka S, Kitamra T, Fuijita M, et al. Value of contrast-enhanced color Doppler sonography in diagnosing hepatocellular carcinoma with special attention to the "color-filled pattern." J Clin Ultrasound 1998;26:207–212.
38. McLarney J, Rucker P, Bender G, et al. Fibrolamellar carcinoma of the liver: radiologic-pathologic correlation. RadioGraphics 1999;19:453–471.
39. Leifer D, Middleton W, Teefey S, et al. Follow-up of patients at low risk for hepatic malignancy with a characteristic hemangioma at US. Radiology 2000;214:167–172.
40. Moody A, Wilson S. Atypical hepatic hemangioma: a suggestive sonographic morphology. Radiology 1993;188:413–417.
41. Mungovan JA, Cronan JJ, Vacarro J. Hepatic cavernous hemangiomas: lack of enlargement over time. Radiology 1994;191:111–113.
42. Nghiem HV, Bogost GA, Ryan JA, et al. Cavernous hemangiomas of the liver: enlargement over time. AJR Am J Roentgenol 1997;169:137–140.
43. Perkins A, Imam K, Smith W, et al. Color and power Doppler sonography of liver hemangiomas: a dream unfulfilled? J Clin Ultrasound 2000;28:159–165.
44. Young L, Yang W, Chan K, et al. Hepatic hemangioma: quantitative color power US angiography—facts and fallacies. Radiology 1998;207:51–57.
45. Brant WE, Floyd JL, Jackson DE, et al. The radiological evaluation of hepatic cavernous hemangioma. JAMA 1987;257:2471–2474.
46. Heilo A, Stenwig A. Liver hemangioma: US-guided 18-gauge core-needle biopsy. Radiology 1997;204:719–722.
47. Beutow PC, Pantongrag-Brown L, Buck JL, et al. Focal nodular hyperplasia of the liver: radiologic pathologic correlation. Radiographics 1996;16:369–388.
48. Di Stasi M, Caturelli E, De Sio I, et al. Natural history of focal nodular hyperplasia of the liver: an ultrasound study. J Clin Ultrasound 1996;24:345–350.
49. Caseiro-Alves F, Zins M, Mahfouz A-E, et al. Calcification in focal nodular hyperplasia: a new problem for differentiation for fibrolamellar hepatocellular carcinoma. Radiology 1996;198: 889–892.
50. Golli M, Tran Van Nhieu J, Mathieu D, et al. Hepatocellular adenoma: color Doppler US and pathologic correlations. Radiology 1994;190:741–744.
51. Wernecke K, Vassallo P, Bick U, et al. The distinction between benign and malignant liver tumors on sonography: value of a hypoechoic halo. AJR Am J Roentgenol 1992;159:1005–1009.
52. Ralls P, Barnes P, Radin D, et al. Sonographic features of amebic and pyogenic abscesses: a blinded comparison. AJR Am J Roentgenol 1987;149:499–501.
53. Ralls P, Quinn M, Boswell WJ, et al. Patterns of resolution in successfully treated hepatic amebic abscess. Radiology 1983;149:541–543.

54. Beggs I. The radiology of hydatid disease. AJR Am J Roentgenol 1985;145:639–648.
55. Durr-E-Sabih, Sabih Z, Khan A. "Congealed waterlily" sign: a new sonographic sign of liver hydatid cyst. J Clin Ultrasound 1996;24:297–303.
56. Görg C, Weide R, Schwerk W, et al. Ultrasound evaluation of hepatic and splenic microabscesses in the immunocompromised patient: sonographic patterns, differential diagnosis, and follow-up. J Clin Ultrasound 1994;22:525–529.
57. Laing F, Jeffrey RJ, Wing V. Biliary dilatation: defining the level and cause by real-time ultrasound. Radiology 1986;160:39–42.
58. Hernanz-Schulman M, Ambrosino M, Freeman P, et al. Common bile duct in children: sonographic dimensions. Radiology 1995;195:193–195.
59. Graham M, Cooperberg P, Cohen M, et al. The size of the normal common hepatic duct following cholecystectomy: an ultrasonographic study. Radiology 1980;135:137–140.
60. White L, Wilson S. Hepatic arterial calcification: a potential pitfall in the sonographic diagnosis of intrahepatic biliary calculi. J Ultrasound Med 1994;13:141–144.
61. Kubaska S, Chew F. Biliary ascariasis. AJR Am J Roentgenol 1997;169:492.
62. Kim OH, Chung HJ, Choi BG. Imaging of choledochal cyst. RadioGraphics 1995;15:69–88.
63. Savader SJ, Benenati JF, Venbrux AC, et al. Choledochal cysts: classification and cholangiographic appearance. AJR Am J Roentgenol 1991;156:327–331.
64. Todani T, Watanabe Y, Narusue M, et al. Congenital bile duct cysts: classification, operative procedure, and review of 37 cases, including cancer arising from choledochal cyst. Am J Surg 1977;134:263–269.
65. Miller WJ, Sechtin AG, Campbell WL, et al. Imaging findings in Caroli's disease. AJR Am J Roentgenol 1995;165:333–337.
66. Majoie CMLM, Reeders JWAJ, Sanders JB, et al. Primary sclerosing cholangitis: a modified classification of cholangiographic findings. AJR Am J Roentgenol 1991;157:495–497.
67. Dodd GI, Niedzwiecki G, Campbell W, et al. Bile duct calculi in patients with primary sclerosing cholangitis. Radiology 1997;203:443–447.
68. Lim JH. Oriental cholangiohepatitis: pathologic, clinical, and radiologic features. AJR Am J Roentgenol 1991;157:1–8.
69. Miller FH, Gore RM, Nemcek AA, Jr, et al. Pancreaticobiliary manifestations of AIDS. AJR Am J Roentgenol 1996;166:1269–1274.
70. Da Silva F, Boudghene F, Lecomte I, et al. Sonography in AIDS-related cholangitis: prevalence and cause of an echogenic nodule in the distal end of the common bile duct. AJR Am J Roentgenol 1993; 160:1205–1207.
71. Soyer P, Bluemke DA, Reichle R, et al. Imaging of intrahepatic cholangiocarcinoma: 1. peripheral cholangiocarcinoma. AJR Am J Roentgenol 1995;165:1427–1431.
72. Bloom C, Langer B, Wilson S. Role of US in the detection, characterization, and staging of cholangiocarcinoma. RadioGraphics 1999;19:1199–1218.
73. Wibulpolprasert B, Dhiensiri T. Peripheral cholangiocarcinoma: sonographic evaluation. J Clin Ultrasound 1992;20:303–314.
74. Soyer P, Bluemke DA, Reichle R, et al. Imaging of intrahepatic cholangiocarcinoma: 2. hilar cholangiocarcinoma. AJR Am J Roentgenol 1995;165:1433–1436.
75. Hann LE, Greatrex KV, Bach AM, et al. Cholangiocarcinoma at the hepatic hilus: sonographic findings. AJR Am J Roentgenol 1997;168:985–989.
76. Neumaier C, Bertolotto M, Perrone R, et al. Staging of hilar cholangiocarcinoma with ultrasound. J Clin Ultrasound 1995;23:173–178.
77. Teefey SA, Baron RL, Bigler SA. Sonography of the gallbladder: significance of striated (layered) thickening of the gallbladder wall. AJR Am J Roentgenol 1991;156:945–947.
78. Rybicki F. The WES sign. Radiology 2000;214:881–882.
79. Hammond D. Unusual causes of sonographic nonvisualization or nonrecognition of the gallbladder: a review. J Clin Ultrasound 1988;16:77–85.
80. Paulson E, Kliewer M, Hertzberg B, et al. Diagnosis of acute cholecystitis with color Doppler sonography: significance of arterial flow in thickened gallbladder wall. AJR Am J Roentgenol 1994;162:1105–1108.
81. Wu C-S, Yao W-J, Hsiao C-H. Effervescent gallbladder: sonographic findings in emphysematous cholecystitis. J Clin Ultrasound 1998;26:272–275.
82. Bloom RA, Libson E, Lebensart PD, et al. The ultrasound spectrum of emphysematous cholecystitis. J Clin Ultrasound 1989;17:251–256.
83. Teefey S, Kimmey M, Bigler S, et al. Gallbladder wall thickening: an in vitro sonographic study with histologic correlation. Acad Radiol 1994;1:121–127.

84. Kane R, Jacobs R, Katz J, et al. Porcelain gallbladder: ultrasound and CT appearance. Radiology 1984;152:137–141.

85. Collett J, Allan R, Chisholm R, et al. Gallbladder polyps: prospective study. J Ultrasound Med 1998;17:207–211.

86. Berk R, van der Vegt J, Lichtenstein J. The hyperplastic cholecystoses: cholesterolosis and adenomyomatosis. Radiology 1983;146:593–601.

87. Raghavendra B, Subramanyam B, Balthazar E, et al. Sonography of adenomyomatosis of the gallbladder: radiologic-pathologic correlation. Radiology 1983;146:747–752.

88. Rooholamini SA, Tehrani NS, Razavi MK, et al. Imaging of gallbladder carcinoma. Radiographics 1994;14:291–306.

89. Li D, Dong B-W, Wu Y, et al. Image-directed and color Doppler studies of gallbladder tumors. J Clin Ultrasound 1994;22:551–555.

90. Wibbenmeyer L, Sharfuddin M, Wolverson M, et al. Sonographic diagnosis of unsuspected gallbladder cancer: imaging findings in comparison with benign gallbladder conditions. AJR Am J Roentgenol 1995;165:1169–1174.

91. Paulson E, Vitellas K, Keogan M, et al. Acute pancreatitis complicated by gland necrosis: spectrum of findings on contrast-enhanced CT. AJR Am J Roentgenol 1999;172:609–613.

92. Fishman EK, Soyer P, Bliss DF, et al. Splenic involvement in pancreatitis: spectrum of CT findings. AJR Am J Roentgenol 1995;164:631–635.

93. vanSonnenberg E, Wittich G, Chon K, et al. Percutaneous radiologic drainage of pancreatic abscesses. AJR Am J Roentgenol 1997;168:979–984.

94. Patel B, Chenoweth J, Parvey H, et al. Complications of chronic pancreatitis: imaging findings. Radiologist 1998;5:227–236.

95. Lee M, Wittich G, Mueller P. Percutaneous intervention in acute pancreatitis. RadioGraphics 1998;18:711–724.

96. Patel B, Chenoweth J, Garvin P, et al. Role of imaging in the diagnosis of chronic pancreatitis and differentiation from carcinoma of the pancreas. Radiologist 1998;5:245–255.

97. Moorthy T, Nalini N, Narendranathan M. Ultrasound imaging in tropical pancreatitis. J Clin Ultrasound 1991;20:389–393.

98. Van Hoe L, Gryspeerdt S, Ectors N, et al. Nonalcoholic duct-destructive chronic pancreatitis: imaging findings. AJR Am J Roentgenol 1998;170:643–647.

99. Luetmer PH, Stephens DH, Ward EM. Chronic pancreatitis: reassessment with current CT. Radiology 1989;171:353–357.

100. Karlson B-M, Ekbom A, Lindgren P, et al. Abdominal US for diagnosis of pancreatic tumor: prospective cohort analysis. Radiology 1999;213:107–111.

101. Angeli E, Venturine M, Vanzulli A, et al. Color Doppler imaging in the assessment of vascular involvement by pancreatic carcinoma. AJR Am J Roentgenol 1997;168:193–197.

102. Procacci C, Graziani R, Bicego E, et al. Intraductal mucin-producing tumors of the pancreas: imaging findings. Radiology 1996;198:249–257.

103. Procacci C, Megibow A, Carbognin G, et al. Intraductal papillary mucinous tumor of the pancreas: a pictorial essay. RadioGraphics 1999;19:1447–1463.

104. de Lima JJ, Javitt M, Mathur S. Mucinous cystic neoplasm of the pancreas. RadioGraphics 1999;19:807–811.

105. Hough DM, Stephens DH, Johnson CD, et al. Pancreatic lesions in von Hippel-Lindau disease: prevalence, clinical significance, and CT findings. AJR Am J Roentgenol 1994;162:1091–1094.

106. Ng C, Loyer E, Iyer R, et al. Metastases to the pancreas from renal cell carcinoma: findings on three-phase contrast-enhanced helical CT. AJR Am J Roentgenol 1999;172:1555–1559.

107. Agrons G, Corse W, Markowitz R, et al. Gastrointestinal manifestations of cystic fibrosis: radiologic-pathologic correlation. RadioGraphics 1996;16:871–893.

108. Subramanyam B, Balthazar E, Horii S. Sonography of the accessory spleen. AJR Am J Roentgenol 1984;143:47–49.

109. Loftus W, Chow L, Metreweli C. Sonographic measurement of splenic length: correlation with measurement at autopsy. J Clin Ultrasound 1999;27:71–74.

110. Paterson A, Frush D, Donnelly L, et al. A pattern-oriented approach to splenic imaging in infants and children. RadioGraphics 1999;19:1465–1485.

111. Masmune A, Okano T, Satake K, et al. Ultrasonic diagnosis of torsion of the wandering spleen. J Clin Ultrasound 1994;22:126–128.

112. Urritia M, Mergo P, Ros L, et al. Cystic lesions of the spleen: radiologic-pathologic correlation. RadioGraphics 1996;16:107–129.

113. Murray JG, Patel MD, Lee S, et al. Microabscesses of the liver and spleen in AIDS: detection with 5-MHz sonography. Radiology 1995;197:723–727.
114. Franquet T, Montes M, Lecumberri FJ, et al. Hydatid disease of the spleen: imaging findings in nine patients. AJR Am J Roentgenol 1990;154:525–528.
115. Goerg C, Schwerk W, Goerg K, et al. Sonographic patterns of the affected spleen in malignant lymphoma. J Clin Ultrasound 1990;18:569–574.
116. Ishida H, Konno K, Ishida J, et al. Isolated splenic metastases. J Ultrasound Med 1997;16:743–749.
117. Goerg C, Schwerk WB. Splenic infarction: sonographic patterns, diagnosis, follow-up, and complications. Radiology 1990;174:803–807.
118. Ros PR, Moser RP, Jr., Dachman AH, et al. Hemangioma of the spleen: radiologic-pathologic correlation in ten cases. Radiology 1987:481–485.
119. Aytac S, Fitoz S, Atasoy C, et al. Multimodality demonstration of primary splenic angiosarcoma. J Clin Ultrasound 1999;27:92–95.
120. Kohr R, Haendiges M, Taube R. Peliosis of the spleen: a rare cause of spontaneous splenic rupture with surgical implications. Am Surgeon 1993;59:197–199.
121. Goletti G, Ghiselli G, Lippolis P, et al. The role of ultrasonography in blunt abdominal trauma: results in 250 consecutive cases. J Trauma 1994;36:178–181.
122. McKenney K. Role of US in the diagnosis of intraabdominal catastrophes. RadioGraphics 1999;19:1332–1339.
123. McGahan JP, Richards J. Blunt abdominal trauma: the role of emergent sonography and a review of the literature. AJR Am J Roentgenol 1999;172:897–903.
124. Shanmuganathan K, Mirvis S, Sherbourne C, et al. Hemoperitoneum as the sole indicator of abdominal visceral injuries: a potential limitation of screening abdominal US for trauma. Radiology 1999;212:423–430.
125. Richards J, McGahan J, Simpson J, et al. Bowel and mesenteric injury: evaluation with emergency abdominal US. Radiology 1999;211:399–403.
126. Stoupis C, Taylor H, Paley M, et al. The rocky liver: radiologic-pathologic correlation of calcified hepatic masses. RadioGraphics 1998;18:675–685.

RENAL, BLADDER, AND ADRENAL ULTRASOUND

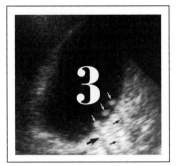

IMAGING TECHNIQUE

KIDNEYS

A renal US examination typically includes sonography of both kidneys, the perirenal areas, the aorta, inferior vena cava (IVC), and the urinary bladder. The American Institute of Ultrasound in Medicine provides guidelines for a satisfactory examination [1]. A sector or curved array transducer using frequencies between 2.25 and 5.0 MHz is recommended. The right kidney is examined from an anterolateral or direct lateral approach with the patient supine or in left lateral decubitus position, using the right lobe of the liver as a sonographic window. The left kidney is often more difficult to visualize because the spleen provides a more limited sonographic window. The left kidney is often obscured by bowel when scanned from the anterior abdomen. Placing the patient in right lateral decubitus position provides access to a more lateral and posterior approach through the spleen and psoas muscle. Multiple images of both kidneys are documented in longitudinal and transverse planes including the upper pole, middle section, and lower pole. Maximum renal lengths are recorded. Renal volumes may be calculated by measuring transverse and anteroposterior (AP) diameters from a mid-kidney transverse image. The standard formula (volume = length × width × AP diameter × 0.52) is utilized. The bladder lumen, wall thickness, and mucosal surface are documented. The retroperitoneum is examined for ureteral dilatation, adenopathy, or other abnormality.

Color flow and spectral Doppler are frequently utilized to confirm patency of the renal artery and vein, parenchymal blood flow, and the vascularity of any lesion detected. Power Doppler allows the most sensitive demonstration of renal vascularity [2,3].

BLADDER

For US examination, the bladder should be moderately distended to stretch the wall and to better visualize the mucosal surface and bladder lumen. Images are obtained in transverse and longitudinal planes. Attention should be directed to the trigone area, ureteral orifices, and prostate gland. Transvaginal scanning will improve evaluation of the bladder in women. Large cystic pelvic masses may be mistaken for the bladder. When this is suspected, the bladder should be emptied by voiding or Foley catheter and rescanned.

ADRENAL GLANDS

The normal adrenal glands may be imaged by US with careful attention to technique and anatomic landmarks.

Although small and tucked away in the retroperitoneum normal and abnormal adrenal glands can be visualized by US in most patients with a little effort and attention to anatomic landmarks. Normal adrenal glands are prominent and easily seen in the third-trimester fetus and the newborn, but require exacting technique to visualize in most adults. Adrenal abnormalities may be detected during routine renal sonography. Careful attention to the location of the adrenal glands is the key to recognizing them on US. The right adrenal gland is truly suprarenal and is best visualized by a posterolateral approach in transverse plane looking for the adrenal gland just above the right kidney, between the liver and right crus of the diaphragm posterior to the IVC as it enters the liver. The left adrenal gland is imaged by a posterolateral approach in coronal plane through the long axis of the left kidney. The left adrenal gland is seen between the upper pole of the left kidney and the aorta. High-resolution, real-time sonography allows visualization of normal adrenal glands in 71–92% of adults [4].

ANATOMY

KIDNEYS

The normal adult kidney is bean-shaped with a smoothly convex, often lobulated, outer border (Fig. 3.1). The kidney is well defined by a thick fibrous capsule outlined by echogenic perirenal fat. This echogenic fat continues into the renal sinus, entering at the anteromedially oriented renal hilum and filling the middle of the kidney. The outer renal cortex is equal to, or slightly less than, the liver and spleen in echogenicity. Renal cortical echogenicity distinctly greater than liver parenchymal echogenicity is highly indicative of impaired renal function [5]. Liver parenchymal echogenicity distinctly greater than renal cortical echogenicity is highly indicative of diffuse hepatocellular fatty infiltration [6]. The cortex that extends centrally into the kidney is called *septal cortex* as it surrounds and separates the less echogenic medullary pyramids. Fusion of septal cortex from adjacent lobes produces a normal, but often bulbous, mass of cortex referred to as a *column of Bertin* (see Fig. 3.3) [7]. Distinct differentiation of cortical and medullary echogenicity is a sign of a

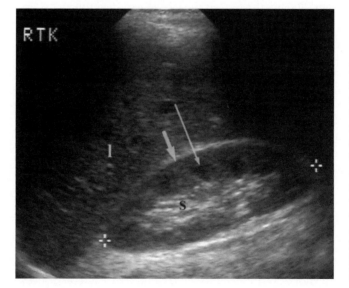

Figure 3.1 *Normal Adult Kidney.* The renal cortex (*short arrow*) is equal in echogenicity to the liver parenchyma (l). The renal pyramids (*long arrow*) are slightly hypoechoic compared to the renal cortex. The septal cortex extends between the medullary pyramids. The central renal sinus (s) is invested with echogenic fat. The contour of the kidney is sharply defined by fat in the perirenal space. The length of the kidney is measured between cursors (+).

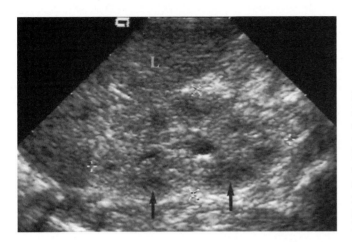

Figure 3.2 *Normal Newborn Infant Kidney.* Longitudinal view of the normal right kidney (*between cursors, +, x*) of a newborn infant demonstrates echogenicity of the cortex to be slightly greater than the echogenicity of the liver (L). The medulla (*arrows*) is significantly less echogenic.

normal kidney. In infants up to 24 months of age, the echogenicity of the cortex is significantly greater than the renal cortex in adults and older children (Fig. 3.2). Its echogenicity commonly exceeds liver parenchymal echogenicity. The medullary pyramids remain echolucent and prominent. This appearance has been mistaken for hydronephrosis.

Persistent fetal lobation is a common renal anatomic variant [8]. The normal kidney is made up of 12–18 separate lobes consisting of a medullary pyramid surrounded by subcapsular and septal cortex [9]. A single lobe drains into a simple calyx. When several lobes drain into a single calyx, the calyx is considered to be a compound calyx. The fetal lobes act as tiny independent kidneys early in fetal life but progressively fuse into a single kidney with maturation. Incomplete lobular fusion is common and results in V-shaped indentations on the renal surface (Fig. 3.3). A prominent indentation between the upper and lower portion of the kidney has been called the *junctional defect* [7]. These normal V-shaped defects should not be mistaken for parenchymal scars.

Calyces unite to form the renal pelvis, which exits the renal sinus at the hilum. The calyces and pelvis are usually collapsed and are not seen as discrete structures within the renal sinus. When patients are well hydrated, high urine output causes mild normal dilatation of the calyces and pelvis. The renal pelvis may also be seen as a prominent fluid-filled structure when it is "extrarenal," that is, primarily outside of the renal sinus. Lower surrounding tissue pressure allows the pelvis to be chronically dilated. These normal variations must be differentiated from hydronephrosis.

The main renal arteries are solitary in 60% of individuals and multiple and smaller in the remainder. The renal arteries arise from the lateral aspects of the aorta approximately 1 cm below the origin of the superior mesenteric artery. The right renal artery passes behind the IVC causing a small but prominent indentation on the posterior wall of the IVC (see Fig. 2.11). The left renal artery has a short direct course to the left kidney. Renal arteries are more commonly multiple when the kidney is malpositioned or malrotated. Supplemental renal arteries may course directly into the polar regions of the kidney without coursing through the renal hilum. Renal veins are usually solitary. The right renal vein is anterior to the right renal artery and courses anterosuperiorly to enter the IVC usually somewhat above the level of the right renal hilum. The left renal vein courses transversely anterior to the aorta to enter the IVC. The left gonadal vein enters the left renal vein just outside the left renal hilum. The right gonadal vein enters the IVC directly just below the junction of right renal vein and IVC.

The Doppler spectrum of the normal renal artery shows continuous forward flow into the kidney with relatively high velocities maintained throughout diastole indicating low intrarenal vascular resistance. Maximum normal peak systolic velocity is **180 cm/sec**. Normal resistive index (RI) is below **0.70**. The Doppler spectrum of the renal vein shows continuous venous flow with slight respiratory undulation.

Doppler spectra can be obtained from tiny intrarenal arteries (interlobar and arcuate arteries), whether they are actually visualized or not, by placing a Doppler sample volume

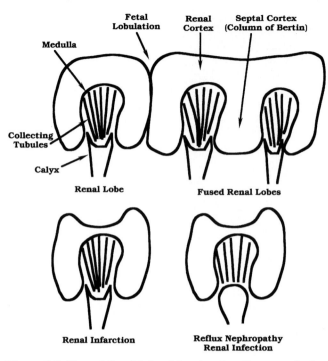

Figure 3.3 *Normal Renal Lobes.* Line drawing illustrates the basic anatomy of the renal lobes. The normal adult kidney is made up of approximately 14 lobes, which are the basic structural unit of the kidney. Each lobe resembles a kernel of corn and consists of subcapsular and septal **cortex** containing glomeruli and a central **medulla** (medullary pyramid) containing collecting tubules and portions of the loops of Henle. The collecting tubules drain urine into calyces. Lack of complete fusion of the renal lobes results in fetal lobulation with a V-shaped defect on the capsular surface marking the junction of the lobes. Fusion of the lobes results in a smooth capsular surface. A **column of Bertin** refers to fusion of the septal cortex of two adjacent lobes. A prominent column of Bertin may be mistaken for a renal mass. The **junctional defect** is a prominent V-shaped defect in the cortical surface that marks the junction of lobes from the upper pole with lobes of the lower pole. Renal parenchymal scarring, occurring as a result of infarction, reflux nephropathy, or renal infection, produces a U-shaped defect that overlies the calyx. The calyx underlying the parenchymal scar is normal in shape with infarction but is blunted as a result of reflux nephropathy or recurrent infection.

at the corticomedullary junction along the borders of the pyramids. The RI, calculated from the spectral display, has diagnostic value in a number of disease states. Like the main renal artery, RI of 0.70 is the upper limit of normal for intrarenal arteries. A number of representative readings should be averaged to determine a single representative value [10].

Characteristics of the normal kidney are summarized in Table 3.1.

The normal adult kidney measures 9–13 cm in length.

BLADDER

The exact shape and appearance of the bladder varies with the degree of distension. When empty or nearly empty, the bladder wall is thick and somewhat irregular due to contraction of the wall musculature and wrinkling of the mucosa. With filling, the wall thins and the mucosa flattens to a smooth, well-defined surface. The normal bladder wall does not exceed 4 mm in thickness when the bladder is distended. The trigone is defined by the slight protuberances of the ureteral orifices and the more inferior urethral opening. The ureteral orifices are most easily located by identifying ureteral jets. Periodic ureteral peristalsis (average rate, 6 waves per minute) squirts jets of urine into the bladder lumen. These jets are seen on gray-scale US as tiny streams of microbubbles, and on color flow US as flashes of color projecting into the bladder lumen (Fig. 3.4) [11]. The urethral orifice is seen as a slight V-shaped depression at the bladder base. Enlargement of the prostate elevates the bladder base. Postvoid bladder volume does not normally exceed 22 mL. Normal

The normal bladder wall measures 4 mm or less.

Ureteral jets are streams of urine propelled into the bladder by ureteral peristalsis. Visualization of a ureteral jet confirms patency of the ureter.

Table 3.1: US Characteristics of Normal Kidneys

Feature	Normal Characteristic

Size [100]	Length:
	Adult: 9–13 cm (decreases with age)
	    Male: 11.4 cm median length
	    Female: 10.9 cm median length
	Volume: (length × width × height × 0.52)
	Adult: Male: range: 109–194 mL
	    151 mL median volume
	Female: range: 91–151 mL
	    122 mL median volume
	Parenchymal thickness: Normal >10 mm

Echogenicity of cortex	Adult: renal parenchyma echogenicity equal to, or slightly less than, normal liver parenchyma Neonate: renal parenchyma echogenicity usually greater than normal liver parenchyma
Echogenicity of medulla	Adult: slightly less than renal cortex Neonate: much less than renal cortex
Surface	Smooth, well-defined, slightly lobulated with V-shaped notches between lobes
Peak systolic velocity in main renal artery	Normal <180 cm/sec
Renal/aortic velocity ratio	Normal <3.5
Resistive index—intrarenal arteries and main renal artery	Adult: Normal <0.70 Child <5 years: Normal commonly >0.70
Systolic rise time (time to early systolic peak) in main renal artery	Normal = 0.05–0.17 sec

urine is anechoic. Reverberation artifact commonly projects into the bladder from the anterior bladder wall. Residual urine after voiding is quantified by the standard formula: volume = width × height × length × 0.52 (Table 3.2).

ADRENAL GLANDS

Adrenal glands are composed of cortex and medulla, which have different embryologic origin, function, and US appearance. The cortex secretes the steroid hormones cortisol, androgens, and aldosterone, whereas the medulla secretes catecholamines. The cortex is hypoechoic to liver parenchyma, whereas the medulla is near isoechoic with fat (Fig. 3.5).

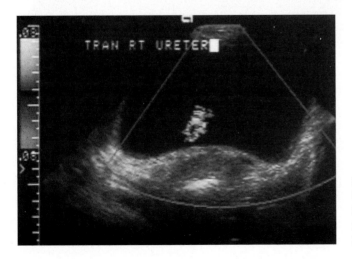

Figure 3.4 *Normal Ureteral Jet.* Ureteral peristalsis produces a flash of color as urine squirts into the bladder lumen (see Color Figure 3.4).

Table 3.2: US Characteristics of Normal Bladder

Feature	Normal Characteristic
Size (bladder volume) Measure length, width, and height. Use formula L × W × H × 0.523 = Volume.	**Post-void volume** Adult: <22 mL Child: <10 mL
Thickness of bladder wall	Adult: <4 mm when distended
	Child: <4 mm when distended
Appearance of bladder wall	Smooth, thin, well defined when distended
	Slightly irregular and thickened when contracted

Adrenal glands are relatively larger in the fetus and newborn because of the presence of the prominent fetal cortex that atrophies by 1 of year of age.

KIDNEYS

CONGENITAL ANOMALIES

Horseshoe Kidney

Horseshoe kidney describes the appearance of congenital fusion of the lower poles of both kidneys [12]. This is the most common renal fusion anomaly with a prevalence of 1:400

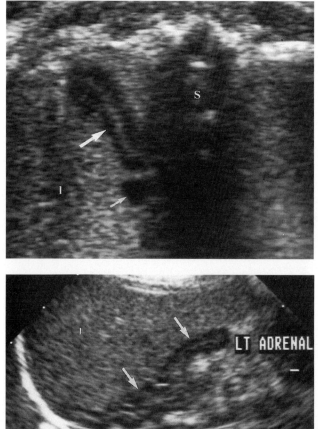

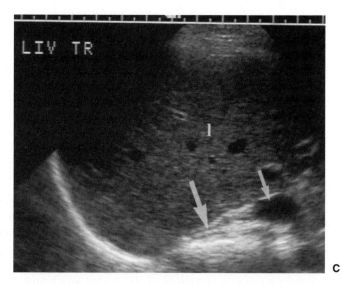

Figure 3.5 *Normal Adrenal Glands.* US images show the normal adrenal glands (*long arrows*) in the fetus at 35 weeks (*A*), the newborn (*B*), and the adult (*C*). The cortex is hypoechoic and the medulla is echogenic. The short arrows indicate the inferior vena cava. l, liver; S, fetal spine.

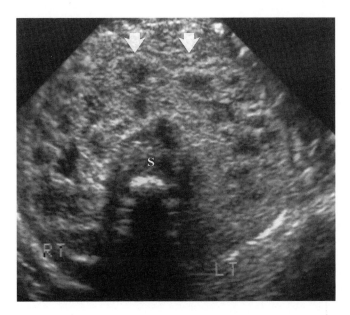

Figure 3.6 *Horseshoe Kidney in an Infant.* Transverse image shows the fusion (*arrows*) of the two kidneys (RT, LT) anterior to the spine (S).

individuals. One-third of affected patients have additional congenital anomalies. Horseshoe kidneys are prone to urinary stasis, infection, calculus formation, hydronephrosis, vesicoureteral reflux, anomalous blood supply, and have increased susceptibility to traumatic injury.

■ The key to US diagnosis is demonstration of the isthmus connecting the kidneys across the midline (Figs. 3.6, 3.7) [12]. The isthmus crosses the midline anterior to the IVC and aorta just below the origin of the inferior mesenteric artery. The isthmus may be functioning renal parenchyma with echogenicity identical to the kidney or it may be thinner and more echogenic fibrous tissue. In 15% of cases, the isthmus may not be demonstrable by US.

■ The kidneys are low in position because the isthmus encounters the inferior mesenteric artery stopping the normal ascent of the kidneys. A definitive sign of low position is the left kidney lying caudal to the inferior tip of the spleen.

■ The long axes of the kidneys are reversed with the lower poles positioned closer together than the upper poles. The kidneys appear curved or bent and the lower poles are ill defined, narrowed, and elongated (Fig. 3.7). The lower poles of the kidneys are not defined on routine longitudinal images. The orientation of the renal pelvis is anterior rather than anteromedial.

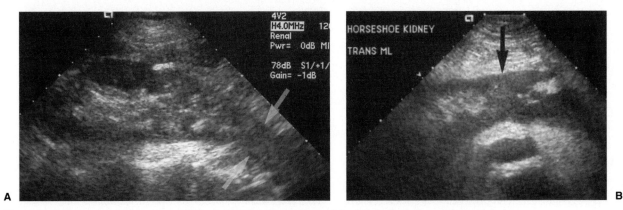

Figure 3.7 *Horseshoe Kidney in an Adult.* A. Longitudinal image of the left kidney shows elongation of the lower pole (*arrows*) without visualization of its lower margin. B. Transverse image over the spine shows the connection of the lower poles (*arrow*) of both kidneys.

Collecting System Duplication

Duplication of the collecting system is the most common congenital anomaly of the urinary tract. Duplication is complete when two separate ureters drain separate portions of one kidney. This anomaly is associated with ureteroceles, obstruction, and reflux. Incomplete duplication ranges from a bifid renal pelvis to duplex ureters that join before entering the bladder through a single orifice. Because non-dilated ureters are seldom demonstrated by US, precise classification is not often possible by US alone.

The Weigert-Meyer rule states that in complete ureteral duplication, the upper pole ureter inserts medial and inferior to the normally located lower pole ureter insertion.

- Two central echogenic sinuses separated by a band of parenchyma suggest some degree of collecting system duplication, statistically most often a bifid pelvis without ureteral duplication.
- With complete duplication, the ureter draining the lower pole collecting system inserts in the normal location at the bladder trigone. The ureter draining the upper pole collecting system always inserts lower and medial to the orifice of the lower pole system. This ectopic location, sometimes outside of the bladder in the prostate or vagina, often results in ureteral obstruction and formation of an ectopic ureterocele. The ectopic ureterocele may mechanically disrupt the valve mechanism of the lower pole ureteral insertion and result in vesicoureteral reflux (VUR).

The upper pole is commonly obstructed, the lower pole commonly refluxes.

STONES AND OBSTRUCTION

Renal Stone Disease

Urolithiasis has its highest prevalence in men aged 20–40 years. Approximately 12% of men and 5% of women experience renal colic caused by stone disease at least once in their lifetimes. Most renal stone disease is idiopathic.

- Both radiopaque and radiolucent calculi produce highly echogenic foci with acoustic shadowing (Fig. 3.8).

Urinary stones smaller than 5 mm are often overlooked by US.

- US reliably demonstrates stones >5-mm size, but smaller stones are commonly not detected [13]. Up to 40% of the small stones present may be missed [14].
- US is inaccurate in measuring stone size.
- Calcifications in renal arteries or within tumors must not be mistaken for renal stones.
- Obstructing stones in the ureter are detected by following the dilated ureter to the point of obstruction (Figs. 3.9, 3.10). Transvaginal or transrectal US are useful adjunctive techniques in the demonstration of distal ureteral calculi [15].

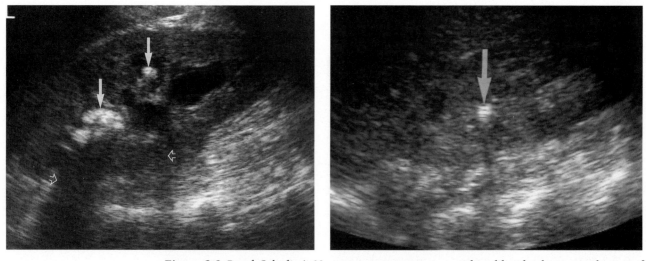

Figure 3.8 *Renal Calculi. A.* Numerous stones are seen within dilated calyces as echogenic foci (*closed arrows*) with acoustic shadowing (*open arrows*). *B.* Solitary stone produces a bright echogenic focus (*arrow*) in the renal sinus and casts an acoustic shadow.

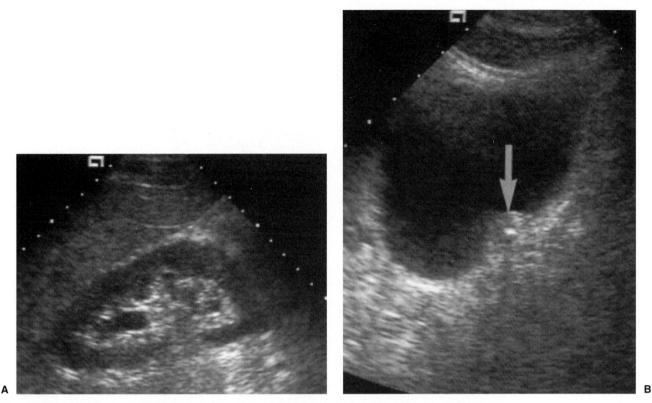

Figure 3.9 *Acute Obstruction with Impacted Distal Ureteral Stone. A.* Acute obstruction produces minimal dilatation of the renal calyces, although the patient experienced severe pain. *B.* Longitudinal image of the bladder reveals a swollen uterovesical junction (*arrow*) with a small impacted stone that shadows.

- A color Doppler "twinkling sign" has been described within or just distal to urinary tract calculi [16]. This appears as a comet tail of alternating bands of red and blue colors. The artifact is useful in identification of calculi and must not be mistaken for blood flow. The artifact is accentuated by increasing Doppler power.

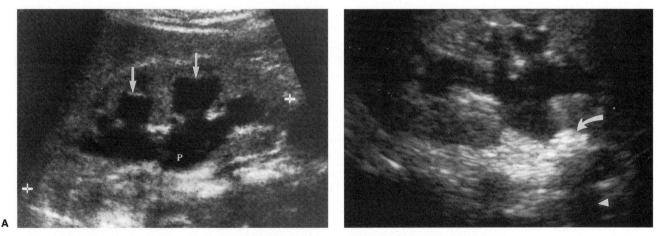

Figure 3.10 *Moderate Hydronephrosis. A.* Rounded calyces filled with urine (*arrows*) connect to the fluid distended pelvis (P). Cursors (+) mark the poles of the kidney. *B.* Hydronephrosis terminates abruptly at a calculus (*arrow*) impacted at the ureteropelvic junction. Note the acoustic shadow (*arrowhead*) emanating from the stone.

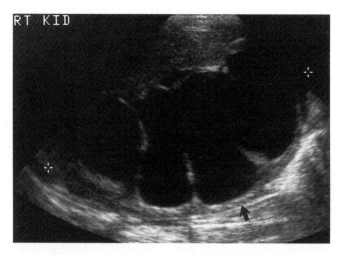

Figure 3.11 *Marked Hydronephrosis.* The renal collecting system is markedly dilated, and the renal parenchyma is thinned (*arrow*), indicating long-standing hydronephrosis. The cause of hydronephrosis in this case was diabetes insipidus. Cursors (+) mark the poles of the kidney.

Hydronephrosis and Obstruction

US demonstration of hydronephrosis is not, by itself, diagnostic of urinary obstruction. Hydronephrosis is an anatomic finding, not a functional one, and is caused by acute and chronic urinary obstruction, VUR, pregnancy, high urine output states (diabetes insipidus), and congenital dilatation of the collecting system (prune belly syndrome). Hydronephrosis may be absent or minimal when obstruction is acute or incomplete (Fig. 3.9), and hydronephrosis may persist for months after obstruction is relieved. Confirmation of functional urinary obstruction must be provided by Doppler US findings, or by additional imaging (intravenous urography, radionuclide studies).

- Dilatation of the calyces, pelvis, and ureter constitutes the anatomic finding of hydronephrosis (Fig. 3.10). Calyces appear rounded and cystic and communicate with the renal pelvis. Well-hydrated normal patients may show mild pelvicalyectasis that is accentuated when the bladder is full. Re-imaging after emptying the bladder shows resolution of this normal dilatation.
- Pelvicalyceal dilatation is most severe when obstruction is long-standing (Fig. 3.11). Chronic obstruction is often associated with diffuse parenchymal atrophy. Proximal obstruction causes greater dilatation than distal obstruction. Acute obstruction, even when complete, often causes only mild hydronephrosis (Fig. 3.9).
- Physiological hydronephrosis is seen in the third trimester of 90% of pregnancies with the right side being more commonly and more severely affected [17].
- Parapelvic cysts mimic the US appearance of hydronephrosis (Fig. 3.12). US differentiation is difficult. The correct diagnosis is confirmed most easily by referring to previous imaging studies that show the presence of renal sinus cysts causing compression and attenuation of the collecting system. Clues to US diagnosis include non-uniform size and appearance of the cysts, the presence of uninvolved areas of the renal sinus, and the observation that the parapelvic cyst does not abut the tip of the medullary pyramid.
- Extrarenal location of the renal pelvis often results in dilatation of the pelvis without associated dilatation of the calyces or ureter. This is a normal variant that should not be mistaken for pathologic hydronephrosis.
- Demonstration of ureteral jets caused by periodic ureteral peristalsis confirms patency of the ureter [11]. Gray scale US shows a stream of low-level echoes extending from the ureteral orifice into the bladder lumen. Color Doppler accentuates detection of this fluid jet (Fig. 3.4).
- Absence of a ureteral jet on the affected side during several minutes of observation confirms complete obstruction [11]. This finding is unreliable in pregnancy [18].
- Intrarenal artery RI >0.70 is highly suggestive of obstruction, provided (a) technique is adequate and waveform is large enough to be clearly measured; (b) the patient is older than 4–5 years (RI is normally >0.70 in children under 5 years); and (c) significant

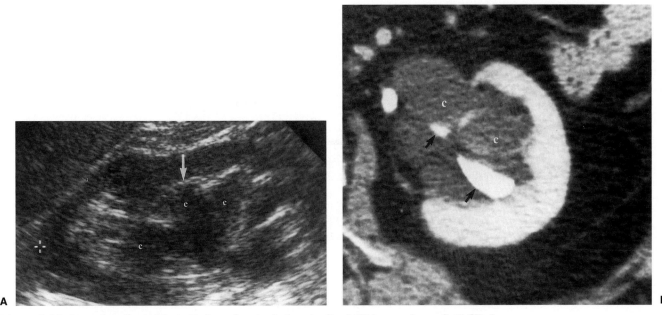

Figure 3.12 *Parapelvic Cysts Mimic Hydronephrosis. A.* Longitudinal US image shows fluid-filled structures (c) in the renal sinus that mimic dilated calyces and pelvis. Note that the dilated "calyx" is separated from the renal parenchyma by a layer of echogenic fat (*arrow*). Compare to the images in Figure 3.10. True dilated calyces directly abut the tip of the medullary pyramid. Cursor (+) marks the upper pole of the kidney. *B.* CT scan shows the parapelvic cysts (c), which compress the contrast-filled collecting system (*arrows*).

medical renal disease is not present. Elevated RI is a more reliable sign of obstruction when the opposite kidney has a normal RI. Obstruction may elevate the intrarenal RI before significant hydronephrosis is present. RI values return to normal after obstruction is relieved, even though pelvicalyectasis may still be present [19].

- Pregnancy-induced hydronephrosis does not typically elevate the intrarenal artery RI. RI >0.70 is highly suggestive of obstructing calculus in a symptomatic pregnant patient [20].
- Urinary obstruction in the newborn may be overlooked on US examinations performed immediately after birth because of dehydration and limited renal function. Infants with antenatal demonstration of fetal pyelectasis are best evaluated at 4–7 days with the examination repeated at 6 weeks [21].

> Hydronephrosis is an anatomic finding that is not always caused by urinary tract obstruction.

Vesicoureteral Reflux and Reflux Nephropathy

VUR is a common problem of childhood associated with frequent urinary tract infections and progressive renal damage if untreated. VUR is seen in adults with neurogenic bladders and bladder outlet obstruction.

- VCUG (voiding cystourethrography) is the imaging method of choice for demonstration of VUR. A normal renal US does not exclude VUR [22].
- VUR is a common cause of fetal and neonatal hydronephrosis. Intermittent, waxing and waning hydronephrosis seen over several minutes of observation suggests VUR [23]. The condition may be unilateral or bilateral.
- Findings of reflux nephropathy include focal renal parenchymal scarring, usually most prominent at the upper pole with associated dilatation of the underlying calyx (see Fig. 3.40). The renal pelvis is spared. Chronic infection progressively scars the kidney and impairs renal growth.
- Serial renal length measurement is a sensitive method of monitoring renal growth in children with VUR [24].

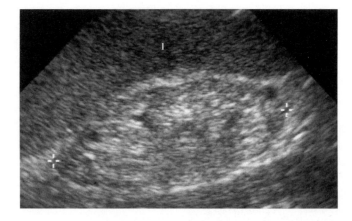

Figure 3.13 *Echogenic End-Stage Kidney.* The kidney (*between cursors, +*) is significantly more echogenic than the adjacent liver parenchyma (l). Differentiation of cortex from medulla, and even from the renal sinus, is lost. The kidney is small, measuring only 7 cm, indicating it is end stage and unlikely to respond to any form of therapy. The patient has chronic renal failure.

Diffuse Renal Parenchymal Disease

Renal Failure
In the clinical setting of impaired renal function, US is used to demonstrate the size and appearance of the kidneys and to detect the rare occurrence of bilateral obstruction presenting with renal failure. US diagnosis of a specific cause of renal failure is exceedingly rare [25].

- Diffuse increased echogenicity of the parenchyma of both kidneys is the US hallmark of diffuse renal parenchymal disease (Fig. 3.13). Corticomedullary differentiation is usually absent.
- End stage kidneys are small and echogenic (Fig. 3.13).
- US is commonly used to guide renal biopsy to provide a specific diagnosis and identify a hopefully treatable cause of renal failure. Kidneys smaller than 9 cm in length in adults are usually end-stage kidneys unresponsive to treatment [25,26]. Biopsy is seldom beneficial to these patients.
- An extracapsular rim of perirenal lucency ("kidney sweat") has been described in 14% of patients with renal failure [27]. The significance of this finding is unknown.

> Small echogenic kidneys are usually a sign of irreversible chronic renal failure.

Diabetic Nephropathy
Diabetes mellitus is the most common cause of chronic renal failure in the United States. Patients develop proteinuria, hypertension, and progressive renal failure over the course of their disease.

- Bilateral renal enlargement (>13 cm length) with normal parenchymal echogenicity is seen early in the course of disease [28].
- With time the kidneys shrink, become diffusely echogenic, and show high (>0.70) intrarenal artery RI.

Human Immunodeficiency Virus–Associated Nephropathy
Nephropathy associated with human immunodeficiency virus (HIV) infection is an important cause of AIDS morbidity. Patients present with rapid deterioration of renal function and proteinuria [29].

> Large echogenic kidneys in a patient with renal failure suggest HIV nephropathy.

- Enlarged kidneys with increased cortical echogenicity are characteristic findings (Fig. 3.14) [30].
- Additional findings include a globular appearance to the kidney, decreased renal sinus fat, and heterogeneous parenchyma with echogenic striations [29].

Echogenic Renal Pyramids
Increased echogenicity of the medullary pyramids is usually a non-specific finding of metabolic disease. Nephrocalcinosis is the most common cause, but numerous other diseases may cause this finding (Table 3.3) [31].

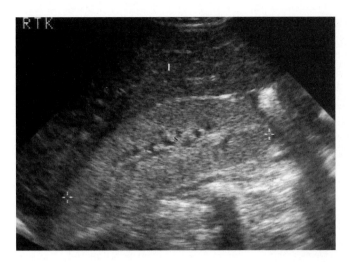

Figure 3.14 *HIV-Associated Nephropathy.* The renal parenchyma (*between cursors,* +) is distinctly more echogenic than the liver parenchyma (l). The renal sinus (s) lacks echogenic fat. Both kidneys measured large (15 cm). These findings are characteristic of HIV nephropathy.

- Echogenicity of the renal pyramids exceeds the echogenicity of the renal cortex (Fig. 3.15). The condition is bilateral. Acoustic shadowing is usually absent. Renal cortical echogenicity is normal.

RENAL TUMORS

Renal Cell Carcinoma

Renal cell carcinoma (RCC) accounts for 90% of solid renal tumors. When a solid renal mass is encountered, the US examination should be extended to examine the retroperitoneum for nodal metastases and should utilize Doppler to look for extension of tumor into the renal vein or IVC. The tumor is often clinically silent until it becomes large. Small "incidental" RCC may be discovered by routine renal US [32].

Table 3.3: *Causes of Increased Echogenicity of the Renal Pyramids*

Infants and Children	*Adults*
Medullary nephrocalcinosis	**Medullary nephrocalcinosis**
Furosemide therapy (for bronchopulmonary dysplasia)	Medullary sponge kidney
Vitamin D therapy (for rickets or hypophosphatemia)	Hyperparathyroidism
Renal tubular acidosis	Renal tubular acidosis
Idiopathic hypercalcemia	Hypercalcemia
Absorptive hypercalciuria	Hypercalciuria
Williams syndrome	**Vascular congestion**
Protein deposition	Sickle hemoglobinopathies
Newborn dehydration	**Urate deposition**
Vascular congestion	Gout
Sickle cell disease	Hyperuricemia
Infection	
Candida	
Cytomegalovirus	
Urate deposition	
Lesch-Nyhan syndrome	
Metabolic diseases	
Glycogen storage disease, type 1	
Fanconi syndrome	
Renal dysplasia	

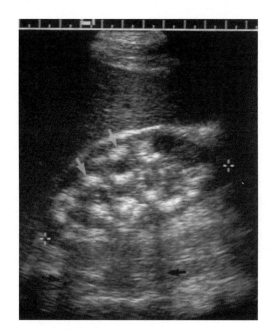

Figure 3.15 *Echogenic Renal Pyramids.* The renal pyramids (*white arrows*) are markedly echogenic (instead of echolucent). Acoustic shadows (*black arrows*) emanate from some of the pyramids in this case of medullary nephrocalcinosis. Cursors (+) mark upper and lower poles of the kidney.

Most solid renal tumors are renal cell carcinomas.

- Most RCC are solid tumors that may be hyperechoic, isoechoic, or hypoechoic compared to renal parenchyma (Fig. 3.16). Tumors commonly have a slightly more heterogeneous echotexture than parenchyma. They cause a focal bulge that distorts the margin of the kidney or impinges on the renal sinus.
- Necrosis, hemorrhage, and cystic degeneration cause intratumoral cystic spaces (Fig. 3.17).
- Calcification is common (up to 18%) and variable in appearance: punctate, coarse, central, peripheral, or curvilinear (Fig. 3.17).
- Cystic forms of RCC most often have thick walls and internal debris [33]. RCC arising within simple cysts are rare and appear as cysts with a mural nodule.
- Multicystic form of RCC has thick walls (>2 mm) and thick septations (Fig. 3.18).

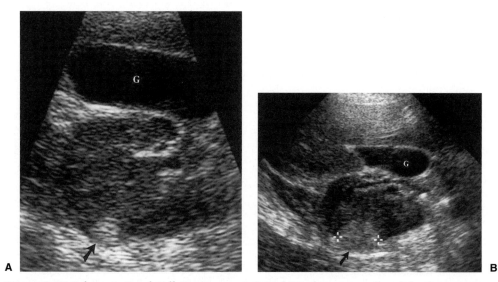

Figure 3.16 *Echogenic Renal Cell Carcinoma. A.* Initial US shows a small, solid echogenic mass (*arrow*) in the renal parenchyma. The lesion resembles angiomyolipoma; however, CT failed to demonstrate intratumoral fat. *B.* US scan 6 months later shows enlargement of the tumor (*arrow, between cursors,* +). Surgical excision confirmed renal cell carcinoma. The gallbladder (G) is seen anterior to the kidney in both images.

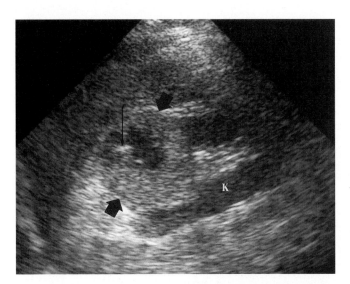

Figure 3.17 *Renal Cell Carcinoma with Hemorrhage and Calcification.* This tumor (*between fat arrows*) expands from the upper pole of the kidney (K) and has central low density representing necrosis and hemorrhage. Punctate calcification (*long arrow*) is also present within the tumor.

- Doppler shows prominent vascularity with high velocity flow in most tumors. Absence of hypervascularity does not exclude malignancy, because some RCC are hypovascular.
- Metastatic lymphadenopathy is visualized as hypoechoic solid nodules near the renal vessels and around and between the aorta and IVC.
- Tumor thrombus within the renal vein or IVC appears as solid tissue enlarging the vein (Fig. 3.19) [34]. Color flow US may show venous blood flow diverting around the tumor thrombus and, sometimes, arterial flow within the tumor thrombus. Venous flow within the vein is absent if the vein is completely occluded.

Angiomyolipoma

Angiomyolipoma (AML) is a common benign renal tumor that contains variable amounts of blood vessels (angio), smooth muscle (myo), and fat (lipoma) [35]. AML is multiple and bilateral in patients with tuberous sclerosis, but is more commonly an isolated lesion discovered incidentally by US. Most tumors are asymptomatic, but large tumors may bleed, especially during pregnancy, or cause flank pain or a palpable mass.

- Tumor appearance depends upon the proportion and distribution of the tumor elements (Fig. 3.20) [36].
- A well-defined, homogeneous hyperechoic lesion is the classic appearance of an AML that is predominantly fat (Fig. 3.21).
- Lesions with minimal fat are typically isoechoic to renal parenchyma [37].

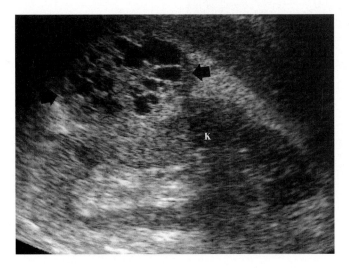

Figure 3.18 *Multicystic Renal Cell Carcinoma.* A multicystic mass (*arrows*) with prominent solid components extends exophytically from the kidney (K). Acoustic enhancement is seen deep to the mass.

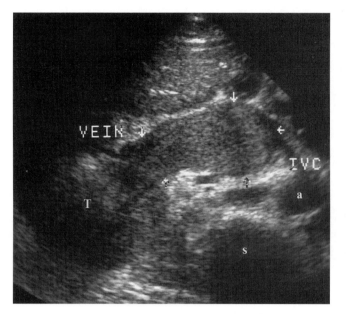

Figure 3.19 *Tumor Invasion of Renal Vein and IVC.* Transverse image shows tumor (T) extending from the right kidney and expanding into the renal vein (*arrows*) and inferior vena cava (IVC). a, aorta; s, spine.

- Tumors may be markedly heterogeneous with a mixture of fat, smooth muscle, and blood vessels (Fig. 3.22).
- Doppler demonstrates internal tumor vascularity in large tumors but often not in small ones. Spectral Doppler shows no specific findings.
- AML is difficult to differentiate from RCC when the renal tumors are small (<3 cm) and echogenic (Fig. 3.21) [38]. Signs that favor RCC over AML include the presence of intratumoral cystic spaces, a peripheral hypoechoic rim, or intratumoral calcification [39,40]. These findings are all rare in AML. Acoustic shadowing is sometimes seen with AML, but not with RCC [39].
- CT confirmation is recommended for lesions discovered on US that are believed to be AML [35,36].
- AML show significant growth when followed by US over time [41].

Calcifications are extremely rare in AML. Small echogenic lesions with calcifications are likely RCC.

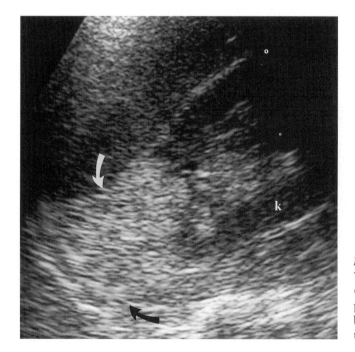

Figure 3.20 *Angiomyolipoma.* This predominantly fatty tumor (*arrows*) extends from the upper pole of the kidney (k) where it becomes indistinguishable from the perirenal fat.

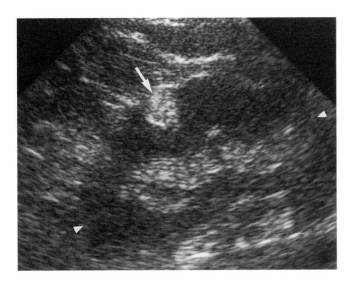

Figure 3.21 *Small Angiomyolipoma.* This tumor was shown by CT to consist almost entirely of fat. US shows a small echogenic mass (*arrow*). Note the similarity to the echogenic renal cell carcinoma shown in Figure 3.16. Arrowheads mark the upper and lower poles of the kidney.

Transitional Cell Carcinoma

Transitional cell carcinoma (TCC) arises from the transitional epithelium that lines the renal collecting system, ureter, and bladder [42]. TCC of the renal pelvis and ureter is much less common than TCC of the bladder. TCC may be papillary (85%) with a frondlike growth pattern or infiltrating with plaque-like lesions, wall thickening, and stricture.

- TCC appears as a central hypoechoic or isoechoic mass that replaces the echogenic renal sinus fat [42].
- Obstruction by the tumor results in focal calyceal or renal pelvis dilatation.
- Infiltrating tumors cause focal thickening of the wall of the collecting system.
- Whereas most tumors are hypovascular, larger and high-grade tumors may show visible vascularity on color Doppler [43].
- Small lesions are easily overlooked with US unless some degree of obstruction is present.
- TCC occasionally have coarse punctate calcifications [44].
- TCC of the ureter appears as intraluminal hypoechoic soft tissue with a variable degree of proximal hydronephrosis [45].

Soft tissue mass within the echogenic central renal sinus suggests TCC.

Renal Lymphoma

The kidney contains no lymphoid tissue, so nearly all cases of renal lymphoma occur by hematogenous dissemination or direct extension in patients with systemic lymphoma. The

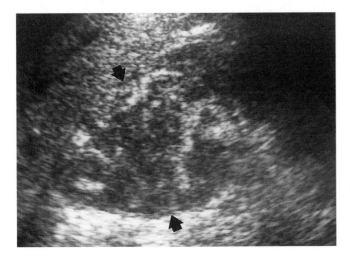

Figure 3.22 *Heterogeneous Angiomyolipoma.* US shows a markedly heterogeneous mass (*between arrows*) reflecting the mixture of tissue elements in this angiomyolipoma.

kidneys are one of the most common sites of extranodal lymphoma. Renal involvement is particularly common in immunocompromised patients [46]. Non-Hodgkin's lymphoma is most common. Most patients have no urinary symptoms.

- Renal lymphoma is typically hypoechoic, homogeneous, and bilateral (75%) [47]. Calcification is extremely rare. Cystic change is also very rare and is seen only in patients with tumor necrosis induced by chemotherapy [46].
- Multiple, small (1–3 cm), bilateral, solid, hypoechoic tumors are most common (60% of cases) [46]. Rarely, the multiple renal lymphomatous masses may be unilateral.
- Direct renal invasion (25–30%) into the renal sinus from contiguous retroperitoneal lymphoma is typically nodular, homogeneous, and hypoechoic. Bulky retroperitoneal adenopathy typically envelops the renal artery and vein, IVC, and aorta. The blood vessels remain patent despite encasement, a finding that is typical of lymphoma.
- Solitary homogeneous hypovascular solid tumor (10–20%) may be indistinguishable from RCC. Solitary lymphoma masses can reach 15 cm in size. A heterogeneous hypervascular lesion with cystic necrosis or calcification favors RCC.
- Disease may invade the perirenal space and surround the kidney with or without directly involving the kidney. This results in a hypoechoic tumor halo partially or completely surrounding the kidney. This pattern of involvement is virtually pathognomonic of lymphoma, but is uncommon.
- Diffuse infiltration of the renal interstitium globally enlarges the kidney with minimal or no alteration of shape or echotexture [47].
- Enlarged retroperitoneal lymph nodes are seen in only 50% of cases.

Renal lymphoma appears as multiple nodules, homogeneous solitary mass, diffuse enlargement, or bulky adenopathy invading the renal sinus.

Renal Leukemia

More than 50% of children and 65% of adults who die of leukemia have renal involvement at autopsy [47]. Acute lymphoblastic leukemia is the most common form to involve the kidney.

- Bilateral, global renal enlargement caused by diffuse, interstitial leukemic infiltration is most common [47]. Corticomedullary differentiation is usually lost.
- Discrete renal masses resemble lymphoma but are uncommon with leukemia.

Metastases to the Kidney

Metastases to the kidney are usually asymptomatic. They are nearly always discovered in patients with a diagnosed malignancy that is already metastatic elsewhere. Lung, breast, and gastrointestinal carcinomas are the most common primary neoplasms [47].

- Metastases to the kidney resemble lymphoma on US (Fig. 3.23) [47].
- Multiple bilateral circumscribed solid renal masses in a patient with associated metastases in other organs are most common [48].
- Solitary renal mass in a patient with a history of non-renal malignancy, but without known metastases, will usually be an RCC. However, metastases to the kidney from colon cancer will often be solitary, large, and cannot be differentiated from RCC without biopsy.

Oncocytoma

Oncocytoma is an uncommon benign solid renal tumor that arises from the proximal tubules. It occurs most often in men in their 60s.

- Well-defined solid mass is the usual appearance. A stellate central scar is characteristic but not pathognomonic. No imaging finding reliably distinguishes this tumor from RCC [49]. Diagnosis is made by surgical excision or biopsy (Fig. 3.24).

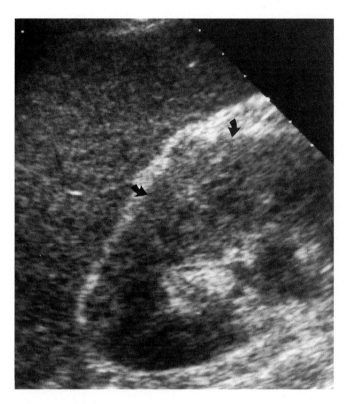

Figure 3.23 *Metastasis to the Kidney.* A subtle mass (*arrows*) causes a focal bulge in the contour of the kidney and disruption of the parenchymal echotexture. This solitary mass proved to be a metastasis from lung carcinoma.

Wilms Tumor

Wilms tumor (also called *nephroblastoma*) is a malignant tumor of childhood that arises from embryonal nephrogenic tissue [50]. Mean age of diagnosis is 3 years. It is the most common solid malignant abdominal tumor found in children. Metastases to lung and liver are most frequent [47].

- The tumor is expansile, replaces renal parenchyma, and forms a pseudocapsule of fibrous tissue and compressed renal parenchyma at its border [47]. Tumors are bilateral in 4–13% of cases [51].
- The tumor is primarily solid (Fig. 3.25) but is typically heterogeneous with hypoechoic and anechoic areas of necrosis and cyst formation [51].

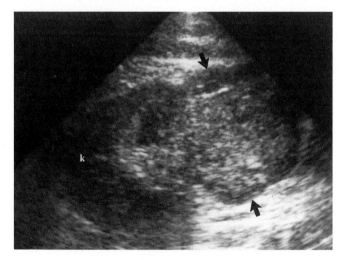

Figure 3.24 *Oncocytoma.* Extending from the kidney (k) is a solid mass (*arrows*) with central echogenicity. It is indistinguishable from a renal cell carcinoma. Surgical excision confirmed benign oncocytoma.

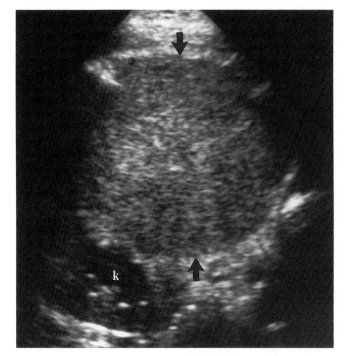

Figure 3.25 *Wilms Tumor.* A well-defined solid mass (*between arrows*) arises from the kidney (k) of a 4-year-old boy.

- Tumor invasion of the renal vein and IVC may occur with findings similar to RCC.
- Calcification is present in 9% of Wilms tumors.
- Echogenic fat is present in some tumors and is not a sign of a benign AML in children as it is in adults [51].

Nephroblastomatosis

Nephroblastomatosis refers to the presence of fetal renal tissue (mesoblastic blastema) in the renal parenchyma of infants and children. Most Wilms tumors and most multilocular cystic nephromas arise from these abnormal rests of benign tissue [52]. Nephroblastomatosis is a common feature of Beckwith-Wiedemann syndrome. The nephrogenic rests may be microscopic, multinodular, or diffusely infiltrating [51,52].

- Enlarged kidneys with loss of corticomedullary differentiation are characteristic of diffusely infiltrating nephroblastomatosis. Renal echogenicity may be normal or increased. Cysts of varying size may be present.
- Multiple homogeneous hypoechoic small masses are a less common appearance. Some nodules may appear hyperechoic.
- Children with documented nephroblastomatosis are followed at regular intervals for progressive enlargement or other signs of developing Wilms tumor [52].

Mesoblastic Nephroma

Mesoblastic nephroma is a benign tumor of infancy, most commonly diagnosed at 2 months of age and rare after 6 months of age [47]. The tumor is infiltrating with benign spindle cells growing between nephrons.

- The tumor is predominantly solid and unencapsulated with indistinct margins. Tumor replaces most of the renal parenchyma.
- Homogeneous solid hypoechoic mass is the most common appearance [47]. Concentric rings of alternating echogenicity have been reported as a characteristic appearance.
- Although necrosis is rare, some tumors develop cystic areas and appear quite heterogeneous.

Renal Pseudotumors
Islands of normal parenchyma may resemble renal tumors.

- Pseudotumors are identical in echogenicity to normal renal parenchyma. Contrast-enhanced CT is definitive in the diagnosis of normal parenchyma when the suspected tumor nodule enhances identical to renal parenchyma.
- Renal cortex may be bulbous at the hilum, so-called "hilar lips."
- Hypertrophied intrarenal cortex extending along the septal columns form prominent islands of tissue between the medullary pyramids [40]. These masses of normal tissue have been called *junctional parenchyma*, *hypertrophied columns of Bertin*, and *cloisons*.

Renal pseudotumors mimic solid renal masses but have echogenicity and vascularity identical to normal renal parenchyma.

RENAL CYSTIC DISEASE

Simple Renal Cyst
Simple renal cysts are by far the most common renal mass lesions. One-half of all adults older than age 50 have simple renal cysts. Although the diagnosis is straightforward and confident when cysts are large, small cysts (<3 cm) sometimes cause difficulty because of volume averaging and when US resolution is poor.

- Simple cysts are definitively diagnosed by US when they have the following features: well-defined thin wall; sharp demarcation with renal parenchyma; anechoic fluid; and accentuated through-transmission (Fig. 3.26).
- These features are more difficult to demonstrate when cysts are small (<3 cm). Excellent US technique is mandatory. When suspected cysts are not clearly demonstrated, consider improving technique by (1) increasing transducer frequency (to improve resolution of the lesion and to improve demonstration of accentuated through-transmission), (2) adjusting the focal (transmit) zone to the level of the lesion, (3) carefully centering the lesion in the US beam (to limit volume-averaging image degradation), (4) adjusting gain to limit false internal echoes, (5) scanning the lesions from different orientation to completely evaluate all aspects of the wall.
- Multiple and bilateral simple cysts occur commonly and must be differentiated from the various forms of polycystic kidney disease. Patients with multiple simple cysts are usu-

Simple renal cysts are anechoic with thin walls and accentuated through-transmission.

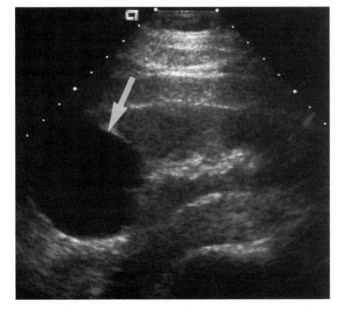

Figure 3.26 *Simple Renal Cyst. Anechoic internal fluid, sharp interface with the renal parenchyma, thin wall, and accentuated through-transmission are features of a simple renal cyst (arrow).*

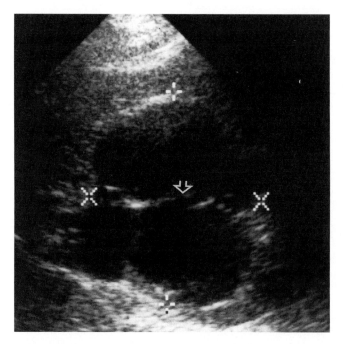

Figure 3.27 *Multilocular Cyst.* The multilocular cyst is indicated by the cursors (+, *x*). A moderately thick septum (*arrow*) separates two of the locules. Blood flow within this septum would favor this lesion being a tumor.

ally older (>50 years), and have a countable number, rather than innumerable, renal cysts. Cysts are generally not found in other organs as they are with autosomal dominant polycystic disease. Multiple simple cysts do not affect renal function.

■ Simple cysts are much less common in children than in adults. However, when a firm US diagnosis of simple cyst is made in a child, no further evaluation or intervention is necessary [53].

Atypical Renal Cysts

Atypical renal cystic lesions are most commonly simple cysts complicated by previous hemorrhage or infection.

Renal cystic lesions that fail to meet the strict criteria for simple renal cyst are considered to be atypical renal cysts [54]. Many of these more complex lesions can still be accurately classified as benign [55,56]. Many are simple cysts that were complicated by hemorrhage or infection (i.e., complicated cysts).

■ **Septations.** Thin, smooth, regular, non-vascular internal septations within a cyst are benign [54]. Thick, nodular septations containing blood vessels are potentially neoplastic (Fig. 3.27).
■ **Thick wall.** Wall thickening may occur when a simple cyst becomes infected or develops internal hemorrhage. Thick walls are also found in abscesses and in cystic renal tumors. These lesions are indeterminate and require further evaluation, usually surgical biopsy [54].
■ **Calcifications.** Thin calcification in the wall of a cyst is benign, provided that all other US criteria for simple cyst are met [54]. Calcification is otherwise a non-specific finding. Thick wall or associated soft tissue mass indicates possible neoplasm.
■ **Echogenic fluid.** Simple cysts have anechoic fluid. Complicated cysts commonly contain echogenic particulate matter resulting from hemorrhage or infection. The echogenic material may be diffusely dispersed within the cyst or show dependent layering (Fig. 3.28). These cysts can be considered benign if the wall is thin and the cyst remains well defined with no solid component.

Multilocular Cystic Nephroma

Multilocular cystic nephroma is an uncommon benign tumor that arises from the same nephrogenic rests that predispose to Wilms tumor [47]. The tumor occurs most commonly in boys younger than age 4 and in women aged 40–60 years [57].

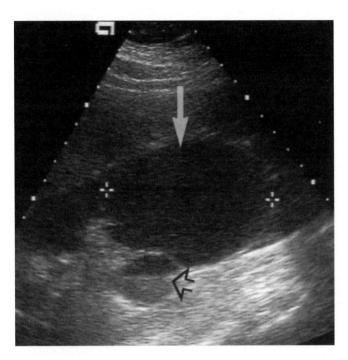

Figure 3.28 *Fluid Layering in Renal Cyst.* Several cysts arise off this kidney. The largest (*large arrow, between cursors, +*) contains fluid with echogenic particulate matter. A smaller cyst shows a fluid-fluid layer (*open arrow*). Both these cysts are simple cysts complicated by hemorrhage.

- The tumors are multicystic with thick walls and septa (Fig. 3.29) [47,58]. Small curvilinear calcifications are occasionally seen in the septa [57]. The tumors are well demarcated from the renal parenchyma.
- Most lesions are 8–10 cm in size but range up to 30 cm.

Autosomal Dominant Polycystic Kidney Disease

The primary anatomic defect of autosomal dominant polycystic kidney disease (ADPKD) is cystic dilatation of the nephrons as well as the collecting tubules. Islands of normal parenchyma are interspersed between cysts. Affected patients develop progressive renal failure and hypertension in middle age. The presence of cerebral aneurysms in 10% of patients results in subarachnoid hemorrhage as a common cause of death.

- The kidneys are progressively replaced and are markedly enlarged by diffuse parenchymal cysts of varying size (Fig. 3.30). The cysts do not communicate with each other or with the calyceal system or pelvis. The condition is always bilateral but may be asymmetric especially in younger patients with less advanced disease.

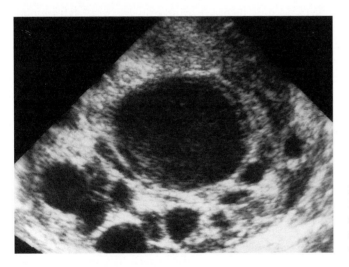

Figure 3.29 *Multilocular Cystic Nephroma.* This renal mass consists of cysts of varying size separated by thick septa and defined by thick walls.

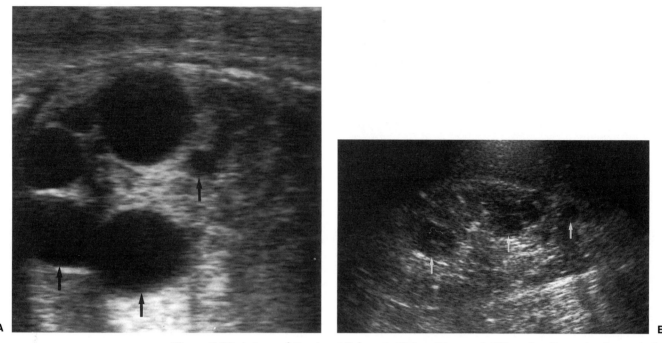

Figure 3.30 *Autosomal Dominant Polycystic Kidney Disease. A.* When the disease is advanced, the renal parenchyma is replaced by numerous non-communicating cysts of varying size (*arrows*). *B.* When the disease is early, the kidneys are of normal size and only a few cysts (*arrows*) are present.

- Hepatic and pancreatic cysts are common and their presence confirms ADPKD.
- Hemorrhage within the cysts is common, causing wall thickening and echogenic internal fluid in affected cysts. Hemorrhage commonly causes flank pain.
- Calcification commonly occurs in cyst walls as a result of hemorrhage. Renal stones are common in this disorder [59].
- In the fetus and young child, the presence of multiple renal cysts confirms the presence of the disease when a parent is known to be affected. The kidneys may be enlarged and echogenic. However, presentation is quite variable and a normal appearance of the kidneys does not exclude the disease.

Autosomal Recessive Polycystic Kidney Disease

Autosomal recessive polycystic kidney disease usually presents in the neonate and is detectable in the fetus. The condition covers a spectrum of abnormality from poor renal function at birth (infantile polycystic kidney disease) to progressive renal failure and hepatic fibrosis in childhood (juvenile polycystic kidney disease) [60]. The primary defect is diffuse tubular and saccular dilatation of the renal collecting tubules. Prognosis depends upon the number of abnormal nephrons present.

- The kidneys are markedly enlarged and strikingly echogenic (Fig. 3.31A) [60]. The marked echogenicity is caused by the numerous sonographic interfaces created by dilatation of the collecting tubules. The peripheral cortex has no collecting tubules and is compressed but otherwise uninvolved, resulting in a characteristic peripheral sonolucent rim [61]. Reniform shape is maintained. Corticomedullary differentiation is absent.
- High-resolution US may visualize tiny cysts and dilated tubules within the renal parenchyma.
- Older children have predominant hepatic fibrosis and less severe renal impairment. The kidneys are less enlarged and show a coarse, more heterogeneous pattern of increased echogenicity (Fig. 3.31B) [62]. Punctate renal parenchymal calcifications are common [63]. The liver shows features of portal hypertension as the hepatic fibrosis progresses.

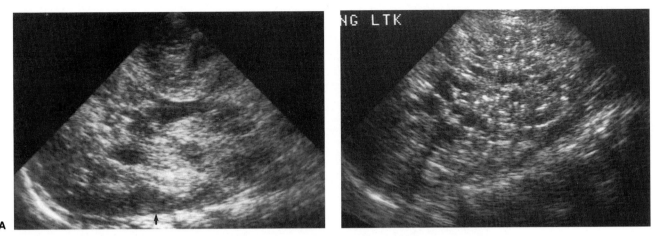

Figure 3.31 *Autosomal Recessive Polycystic Kidney Disease (ARPKD)*. A. Longitudinal image of a kidney in a newborn infant reveals massive enlargement with marked increase in central echogenicity. The peripheral sonolucent rim (*arrow*) of compressed cortex is characteristic. B. The kidney of a 5-year-old boy with ARPKD is mildly enlarged and heterogeneous with visible small cysts. The child had moderately severe liver disease.

Acquired Renal Cystic Disease Associated with Hemodialysis

Patients with end-stage renal disease on chronic hemodialysis are prone to develop multiple renal cysts and RCC in their native kidneys [64]. The disease is progressive and increases in prevalence with length of time on hemodialysis [65]. It occurs in 10–20% of patients on hemodialysis for 1–3 years and in up to 90% of patients treated with hemodialysis for longer than 10 years. RCC develops in approximately 5% of patients [65]. After renal transplantation the cysts reduce in size and number but the risk of malignancy persists [66]. Affected patients lack a history of polycystic kidney disease.

- The kidneys are initially small and echogenic reflecting end-stage renal disease.
- As the time on hemodialysis treatment lengthens, cysts form primarily in the cortex and vary in size up to 2–3 cm [65]. As cyst formation progresses, the kidneys enlarge.
- The cysts are fragile and may develop internal or perirenal hemorrhage [64].
- Calcifications within cyst walls and in the renal parenchyma are common [66].
- The presence or development of a solid tumor is highly suggestive of RCC.

Von Hippel-Lindau Disease

Von Hippel-Lindau disease (VHL) is an uncommon, autosomal-dominant, neurocutaneous disorder characterized by cerebellar hemangioblastomas, retinal angiomas, multiple visceral cysts, RCC, and pheochromocytoma [67]. Because RCC develops in 24–45% of patients with VHL, periodic surveillance of the kidneys is often recommended [68]. RCC may develop as early as age 15. Renal cysts are found in 59–85% of patients. Central nervous system and eye manifestations are usually evident at the time of discovery of renal disease.

- Renal cysts in VHL show a continuum of appearance from simple cyst to thick-walled cyst to cystic tumor with papillary projections and small solid nodules [67]. Simple cysts grow slowly (5 mm/year) and may involute [68]. Extensive renal cystic disease mimics ADPKD and may progress to renal failure. End-stage kidneys should be removed because of risk of RCC.
- Most RCC arise *de novo* as a solid renal tumor that grows rapidly (up to 2.2 cm/year) [68]. Some RCC have a cystic appearance. Any distinct solid element within a cystic lesion in a patient with VHL is likely to be RCC [67].
- Adrenal pheochromocytoma is found in 7–18% of patients.

Cysts in the kidneys and in the pancreas occur in both ADPKD and VHL.

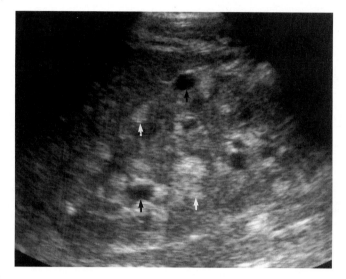

Figure 3.32 *Tuberous Sclerosis.* The renal parenchyma contains numerous small cysts (*black arrows*) and numerous echogenic nodules (*white arrows*) representing fat in multiple angiomyolipomas.

- Cysts in the pancreas are a feature of VHL found in high prevalence (93%) in some families and absent in others [67]. Pancreatic cysts vary in size from 1–2 mm up to 10 cm and may completely replace the pancreas.

Tuberous Sclerosis

Tuberous sclerosis is another uncommon, autosomal-dominant, neurocutaneous disorder with renal manifestations. Clinical features include adenoma sebaceum, mental handicap, epilepsy, retinal hamartomas, cortical tubers, and subependymal nodules. Renal lesions consist of multiple bilateral renal cysts and AMLs [69]. The renal lesions have no malignant potential.

- Cysts are bilateral and vary in size and number (Fig. 3.32) [69].
- AMLs are characteristically bilateral and infiltrative [69]. They vary in size from 1–2 mm up to several cm. The fatty component of the tumors causes foci of high echogenicity and a markedly heterogeneous echotexture to both kidneys (Fig. 3.32). Tumors may enlarge and bleed during pregnancy.

Multicystic Dysplastic Kidney

Classic multicystic dysplastic kidney (MCDK) results from complete ureteral obstruction in early fetal life [60]. Complete obstruction in classic MCDK results from atresia of the upper third of the ureter [70]. The pelvis and calyces never form. The affected kidney does not function and renal parenchyma is completely replaced by cysts. When *in utero* obstruction is incomplete, hydronephrosis develops, cystic dysplastic change is less severe, and residual renal function is present. This condition is not heritable. When bilateral, it is fatal at birth.

- Classic MCDK appears as multiple non-communicating cysts of varying size completely replacing all parenchyma (Fig. 3.33A) [60]. No renal pelvis or calyces are present [70]. The kidney is markedly enlarged at birth but will progressively shrink to a small nubbin that commonly calcifies [71,72]. No renal function is present on radionuclide imaging.
- In the hydronephrotic form of MCDK, dilated renal pelvis and calyces are identifiable (Fig. 3.33B). Multiple cysts of varying size replace most, but not all, of the renal parenchyma. Islands of heterogeneous dysplastic solid renal tissue are also seen. Radionuclide studies show limited renal function.
- Atypical forms of MCDK include a single or few large cysts replacing the kidney (Fig. 3.33C).

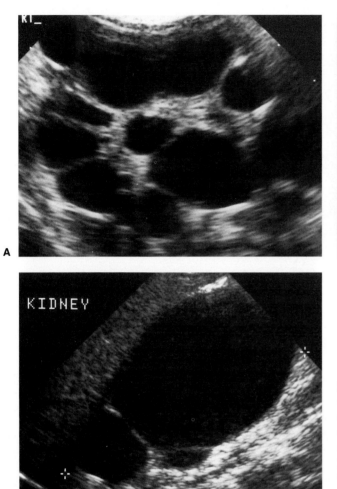

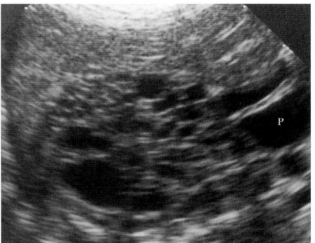

Figure 3.33 *Multicystic Dysplastic Kidney. A.* The classic multicystic dysplastic kidney consists of cysts of varying size replacing all of the renal parenchyma. This kidney showed no function on radionuclide scan. *B.* Transverse image shows the hydronephrotic form consisting of advanced hydronephrosis with a recognizable renal pelvis (P) and extensive cystic dysplasia of the parenchyma. Radionuclide imaging showed very limited renal function. *C.* The variant form of multicystic dysplastic kidney consists of a few large cysts replacing all of the renal parenchyma (*between cursors, +*).

- The opposite kidney commonly (30–41%) shows a developmental anomaly, more often congenital ureteropelvic (UPJ) obstruction.

Renal Dysplasia

Renal dysplasia describes the presence of primitive mesenchymal tissue, cartilage, and cysts of varying size in the parenchyma of a kidney obstructed early in fetal life [73]. Dysplastic tissue is functionless tissue. Overall renal function is determined by the number of normal nephrons present relative to the amount of dysplastic tissue present. The timing and severity of renal obstruction in fetal life determine the severity of renal dysplasia. Dyplasia may develop as a result of any cause of fetal renal obstruction including such entities as congenital ureteropelvic or uterovesical junction (UVJ) obstruction, posterior urethral valves, or ectopic ureterocele.

- Cysts are a primary feature of renal dysplasia seen in the newborn. Cysts vary in number from one to many and in size from 1 mm up to 3 cm or larger [73]. The more proximal and severe the obstruction, the greater the number and size of the cysts.
- Solid renal dysplasia decreases the volume of renal parenchyma and increases its echogenicity. Globally dysplastic, functionless kidneys are tiny and echogenic. Segmental areas of dysplasia show limited echogenic solid tissue and cysts. Renal dysplasia may produce a solid renal mass (Fig. 3.34).
- MCDK is on the most severe end of the spectrum of renal dysplasia.

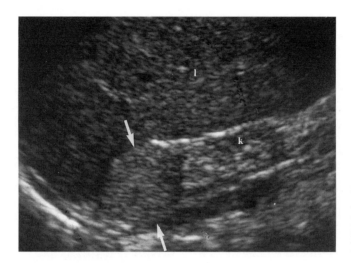

Figure 3.34 *Solid Renal Dysplasia.* A focus of renal dysplasia produced a solid mass (*arrows*) in the kidney (k) of a child. l, liver.

RENAL INFECTION

Acute Pyelonephritis

In adults, the diagnosis of acute renal infection is usually based on clinical and laboratory findings and imaging is utilized primarily to detect complications. In children, the clinical diagnosis is commonly equivocal and imaging is used to confirm the diagnosis. Acute pyelonephritis is most common in young women, aged 15–35 years. Patients who respond to therapy require no imaging.

- Renal US is commonly normal in uncomplicated acute pyelonephritis.
- Renal involvement by infection may be focal, multifocal, or diffuse. The kidney becomes diffusely or focally swollen. Corticomedullary differentiation is lost. The margin of the kidney becomes indistinct.
- Affected areas are usually hypoechoic because of edema fluid (Fig. 3.35A). If interstitial hemorrhage occurs, affected areas become hyperechoic (Fig. 3.35B).
- Inflammation and edema constrict renal arterioles in affected areas and result in segments of reduced perfusion. Color or power Doppler flow imaging shows single or multiple foci of decreased or absent blood flow, often in a wedge-shaped pattern [74]. These areas of decreased perfusion correspond to areas of decreased enhancement seen on CT. Power Doppler is more sensitive than color Doppler in showing subtle areas of abnormality.

> Acute pyelonephritis causes wedge-shaped areas of subtle decreased or increased echogenicity with associated decreased blood flow.

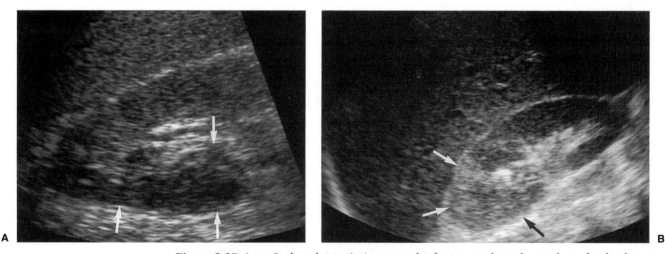

Figure 3.35 *Acute Pyelonephritis. A.* Acute renal infection produces hypoechoic, focal, edematous swelling of the renal parenchyma (*arrows*). *B.* Acute renal infection with interstitial hemorrhage produces hyperechoic focal swelling of the renal parenchyma (*arrows*).

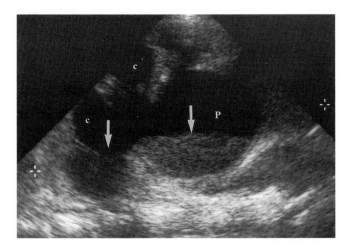

Figure 3.36 *Pyonephrosis.* Pus produces fluid layers (*arrows*) within the dilated collecting system of a 5-year-old boy with infection complicating congenital, ureteropelvic junction obstruction. c, dilated calyces; P, dilated renal pelvis. Cursors (+) measure size of the kidney.

Pyonephrosis

Pyonephrosis describes the presence of purulent material within an obstructed collecting system [75]. Most patients are acutely symptomatic, although an indolent presentation is prevalent (15%). Relief of obstruction and treatment of infection are critical to prevention of septic shock and rapidly progressive renal parenchymal destruction.

Infection of an obstructed kidney necessitates emergency drainage.

- The collecting system is dilated and contains layering echogenic debris, and, sometimes, calculi or gas (Fig. 3.36).
- The wall of the collecting system is often thickened.
- The renal parenchyma may show any of the signs of acute pyelonephritis or abscess.
- An echogenic, nonshadowing, mobile mass within the collecting system suggests a fungus ball (a mycetoma) (Fig. 3.37), caused by chronic fungal infection [76].

Renal and Perirenal Abscess

Abscess results from areas of pyelonephritis that progress to parenchymal necrosis, or from infection of cysts. Most renal abscesses extend into the perirenal space. Rupture of pyonephrosis may also result in perirenal abscess.

- Poorly marginated, thick-walled, hypoechoic mass with internal debris and acoustic enhancement is characteristic (Fig. 3.38A) [75]. The mass may appear echogenic and solid depending on the nature of its contents. Abscesses may be solitary, multiple, or small (microabscesses) with a tendency to coalesce into a single cavity.
- Stones or gas may be present within or near the abscess (Fig. 3.38B).

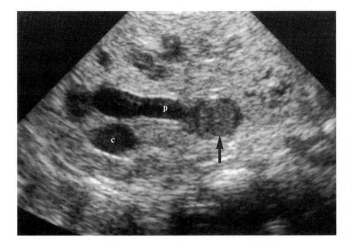

Figure 3.37 *Fungus Ball.* Transverse image of the kidney of a 2-month-old premature infant with systemic *Candida albicans* infection shows dilated pelvis (p) and calyces (c) that contain echogenic urine and a discrete mobile fungus ball (*arrow*). The fungus ball caused partial urinary obstruction. Fungus balls consist of fungal hyphae mixed with inflammatory cells and debris.

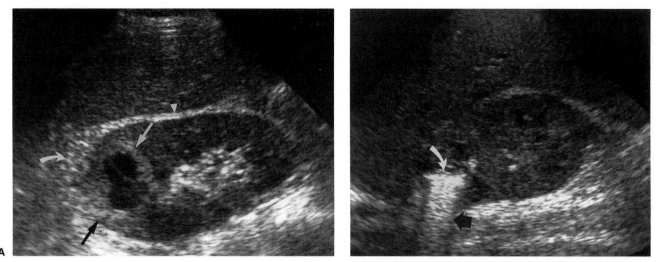

Figure 3.38 *Renal Abscess. A.* An intrarenal abscess produces a thick-walled mass (*straight arrows*) containing echogenic fluid within the kidney. The perirenal space contains mostly normal echogenic fat (*arrowhead*) and an area of inflammatory infiltration (*curved arrow*) but no distinct fluid collection. *B.* This renal abscess contains a large pocket of air (*white arrow*) that produces characteristic intense reverberation artifact (*black arrow*).

- Extrarenal extension is suggested by a hypoechoic perirenal mass (Fig. 3.39).
- US is commonly used to guide aspiration for culture and catheter drainage.

Emphysematous Pyelonephritis

Emphysematous pyelonephritis is a rare and serious complication of urinary tract infection with extensive necrosis and gas formation in the renal parenchyma. Most patients (90%) have diabetes mellitus and 20% have associated urinary tract obstruction [77,78]. Patients are acutely ill with fever and flank pain. *Escherichia coli* is the most common causative organism. Gas formation results from fermentation of glucose in the urine by the infecting bacteria.

- High-amplitude echoes with reverberation or comet tail echoes characteristic of air (Fig. 3.39) emanate from the renal parenchyma or perirenal space [78]. Extensive emphysema may completely obscure the affected kidney.
- Plain film radiographs or CT confirm the presence of air in the renal parenchyma. Gas confined to the collecting system or within a discrete abscess is a less ominous finding than diffuse gas in the renal parenchyma [79].

Chronic Pyelonephritis/Reflux Nephropathy

Chronic pyelonephritis may be the end stage of reflux nephropathy or occur as the result of recurring infection associated with calculi and chronic obstruction [76]. Patients at risk include those with neurogenic bladders, ileal conduits, and recurrent renal stone disease.

Parenchymal scars are concave (U-shaped) depressions of the midportion of the renal lobes overlying the calyx. Fetal lobulation produces V-shaped depressions between the lobes.

- Focal parenchymal scars with an underlying blunted calyx are the hallmark finding (Fig. 3.40). The polar regions are most often affected.
- The affected kidney is often reduced in size and is lobulated in contour with focal parenchymal thinning, usually most pronounced at the poles.
- Compensatory hypertrophy in uninfected areas may result in bulbous islands of normal tissue that resemble tumors.

Xanthogranulomatous Pyelonephritis

Xanthogranulomatous pyelonephritis is a rare form of chronic renal infection with progressive destruction of renal tissue and replacement by a cellular infiltrate of lipid-laden mac-

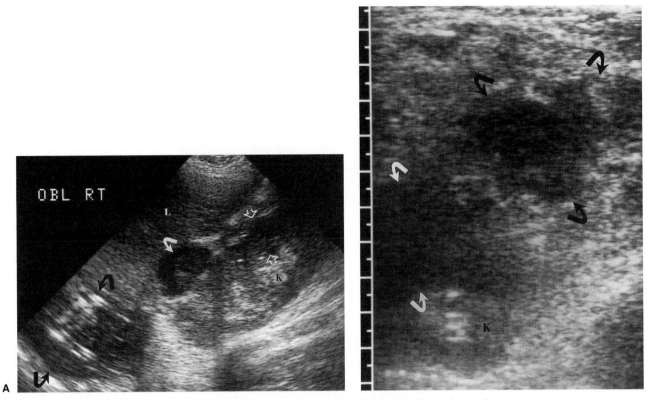

Figure 3.39 *Perirenal Abscess. A.* The kidney (K) shows inflammatory changes that extend into the perirenal space (*open arrows*). A discrete perirenal abscess (*white arrow*) spread to the liver by tracking along the retroperitoneum to the bare area, forming a hepatic abscess (*black arrows*). L, liver. *B.* In another patient a perirenal abscess (*white arrows*) extended into the muscles and soft tissues of the back (*black arrows*). K, left kidney.

rophages [76]. Most patients are middle-aged women who present with recurrent flank pain and fever.

- The process is unilateral and may be diffuse, focal, or segmental (Fig. 3.41).
- The kidney enlarges but maintains its reniform shape.
- An obstructing calculus is commonly present (70%) [47].
- Multiple hypoechoic areas represent purulent cavities in the affected areas of the kidney.

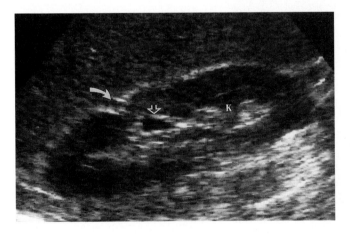

Figure 3.40 *Chronic Pyelonephritis.* Longitudinal image of the kidney (K) demonstrates a focal parenchymal scar (*curved arrow*) with an underlying dilated calyx (*open arrow*).

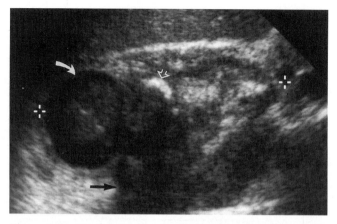

Figure 3.41 *Xanthogranulomatous Pyelonephritis (XGP).* Longitudinal image of the kidney (*between cursors, +*) in a patient with chronic urinary tract infection shows an obstructing calculus (*open arrow*) with acoustic shadow (*black arrow*) and a low density complex hypoechoic mass (*curved white arrow*). The kidney had minimal function on a radionuclide scan and was surgically removed, resolving the chronic infection. Pathology confirmed XGP.

Renal Tuberculosis

Renal tuberculosis is a delayed complication of pulmonary tuberculosis, occurring as long as 10–15 years after the initial infection [76]. Patients present with hematuria or sterile pyuria. The pathologic effects of tuberculous infection include granuloma formation, parenchymal destruction, fibrosis, stricture, and calcification.

- Hypoechoic parenchymal masses are granulomas or chronic abscess cavities.
- Parenchymal scarring and calcification are typical findings.
- Calyceal clubbing and hydronephrosis result from papillary necrosis and obstruction caused by strictures in the collecting system.
- The kidney can become a functionless hydronephrotic sac (Fig. 3.42) or a shrunken calcified mass.

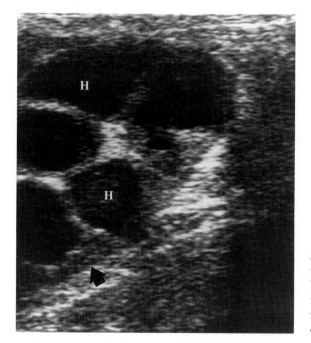

Figure 3.42 *Renal Tuberculosis.* Chronic renal tuberculosis with ureteral stricture has resulted in an end-stage, minimally functioning kidney with marked hydronephrosis (H) and thinned renal parenchyma (*arrow*).

Renal Hydatid Disease

The kidneys are affected in only 3% of patients with hydatid disease [80]. Renal lesions are usually asymptomatic, although they may cause hematuria or pain. The disease may be suspected in patients living in or traveling to endemic cattle and sheep raising areas of northern and eastern Africa, Asia, New Zealand, Australia, South America, and the Mediterranean coast. Complications include secondary infection and rupture of the cyst into the perinephric space or collecting system. Diagnosis is confirmed by immunoelectrophoresis.

- Multilocular cysts with curvilinear internal septa and floating internal echoes are characteristic [80]. The internal echoes are produced by "hydatid sand," which consists of parasite parts and debris. Septa are produced by the walls of daughter cysts. Most cysts are located at the upper or lower poles.
- Cyst walls and septa become thickened and commonly calcify. Hydatid sand may completely fill the cyst and mimic a solid lesion.

VASCULAR ABNORMALITIES

Renal Vein Thrombosis

Thrombosis of the renal vein may be primary, caused by intrinsic renal disease (glomerulonephritis, pyelonephritis, lupus nephritis) or, more commonly, is secondary to other diseases (RCC invasion of the renal vein, pancreatitis, systemic hypercoagulable states, acute dehydration, extension of IVC thrombosis) [81]. Clinical findings include hematuria, proteinuria, and flank pain. The condition may be clinically silent. US findings depend upon whether the thrombosis is acute or gradual, complete or partial [81,82].

- Echogenic clot is visualized in an enlarged renal vein (Fig. 3.19). In acute stage the clot may be isoechoic with flowing blood on gray scale US.
- Color flow shows absent venous flow with complete occlusion, or flow around the clot with partial occlusion.
- Acute complete thrombosis causes marked renal edema seen as renal enlargement with decreased parenchymal echogenicity.
- With partial occlusion, renal swelling is less prominent.
- Venous collateral formation and enlargement begin at 24 hours and peak at 2 weeks following thrombosis.
- Left renal vein collaterals are more prominent and include enlarged ureteral, gonadal, adrenal, and inferior phrenic veins.
- Right renal vein collaterals are limited to the ureteral vein.
- Lumbar, azygos, perivesical, and portal vein collaterals may become enlarged via ureteral vein connections.
- Intrarenal artery Doppler resistance index is commonly, but not always, elevated (>0.70). Absent or reversed diastolic flow may be seen with renal vein thrombosis (40% of cases) [82].

Renal Artery Stenosis

When a complete examination is possible, Doppler US is highly accurate in the diagnosis of renal artery stenosis. Unfortunately, complete diagnostic evaluation with US is difficult because of problems with patient body habitus, breath holding, and overlying bowel gas. Technically satisfactory examinations are reportedly performed in 0–75% of cases [2]. In any case, the examination is time-consuming and highly operator dependent. Breath-hold, gadolinium-enhanced, magnetic resonance angiography is superior to US in detection of significant stenosis and in the demonstration of accessory renal arteries [83]. A variety of criteria have been utilized for US diagnosis of significant stenosis.

- Thickening and calcification of the wall of the renal artery indicate the presence of atherosclerotic plaque, but not necessarily significant stenosis [2].

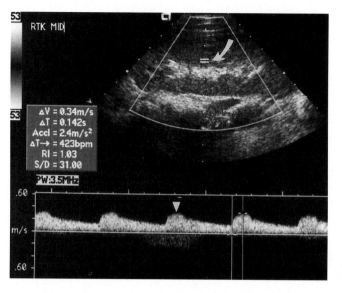

Figure 3.43 *Renal Artery Stenosis.* Doppler spectrum obtained from an intrarenal artery shows a tardus-parvus waveform. The peak systolic velocity (*arrowhead*) is late and reduced in velocity. The curved arrow shows the position of the Doppler sample volume.

- The beaded appearance characteristic of fibromuscular dysplasia may be visualized on gray-scale US of the main renal artery [2].
- Early systolic acceleration <3 m/sec^2 indicates significant stenosis.
- Renal:aortic ratio >3.5 is 75% sensitive for 75% stenosis. The renal:aortic ratio is calculated by dividing the highest renal artery velocity by the highest aortic velocity obtained at the level of the renal arteries.
- Peak systolic velocity >200 cm/sec in the renal artery indicates significant stenosis.
- Turbulent flow with spectral broadening and flow reversal is present downstream from the stenosis.
- Tardus-parvus spectral waveform is present in the distal renal artery with high-grade (>80%) proximal stenosis (Fig. 3.43). The rise to peak systolic velocity is slow (tardus) and the peak systolic velocity is decreased (parvus).

Renal Artery Occlusion

Occlusion of the renal artery occurs with embolus, thrombosis, trauma, or surgical error. Occlusion of the main renal artery results in global infarction whereas occlusion of an accessory or branch renal artery results in focal or segmental infarction.

- With acute global infarction, the appearance of the kidney remains normal on gray-scale US.
- Color Doppler shows the occluded stump of the renal artery with no blood flow (~60%) [2].
- Intrarenal arteries may show no detectable Doppler signals (~80%) or a severe tardus-parvus spectrum (~20%) [2].
- Focal or segmental arterial occlusion results in a wedge-shaped area of decreased or increased echogenicity indistinguishable from acute pyelonephritis.
- Power Doppler imaging is the most sensitive for demonstration of the corresponding area of hypoperfusion [84].

Arteriovenous Fistula

Most often, intrarenal arteriovenous fistulas (AVF) occur as a complication of renal biopsy or other penetrating trauma.

- Color flow US shows a bright focus of high-velocity blood flow. Tissue vibration artifact may be prominent [2].
- The draining vein is enlarged, particularly if the AVF is long-standing.
- High-velocity, highly turbulent flow is present at the site of the AVF.
- The supplying artery shows a very low resistance spectral pattern (RI <0.40).
- The draining vein spectrum shows arterial pulsations.

BLADDER

THICKENING OF THE BLADDER WALL

The bladder wall is thickened when it exceeds 4 mm in diameter with the bladder distended. Thickening is commonly the result of hypertrophy of the detrusor muscle that causes marked irregularity (trabeculation) of the luminal surface of the bladder wall (Fig. 3.44) (Box 3.1).

- **Neurogenic bladder** is a cause of bladder wall thickening, trabeculation, incomplete bladder emptying, ureteral dilatation, and stone formation. A "Christmas tree" appearance of the bladder with several areas of focal constriction of the bladder lumen is characteristic of long-standing neurogenic bladder.
- **Bladder outlet obstruction** caused by prostatic enlargement is a common cause of bladder wall thickening. The enlarged prostate is evident. Other causes of outlet obstruction include posterior urethral valves, urethral stricture, and ectopic ureterocele.
- **Cystitis** is caused by infection, radiation, and chemotherapy. The bladder may appear normal, or show focal or diffuse wall thickening. Floating debris is commonly present in the bladder lumen.
- **Bladder augmentation procedures** are performed to prevent progressive renal damage in patients with small capacity bladders and high intravesical pressures. A bowel loop is opened and transposed to the bladder dome to increase bladder capacity. The bowel wall is commonly irregular in thickness and shape and may show peristalsis. Secreted mucus mixes with urine to produce echogenic particles and debris in the bladder lumen.

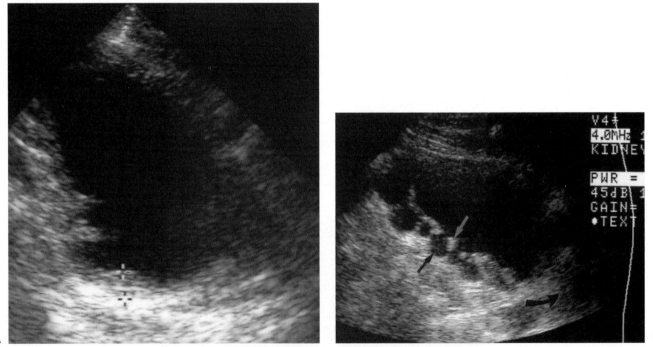

Figure 3.44 *Thickened Bladder Wall.* Two patients with neurogenic bladders have thickened bladder walls. *A.* The bladder wall is thickened to 11 mm (*between cursors,* +). Thickening of the bands of the detrusor muscle causes the irregularity of the mucosa surface of the bladder. *B.* Mucosal herniation through the hypertrophied muscle bands (*white arrow*) causes the formation of numerous saccules (*black arrow*) in the thickened bladder wall. The curved arrow indicates an enlarged prostate.

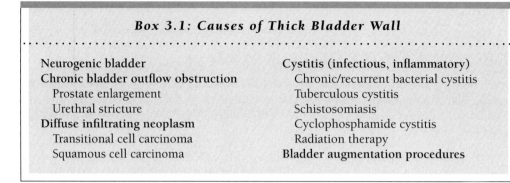

Box 3.1: Causes of Thick Bladder Wall

Neurogenic bladder
Chronic bladder outflow obstruction
   Prostate enlargement
   Urethral stricture
Diffuse infiltrating neoplasm
   Transitional cell carcinoma
   Squamous cell carcinoma

Cystitis (infectious, inflammatory)
   Chronic/recurrent bacterial cystitis
   Tuberculous cystitis
   Schistosomiasis
   Cyclophosphamide cystitis
   Radiation therapy
Bladder augmentation procedures

EMPHYSEMATOUS CYSTITIS

In patients with diabetes, chronic bladder outlet obstruction, or chronic infection, bacterial infection may produce air in the bladder wall or lumen. *E. coli* and *Enterobacter aerogenes* are the most common causative organisms.

- The bladder wall is diffusely thickened and markedly echogenic [79]. Reverberation and comet tail artifacts are produced by focal collections of air.
- CT and plain film radiography confirm the presence of air in the bladder wall and bladder lumen.

BLADDER DIVERTICULI

Bladder diverticuli are congenital or acquired herniations of bladder mucosa through the muscle of the bladder wall [85].

- Fluid-filled perivesical masses communicate with the bladder lumen through a small orifice (Fig. 3.45).
- If the orifice is not clearly seen, compression of the bladder during color Doppler examination shows a jet of urine flow into the diverticulum.
- Stasis of urine within the diverticulum may result in echogenic urine and stones within the diverticulum. TCC may arise within a bladder diverticulum.

INTRALUMINAL OBJECTS

A variety of iatrogenic and pathologic structures may be seen within the bladder lumen.

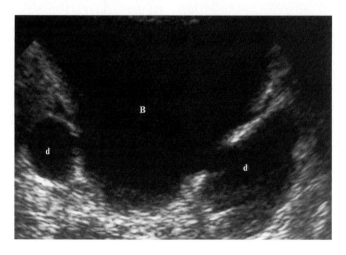

Figure 3.45 *Bladder Diverticuli.* Transverse image of the bladder (B) demonstrates bilateral diverticuli (d) that communicate with the parent bladder via small openings. When the bladder empties, the neck of the diverticulum may close, resulting in the diverticulum remaining filled with urine.

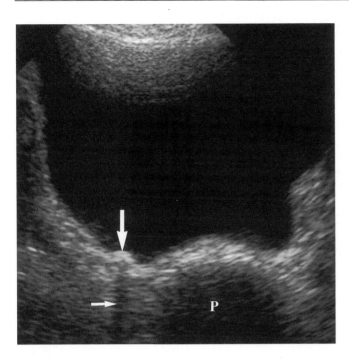

Figure 3.46 *Bladder Calculus.* Transverse image of the bladder shows an echogenic focus (*large arrow*) with acoustic shadowing (*small arrow*) lying on the dependent bladder wall. The stone was observed to move when the patient rolled into the decubitus position. Enlargement of the prostate (P) resulted in urinary stasis within the bladder, predisposing to stone formation.

- **Bladder calculi** appear as mobile hyperechoic foci with acoustic shadowing (Fig. 3.46).
- **Blood clots** appear as moderately echogenic nodules that commonly adhere to the bladder wall (Fig. 3.47). Absence of blood flow on color flow US distinguishes clots from tumors. Fluid-fluid levels from layering blood and urine are commonly present. Most patients have gross hematuria.
- **Foley catheter balloons** will be seen even when the bladder is empty. Air within the Foley balloon produces a bright interface with shadowing.
- **Ureteral stents** are identified as coiled hyperechoic tubes. The walls of the stent produce parallel curving echogenic lines.
- **Foreign bodies** are of any shape and may be mobile or adherent to the bladder wall.

Foley catheters are recognized by their characteristic nipple-on-a-ball appearance.

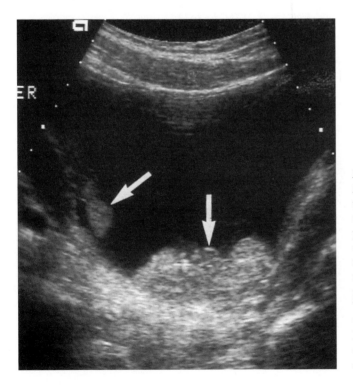

Figure 3.47 *Blood Clots in the Bladder.* Blood clots appear as moderately echogenic masses (*arrows*) within the bladder in a patient with gross hematuria caused by renal trauma. Documenting free movement of these masses with changes in patient position confirms blood clots. When blood clots are adherent to the bladder wall, showing a lack of blood flow by use of color Doppler aids in differentiation from tumors.

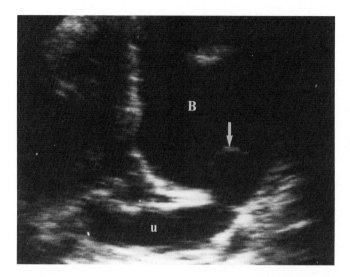

Figure 3.48 *Simple Ureterocele.* Longitudinal image of a distended bladder (B) shows the cystic protrusion (*arrow*) of a dilated distal ureter (u) into the bladder lumen. The wall of the ureterocele includes the wall of the ureter and the mucosa of the bladder. The ureterocele changes in size and appearance with ureteral peristalsis.

URETEROCELE

Ureteroceles are balloon-like dilatations of the terminal ureter caused by obstruction of the ureteral orifice. Urinary stasis increases the risk of infection and stone formation [86].

- **Simple ureteroceles** occur at the normal location of the ureteral orifice and are seen as thin-walled cystic masses (Fig. 3.48). Ureteral peristalsis causes the ureteroceles to periodically distend and collapse. The degree of obstruction is usually mild with dilatation confined to the terminal ureter. More severe obstruction causes dilatation of the proximal ureter and occasionally pelvicalyectasis.
- **Ectopic ureteroceles** occur with complete duplication of the collecting system at the ectopic location of the upper pole ureter insertion. Large ectopic ureteroceles may obstruct the contralateral ureter or the urethral orifice. Ectopic ureteroceles are more varied in appearance (Fig. 3.49). Some contain anechoic urine whereas others are intensely echogenic due to urine precipitates and complications of obstruction.

BLADDER TRANSITIONAL CELL CARCINOMA

Bladder TCC is the most common neoplasm of the urinary tract [42]. Most (90%) bladder tumors are TCC. Papillary bladder TCC are often multiple (30%) and usually (80%) superficial and low stage. Invasive TCC is solitary and high grade. Synchronous tumors are present in the upper tracts in 2–3% of patients with bladder TCC.

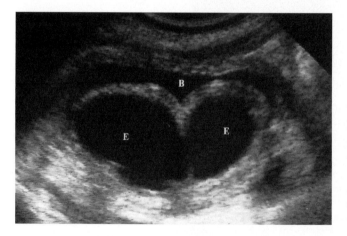

Figure 3.49 *Ectopic Ureteroceles.* Transverse image of the bladder (B) of an infant reveals bilateral ectopic ureteroceles (E). Both kidneys showed complete duplication of the collecting system with hydronephrotic upper pole moieties that terminated in these ectopic ureteroceles.

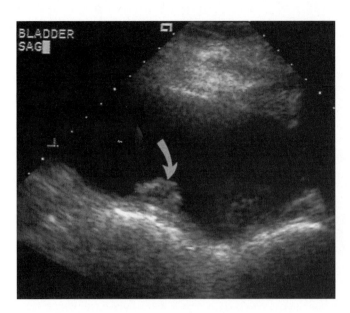

Figure 3.50 *Polypoid Transitional Cell Carcinoma.* Longitudinal image of the bladder shows a broad-based polypoid projection (*arrow*) from the otherwise smooth bladder mucosa. Color flow (not shown) revealed blood flow within the polypoid mass. Transurethral resection confirms a superficial transitional cell carcinoma.

- Smooth or papillary hypoechoic soft tissue mass projects into the bladder lumen (Fig. 3.50) [42].
- Focal or diffuse thickening of the wall occurs with infiltrating tumors (Fig. 3.51).
- Whereas most tumors are hypovascular, larger and high-grade tumors may show visible vascularity on color Doppler [43].
- Blood clots may be present in the bladder lumen. Hydronephrosis and hydroureter result from involvement of the ureteral orifice.

URACHAL ANOMALIES

The urachus is a vestigial remnant of the embryonic allantois. The normal urachus is a fibrous cord (also called the *median umbilical ligament*) that extends anterior to the peritoneum along the midline anterior abdominal wall from the umbilicus to the apex of the bladder [87]. Failure of complete closure of the urachus results in cystic and tubular masses. Infection may complicate any of the urachal anomalies.

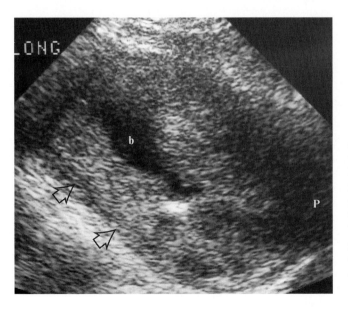

Figure 3.51 *Diffusely Infiltrating Transitional Cell Carcinoma.* Longitudinal image shows marked circumferential thickening (*arrows*) of the bladder wall with a markedly contracted bladder lumen (b). Biopsy revealed an aggressive, diffusely infiltrative transitional cell carcinoma. A portion of the prostate (P) is visible.

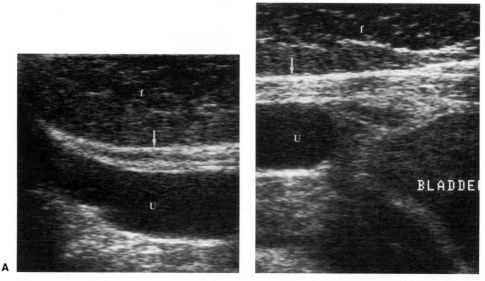

Figure 3.52 *Urachal Cyst.* Longitudinal images (*A, B*) show an anechoic, fluid-filled tubular structure (U) in the midline intimately applied to the inner surface of the anterior abdominal wall (*arrow*) between the bladder and the umbilicus. f, subcutaneous fat.

- **Patent urachus** is vesicocutaneous fistula that extends from the dome of the bladder to the umbilicus. US shows a small diameter tubular structure in the midline anterior abdominal wall.
- **Vesicourachal diverticulum** is a closed sac that extends from the anterior bladder dome to the anterior abdominal wall.
- **Urachal cysts** are found closely applied to the midline anterior abdominal wall between the umbilicus and the bladder. Cyst contents are usually anechoic and may be spherical or tubular in shape (Fig. 3.52).
- **Urachal sinus** is a tubular tract that extends caudally from the umbilicus and ends blindly on the midline anterior abdominal wall.

ADRENAL GLANDS

ADRENAL ADENOMA

Benign, nonhyperfunctioning adrenal adenomas are common incidental findings on imaging studies. Hyperfunctioning adenomas produce endocrine syndromes (Cushing's disease, Conn's syndrome). Lesions can be accurately characterized as benign or potentially malignant by non-contrast CT or chemical-shift MR but not reliably by US [88].

- Most adrenal adenomas are homogeneous, solid, well defined, and less than 5 cm in size (Fig. 3.53). Adenomas are bilateral in up to 10% of patients.
- Hemorrhage, necrosis, and calcification may occur in benign adenomas, but these findings are more characteristic of carcinoma [89].

ADRENAL CARCINOMA

Carcinoma of the adrenal cortex is a rare but aggressive lesion. Approximately one-half of the tumors secrete hormone, most commonly producing Cushing's syndrome. Metastases go to bone, liver, lung, and lymph nodes.

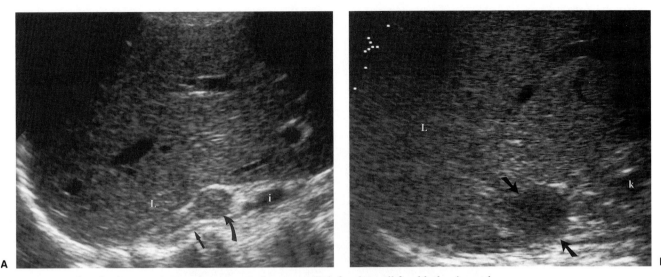

Figure 3.53 *Adrenal Adenoma. A.* Transverse image shows a well-defined, small focal bulge (*curved arrow*) in the right adrenal gland. In an asymptomatic patient, this finding is most indicative of benign adrenal adenoma. Note the anatomic landmarks used for identification of the right adrenal gland. i, inferior vena cava; L, right lobe of the liver; straight arrow, right crus of the diaphragm. *B.* Longitudinal image obtained from a patient with Cushing's disease shows a homogeneous solid mass (*arrows*) above the right kidney (k). L, liver.

- Tumors are usually large (>5 cm) and necrotic at presentation. Calcifications are common (30%) [90]. Up to 10% are bilateral [91].
- The tumor may invade the renal vein or IVC producing findings similar to those found with RCC.

ADRENAL METASTASES

Metastases to the adrenal gland arise most commonly from lung, breast, colon and renal cancer, or melanoma.

- Lesions smaller than 3 cm are homogeneous, solid, round, and indistinguishable by US from benign adenoma.
- Lesions larger than 3 cm are typically heterogeneous with necrosis, hemorrhage, calcification, and poorly defined borders (Fig. 3.54).

PHEOCHROMOCYTOMA

Pheochromocytoma secretes catecholamines and typically presents with paroxysmal hypertension. However, atypical presentation is common and the tumor may not be suspected clinically. Approximately 10% of lesions are malignant and 10% are extra-adrenal. Pheochromocytoma is found in 7–18% of patients with VHL [67]. Tumors in VHL are often multiple, bilateral (50–80%), and extra-adrenal. Pheochromocytoma shows a broad spectrum of US findings [92].

- Most lesions (two-thirds) are purely solid with either homogeneous (~50%) or heterogeneous (~50%) echogenicity [92]. Compared to renal parenchyma, tumors may be isoechoic, hypoechoic, or hyperechoic (Fig. 3.55).
- One-third of lesions are partially or near completely cystic [92]. Cystic lesions contain echogenic fluid and have thick walls and visible solid components.
- US is unable to differentiate benign from malignant pheochromocytomas [92].

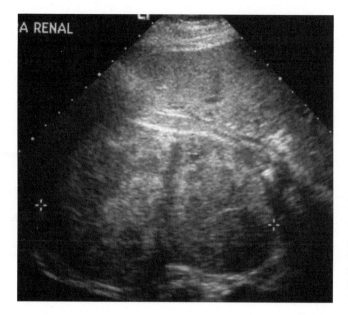

Figure 3.54 *Metastasis to Adrenal Gland.* A large, heterogeneous, solid mass (*between cursors, +*) arises from the right adrenal area, displacing the liver anteriorly. This was a metastasis from malignant melanoma to the adrenal gland.

■ Percutaneous biopsy of pheochromocytoma may result in hypertensive or hypotensive crisis [93].

ADRENAL HEMORRHAGE

Adrenal hemorrhage occurs in stressed newborns, patients on anticoagulant therapy, and following blunt trauma, surgery, childbirth, myocardial infarction, liver transplantation, sepsis, or burns [94]. Hemorrhage may be unilateral or bilateral.

■ Oval heterogeneous mass replaces the adrenal gland. Size varies up to 4–6 cm.
■ The mass shows the evolution characteristic of hematoma on serial follow-up. Acutely the mass is echogenic. With time the mass becomes heterogeneous, hypoechoic and cystic, and shrinks (Fig. 3.56).

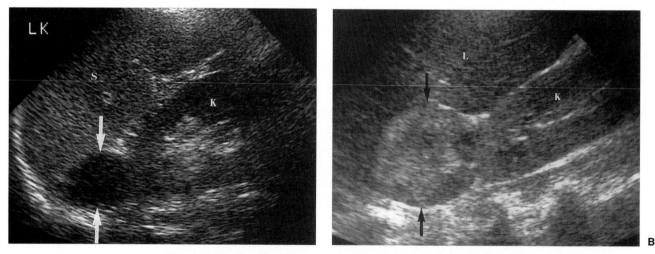

Figure 3.55 *Pheochromocytoma. A.* Longitudinal image through the spleen (S) and left kidney (K) of a patient with von Hippel-Lindau syndrome reveals a homogeneous, hypoechoic, solid left adrenal mass (*arrows*). *B.* Longitudinal image through the liver (L) and right kidney (K) of a patient with severe hypertension reveals a heterogeneous, hyperechoic, solid right adrenal mass (*arrows*). Both lesions were confirmed to be pheochromocytomas.

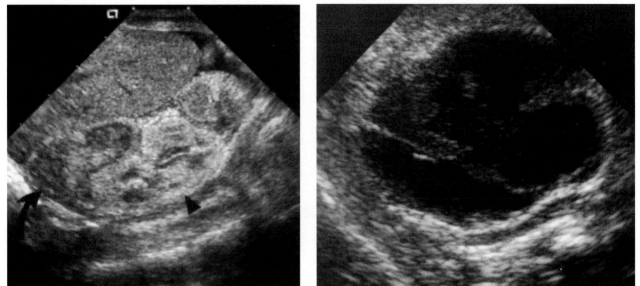

Figure 3.56 *Adrenal Hemorrhage. A.* Longitudinal image in a 30-week-gestation, premature infant shows acute hemorrhage into the right adrenal gland (*curved arrow*). The right kidney (*arrowhead*) is compressed by the hemorrhage. *B.* Transverse image of the adrenal obtained for follow-up of adrenal hemorrhage in another infant shows the lucency that characteristically develops within adrenal hemorrhage in 2–3 weeks.

- Adrenal hemorrhage following blunt trauma has a strong predilection for the right side [95].

ADRENAL CYSTS

Four types of adrenal cysts are encountered [96]. Approximately equally common are endothelial cysts (45%) and post-hemorrhage pseudocysts (39%). True epithelial cysts and parasitic cysts are rare. Cysts may hemorrhage internally or become secondarily infected [97].

- Cysts are well marginated with anechoic contents unless hemorrhage or infection has occurred [90].
- Most adrenal cysts have a visible wall 3 mm or less in thickness [98].
- Avascular internal septations are characteristic of post-hemorrhage pseudocysts. Calcification in the wall of old pseudocysts is common.
- Distinct, vascularized solid components suggest a malignant lesion (carcinoma or metastasis).

ADRENAL MYELOLIPOMAS

Myelolipomas are rare benign tumors containing mature fat and bone-marrow elements. Hemorrhage into the tumor may occur [99].

- Tumors are typically intensely echogenic because of their fat content (Fig. 3.57). Hypoechoic regions represent myeloid content. They are easily overlooked on US because they blend in with retroperitoneal fat. CT confirmation of fat content is diagnostic [99].

NEUROBLASTOMA

Neuroblastoma is the most common extracranial malignancy in infants.

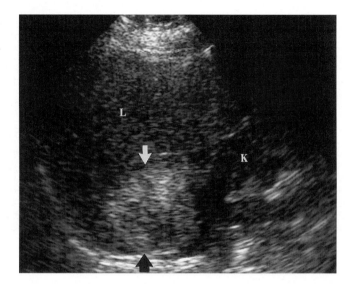

Figure 3.57 *Adrenal Myelolipoma.* Longitudinal image demonstrates the high echogenicity of this tumor (*between black and white arrows*) containing mostly fat. Because they blend in with retroperitoneal fat, these lesions are easily missed during US examination. K, right kidney; L, liver.

- Lesions are large, solid, poorly encapsulated, and commonly cross the midline (Fig. 3.58).
- Calcifications are found in 50% of tumors.
- The tumor commonly encases blood vessels and may extend into the spinal canal.

ADRENAL HYPERPLASIA

Bilateral adrenal hyperplasia accounts for approximately 20% of adrenal endocrine syndromes.

- Hyperplasia diffusely enlarges the adrenal glands without a discrete mass. The limbs exceed 1-cm diameter and are elongated [91].

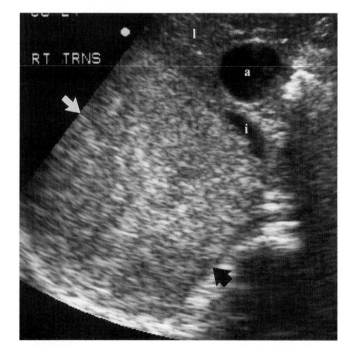

Figure 3.58 *Neuroblastoma.* Transverse image shows a large solid mass (*arrows*) arising from the right adrenal and compressing the liver (l) and inferior vena cava (i). a, aorta.

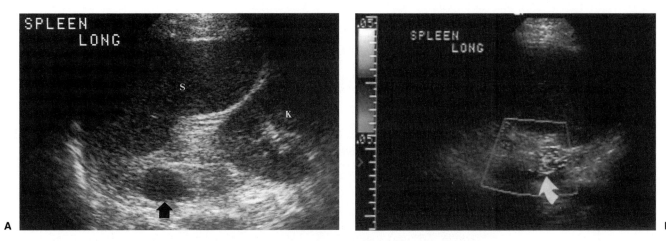

Figure 3.59 *Varix Mimics an Adrenal Mass.* This patient was referred for biopsy of a left adrenal mass seen on a CT of the abdomen performed without contrast because the patient had impaired renal function. *A.* US revealed a homogeneous, hypoechoic, left suprarenal mass (*arrow*). K, left kidney; S, spleen. *B.* Color Doppler confirmed the "mass" was a varix (*arrow*) formed because of the patient's portal hypertension (see Color Figure 3.59).

ADRENAL CALCIFICATION

The adrenal gland may become completely or partially calcified as a result of previous adrenal hemorrhage, or late in adrenal involvement by tuberculosis or histoplasmosis. Destruction of 90% or more of the adrenal cortex by these infections may result in adrenal insufficiency (Addison's disease) [91].

- Coarse or punctate calcifications produce bright echodensities with acoustic shadowing. No adrenal parenchyma may be evident.
- **Wolman's disease** is a rare lipid storage disorder characterized by large adrenal glands with punctate calcification. Marked hepatosplenomegaly is usually present.

PITFALLS IN ADRENAL IMAGING

Because the adrenal glands are small and surrounded by numerous other structures, non-adrenal structures are commonly mistaken for adrenal masses (Fig. 3.59). Tortuous splenic vessels, portosystemic collateral vessels, renal, splenic, and pancreatic masses, adenopathy, gastric diverticuli, and portions of the stomach may all mimic adrenal masses.

REFERENCES

1. American Institute of Ultrasound in Medicine. Standards and guidelines for performance of the renal and retroperitoneal examination. Bethesda, Maryland: AIUM, 1990.
2. Hèlènon O, Rody FE, Correas J-M, et al. Color Doppler US of renovascular disease in native kidneys. RadioGraphics 1995;15:833–854.
3. Hèlènon O, Correas J-M, Chabriais J, et al. Renal vascular Doppler imaging: clinical benefits of power mode. RadioGraphics 1998;18:1441–1454.
4. Marchal G, Gelin J, Verbeken E, et al. High resolution real-time sonography of the adrenal glands: a routine examination. J Ultrasound Med 1986;5:65–68.
5. Platt J, Rubin J, Bowerman R, et al. The inability to detect kidney disease on the basis of echogenicity. AJR Am J Roentgenol 1988;151:317–319.
6. Wilson S, Rosen I, Chin-Sang H, et al. Fatty infiltration of the liver: an imaging challenge. J Can Assoc Radiol 1982;4:227–232.
7. Yeh HC, Halton KP, Shapiro RS, et al. Junctional parenchyma: revised definition of hypertrophic column of Bertin. Radiology 1992;185:725–732.

8. Patriquin H, Lefaivre J-F, Lafortune M, et al. Fetal lobation—an anatomo-ultrasonographic correlation. J Ultrasound Med 1990;9:191–197.

9. Hodson J. The lobar structure of the kidney. Br J Urol 1972;44:246–261.

10. Keogan M, Kliewer M, Hertzberg B, et al. Renal resistive indexes: variability in Doppler US measurement in a healthy population. Radiology 1996;199:165–169.

11. Burge H, Middleton W, McClennon B, et al. Ureteral jets in healthy subjects and in patients with unilateral ureteral calculi: comparison with color Doppler ultrasound. Radiology 1991;180:437–442.

12. Strauss S, Dushnitsky T, Peer A, et al. Sonographic features of horseshoe kidney: review of 34 patients. J Ultrasound Med 2000;19:27–31.

13. Middleton WD, Dodds WJ, Lawson TL, et al. Renal calculi: sensitivity for detection with ultrasound. Radiology 1988;167:239–244.

14. Vrtiska T, Hattery R, King B, et al. Role of ultrasound in medical management of patients with renal stone disease. Urol Radiol 1992;14:131–138.

15. Yoon D-Y, Bae S-H, Choi C-S. Transrectal ultrasonography of distal ureteral calculi: comparison with intravenous urography. J Ultrasound Med 2000;19:271–275.

16. Aytaç S, Özcan H. Effect of color Doppler system on the twinkling sign associated with urinary tract calculi. J Clin Ultrasound 1999;27:433–439.

17. Boridy I, Maklad N, Sandler C. Suspected urolithiasis in pregnant women: imaging algorithm and literature review. AJR Am J Roentgenol 1996;167:869–875.

18. Wachsberg R. Unilateral absence of ureteral jets in the third trimester of pregnancy: pitfall in color Doppler US diagnosis of urinary obstruction. Radiology 1998;209:279–281.

19. Platt J, Ellis J, Rubin J. Role of renal Doppler imaging in the evaluation of acute renal obstruction. AJR Am J Roentgenol 1995;164:379–380.

20. Hertzberg B, Carroll B, Bowie J, et al. Doppler US assessment of maternal kidneys: analysis of intrarenal resistivity indexes in normal pregnancy and physiologic pelvicaliectasis. Radiology 1993;186:689–692.

21. Clautice-Engle T, Anderson N, Allan R, et al. Diagnosis of obstructive hydronephrosis in infants: comparison sonograms performed 6 days and 6 weeks after birth. AJR Am J Roentgenol 1995;164:963–967.

22. Stokland E, Hellstrom M, Hansson S, et al. Reliability of ultrasonography in identification of reflux nephropathy in children. BMJ 1994;309:235–239.

23. Weinberg B, Yeung N. Sonographic sign of intermittent dilatation of the renal collecting system in 10 patients with vesicoureteral reflux. J Clin Ultrasound 1998;26:65–68.

24. Pruthi R, Angell S, Dubocq F, et al. The use of renal parenchymal area in children with high grade vesicoureteral reflux. J Urol 1997;158:1232–1235.

25. Hricak H, Cruz C, Romanski R, et al. Renal parenchymal disease: sonographic-histologic correlation. Radiology 1982;144:141–147.

26. Roger S, Beale A, Cattell W, et al. What is the value of measuring renal parenchymal thickness before renal biopsy? Clin Radiol 1994;49:45–49.

27. Yassa N, Peng M, Ralls P. Perirenal lucency ("kidney sweat"): a new sign of renal failure. AJR Am J Roentgenol 1999;173:1075–1077.

28. Rodreguez-de-Velasquez A, Yoder I, Velasquez P, et al. Imaging the effects of diabetes on the genitourinary system. RadioGraphics 1995;15:1051–1068.

29. Di Fiori J, Rodrigue D, Kaptein E, et al. Diagnostic sonography of HIV-associated nephropathy: new observations and clinical correlation. AJR Am J Roentgenol 1998;171:713–716.

30. Rao T, Filippone E, Nicastri A, et al. Associated focal and segmental glomerulosclerosis in the acquired immunodeficiency syndrome. N Engl J Med 1984;290:19–23.

31. Jequier S, Kaplan B. Echogenic renal pyramids in children. J Clin Ultrasound 1991;19:85–92.

32. Porena M, Vaspasiani G, Rosi P, et al. Incidentally detected renal cell carcinoma: role of ultrasonography. J Clin Ultrasound 1992;20:395–400.

33. Roberts SI, Winick A, Santi M. Papillary renal cell carcinoma: diagnostic dilemma of a cystic renal mass. RadioGraphics 1997;17:993–998.

34. Habboub HK, Abu-Yousef MM, Williams RD, et al. Accuracy of color Doppler sonography in assessing venous thrombus extension in renal cell carcinoma. AJR Am J Roentgenol 1997;168:267–271.

35. Wagner BJ, Wong-You-Cheong JJ, Davis CJ, Jr. Adult renal hamartomas. RadioGraphics 1997;17:155–169.

36. Hèlènon O, Merran S, Paraf F, et al. Unusual fat-containing tumors of the kidney: a diagnostic dilemma. RadioGraphics 1997;17:129–144.

37. Jinzaki M, Tanimoto A, Narimatsu Y, et al. Angiomyolipoma: imaging findings in lesions with minimal fat. Radiology 1997;205:497–502.

38. Forman H, Middleton W, Melson G, et al. Hyperechoic renal cell carcinomas: increase in detection at US. Radiology 1993;188:431–434.

39. Siegel CL, Middleton WD, Teefey SA, et al. Angiomyolipoma and renal cell carcinoma: US differentiation. Radiology 1996;198:789–793.

40. Yamashita Y, Ueno S, Makita O, et al. Hyperechoic renal tumors: anechoic rim and intratumoral cysts in US differentiation of renal cell carcinoma from angiomyolipoma. Radiology 1993;188:179–182.

41. Lemaitre L, Robert Y, Dubrulle F, et al. Renal angiomyolipoma: growth followed up with CT and/or US. Radiology 1995;197:598–602.

42. Wong-You-Cheong J, Wagner B, Davis CJ. Transitional cell carcinoma of the urinary tract: radiologic-pathologic correlation. RadioGraphics 1998;18:123–142.

43. Horstman W, McFarland R, Gorman J. Color Doppler sonographic findings in patients with transitional cell carcinoma of the bladder and renal pelvis. J Ultrasound Med 1995;14:129–133.

44. Dinsmore B, Pollack H, Banner M. Calcified transitional cell carcinoma of the renal pelvis. Radiology 1988;167:401–404.

45. Hadas-Halpern I, Farkas A, Patlas M, et al. Sonographic diagnosis of ureteral tumors. J Ultrasound Med 1999;18:639–645.

46. Urban B, Fishman E. Renal lymphoma: CT patterns with emphasis on helical CT. RadioGraphics 2000;20:197–212.

47. Pickhardt P, Lonergan G, Davis CJ, et al. Infiltrative renal lesions: radiologic-pathologic correlation. RadioGraphics 2000;20:215–243.

48. Choyke PL, White EM, Zeman RK, et al. Renal metastases: clinicopathologic and radiologic correlation. Radiology 1987;162:359–363.

49. Davidson AJ, Hayes WS, Hartman DS, et al. Renal oncocytoma and carcinoma: failure of differentiation with CT. Radiology 1993;186:693–696.

50. Green D, D'Angio G, Beckwith J, et al. Wilms tumor. CA Cancer J Clin 1996;46:46–63.

51. Lonergan G, Martinez-Leon M, Agrons G, et al. Nephrogenic rests, nephroblastomatosis, and associated lesions of the kidney. RadioGraphics 1998;18:947–968.

52. White K, Dirks D, Bove K. Imaging of nephroblastomatosis: an overview. Radiology 1992;182:1–5.

53. McHugh K, Stringer D, Hebert D, et al. Simple renal cysts in children: diagnosis and follow-up with US. Radiology 1991;178:383–385.

54. Bosniak MA. The current radiological approach to renal cysts. Radiology 1986;158:1–10.

55. Bosniak MA. The small (<3.0 cm) renal parenchymal tumor: detection, diagnosis, and controversies. Radiology 1991;179:307–317.

56. Bosniak MA. Problems in the radiologic diagnosis of renal parenchymal tumors. Urol Clin North Am 1993;20:217–230.

57. Agrons GA, Wagner BJ, Davidson AJ, et al. Multilocular cystic renal tumor in children: radiologic-pathologic correlation. RadioGraphics 1995;15:653–669.

58. Hartman DS, Davis CJ, Sanders RC, et al. The multiloculated renal mass: considerations and differential features. Radiographics 1987;7:29–52.

59. Levine E, Grantham J. Calcified renal stones and cyst calcifications in autosomal dominant polycystic kidney disease: clinical and CT study in 84 patients. AJR Am J Roentgenol 1992;159:77–81.

60. Hayden CJ, Swischuk L. Renal cystic disease. Semin Ultrasound CT MR 1991;12:361–373.

61. Jain M, LeQuesne GW, Bourne A, et al. High-resolution ultrasonography in the differential diagnosis of cystic diseases of the kidney in infancy and childhood: preliminary experience. J Ultrasound Med 1997;16:235–240.

62. Blickman JG, Bramson RT, Herrin JT. Autosomal recessive polycystic kidney disease: long-term sonographic findings in patients surviving the neonatal period. AJR Am J Roentgenol 1995;164:1247–1250.

63. Lucaya J, Enriquez G, Nieto J, et al. Renal calcifications in patients with autosomal recessive polycystic kidney disease: prevalence and cause. AJR Am J Roentgenol 1993;160:359–362.

64. Levine E, Slusher SL, Grantham JJ, et al. Natural history of acquired renal cystic disease in dialysis patients: a prospective longitudinal CT study. AJR Am J Roentgenol 1991;156:501–506.

65. Heinz-Peer G, Schoder M, Rand T, et al. Prevalence of acquired cystic kidney disease and tumors in native kidneys of renal transplant recipients: a prospective US study. Radiology 1995;195:667–671.

66. Cochran S. Imaging the complications of dialysis. The Radiologist 1997;4:13–22.
67. Choyke PL, Glenn GM, Walther MM, et al. Von Hippel-Lindau disease: genetic, clinical, and imaging features. Radiology 1995;194:629–642.
68. Choyke P, Glenn G, Walther M, et al. The natural history of renal lesions in von Hippel-Lindau disease: a serial CT study in 28 patients. AJR Am J Roentgenol 1992;159:1229–1234.
69. Narla L, Slovis T, Watts F, et al. The renal lesions of tuberous sclerosis (cysts and angiomyolipoma): screening with sonography and computerized tomography. Pediatr Radiol 1988;20:491–493.
70. Mellins H. Cystic dilatations of the upper urinary tract: a radiologist's developmental model. Radiology 1984;153:291–301.
71. Vinocur L, Slovis T, Perlmutter A, et al. Follow-up studies of multicystic dysplastic kidneys. Radiology 1988;167:311–316.
72. Strife JL, Souza AS, Kirks DR, et al. Multicystic dysplastic kidney in children: US follow-up. Radiology 1993;186:785–788.
73. Sanders R, Nussbaum A, Solez K. Renal dysplasia, sonographic findings. Radiology 1988;167:623–626.
74. Dacher J-N, Pfister C, Monroc M, et al. Power Doppler sonographic pattern of acute pyelonephritis in children: comparison with CT. AJR Am J Roentgenol 1996;166:1451–1455.
75. Lowe LH, Zagoria RJ, Baumgartner BR, et al. Role of imaging and intervention in complex infections of the urinary tract. AJR Am J Roentgenol 1994;163:363–367.
76. Kenney PJ. Imaging of chronic renal infections. AJR Am J Roentgenol 1990;155:485–494.
77. Patel N, Lavengood R, Fernandes M, et al. Gas-forming infections in genitourinary tract. Urology 1992;39:341–345.
78. Kirpekar M, Cooke K, Abiri M, et al. US case of the day. RadioGraphics 1997;17:1601–1603.
79. Joseph RC, Amendola MA, Artze ME, et al. Genitourinary tract gas: imaging evaluation. RadioGraphics 1996;16:295–308.
80. Migaleddu V, Conti M, Canalis G, et al. Imaging of renal hydatid cysts. AJR Am J Roentgenol 1997;169:1339–1342.
81. Witz M, Kantarovsky A, Morag B, et al. Renal vein occlusion, a review. J Urol 1996;155:1173–1179.
82. Platt J, Ellis J, Rubin J. Intrarenal arterial Doppler sonography in the detection of renal vein thrombosis of the native kidney. AJR Am J Roentgenol 1994;162:1367–1370.
83. De Cobelli F, Venturini M, Vanzulli A, et al. Renal arterial stenosis: prospective comparison of color Doppler US and breath-hold, three-dimensional, dynamic, gadolinium-enhanced MR angiography. Radiology 2000;214:373–380.
84. Clautice-Engle T, Jeffrey RJ. Renal hypoperfusion: value of power Doppler imaging. AJR Am J Roentgenol 1997;168:1227–1231.
85. Maynor C, Kliewer M, Hertzberg B, et al. Urinary bladder diverticula: sonographic diagnosis and interpretive pitfalls. J Ultrasound Med 1996;16:189–194.
86. Fernbach SK, Feinstein KA. Abnormalities of the bladder in children: imaging findings. AJR Am J Roentgenol 1994;162:1143–1150.
87. Knati N, Enquist E, Javitt M. Imaging of the umbilicus and periumbilical region. RadioGraphics 1998;18:413–431.
88. McNicholas MMJ, Lee MJ, Mayo-Smith WW, et al. An imaging algorithm for the differential diagnosis of adrenal adenomas and metastases. AJR Am J Roentgenol 1995;165:1453–1459.
89. Newhouse J, Heffess C, Wagner B, et al. Large degenerated adrenal adenomas: radiologic-pathologic correlation. Radiology 1999;210:385–391.
90. Cirillo R, Bennett W, Vitellas K, et al. Pathology of the adrenal gland: imaging features. AJR Am J Roentgenol 1998;170:429–435.
91. Dunnick NR. Adrenal imaging: current status. AJR Am J Roentgenol 1990;154:927–936.
92. Schwerk WB, Görg C, Görg K, et al. Adrenal pheochromocytomas: a broad spectrum of sonographic presentation. J Ultrasound Med 1994;13:517–521.
93. Casola G, Nicolet V, vanSonnenberg E, et al. Unsuspected pheochromocytoma: risk of blood-pressure alterations during percutaneous adrenal biopsy. Radiology 1986;159:733–735.
94. Kawashima A, Sandler C, Ernst R, et al. Imaging of nontraumatic hemorrhage of the adrenal gland. RadioGraphics 1999;19:949–963.
95. Nimkin K, Teeger S, Wallach MT, et al. Adrenal hemorrhage in abused children: imaging and postmortem findings. AJR Am J Roentgenol 1994;162:661–663.

96. Tung G, Pfister R, Papanicolaou N, et al. Adrenal cysts, imaging and percutaneous aspiration. Radiology 1989;173:107–110.
97. Otal P, Escourrou G, Mazerolles C, et al. Imaging features of uncommon adrenal masses with histopathologic correlation. RadioGraphics 1999;19:569–581.
98. Rozenblit A, Morehouse HT, Amis ES, Jr. Cystic adrenal lesions: CT features. Radiology 1996;201:541–548.
99. Rao P, Kenney PJ, Wagner BJ, et al. Imaging and pathologic features of myelolipoma. Radiographics 1997;17:1373–1385.
100. Emamian S, Nielsen M, Pedersen J, et al. Kidney dimensions at sonography: correlation with age, sex, and habitus is 665 adult volunteers. AJR Am J Roentgenol 1993;160:83–86.

Ultrasound of the Gastrointestinal Tract

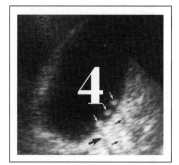

Patients are commonly referred for US examination of the abdomen because of vague and non-specific symptoms such as abdominal pain or abdominal distention. The gastrointestinal (GI) tract is a common site of disease in these patients [1]. Rather than being "between the transducer and what we want to see," the GI tract is what we want to see. Nonetheless, examination of the GI tract by US is challenging because of obscuring bowel gas and confusing artifacts.

Imaging Technique

In the setting of acute abdominal pain, US examination should include the GI tract as well as the solid organs of the abdominal cavity. In women, transvaginal US should be added if transabdominal US is not conclusive. Graded compression US is utilized to examine the intestinal tract [2]. The patient is asked to localize the area of maximal pain or tenderness and attention is focused on that area. A linear array 7-to 10-MHz transducer is utilized. In large patients a 5-MHz linear or curved array transducer may be needed. Color Doppler US greatly aids in the detection of inflammation.

Anatomy

The GI tract has a recognizable "gut signature" that identifies bowel during US examination. Although the wall of the intestinal tract has 5 histologic layers, a 3-layer pattern is usually demonstrated by US (Fig. 4.1). The innermost mucosa and submucosa are seen as a distinct echogenic rind that surrounds the gut lumen. The inner circular and outer longitudinal layers of the muscularis propria produce a central hypoechoic muscle layer on US. The outer adventitia/serosa and surrounding fat produce an outer echogenic layer.

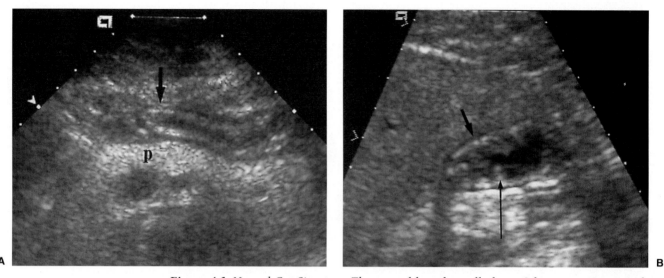

A   B

Figure 4.1 *Normal Gut Signature.* The normal bowel usually has a 3-layer appearance with an echogenic inner layer of mucosa and submucosa, a hypoechoic middle layer of muscle wall, and a thin echogenic outer layer of serosa. Contents of the gut lumen are variable in appearance. *A.* The gastric antrum (*arrow*) is commonly visualized as it crosses anterior to the pancreas (p). *B.* The gastric antrum in another patient is distended with mixed echogenicity fluid and shows echogenic mucosal folds (*long arrow*). The distended bowel has a thinner hypoechoic muscle zone (*short arrow*).

Thus the usual gut signature shown by US is two echogenic layers separated by a hypoechoic muscle layer that define the wall of the GI tract. The lumen of the gut may contain fluid, food, stool, and air in varying combinations at different locations. Portions of the GI tract are identified by location, appearance, peristaltic activity, and luminal contents.

The stomach is a large sac in the left upper quadrant and epigastrium. It commonly contains fluid and air and, if the patient has recently eaten, food. The antrum extends across the pancreas to the duodenum. The duodenal bulb is commonly just inferior to the gallbladder. The third portion of the duodenum is the only portion of the GI tract that extends posterior to the superior mesenteric artery (SMA) and vein (SMV). The jejunum and ileum occupy the central abdomen. The jejunum is identified by its regular folds, the valvulae conniventes, that produce a "keyboard" pattern seen when fluid is in the lumen (Fig. 4.2). The ileum lacks folds and has a flat featureless wall pattern.

The normal appendix is a narrow tube approximately 10 cm in length (Fig. 4.3). It arises from the tip of the cecum approximately 3 cm below the ileocecal valve. The base of the appendix has a constant relationship to the tip of the cecum, but the remainder of the

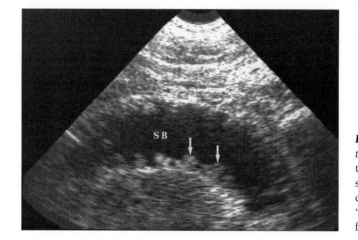

Figure 4.2 *Typical Keyboard Pattern of Jejunal Folds.* A fluid distended loop of jejunum (SB) shows the folds of the valvulae conniventes as a row of echogenic "piano keys" (*arrows*) extending from its wall.

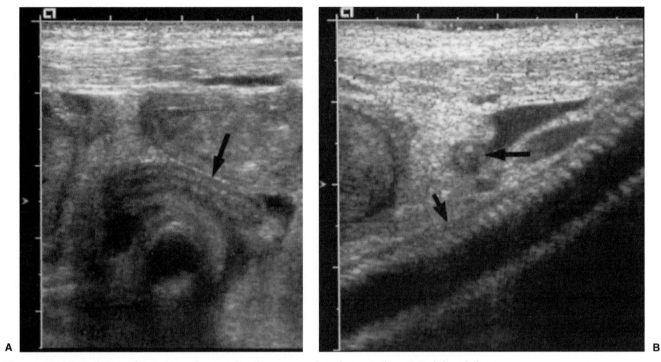

Figure 4.3 *Normal Appendix.* A normal appendix (*longer arrow*) is shown in long axis (*A*) and short axis (*B*). This patient has an iliac artery graft (*shorter arrow*).

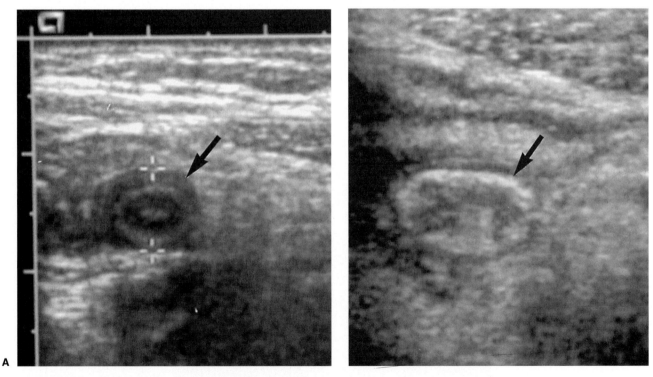

Figure 4.4 *Ileum versus Appendix. A.* In transverse section, the appendix (*arrow, between cursors, +*) is round and smaller. *B.* In transverse section, the distal ileum (*arrow*) is oval and larger.

appendix is free and variably located. It may be behind or below the cecum, behind or in front of the distal ileum, in the pelvis, or occasionally in the left side of the abdomen. The great variability in location influences the clinical presentation of acute appendicitis.

In short axis section the appendix is round, whereas the ileum and colon are oval or elliptical (Fig. 4.4). The colon is identified by its larger size, haustral pattern, and stool content. Stool is heterogeneous in echotexture and liquid, semi-solid, or solid in consistency. Stool commonly contains tiny gas bubbles that produce bright echoes at varying depths.

Doppler routinely shows little or no signal from the gut wall. Increased signal is highly indicative of the increased vascularity of an acute inflammatory process or a neoplasm [3,4].

WALL THICKENING

The normal bowel wall is 2–5 mm in thickness depending upon distention (Fig. 4.1). Wall thickening is nearly always pathologic but is often a non-specific finding. More precise diagnosis is made by detailed examination and correlation with clinical findings [5]. Benign wall thickening produces a target or bull's-eye appearance and is usually uniform and symmetric (Figs. 4.5, 4.6). Any wall thickening, focal or diffuse, that exceeds 25 mm in thickness is more likely to be malignant. Masses demonstrate focal, asymmetric wall thickening, and may extend intraluminally or be exophytic (Fig. 4.7). Differential diagnosis of thickening of the wall of the small bowel and colon is listed in Boxes 4.1 and 4.2 [5].

CROHN'S DISEASE

US can demonstrate characteristic features of Crohn's disease [5].

- Circumferential thickening of the wall of affected bowel >5 mm is indicative of the presence of disease.
- Strictures show marked thickening of the bowel wall with fixed narrowing of the lumen. Dilatation of proximal bowel and hyperperistalsis may be evident [6].
- Mesenteric lymphadenopathy appears as multiple oval hypoechoic masses.
- Skip areas of normal bowel are seen between affected segments.
- The distal ileum is nearly always involved.
- Increased blood flow may be demonstrated in areas of wall thickening, reflecting active inflammation [4].

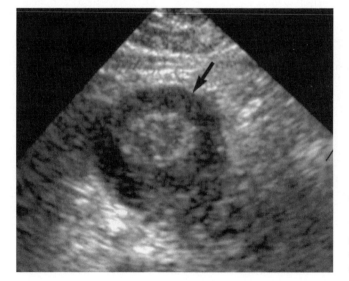

Figure 4.5 *Benign Gastric Wall Thickening.* The wall of the gastric antrum (*arrow*) as seen in short axis view is diffusely and symmetrically thickened by adjacent acute pancreatitis.

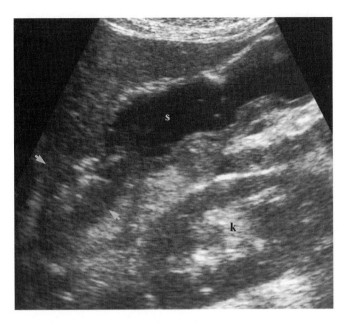

Figure 4.6 *Wall Thickening Caused by Duodenitis.* The stomach (s) is distended with fluid reflecting partial gastric outlet obstruction. The wall of the duodenum (*arrows*) is circumferentially thickened to >10 mm. k, right kidney.

LYMPHOMA OF THE GASTROINTESTINAL TRACT

The GI tract is the most common site of extra-nodal involvement by non-Hodgkin's lymphoma. Most commonly involved sites are the stomach, small bowel, cecum, and remainder of the colon.

- Profound circumferential thickening of the wall is characteristic. Thickening up to 4 cm is common.
- Thickening may be nodular and asymmetric.
- Enlarged mesenteric and retroperitoneal nodes are common.
- Peristalsis is characteristically preserved with a notable lack of bowel obstruction despite marked involvement.

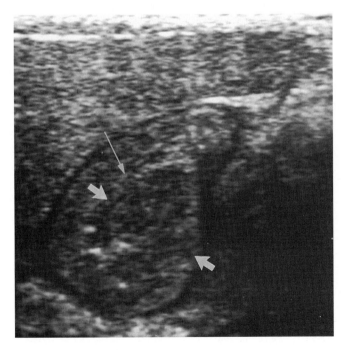

Figure 4.7 *Wall Thickening Caused by Leiomyoma.* The wall of the duodenum shows asymmetric thickening (*between arrows*) of the hypoechoic muscle layer. The lumen (*long skinny arrow*) is compressed and distorted by the mass. Surgical resection confirmed a small leiomyoma.

Box 4.1: Causes of Wall Thickening of the Small Bowel

Wall edema
  Postoperative
  Cirrhosis/ascites
  Hypoproteinemia
Inflammatory bowel disease
  Crohn's disease
  Acute ileitis (*Yersinia, Campylobacter*)
  Extraintestinal inflammatory conditions
    Pancreatitis
    Endometriosis

Malignancy
  Lymphoma
  Peritoneal carcinomatosis
Mesenteric ischemia/infarction
  Thrombosis of mesenteric veins
  Thrombosis of mesenteric arteries
Small bowel disease/malabsorption
  Celiac disease
  Whipple's disease
Benign intestinal tumors (adenoma, lipoma)

Adapted from Ledermann HP, Börner N, Strunk H, et al. Bowel wall thickening on transabdominal sonography. AJR Am J Roentgenol 2000;174:107–117.

COLITIS

Pseudomembranous (*Clostridium difficile*) colitis has become increasingly common in the hospital setting, causing antibiotic therapy–related diarrhea [7]. Ischemic colitis and other forms of infectious and noninfectious colitis have similar findings [8].

- Gross edema of the submucosa is reflected in marked thickening and decreased echogenicity of the inner hyperechoic layer of the colon.
- The swollen submucosa may be folded into a gyral pattern.
- Intraluminal gas is strikingly absent.
- Most patients (64–77%) have accompanying ascites.

ACUTE DIVERTICULITIS

Acute diverticulitis of the colon is a common cause of acute abdominal pain in older patients. Most present with left lower quadrant pain, fever, and leukocytosis [9,10].

- The involved segment of colon shows concentric hypoechoic thickening, predominantly involving the muscle layer.

Box 4.2: Causes of Wall Thickening of the Colon

Inflammation
  Diverticulitis
  Inflammatory bowel disease
    Crohn's disease
    Ulcerative colitis
  Pseudomembranous colitis
  Appendicitis
  Extracolonic inflammatory conditions
    Endometriosis

Malignancy
  Colon carcinoma
  Lymphoma
  Peritoneal carcinomatosis
Edema
  Postoperative
  Cirrhosis/ascites
  Hypoproteinemia
Ischemia/infarction
  Ischemic colitis
  Colon infarction

Adapted from Ledermann HP, Börner N, Strunk H, et al. Bowel wall thickening on transabdominal sonography. AJR Am J Roentgenol 2000;174:107–117.

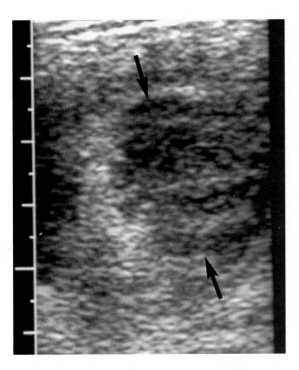

Figure 4.8 *Colon Carcinoma.* A 3-cm colon carcinoma causes a poorly defined, hypoechoic, somewhat spiculated mass (*between arrows*) on US examination.

- Inflamed diverticuli commonly contain impacted fecaliths or gas and appear as bright echogenic foci with ring-down artifact adjacent to the thickened bowel.
- Pericolonic inflammation produces poorly defined hypoechoic areas adjacent to the involved bowel.
- Pericolonic abscesses are seen as loculated fluid collections containing anechoic or echogenic fluid and, sometimes, gas.
- Echogenic or hypoechoic linear tracts in the colon wall or extending to bladder, vagina, or other bowel suggests fistulae and sinus tracts.
- Thickening and inflammation of the colonic mesentery are sometimes evident.

COLON CARCINOMA

Although US is not the method of choice for colon cancer detection, tumors may be identified unexpectedly in patients presenting with acute or chronic symptoms [11].

- Colon cancer may present as a bulky mass up to 10 cm or more in size. On US the mass is usually hypoechoic with irregular, lobulated, or ill-defined contours (Fig. 4.8).
- Intraluminal gas is commonly seen eccentrically located around the tumor.
- Segmental, circumferential, or eccentric thickening of the colon wall may also represent colon cancer (Fig. 4.9).
- Colonic obstruction may be evident with colon and small bowel dilatation.

BOWEL OBSTRUCTION

US may provide evidence of the presence and cause of bowel obstruction [12]. US is particularly good at demonstrating fluid-filled, dilated bowel loops when the abdomen is gasless and difficult to evaluate on plain film radiography. Gas-filled bowel loops seriously impair US assessment. US evaluation of adynamic ileus is limited because large amounts of gas are usually present in the bowel lumen.

- Continuous distention of a loop of bowel with abrupt transition to non-distended bowel is evidence of bowel obstruction.

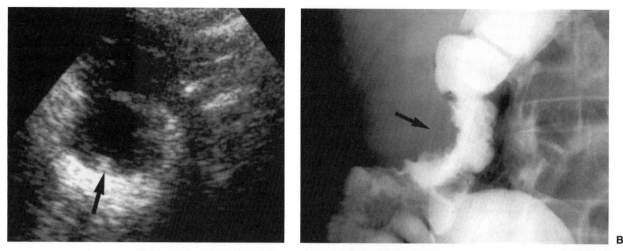

Figure 4.9 *Colon Carcinoma.* *A.* This irregular dumbbell-shaped mass (*arrow*) in the right upper quadrant of the abdomen was initially thought to be a gallbladder carcinoma. *B.* Subsequent barium enema revealed the classic constricting spiculated mass (*arrow*) of a colon carcinoma.

- Peristalsis is increased and luminal contents show an ineffective to-and-fro motion.
- US may demonstrate a mass or stricture at the site of obstruction.

HYPERTROPHIC PYLORIC STENOSIS

The differential diagnosis of vomiting in the first two months of infancy includes hypertrophic pyloric stenosis (HPS), pylorospasm, malrotation with Ladd's bands or midgut volvulus, duodenal atresia, and gastroesophageal reflux. Barium studies are preferred in the diagnosis of gastroesophageal reflux and confirmation of malrotation. US is the examination of choice for HPS [13].

The US examination is performed with fluid in the stomach and the infant in right posterior oblique position. This position places fluid in the antropyloric region for optimal visualization. The infant can be fed glucose solution if the stomach is empty. However, excessive feeding must be avoided because overdistention of the stomach displaces the pylorus posteriorly and makes examination more difficult [14]. Imaging is performed in the epigastrium along the edge of the liver. The fluid-filled antrum is tracked to the pylorus. The pylorus is carefully evaluated in transverse and longitudinal section for documentation of muscle thickness and length of the pyloric channel, and observation for peristalsis and fluid movement through the pylorus.

NORMAL PYLORUS

The normal pylorus is significantly more difficult to identify than the abnormally thickened pylorus (Fig. 4.10).

- Muscle thickness <2 mm in transverse plane is unequivocally normal. The circular muscle may be so thin that it is difficult to measure.
- The length of the pyloric channel is short, often <10 mm. It may be so short that it, too, is difficult to measure.
- Peristaltic activity is observed to pass through the antrum and open the pylorus, allowing passage of fluid through the pylorus into the duodenum.

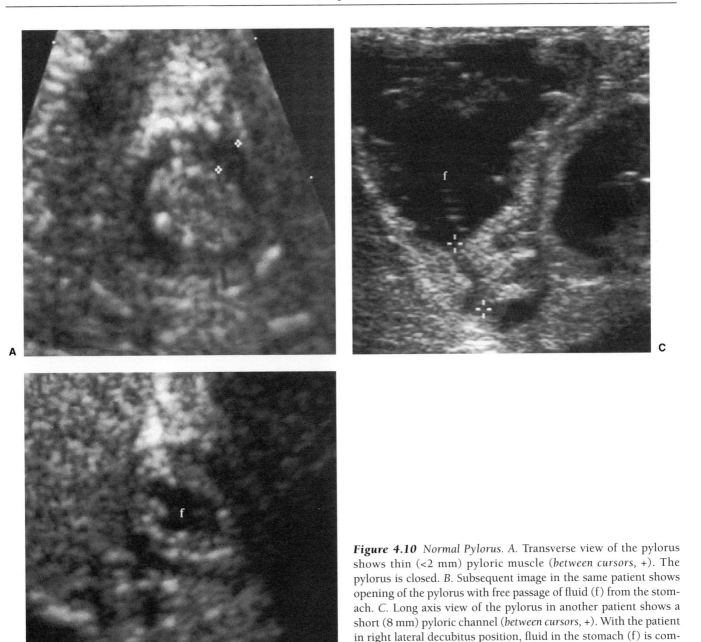

Figure 4.10 *Normal Pylorus. A.* Transverse view of the pylorus shows thin (<2 mm) pyloric muscle (*between cursors,* +). The pylorus is closed. *B.* Subsequent image in the same patient shows opening of the pylorus with free passage of fluid (f) from the stomach. *C.* Long axis view of the pylorus in another patient shows a short (8 mm) pyloric channel (*between cursors,* +). With the patient in right lateral decubitus position, fluid in the stomach (f) is compelled against the pylorus.

HYPERTROPHIC PYLORIC STENOSIS

Hypertrophy of the circular muscle of the pylorus constricts the pyloric channel, resulting in gastric outlet obstruction and projectile nonbilious vomiting. HPS most often affects infants 2–6 weeks old. Rarely, the condition presents at birth or as late as 5 months of age. Boys are affected five times more frequently than girls. In the United States, HPS is usually treated surgically with longitudinal pyloromyotomy.

- The pyloric muscle is thickened and the pyloric channel is elongated (Fig. 4.11).
- On short axis images, the abnormal pylorus resembles a bull's eye with hypoechoic thickened muscle surrounding central echogenic submucosa.
- Muscle thickness >3 mm is diagnostic of HPS [14]. Muscle thickness is measured from the echogenic submucosa to the outer edge of the hypoechoic muscle band [15]. Care

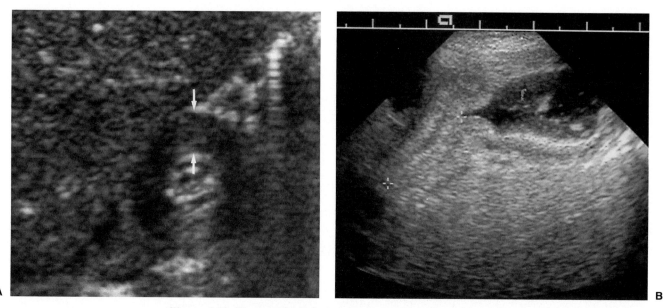

Figure 4.11 *Hypertrophic Pyloric Stenosis. A.* Transverse image of the pylorus shows the characteristic doughnut or bull's-eye appearance of thickened pyloric muscle. The muscle measured 5.6 mm in thickness (*between arrows*). In more than 20 minutes of examination time, the pylorus never opened. *B.* Longitudinal image of the pylorus in another patient shows an 18.5-mm length (*between cursors,* +) of the pyloric channel. Fluid in the stomach (f) outlines a prominent "shoulder sign" produced by the thickened pyloric muscle and a "tit" sign of fluid extending into the contracted pyloric channel.

must be taken to make measurement in true transverse plane to the pylorus. Oblique planes falsely increase the apparent muscle thickness [14].

- Length of the pyloric channel greater than 12 mm is indicative of HPS. Pyloric channel length is measured along the persistently contracted portion of the pylorus [15].
- No peristalsis or passage of fluid through the pylorus is observed. Gastric peristalsis through the antrum ends abruptly at the pylorus.
- A "shoulder sign" may be seen as the bulging impression of hypertrophied muscle on the wall of the gastric antrum.
- The "antral nipple sign" describes the prolapse of folded pyloric mucosa into the fluid-filled antrum [16]. A "tit" sign is produced by fluid extending into the contracted pylorus (Fig. 4.11B).
- Anisotropic effect causes increased echogenicity of the muscle band in transverse section at 6 and 12 o'clock positions. This artifact creates difficulty in muscle measurement [14,17].
- The thickness of the pyloric muscle returns to normal within 2–12 weeks after surgery.

PYLOROSPASM

Pylorospasm is a cause of projectile vomiting in infancy and must be considered in the differential diagnosis of HPS. Pylorospasm is treated with watchful waiting or, occasionally, with antispasmodics [18].

- US findings of pylorospasm overlaps those of the HPS.
- Although the pyloric channel may be closed for a large portion of the examination, it is eventually observed to open.
- Most authors report the thickness of the muscle wall in pylorospasm is <3 mm.
- A recent study of 34 patients with pylorospasm reported mean thickness of the muscle wall as 3.8 mm with mean pyloric channel length of 14.4 mm [18]. These data have not been confirmed.

■ The major clue to diagnosis of pylorospasm is the variability of the appearance and thickness of pyloric muscle visualized during the US examination [18].

GASTROESOPHAGEAL REFLUX

Gastroesophageal reflux also presents with vomiting in infancy. Barium esophagram is the diagnostic study of choice, but US may be utilized [19].

■ The transducer is placed in the epigastrium below the xiphoid to visualize the gastroesophageal junction and distal esophagus.
■ Fluid is seen refluxing into the distal esophagus from the stomach. Fluid may be anechoic or mixed with gas bubbles [19].

MALROTATION

Malrotation of the midgut may obstruct the duodenum and result in a vomiting infant. A narrowed base of the small bowel mesentery predisposes to midgut volvulus. Approximately 90% of affected infants present with obstruction in the first month of life.

■ Transverse examination in the epigastrium demonstrates the SMV lying anterior or to the left of the SMA [20]. The SMV normally is positioned to the right of the SMA.
■ The duodenum is obstructed from volvulus or from peritoneal bands (Ladd's bands) that cross the second or third portion of the duodenum. The stomach and proximal duodenum are dilated and fluid-filled.
■ Barium upper GI series confirms the malrotation and abnormal position of the ligament of Treitz.

ACUTE APPENDICITIS

Acute appendicitis is the most common cause of emergency abdominal surgery [21]. Diagnosis is routinely made by careful clinical examination. However, approximately 20% of patients have an atypical presentation. Imaging diagnosis is indicated in any patient in whom the diagnosis is uncertain.

Acute appendicitis most often results from obstruction of the lumen of the appendix by appendicoliths, lymph nodes, tumors, foreign bodies, or parasites [21]. Continued secretion of mucus causes luminal dilatation and increased intraluminal pressures causing pain and often progressing to ischemia and perforation. Classic presentation (50–60% of patients) is right lower quadrant abdominal pain with nausea, vomiting, and leukocytosis. The presence of fever is evidence of perforation. Peak age is 10–30 years.

Both US and CT are used with high accuracy in the diagnosis of acute appendicitis [22,23]. US is usually considered the imaging method of choice in children and in women with active menstrual cycles [24]. US provides the capacity to offer an alternative diagnosis such as hemorrhagic ovarian cyst in patients who do not have appendicitis. In men, in older patients (>45 years), in obese patients, and in patients with symptoms longer than 2–3 days, CT is usually chosen for imaging diagnosis [21,24].

NORMAL APPENDIX

Visualization of the normal appendix is exceptionally operator- and technique-dependent and is not always possible. Studies indicate visualization of a normal appendix in 10–56% of patients with higher percentages reported in children [23,25]. When the normal appendix is identified, it should be examined from cecal junction to bulbous blind-ending tip.

- The normal appendix is a small, blind-ended, tubular structure that arises from the tip of the cecum (Figs. 4.3, 4.4). In cross section, the appendix is rounder than the nearby ovoid ileum and cecum. The appendix does not demonstrate peristalsis. The lumen may be collapsed or it may contain stool or air.
- Gas within the lumen of the appendix is a normal finding. In a study of 457 patients, gas was seen in the lumen of 86% of normal patients and in only 15% of patients with acute appendicitis [26]. When the appendix is air-filled it may be recognized by its proximal interface that is round and of short diameter.
- The normal appendix is identified by first finding the cecal tip. The cecum is usually the most lateral structure in the right lower quadrant. It is oriented in the long axis of the body and is larger than adjacent small bowel. The cecum is ellipsoid in shape in all imaging planes. Gas bubbles are usually present in semisolid stool within the cecum. Gas in stool produces a stippled pattern of small echoes at varying depths.
- The terminal ileum is medial to and smaller than the cecum (Fig. 4.4). It may contain gas or liquid and routinely demonstrates peristalsis.
- The appendix may be seen anterior to the iliac vessels or overlying the iliacus muscle, occupying the shallow concavity of the iliac bone.
- The normal appendix is less than 6 mm in diameter and is at least partially compressible. The appendix has a typical target appearance with hypoechoic outer zone representing the muscularis propria and a thin, inner, hyperechoic, submucosal layer surrounding the usually collapsed lumen (Figs. 4.3, 4.4A).
- The normal appendix shows little or no flow on color Doppler [27].

ACUTE APPENDICITIS

The US criteria for acute appendicitis apply to acutely symptomatic patients with abdominal pain.

- US diagnosis of acute appendicitis is made when the visualized appendix exceeds 6 mm in diameter and is noncompressible (Fig. 4.12) [2,28]. Measurements of the size of the

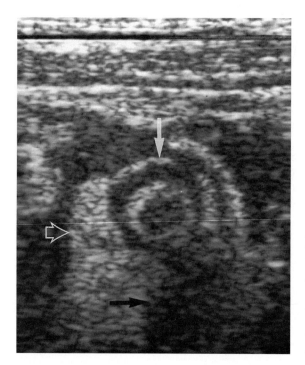

Figure 4.12 *Acute Appendicitis.* Transverse image reveals an 8-mm diameter, non-compressible appendix (*white arrow*). Also evident is increased prominence of the periappendiceal fat (*open arrow*) representing inflammatory change and a hypoechoic periappendiceal mass (*black arrow*) representing a small contained rupture confirmed at surgery.

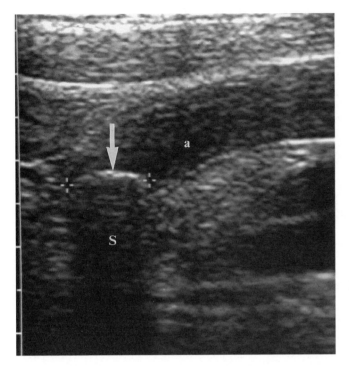

Figure 4.13 *Appendicolith.* An obstructing appendicolith (*white arrow, between cursors, +*) casts an acoustic shadow (S) and obstructs and dilates the appendix (a) resulting in acute appendicitis.

appendix are made from outer wall to outer wall. Anechoic or hypoechoic fluid is commonly seen in the lumen because the appendix is obstructed [25].

■ Identification of an appendicolith is another criterion for a positive examination (Fig. 4.13). Appendicoliths are intestinal concretions that form around some indigestible hard substance in the gut. These calculi may obstruct the appendix. The presence of an appendicolith in a patient with acute abdominal pain is 90% predictive of acute appendicitis and is associated with a 50% incidence of appendix perforation [24]. Appendicoliths appear as discrete echogenic nodules that cast acoustic shadows. They are seen

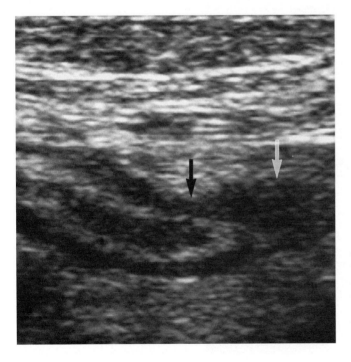

Figure 4.14 *Acute Appendicitis Confined to Tip.* Image in long axis of the appendix shows acute inflammation of the appendiceal tip (*black arrow*) with adjacent small phlegmon (*white arrow*).

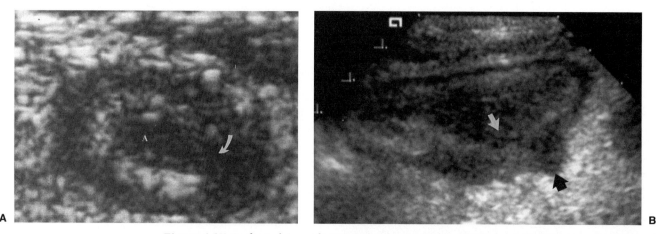

Figure 4.15 *Perforated Appendicitis. A.* Transverse image of the appendix (A) shows focal loss of visualization of the echogenic ring of submucosa (*arrow*) representing focal necrosis. *B.* Image in the long axis of the appendix in another patient shows long segment loss of visualization of the submucosa (*white arrow*) and a focal perforation (*black arrow*).

within the lumen of the appendix or within a periappendiceal inflammatory mass. Appendicoliths are variable in size (5–20 mm) and shape and occasionally are multiple.

- Gas may be present within the inflamed appendix released by gas-forming infection (15% of cases) [26]. Gas with ring down and acoustic shadowing increases the difficulty of identifying the appendix but is commonly limited to only a portion of the appendix [29].
- Appendicitis may be confined to its tip (4–5% of cases) (Fig. 4.14) with normal appearing more proximal appendix [30].
- Gangrenous or perforating appendicitis shows loss of visualization of the echogenic submucosa due to necrosis (Fig. 4.15).

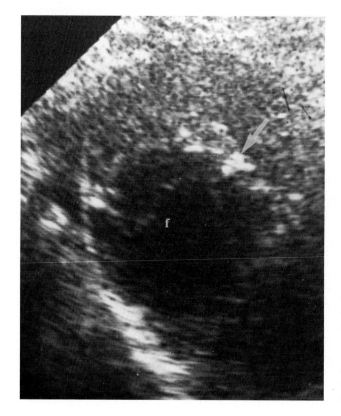

Figure 4.16 *Chronic Appendiceal Abscess.* A fluid-filled mass (f) with a calcified wall (*arrow*) located in the right lower quadrant was found at surgery to be a chronic appendiceal abscess. A mucocele of the appendix may have a similar appearance.

- Edema of the periappendiceal tissues causes increased prominence of the echogenic surrounding fat (Fig. 4.12).
- Periappendiceal mass with poorly defined borders represents phlegmon or abscess. Loculated fluid collections are usually abscesses associated with perforated appendicitis; however, loculated fluid collections may also be seen with nonperforated appendicitis. Untreated appendicitis may result in a chronic walled-off abscess (Fig. 4.16).
- Hyperemia in the wall of the appendix on color Doppler US is strong evidence of acute appendicitis, especially when the appendix is minimally dilated [27]. The normal appendix shows little or no color Doppler signal in its wall.
- In most cases of acute appendicitis, the appendix does not exceed 10–12 mm in diameter. However, in some cases the appendix may be greatly enlarged up to 15–20 mm and may be misidentified as small bowel. Identification of a blind-ended tip confirms an abnormal appendix [29].
- Acute appendicitis resolves spontaneously in a small percentage of cases [31,32]. These patients have sonographic features of acute appendicitis, but their clinical course usually dictates conservative, non-surgical treatment [21].
- Mesenteric lymphadenopathy appears as multiple oval or round nodules isoechoic or hypoechoic to muscle. Adenopathy is found in association with nonperforating appendicitis (20% of cases), perforating appendicitis (5% of cases), and in absence of appendicitis (14% of cases) [25].
- Tumors are an unusual cause of acute appendicitis (Fig. 4.17). The most common tumors of the appendix are carcinoid tumor and adenocarcinoma. A focal mass or an unusual appearance to the appendix is a clue to diagnosis.

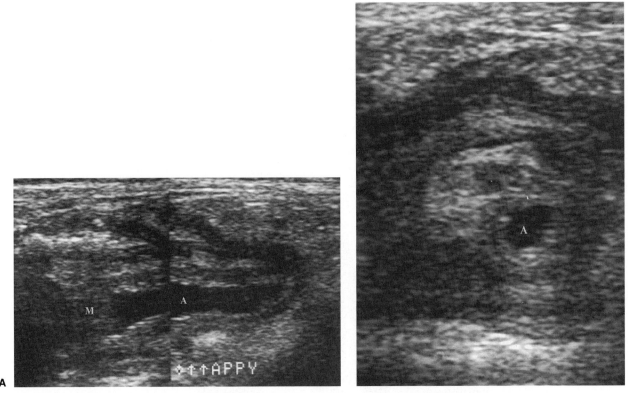

Figure 4.17 *Adenocarcinoma Causes Acute Appendicitis.* Images in the long (A) and short (B) axis of the appendix (A) show marked thickening and irregularity of the wall. The patient is a 65-year-old woman presenting with right lower quadrant pain. The patient is unusually old to present with acute appendicitis. A hypoechoic mass (M) obstructs the appendix. Adenocarcinoma was shown at surgery to be the cause of acute appendicitis.

MUCOCELE OF THE APPENDIX

Mucocele of the appendix describes a dilated lumen of the appendix caused by chronic obstruction with progressive accumulation of mucus within the lumen. It is a rare condition but is easily recognized by US. Patients may be asymptomatic or present with acute or chronic abdominal pain. Rupture of a mucocele of the appendix seeds the peritoneal cavity with mucin-producing cells resulting in pseudomyxoma peritonei [33].

- US shows a well-encapsulated, oblong, tubular, cystic mass, usually in the right lower quadrant of the abdomen. The wall of the mass is usually thin (<6 mm).
- Internal fluid may be anechoic, but is more commonly echogenic with floating particulate matter.
- Calcification may occur in the wall of the mucocele.

INTUSSUSCEPTION

Intussusception occurs when a segment of bowel telescopes into the lumen of an adjacent, downstream segment of bowel. It is one of the most common causes of acute abdomen in infancy, occurring most often between the ages of 6 months and 2 years. Nearly all cases in this age group are idiopathic. Most cases are ileocolic (75–95%). The distal ileum telescopes into the ascending colon. Other forms include ileoileocolic, ileoileal, and colocolic. In approximately 10% of cases in children, especially children older than 3 years, and in nearly all adults, a lead point is responsible for the intussusception. The lead point may be a Meckel's diverticulum, enlarged lymph nodes, malignant tumor, polyp, lipoma, enteric duplication cyst, inflammatory mass of appendicitis, or ectopic pancreas [34].

US has replaced the barium enema as the diagnostic method of first choice, especially in children [35]. US has high sensitivity (98–100%) and specificity (88–100%), and offers the advantage of providing an alternate diagnosis when intussusception is not present.

An understanding of the anatomy of intussusception is required to interpret the US findings (Fig. 4.18) [35]. The receiving loop (the **intussuscipiens**) contains the folded donor loop (the **intussusceptum**). The intussusceptum has two components, an inner entering limb and an outer returning limb. The mesentery of the intussusceptum is dragged into the intussusception between the entering limb and the returning limb. The center of the mass of the intussusception contains the entering limb surrounded by the echogenic

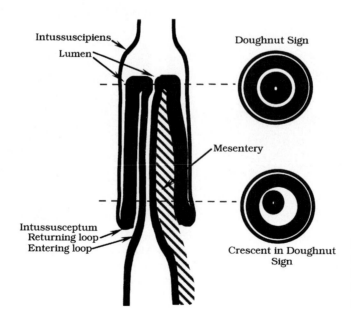

Figure 4.18 *Anatomy of Intussusception.* Diagram illustrates the anatomy of intussusception in long (*left*) and short (*right*) axis.

fat of its mesentery. The wall of the entering limb is usually of normal thickness. A thick, hypoechoic, outer ring of the mass of the intussusception is formed by the returning limb, which is encircled by the wall of the intussuscipiens. The wall of the intussuscipiens is of normal thickness, while the wall of the returning limb of the intussusceptum is thickened. Compression of the entrapped mesentery impairs venous return, resulting in edematous thickening of the bowel wall of the returning limb. Impairment of arterial supply leads to bowel necrosis. Only the blood supply of the intussusceptum is affected. The blood supply of the intussuscipiens is unimpaired and its wall does not become edematous.

INTUSSUSCEPTION

Scanning the mass of the intussusception in different anatomic planes produces characteristic appearances described with vivid names. In the descriptions listed, *longitudinal* refers to the long axis of the intussusception mass and *axial* refers to the short axis of the mass.

- Intussusception creates a large abdominal mass (~5 × 3 cm) that is usually easily visualized by US [35]. In the common ileocolic intussusception the mass is subhepatic in location.
- Doughnut sign (Fig. 4.19). In axial plane, a thick, hypoechoic, outer ring surrounds a hypoechoic central mass, creating the appearance of a doughnut. The thicker outer ring is made up of the thickened wall of the returning limb of the intussusceptum and the thinner outer wall of the intussuscipiens. The central mass varies in appearance with location.
- Crescent in doughnut sign (Fig. 4.20). On axial scans the appearance of intussusception changes from the apex to the base of the mass. The changing appearance is caused by the progressive increase in volume of enclosed mesentery from apex to base. At the leading edge of the intussusception (the apex), the amount of mesentery present is minimal. Axial scans show a hypoechoic center surrounded by a thick hypoechoic ring (doughnut sign). As scan level progresses toward the base, the volume of echogenic trapped mesentery increases. At the trailing edge of the mass (the base), the amount of crescentic-shaped, echogenic mesentery is maximal, creating a crescent in doughnut appearance [36].
- Sandwich sign (Fig. 4.21). In longitudinal plane, the arrangement of the entrapped mesentery and the exact plane of section determine the appearance of the intussusception. An appearance of three parallel hypoechoic bands separated by two parallel hyperechoic bands has been termed the *sandwich sign*. The hyperechoic bands represent the

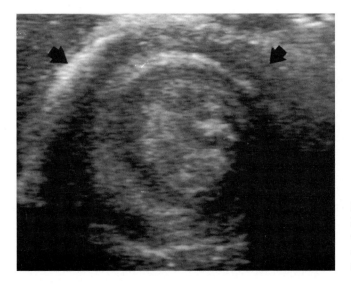

Figure 4.19 *Intussusception—Doughnut Sign.* In short axis view, the mass of the intussusception (*arrows*) resembles a doughnut.

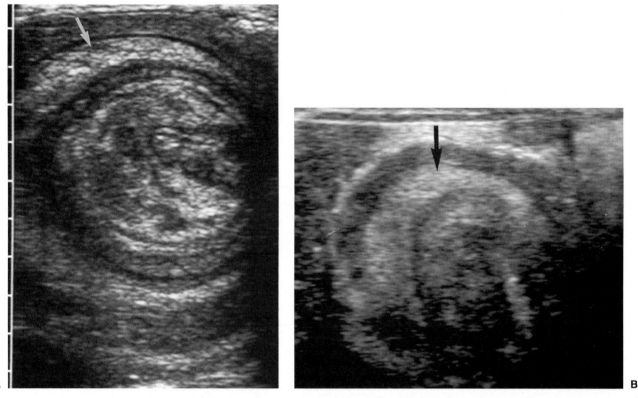

Figure 4.20 *Intussusception—Crescent in Doughnut Sign.* In short axis view, the amount of trapped mesentery increases as the base of the intussusception is approached. The trapped mesentery has a crescent appearance (*arrows*), as demonstrated in two patients, *A* and *B*.

   entrapped mesentery, which separates the central hypoechoic entering limb from the thickened edematous returning limb of the intussusceptum.

- Pseudokidney sign (Fig. 4.22). The intussusception mass may resemble a kidney, particularly if the mass is curved or the plane of imaging is slightly oblique. The enveloped mesentery produces an echogenic "renal sinus" within the hypoechoic thickened walls of bowel that resemble the "renal parenchyma" [37].

- Enlarged lymph nodes produce focal oval or round hypoechoic masses within the entrapped echogenic mesentery.

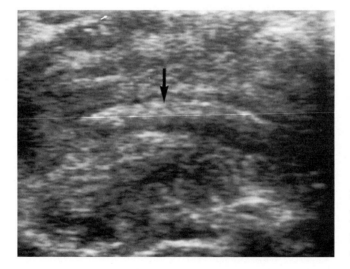

Figure 4.21 *Intussusception—Sandwich Sign.* Trapped mesentery (*arrow*) is "sandwiched" between layers of the intussusception in long axis view.

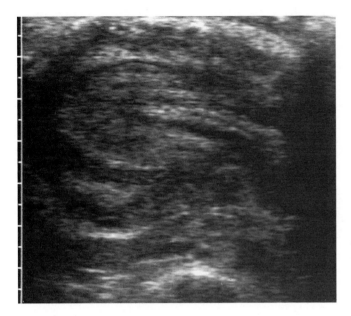

Figure 4.22 *Intussusception—Pseudokidney Sign.* The layers of the intussusception resemble a kidney in this oblique long axis view.

- Gas bubbles trapped within the lumen produce hyperechoic dots with ring down or shadowing.
- Peritoneal fluid trapped between the serosal layers of the intussuscipiens and the everted limb of the intussusceptum is evidence of ischemia and need for surgical reduction [38].
- Color flow US is useful in assessing the reducibility of intussusception [39]. The presence of color signal within the intussusception is a good predictor of reducibility by enema (Fig. 4.23). The absence of color blood flow signal in the intussusception indicates that the chance for non-operative reduction is decreased and that surgical reduction may be needed. The absence of blood flow on Doppler US does not correlate well with the presence of necrosis in the intussusception [40].

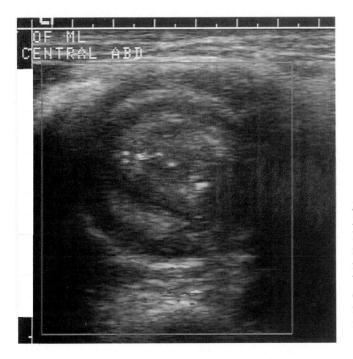

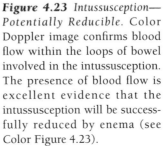

Figure 4.23 *Intussusception—Potentially Reducible.* Color Doppler image confirms blood flow within the loops of bowel involved in the intussusception. The presence of blood flow is excellent evidence that the intussusception will be successfully reduced by enema (see Color Figure 4.23).

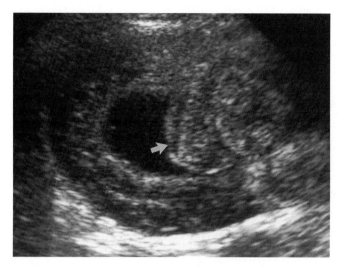

Figure 4.24 *Intussusception Caused by a Leading Mass.* A colo-colonic intussusception in a 50-year-old woman was induced by this heterogeneous cecal mass (*arrow*) identified by US. Pathology revealed a benign mucinous cystadenoma.

- In older children and adults, a careful search should be made for a lead-point mass responsible for the intussusception (Fig. 4.24).
- Copious feces in the colon may resemble the appearance of intussusception. Differentiation is made by recognizing that the hypoechoic rim of colon wall surrounding the echogenic feces is thin (<5–6 mm) rather than thick [41].
- Rarely, intussusception will reduce spontaneously [42].
- Treatment by enema, using barium, water-soluble contrast media, water, electrolyte solutions, or air guided by fluoroscopy or US, has been shown to be effective [35,43].

DISEASE OF THE MESENTERY AND OMENTUM

Masses in the mesentery and omentum are usually easily demonstrated by US examination. A specific diagnosis can often be made based upon the US findings and clinical evaluation.

The small bowel mesentery is a fan-shaped structure that connects the jejunum and ileum to the posterior abdominal wall. It extends from the right lower quadrant region of the terminal ileum to the left upper quadrant ligament of Treitz. Whereas the root of the mesentery is approximately 15 cm in length, its accordion folds suspend approximately 25 feet of small bowel [44]. It is easiest to recognize when ascites is present and bowel loops are suspended in fluid. The mesentery consists of two layers of peritoneum that encase arteries, veins, lymphatic channels, lymph nodes, and a variable amount of fat. Masses may arise from any component of the mesentery. The normal mesentery is approximately 15 mm in thickness [45].

The lesser omentum is a fold of mesentery that extends from the liver to the lesser curvature of the stomach. It is made up of the hepatogastric and hepatoduodenal ligaments and forms a portion of the anterior boundary of the lesser sac. The greater omentum extends from the greater curvature of the stomach as an apron-like, 4-layer fold of peritoneum between the anterior abdominal wall and the intestinal tract. The greater omentum crosses the transverse colon and descends in front of the viscera.

LYMPHADENOPATHY

Normal mesenteric lymph nodes are less than 5 mm in diameter [6]. Lymphadenopathy may occur with infection, inflammation, or neoplasm.

- Enlarged lymph nodes appear as hypoechoic, solid, well-defined oval or round masses (>5 mm size) in the mesentery in close proximity to mesenteric blood vessels.
- Mesenteric adenitis mimics acute appendicitis, especially in children.

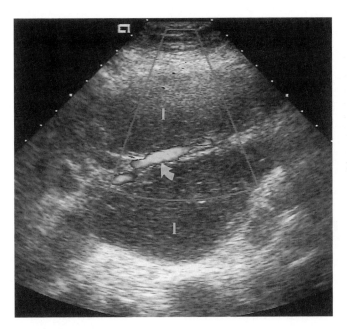

Figure 4.25 *Sandwich Sign of Mesenteric Lymphoma.* A mesenteric artery (*arrow*) is sandwiched between two homogeneous hypoechoic masses of lymphoma (l) (see Color Figure 4.25).

LYMPHOMA

Non-Hodgkin's lymphoma more commonly involves the mesentery. Mural involvement of small bowel usually extends from its mesenteric border [44].

- Lymphoma in the mesentery may appear as discrete enlarged lymph nodes.
- Confluent adenopathy forms round or cake-like hypoechoic masses that may be well defined and lobulated in contour or ill defined.
- Encasement of mesenteric vessels produces a "sandwich sign" of blood vessels between two layers of flattened, bread-like confluent adenopathy (Fig. 4.25) [44].
- Retroperitoneal adenopathy is usually also present.

DESMOIDS

Desmoids are benign, dense, fibrous neoplasms that arise from the fascial sheath of striated muscle [46]. Desmoid tumors are also classified as aggressive fibromatosis. Although benign, they are locally aggressive and recur after surgical resection in 25–65% of cases. Desmoid tumors are found in association with Gardner's syndrome or as isolated lesions [47].

- Desmoids appear as well-defined solid masses.
- Echogenicity varies with cellular composition as well as inclusion of fat and blood vessels within the mass. Appearance varies from homogeneous and hypoechoic to heterogeneous and echogenic.

MESENTERIC CARCINOID TUMOR

Carcinoid tumor is the most common malignant tumor of the jejunum and ileum. Metastases to the mesentery are present in 40–80% of cases.

- Mesenteric involvement appears as an ill-defined, hypoechoic, retractile mass with stellate margins.

MESENTERIC/OMENTAL CYST

The most common cyst of the mesentery or omentum is a lymphangioma [48]. Lymphangiomas are congenital lesions produced by failure of lymphatic tissue to communicate with lymphatic drainage channels. Lesions tend to progressively enlarge over time.

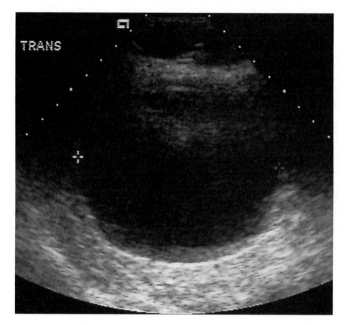

Figure 4.26 *Omental Cyst.* A thin-walled, unilocular, 10-cm cyst (*between cursors, +*) moved freely with the omentum within the peritoneal cavity.

- Lymphangiomas appear as large, thin-walled cysts (Fig. 4.26) that are usually multiloculated [49].
- Internal fluid may be anechoic, or may contain internal echoes dispersed evenly through the fluid or layering with fluid-fluid levels. Internal echoes represent hemorrhage, internal debris, or fatty material (Fig. 4.27).
- Cysts in the mesentery are seen between loops of bowel.
- Cysts in the omentum are located adjacent to the anterior abdominal wall and displace bowel posteriorly.
- Partial small bowel obstruction may be present.

ENTERIC DUPLICATION CYST

The wall of an enteric duplication cyst contains all the elements of normal bowel wall.

- US shows an anechoic cyst with a multilayered thick wall similar in appearance to bowel wall [48].

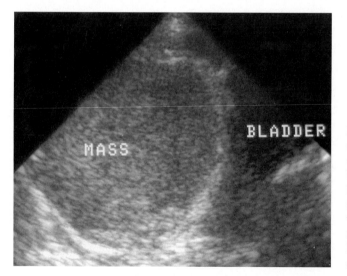

Figure 4.27 *Cystic Lymphangioma.* A large cystic lymphangioma (MASS) arising in the small bowel mesentery of 2-year-old boy presented as an abdominal mass. US reveals a cystic mass with internal echoes. The internal echoes are indicative of prior hemorrhage that was confirmed at pathological examination.

ENTERIC CYSTS

Enteric cysts are lined by GI mucosa but lack the smooth muscle component in the wall that characterizes enteric duplication cysts [48].

■ Enteric cysts have thin smooth walls and contain anechoic serous fluid [49].
■ Most are unilocular, although some contain a few thin septations.

PANCREATIC FLUID COLLECTIONS

Pancreatitis-associated fluid collections commonly dissect into the small bowel mesentery and may extend into the omentum.

■ Fluid collections in the mesentery are found in association with findings of acute pancreatitis and fluid collections elsewhere in the abdomen.

PSEUDOCYSTS

Pseudocysts are cystic masses with a thick fibrous wall that lacks a cellular lining [48]. They result from incomplete resolution of a mesenteric or omental abscess or hematoma and contain hemorrhagic or purulent debris.

■ Pseudocysts are thick walled and usually septated [49].
■ Internal contents are echogenic with floating debris and usually fluid-fluid levels.

BENIGN CYSTIC TERATOMA

Cystic teratomas are usually discovered in children. The mesentery and omentum are uncommon locations.

■ Cystic teratomas contain multiple tissue types that produce cystic and solid components. Cystic areas are usually anechoic.
■ Calcifications are common and produce focal echogenicities with acoustic shadowing.

REFERENCES

1. Carrico C, Fenton L, Taylor G, et al. Impact of sonography on the diagnosis and treatment of acute lower abdominal pain in children and young adults. AJR Am J Roentgenol 1999;172:513–516.
2. Puylaert J, Rutgers P, Lalisang R, et al. A prospective study of ultrasonography in the diagnosis of appendicitis. N Engl J Med 1987;317:666–669.
3. Jeffrey RJ, Sommer F, Debatin J. Color Doppler sonography of focal gastrointestinal lesions: initial clinical experience. J Ultrasound Med 1994;13:473–478.
4. Quillin S, Siegel M. Gastrointestinal inflammation in children: color Doppler ultrasonography. J Ultrasound Med 1994;13:751–756.
5. Ledermann H, Börner N, Strunk H, et al. Bowel wall thickening on transabdominal sonography. AJR Am J Roentgenol 2000;174:107–117.
6. Puylaert J. Mesenteric adenitis and acute terminal ileitis: US evaluation using graded compression. Radiology 1986;161:691–695.
7. Downey D, Wilson S. Pseudomembranous colitis: sonographic features. Radiology 1991; 180:61–64.
8. Truong M, Atri M, Bret P, et al. Sonographic appearance of benign and malignant conditions of the colon. AJR Am J Roentgenol 1998;170:1451–1455.
9. Wilson S, Toi A. The value of sonography in the diagnosis of acute diverticulitis of the colon. AJR Am J Roentgenol 1990;154:1199–1202.
10. Verbanck J, Lambrecht S, Rutgeerts L, et al. Can sonography diagnose acute colonic diverticulitis in patients with acute intestinal inflammation? A prospective study. J Clin Ultrasound 1989;17:661–666.
11. Lim J. Colorectal cancer: sonographic findings. AJR Am J Roentgenol 1996;167:45–47.

12. Lim J, Ko Y, Lee D, et al. Determining the site and causes of colonic obstruction with sonography. AJR Am J Roentgenol 1994;163:1113–1117.
13. Hernanz-Schulman M, Sells L, Ambrosino M, et al. Hypertrophic pyloric stenosis in the infant without a palpable olive: accuracy of sonographic diagnosis. Radiology 1994;193:771–776.
14. Swischuk L, Hayden CJ, Stansberry S. Sonographic pitfalls in imaging of the antropyloric region in infants. Radiographics 1989;9:437–447.
15. Blumhagen J, Maclin L, Krauter D, et al. Sonographic diagnosis of hypertrophic pyloric stenosis. AJR Am J Roentgenol 1988;150:1367–1370.
16. Hernanz-Schulman M, Dinauer P, Ambrosino M, et al. The antral nipple sign of pyloric mucosal prolapse: endoscopic correlation of a new sonographic observation in patients with pyloric stenosis. J Ultrasound Med 1995;14:283–287.
17. Spevak M, Ahmadjian J, Kleinman P, et al. Sonography of hypertrophic pyloric stenosis: frequency and cause of nonuniform echogenicity of the thickened pyloric muscle. AJR Am J Roentgenol 1992;158:129–132.
18. Cohen H, Zinn H, Haller J, et al. Ultrasonography of pylorospasm: findings may simulate hypertrophic pyloric stenosis. J Ultrasound Med 1998;17:705–711.
19. Westra S, Wolf B, Staalman C. Ultrasound diagnosis of gastroesophageal reflux and hiatal hernia in infants and young children. J Clin Ultrasound 1990;18:477–485.
20. Weinberger E, Winters W, Liddell R, et al. Sonographic diagnosis of intestinal malrotation in infants: importance of relative positions of the superior mesenteric vein and artery. AJR Am J Roentgenol 1992;159:825–828.
21. Birnbaum B, Wilson S. Appendicitis at the millennium. Radiology 2000;215:337–348.
22. Balthazar E, Birnbaum B, Yee J, et al. Acute appendicitis: CT and US correlation in 100 patients. Radiology 1994;190:31–35.
23. Rioux M. Sonographic detection of the normal and abnormal appendix. AJR Am J Roentgenol 1992;158:773–778.
24. Gore R, White E, Port R, et al. Acute appendicitis: a practical approach. Radiologist 1994;1:1–10.
25. Sivit C. Diagnosis of acute appendicitis in children: spectrum of sonographic findings. AJR Am J Roentgenol 1993;161:147–152.
26. Rettenbacher T, Hollerweger A, Macheiner P, et al. Presence or absence of gas in the appendix: additional criteria to rule out or confirm appendicitis—evaluation with US. Radiology 2000;214:183–187.
27. Lim H, Lee W, Kim T, et al. Appendicitis: usefulness of color Doppler US. Radiology 1996;201:221–225.
28. Abu-Yousef M, Bleichen J, Maher J, et al. High-resolution sonography of acute appendicitis. AJR Am J Roentgenol 1987;149:53–58.
29. Jeffrey RB, Jr, Jain KA, Nghiem HV. Sonographic diagnosis of acute appendicitis: interpretive pitfalls. AJR Am J Roentgenol 1994;162:55–59.
30. Lim H, Lee W, Lee S, et al. Focal appendicitis confined to the tip: diagnosis at US. Radiology 1996;200:799–801.
31. Cobben L, van Otterloo A, Puylaert J. Spontaneously resolving appendicitis: frequency and natural history in 60 patients. Radiology 2000;215:349–352.
32. Migraine S, Atri M, Bret P, et al. Spontaneously resolving acute appendicitis: clinical and sonographic documentation. Radiology 1997;205:55–58.
33. Madwed D, Mindelzun R, Jeffrey RB, Jr. Mucocele of the appendix: imaging findings. AJR Am J Roentgenol 1992;159:69–72.
34. Miller S, Landes A, Dautenhahn L, et al. Intussusception: ability of fluoroscopic images obtained during air enemas to depict lead points and other abnormalities. Radiology 1995;197:493–496.
35. del-Pozo G, Albillos J, Tejedor D, et al. Intussusception in children: current concepts in diagnosis and enema reduction. Radiographics 1999;19:299–319.
36. del-Pozo G, Albillos J, Tejedor D. Intussusception: US findings with pathologic correlation—the crescent-in-doughnut sign. Radiology 1996;199:688–692.
37. Anderson D. The pseudokidney sign. Radiology 1999;211:395–397.
38. del-Pozo G, Gonzalez-Spinola J, Gomez-Anson B, et al. Intussusception: trapped peritoneal fluid detected with US—relationship to reducibility and ischemia. Radiology 1996;201:379–383.
39. Lim H, Bae S, Lee K, et al. Assessment of reducibility of ileocolic intussusception in children: usefulness of color Doppler sonography. Radiology 1994;191:781–785.
40. Kong M, Wong H, Lin S, et al. Factors related to detection of blood flow by color Doppler ultrasonography in intussusception. J Ultrasound Med 1997;16:141–144.

41. Verschelden P, Filiatrault D, Garel L, et al. Intussusception in children: reliability of US in diagnosis. Radiology 1992;184:741–744.

42. Swischuk L, John S, Swischuk P. Spontaneous reduction of intussusception: verification with US. Radiology 1994;192:269–271.

43. McAlister W. Intussusception: even Hippocrates did not standardize his technique of enema reduction. Radiology 1998;206:595–598.

44. Meyers M, Oliphant M, Berne A, et al. The peritoneal ligaments and mesenteries: pathways of intraabdominal spread of disease. Radiology 1987;163:593–604.

45. Derchi L, Solbiati L, Rizzato G, et al. Normal anatomy and pathologic changes of the small bowel mesentery: US appearance. Radiology 1987;164:649–652.

46. Eistein DM, Tagliabue JR, Desai RK. Abdominal desmoids: CT findings in 25 patients. AJR Am J Roentgenol 1991;157:275–279.

47. Forte MD, Brant WE. Spontaneous isolated mesenteric fibromatosis. Diseases Colon Rectum 1988;31:315–317.

48. Stoupis C, Ros PR, Abbitt PL, et al. Bubbles in the belly: imaging of cystic mesenteric or omental masses. Radiographics 1994;14:729–737.

49. Ros P, Olmstead W, Moser RJ, et al. Mesenteric and omental cysts: histologic classification with imaging correlation. Radiology 1987;164:327–332.

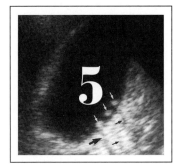

FEMALE PELVIS ULTRASOUND

Sonography plays the primary role in imaging of the female pelvis. CT and MR are supplemental techniques used when the US examination is equivocal and in the staging of pelvic malignancy. Primary indications for female pelvic US examination are pelvic pain, abnormal vaginal bleeding, and suspicion of pelvic mass. Additional indications include evaluation of precocious puberty, infertility, and early cancer detection.

IMAGING TECHNIQUE

US examination of the pelvis is routinely performed both transabdominally with a full bladder and transvaginally with the bladder empty. Additional examination techniques include the translabial imaging and sonohysterography.

Examination is often begun using the **transabdominal** (TA) approach. The patient is asked to fill her bladder by drinking several glasses of fluid and by not urinating for at least 1 hour prior to examination. The patient lies supine on the examination table. A 3.5–5.0-MHz sector transducer is placed on the lower abdomen just above the symphysis pubis and the pelvic organs are examined through the window of the distended bladder. Bladder filling is ideal when the bladder dome is just above the uterine fundus. Overdistention compresses the normal anatomy and displaces masses and fluid out of the pelvis. Underdistention limits visualization. Images are obtained in sagittal and transverse planes. To optimally image the uterus, the transducer is aligned with the long axis of the uterus, which is often angled right or left from the midline cervix. The ovaries and adnexa are often best seen by sliding the transducer to the contralateral side and angling back toward the ovary of interest. Measurements are obtained of the uterus, ovaries, and any masses detected in three orthogonal planes. Volumes may be calculated using the formula: volume = length × width × height × 0.52. The TA technique provides the best overview of the pelvis, and is best for examining large masses, but is less comfortable for the patient because of the distended bladder.

For **transvaginal** (TV) examination, the patient is asked to empty her bladder and lie supine with her legs flexed. Folded sheets or pads are placed under her buttocks to elevate her pelvis above the examination table to allow room for transducer manipulation. Alternatively, the patient may be examined on a pelvic examination table with her feet in stirrups. A 4.0–7.0-MHz TV US probe is coated with gel and is covered with a sterile condom that is also coated with gel. The probe may be placed in the vagina by the patient, the sonographer, or the sonologist. Prudence dictates that a woman should be in the room at all times during a vaginal sonogram, either as the examiner or as a chaperone [1]. The uterus is examined for size, shape, contour, orientation, and appearance of the myometrium, endometrium, and cervix. The ovaries are documented for size, shape, contour, echogenicity, and position. Any masses or abnormalities are evaluated for origin, echotexture, size, shape, and relationship to other organs. The cul-de-sac is examined for fluid and masses. Loops of bowel in the pelvis are inspected for peristalsis and wall thickening.

The TV technique offers better tissue characterization because of the ability to use high-frequency transducers. However, the field of view is limited and large masses may be overlooked. If TV examination is performed first, the pelvis should always be examined transabdominally, even if the bladder is empty, to check for abnormalities outside the TV field of view.

The **translabial** approach is particularly useful for examination of the vagina and cervix, and is an effective alternative for any patient unwilling or unable to undergo TV examination [2]. A 3.5–5.0-MHz sector transducer, covered with a transducer sheath and generously coated with gel, is placed on the labia. Examination is performed in sagittal and coronal planes along the long axis of the vagina.

A **transrectal** approach to pelvic US may also be used especially in patients unwilling or unable to undergo TV US. The transrectal approach offers similar advantages of placing the transducer closer to the organs of interest allowing higher frequency transducers with better resolution.

Sonohysterography (SHG) is a useful technique to examine the endometrium and uterine cavity [3–5]. The examination is easiest to perform with the patient on a pelvic examination table with her feet in stirrups. A speculum is used to visualize and cleanse the cervix with antiseptic solution. A 5-F pediatric feeding tube or a balloon SHG catheter, prefilled with sterile saline solution, is placed into the cervix. If a balloon catheter is used, the balloon is distended in the cervical canal with 3–5 mL of water, not air. The speculum is removed and a TV US transducer is placed into the vagina. Using direct US visualization, saline is injected to distend the uterine cavity, detect polypoid masses, and to assess the appearance and thickness of the endometrium.

ANATOMY

The size and shape of the **uterus** vary with age and parity. The uterus of the neonate, stimulated by maternal hormones as a fetus, is up to 1 cm longer and 1 cm larger in diameter than the uterus of a young child. The cervix is commonly twice as long and twice as thick as the body. By the end of the first year of life the uterus has become smaller and is sausage shaped. With puberty, the uterus assumes a pear shape with the body twice as large as the cervix. The uterus enlarges with multiparity and atrophies following menopause. Normal uterine dimensions are listed in Table 5.1.

The surface of the uterus is smooth and well defined (Fig. 5.1). A slightly indented isthmus separates the body from the cervix. The cervix is fixed in the midline of the pelvis,

Table 5.1: Normal Dimensions of the Uterus	
Stage of Life	*Normal Dimensions (cm)*
Neonate	$4 \times 2 \times 2$
Child (pre-pubertal)	$3 \times 1 \times 1$
Woman (nulliparous)	$8 \times 4 \times 4$
Woman (multiparous)	$9 \times 5 \times 5$
Woman (postmenopausal)	$7 \times 2 \times 2$

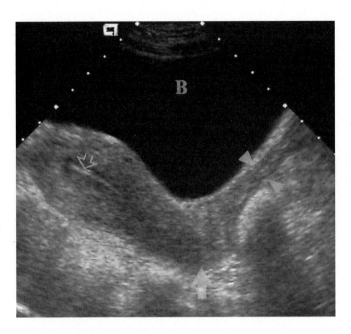

Figure 5.1 *Normal Uterus—Transabdominal.* Longitudinal scan through the urine-filled bladder (B) demonstrates a normal adult uterus with smooth contours, pear shape, and well-defined bright endometrial echo (*open arrow*). The cervix (*arrow*) is recognized at the junction of imaginary lines drawn through the long axis of the uterus and the long axis of the vagina (*between arrowheads*). This uterus is anteverted.

but the body is often "flexed" and angled ("verted") with respect to the cervix. The uterus is most commonly **anteflexed** and **anteverted**, lying on the bladder dome. A **retroflexed** uterus is bent at the isthmus with the body folded backwards on the cervix (Fig. 5.2). A **retroverted** uterus is straight but directed posteriorly. The body may also be angled toward the right or left pelvic sidewalls.

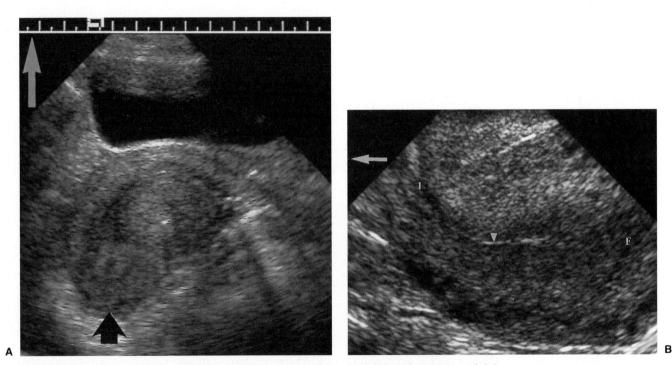

Figure 5.2 *Normal Uterus—Retroflexed.* Longitudinal transabdominal (*A*) and transvaginal (*B*) images demonstrate a normal retroflexed uterus. The uterus is flexed at the uterine isthmus (I) with the fundus (F, *black arrow*) directed posteriorly. The endometrium (*arrowhead*) is thin in the early proliferative phase. The large arrows indicate the direction of "up" when scanning transabdominally and transvaginally in longitudinal plane.

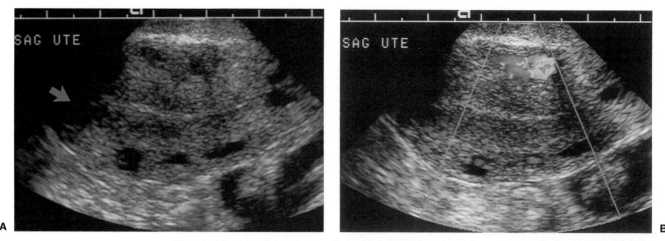

Figure 5.3 *Normal Arcuate Vessels.* Longitudinal transvaginal gray-scale (*A*) and corresponding color Doppler (*B*) images show prominent but normal arcuate vessels that divide the middle from the outer layer of myometrium. Visibility of these vessels varies greatly from patient to patient. This uterus is anteverted. The arrow shows the location of the fundus.

The **myometrium** is medium in echogenicity and granular in echotexture. Three layers of myometrium can often be recognized. The inner **junctional myometrium** is thin, compressed, hypovascular, and mildly hypoechoic compared to the thick homogeneous middle layer. The arcuate vessels, which are often prominent, divide the middle layer from the slightly hypoechoic outer layer (Fig. 5.3). Calcification of the arcuate arteries occurs in older women and diabetics (Fig. 5.4).

The **endometrium** varies in thickness and appearance with the degree of stimulation by hormones, primarily estrogens and progesterones (Table 5.2). In the neonate, because of maternal hormones, the endometrium is brightly echogenic but thin. In the prepubertal child, the endometrium remains thin and is nearly isoechoic with the myometrium. Following puberty, the endometrial appearance varies with the menstrual cycle [6]. In the **proliferative phase** (Fig. 5.5A), prior to ovulation, the endometrium assumes a three-layer appearance as it thickens to 4–8 mm. The central line, which defines the endometrial cavity, is echogenic. The proliferating **functional layer**, which will slough with menstruation, is hypoechoic. The outer **basal layer**, which remains intact throughout the menstrual cycle, is echogenic and surrounded by the hypoechoic junctional zone of the myometrium. In the **secretory phase**, following ovulation, the functional layer continues to thicken and becomes echogenic (Fig. 5.5B). The entire double-layer thickness of the endometrium in the secretory phase is 7–14 mm. During menstruation, the functional layer is lost and the

Because the appearance of the ovaries and uterus varies dramatically with the menstrual cycle, patients should always be queried as to their menstrual history and the date of their last menstrual period.

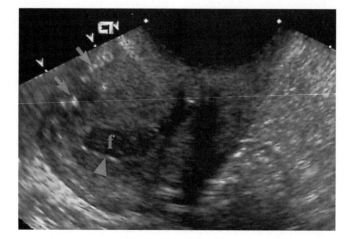

Figure 5.4 *Calcified Arcuate Arteries.* Transvaginal image of the uterus of an 85-year-old woman reveals calcification in the arcuate arteries (*arrows*). These calcifications occur as a result of atherosclerosis. This patient also has a small amount of fluid (f) in the uterine cavity. The thin, well-defined endometrial stripe (*arrowhead*) indicates the endometrium is benign and atrophic. Clinical evaluation is needed to look for evidence of cervical carcinoma.

Table 5.2: Normal Endometrial Appearance and Thickness

Phase	Normal Thickness (mm)	Appearance
Proliferative phase (pre-ovulation)	4–8	Triple layer (hyper-hypo-hyper)
Secretory phase (post-ovulation)	7–14	Uniform hyperechoic
Menstrual phase	1–2	Thin, broken echogenic line
Postmenopausal without bleeding	<8	Uniform hyperechoic
Postmenopausal with bleeding	<5 = endometrial atrophy >5 = risk of carcinoma	Uniform hyperechoic
Postmenopausal on hormone replacement therapy	Add 1–2 mm to values listed for postmenopausal women	Uniform hyperechoic

Endometrial thickness is measured perpendicular to the long axis of the uterine cavity and includes both the anterior and posterior endometrial layers. Any fluid in the endometrial cavity and the hypoechoic junctional zone myometrium is not included in the measurement.

remaining basal endometrium appears as a thin, broken, irregular echogenic line. Following menopause, the endometrium atrophies, thins (to <4 mm), and becomes less echogenic. Hormone replacement therapy in the postmenopausal woman will stimulate the endometrium. Unopposed estrogen has the greatest effect. Sequential hormone replacement, with estrogen followed by progesterone, causes the endometrium to change to an appearance very similar to the premenopausal woman.

The **fallopian tubes** extend laterally from the uterus in the free edge of the broad ligament. Each is 7–12 cm in length and consists of an **intramural** portion traversing the myometrium, a cord-like **isthmus**, a wider and tortuous **ampullary** portion, and the funnel-shaped, fimbriated **infundibulum** that opens into the peritoneal cavity. The fallopian tubes are not appreciated on US unless they are dilated or when peritoneal fluid defines the edge of the broad ligament.

The **ovaries** are elliptical in shape and lobulated in contour. Follicles project from the outer cortex, and the stroma and blood vessels occupy the inner medulla (Fig. 5.6). The ovaries are attached to the uterus by a fold of the broad ligament called the ovarian ligament, and to the pelvic sidewall by the suspensory ligament of the ovary. The fallopian tubes in the broad ligament and the mesosalpinx drape over the ovary. The ovaries are

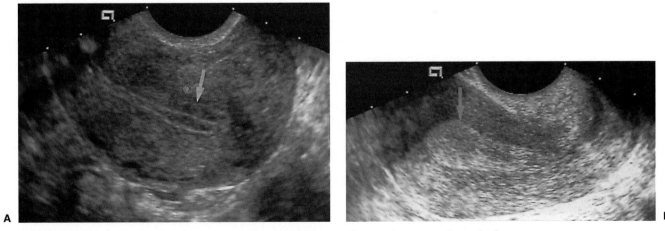

Figure 5.5 Physiologic Changes in the Endometrium. A. Proliferative phase endometrium (*arrow*) of the first half of the menstrual cycle has a triple-layer appearance. The outer (basal layer) endometrium is echogenic. The inner functional endometrium is hypoechoic, and the line demarcating the uterine cavity is echogenic. *B.* Secretory phase endometrium (*arrow*) of the second half of the menstrual cycle is uniformly echogenic and thickens to 7–14 mm.

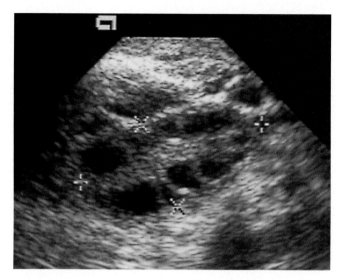

Figure 5.6 *Normal Ovary. A normal ovary (marked by calipers) is shown in this transvaginal image. Normal follicles outline the periphery of the ovary, whereas echogenic stroma is seen centrally.*

imaged in a shallow fossa anterior to the internal iliac vessels and medial to the external iliac vessels. The ovaries are displaced cephalad by increasing bladder distention. When the uterus is positioned toward the pelvic sidewall, the ipsilateral ovary is frequently located cephalad to the fundus. When the uterus is retroverted, the ovaries are usually ventral to the uterus at the level of the uterine body.

The size and appearance of the ovaries change with age and with phase of the menstrual cycle (Table 5.3) [6]. In children younger than 8 years of age, the ovaries are homogeneous and solid [7]. Occasionally small follicles (<9 mm) are present. Normal **follicles** appear as anechoic, thin-walled cysts on the periphery of the ovary. In the follicular (proliferative) phase of the menstrual cycles, elevated levels of follicle-stimulating hormone and luteinizing hormone stimulate the development and enlargement of a variable number of follicles [6]. One follicle becomes dominant and matures as the Graafian follicle. This **dominant follicle** reaches a size of 20–25 mm, whereas most of the other follicles involute. Ovulation occurs when the dominant follicle ruptures, releasing the ovum and 15–25 ml of fluid into the peritoneal cavity. Mid-cycle pain, "mittelschmertz," coincides with ovulation. The **corpus luteum** develops at the site of the ruptured dominant follicle. Blood clot and fibroblasts invade the collapsed follicle, which becomes intensely vascular and reforms a lymph and blood-filled cyst. The corpus luteum produces progesterone that supports the secretory endometrium to allow successful implantation if fertilization of the ovum occurs. The corpus luteum will degenerate in 14 days in the absence of an intervening pregnancy.

Size of the ovary is evaluated by measurement and calculation of volume using the standard formula (length × width × height × 0.52). Normal values are given in Table 5.3 [8–10]. The ovaries shrink with age after menopause [10].

Table 5.3: Normal Size of the Ovaries

Phase of Life	Mean Volume (cc)	Upper Limit of Normal Volume (cc)
0–3 months	1	4
3 months–2 years	1	3
Premenarchal (3–15 years)	3	9
Menstrual female	10	22
Postmenopausal	6	14
>15 years after menopause	2	4

Adapted from Cohen H, Shapiro M, Mandel F, et al. Normal ovaries in neonates and infants: a sonographic study of 77 patients 1 day to 24 months old. AJR Am J Roentgenol 1993;160:583–586; Cohen H, Tive H, Mandel F. Ovarian volumes measured by US: bigger than we think. Radiology 1990;177:189–192; and Tepper R, Zalel Y, Markov S, et al. Ovarian volume in postmenopausal women—suggestions to an ovarian size nomogram for menopausal age. Acta Obstet Gynecol Scand 1993;74:208–211.

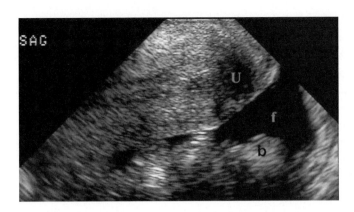

Figure 5.7 *Normal Fluid in the Cul-de-Sac.* Anechoic fluid (f) is seen in the cul-de-sac posterior to the uterus (U). The fluid outlines loops of small bowel (b).

The ovaries have a dual blood supply from the ovarian artery and from an adnexal branch of the uterine artery. Spectral Doppler shows high resistance flow in the first half of the menstrual cycle and low resistance flow in the second half after formation of the corpus luteum. The ovaries are hypovascular after menopause with flow detected only in the main ovarian artery.

The cul-de-sac frequently contains a small volume of fluid (~10 cc) that is best seen on TV US. A small volume of fluid is normal and physiologic (Fig. 5.7). The volume of fluid is increased with ovulation.

The normal **vagina** is a muscular tube in the midline of the pelvis extending from the vestibule of the external genitalia to the cervix. The cervix projects into the vaginal apex and is surrounded by vaginal recesses called the *fornices*. On sagittal images, the vagina appears as a tubular structure with hypoechoic muscular walls and a bright linear central echo caused by the apposing surfaces of the vaginal mucosa (Fig. 5.1). On transverse images (Fig. 5.8), the vagina appears as a flattened oval or flattened H-shaped structure with folds of vaginal mucosa laterally and the urethra coursing prominently in the anterior vaginal wall.

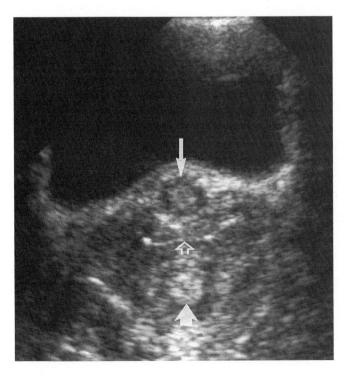

Figure 5.8 *Normal Urethra and Vagina.* Low transverse image shows the urethra (*long arrow*) in the anterior wall of the vagina. The muscular walls of the vagina appear hypoechoic compared to the echogenic line (*open arrow*) that marks the collapsed lumen and mucosa. The rectum (*short arrow*) is posterior.

> ### Box 5.1: Causes of Thickening of the Endometrium
>
> Secretory phase endometrium
> Decidual reaction of pregnancy
>   Early intrauterine pregnancy
>   Ectopic pregnancy
>   Incomplete abortion
>
> Gestational trophoblastic disease
> Endometrial hyperplasia
> Endometrial polyps
> Endometrial carcinoma
> Intrauterine adhesions

UTERUS

ENDOMETRIAL ABNORMALITIES

Measuring Endometrial Thickness

Recurrence of vaginal bleeding in postmenopausal women is a common and potentially ominous complaint, with cancer as the cause of approximately 10% of cases. The majority of cases are caused by benign conditions including endometrial atrophy, hyperplasia, and polyps (Box 5.1). Conventional teaching has been that every postmenopausal woman with vaginal bleeding should undergo dilatation and curettage to sample the endometrium. US has provided a method of visualizing the endometrium and of being more selective in identifying patients for biopsy. US is used to assess the appearance and measure the thickness of the endometrium.

To properly use established criteria for basing the decision to biopsy on the thickness of the endometrium, the endometrium must be measured correctly. Endometrial thickness measurements are made "double layer" and include both the anterior and posterior endometrium (Fig. 5.9). The measurement is made perpendicular to the long axis of the uterine cavity where the endometrium is thickest and excludes any fluid in the cavity and the hypoechoic junctional myometrium. TV measurements are the most accurate. SHG aids in evaluation of the endometrium by outlining the endometrium surface and defining any polypoid protrusions [11]. A thin endometrium (<4 mm) or diffuse, smooth, regular thickening of the endometrium is the best predictor of benignancy [12]. Endometrial masses, irregular thickening, or focal thickening requires biopsy to exclude malignancy. In some patients, especially women with leiomyoma, the endometrium is distorted and is not adequately visualized for accurate measurement (~3% of patients) [13]. These women should undergo SHG or biopsy for diagnosis.

Criteria for biopsy as recommended by most authors is to biopsy patients with postmenopausal bleeding if the double-layer endometrial thickness exceeds 5 mm [13,14]. In

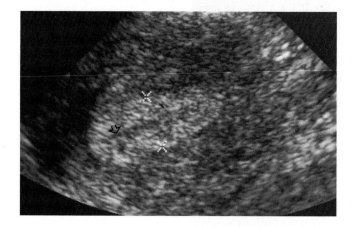

Figure 5.9 *Measuring Endometrial Thickness.* Transvaginal image shows two well-defined endometrial layers separated by the dark line demarcating the endometrial cavity (*arrow*). Measurement (*calipers, x*) is made perpendicular to the long axis of the uterine cavity and includes the thickness of both layers of the endometrium. This postmenopausal patient has benign endometrial hyperplasia.

patients who are asymptomatic, that is, specifically, without vaginal bleeding, the endometrium is considered normal up to 8 mm. Endometrial thickness >15 mm in a postmenopausal patient is very high risk for malignancy.

Hormone Replacement Therapy

In postmenopausal women, hormone replacement therapy is commonly prescribed to abate menopausal symptoms and to prevent osteoporosis. The supplemental hormones have a small but notable effect on the appearance of the endometrium [15].

- Unopposed estrogen therapy and concurrent estrogen and progesterone therapy increase endometrial thickness by 1.0–1.5 mm.
- Sequential estrogen-progesterone therapy increases stripe thickness by 3.0 mm.

Endometrial Atrophy

Atrophy of the endometrium is the most common cause of postmenopausal bleeding (~60% of cases). The endometrium becomes inactive and atrophies as estrogen stimulation diminishes with menopause.

- Uniform thin endometrium (<5 mm) (Figs. 5.4, 5.10).
- Cystic changes may occur and result in thickening of the endometrium.
- Blood flow on Doppler US is minimal or absent.

Endometrial Hyperplasia

Endometrial hyperplasia is a proliferation of endometrial glands, which increase in size and assume an irregular shape. The hyperplasia is caused by unopposed stimulation of the endometrium by estrogen. Hormone replacement therapy with only estrogen is the most common cause of hyperplasia in postmenopausal women. In premenopausal women, causes include recurring anovulatory cycles, polycystic ovary disease, and obesity. Hyperplasia may be focal or diffuse, and is classified as adenomatous, cystic, or atypical adenomatous. Up to 25% of patients with endometrial hyperplasia with atypia will eventually develop endometrial cancer.

> The endometrium is considered abnormally thickened if it exceeds 14 mm in a premenopausal women, 5 mm in a postmenopausal woman with vaginal bleeding, or 8 mm in a postmenopausal woman without vaginal bleeding.

- Diffuse or focal smooth thickening of the echogenic endometrium (Fig. 5.9).
- Cystic changes are common.
- Atypical hyperplasia often appears heterogeneous and irregular (Fig. 5.11).

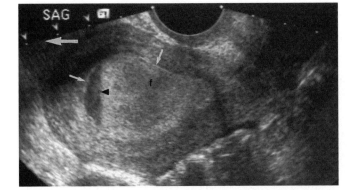

Figure 5.10 *Endometrial Atrophy and Cervical Stenosis.* Echogenic fluid (f) fills and distends the uterine cavity and shows a fluid-fluid level (*black arrowhead*). The large white arrow indicates the direction of "up" on this transvaginal image. The endometrium (*small white arrows*) is thin and regular with double-layer thickness of 2 mm indicating endometrial atrophy in this 65-year-old patient. The fluid in the uterine cavity is excluded from the endometrial measurement. Further clinical evaluation confirmed cervical stenosis.

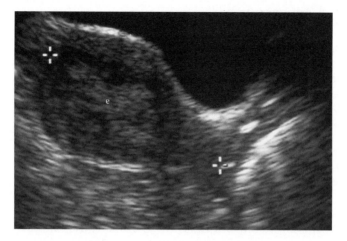

Figure 5.11 *Atypical Endometrial Hyperplasia.* The endometrium (e) is irregularly thickened, lobulated in contour, and has an ill-defined margin. Endometrial biopsy revealed endometrial hyperplasia with atypia. This is a transabdominal image in sagittal plane. Cursors (+) mark the extent of the uterus.

Endometrial Polyps

Endometrial polyps are localized, pedunculated, or broad-based growths of endometrial tissue that commonly cause bleeding. Polyps peak in prevalence in the fifth decade of life, but may be a cause of infertility in younger patients. Approximately 20% present after menopause. On routine TV sonography, the polyps appear as a non-specific echogenic thickening of the endometrium. However, when fluid is naturally present in the endometrial cavity or is introduced during SHG, an oval echogenic mass of intraluminal endometrium is evident. Treatment is resection by dilatation and curettage or by hysteroscopy.

- Focal polypoid thickening of the endometrium (Fig. 5.12) [16].
- Polyps may be pedunculated on a narrow stalk or broad-based (Fig. 5.13).
- Vascular pedicle is demonstrable on color Doppler US.
- Echogenicity is uniform, hyperechoic relative to myometrium and isoechoic to endometrium.
- Cystic areas are occasionally present within the polyp.
- Polyps are differentiated from submucosal leiomyomas by the uniform high echogenicity of the polyp (Fig. 5.13) [17].
- Multiple polyps are present in 20% of cases.

Endometrial Carcinoma

Endometrial carcinoma is the most common gynecologic malignancy, occurring in 3% of American women. Most cases (80%) occur in postmenopausal women and most present with abnormal vaginal bleeding. Endometrial carcinoma is the cause of 7–30% of postmenopausal bleeding. US shows thickening of the endometrium that is often indistinguishable from hyperplasia and polyps. Signs that suggest cancer include inho-

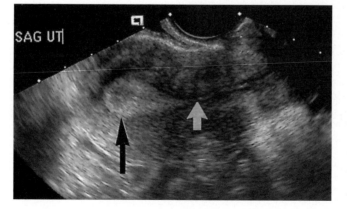

Figure 5.12 *Endometrial Polyp.* Focal, smooth, echogenic thickening of the endometrium (*long black arrow*) is contrasted with a long segment of thin endometrium (*short white arrow*). This appearance suggests an endometrial polyp. Diagnosis can be confirmed with a sonohysterogram.

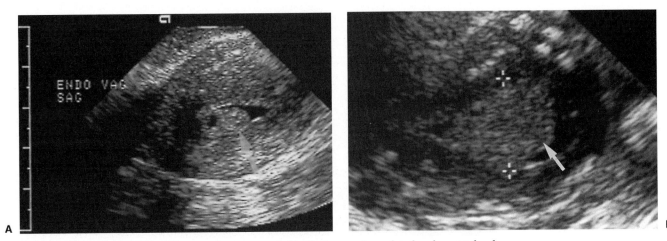

A   B

Figure 5.13 *Endometrial Polyps.* Two sonohysterograms (*A, B*) show pedunculated endometrial polyps (*arrows*) outlined by fluid instilled into the endometrial cavity. Note the high echogenicity of the polyp equal to that of the endometrium. Compare to the low echogenicity of the submucosal leiomyomas in Figure 5.16. Calipers (+) measure the size of the polyp in B.

mogeneous echogenicity, irregular and poorly defined margins, and invasion of the myometrium [18].

- Thickened endometrium is a hallmark sign. Endometrial thickening >15 mm in post-menopausal women has a high risk of malignancy.
- The endometrium is usually diffusely or partially echogenic (80–90%).
- The endometrium is unevenly thickened and irregular in contour in 60–70% (Fig. 5.14).
- Smooth, uniform, endometrial thickening indistinguishable from endometrial hyperplasia is present in 30–40%.
- Poorly defined endometrium that is difficult to visualize suggests carcinoma (Fig. 5.15).
- Cystic changes are present in 24%.

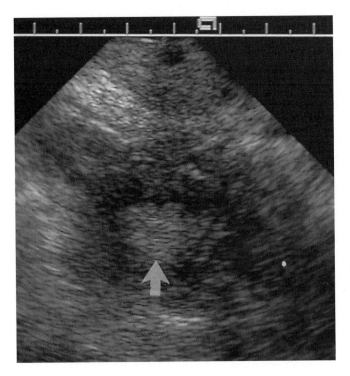

Figure 5.14 *Endometrial Carcinoma.* The endometrium (*arrow*) is thickened (to 12 mm) and is irregular in contour. Echogenicity is that of normal endometrium. Biopsy confirmed endometrial carcinoma. This transvaginal US image is in coronal plane.

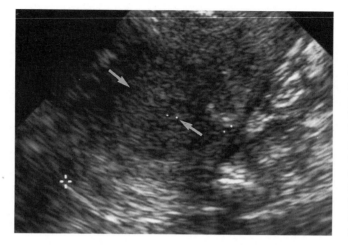

Figure 5.15 Endometrial Carcinoma. This postmenopausal patient presented with new onset uterine bleeding. On transvaginal US, the endometrium (*between arrows*) is low in echogenicity, very poorly defined, and thickened (>15 mm). This appearance is highly predictive of endometrial carcinoma, which was confirmed at biopsy. The cursor (+) marks the fundus of the uterus.

- Some carcinomas are polypoid with a broad base.
- Lack of distensibility of the endometrial canal may be evident on SHG [17].
- Calcification is rare.

Tamoxifen-Related Endometrial Changes

Tamoxifen is an antiestrogen chemotherapeutic agent used in patients with breast cancer [19]. Although it is used for its antiestrogen, tumor-suppressive effects, the drug has proliferative effects on the endometrium and may promote endometrial tumor growth. Histologic changes reported with tamoxifen therapy include endometrial hyperplasia, endometrial polyps, and endometrial carcinoma [20,21]. Cystic change is characteristic. Thickness of the endometrium increases with duration of tamoxifen therapy especially after 5 years.

- The endometrium is irregularly thickened (usually >8 mm in postmenopausal patients).
- Multicystic changes in the thickened endometrium is characteristic.
- Endometrial polyps are common (33%).

Submucosal Leiomyoma

Leiomyomas located just beneath the endometrium are prone to ulceration and bleeding. They compress the endometrium, may bulge into the endometrial cavity, and may become a polypoid mass within the endometrial cavity. SHG is used to characterize the size and intraluminal extent of the mass so that surgical resection can be optimally planned using either a TA or hysteroscopic approach.

- Hypoechoic mass just beneath the endometrium (Fig. 5.16).
- The mass may cause acoustic shadowing.
- The mass compresses the endometrium and may project into the endometrial cavity.
- Vascularity, demonstrated by color Doppler, helps to differentiate leiomyomas from blood clots.
- Low and heterogeneous echogenicity differentiates leiomyomas from echogenic endometrial polyps (Fig. 5.16) [17].
- Leiomyomas commonly calcify.

Intrauterine Device

Intrauterine devices (IUDs) are currently in less common use because of complications of endometritis, ectopic pregnancy, and uterine perforation. US is effectively used to document IUD location when the IUD string is lost or to confirm proper IUD placement.

- IUDs are seen as brightly echogenic structures in uterine cavity. The appearance depends upon the type of IUD.
- The normal location for an IUD is centered in the uterine cavity near the fundus.

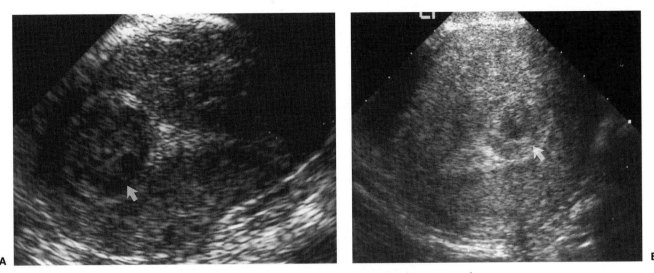

Figure 5.16 *Submucosal Leiomyomas.* Sonograms on two patients (*A*, *B*) show the characteristic low echogenicity of submucosal leiomyomas (*arrows*) that protrude into the uterine cavity. Compare with the appearance of endometrial polyps in Figure 5.12.

- Copper-wrapped IUDs are intensely echogenic and cause comet tail artifacts (Fig. 5.17). Most are in the shape of a 7 or a T.
- Lippes loops have a regular pattern of repeating echogenic foci that cast acoustic shadows.

Fluid in the Endometrial Canal

A small volume of anechoic fluid in the endometrial canal is common in postmenopausal women (Fig. 5.4). It usually reflects cervical stenosis, or results from hormone replacement therapy [22]. According to one study, if the single layer endometrium measures 3 mm or less (<6 mm double layer), the endometrium is atrophic and inactive, so no further evaluation of the endometrium is necessary (Figs. 5.4, 5.10) [23]. Patients should be examined clinically for evidence of cervical carcinoma.

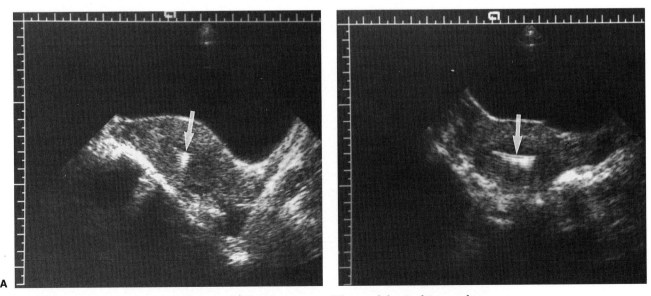

Figure 5.17 *Copper-Wrapped IUD.* Longitudinal (*A*) and transverse (*B*) transabdominal images demonstrate the characteristic appearance of a copper-wire-wrapped IUD (*arrows*) in normal location in the uterine cavity. Note the comet tail artifacts deep to the IUD.

Intrauterine Adhesions

Adhesions are formed by scarring that fastens the walls of the uterus together and obliterates part or all of the uterine cavity [24]. Patients with a history of repeated uterine instrumentation or uterine infections are at highest risk. Patients present with amenorrhea or repeated spontaneous abortion.

- Adhesions appear as an irregular hypoechoic bridge that interrupts the endometrium and is in continuity with the myometrium. Size, shape, and extent are variable.
- Adhesions are best seen when fluid is present in the endometrial cavity either naturally or during SHG.

Endometritis

Endometritis occurs within the spectrum of pelvic inflammatory disease (PID). Puerperal endometritis is most common 2–5 days after delivery.

- The endometrium is thickened and edematous.
- Fluid is usually found in the endometrial cavity. It is commonly echogenic and layers producing fluid-fluid levels.
- Gas in the endometrial cavity is found in 15% of patients. This is not a specific finding in the postpartum patient. In women with uncomplicated vaginal deliveries, gas may be found in the endometrial cavity in 19% of women during the first 3 postpartum days and in 7% of women for 3 weeks postpartum [25].

MYOMETRIAL ABNORMALITIES

Leiomyomas

Leiomyomas are the most common tumor of the female pelvis, occurring in up to 40% of women older than age 35 [26] years. The tumors are composed of smooth muscle with variable amount of fibrous connective tissue. Most leiomyomas cause no symptoms, but they can cause menorrhagia, dysmenorrhea, irregular uterine bleeding, pelvic pain, infertility, and the discomfort of a large pelvic mass. Tumors grow in response to estrogen and typically enlarge during pregnancy and regress after menopause. Tumor location is described as intramural, submucosal (beneath the endometrium), or subserosal (on the surface of the uterus).

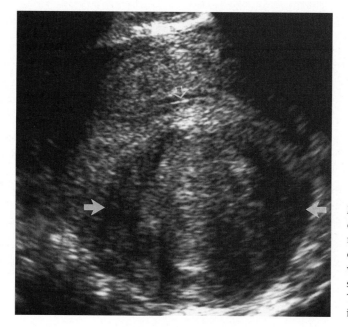

Figure 5.18 Leiomyoma. Leiomyoma appears as a hypoechoic mass (*between arrows*) in the wall of the uterus. Fibrous areas within the leiomyoma cause streaks of acoustic shadowing. The endometrium (*open arrow*) is bowed around the leiomyoma.

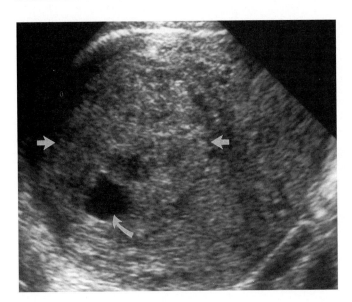

Figure 5.19 *Cystic Change in Leiomyoma.* An intramural leiomyoma (*between arrows*) with echogenicity slightly greater than normal myometrium shows an area of cystic necrosis (*curved arrow*).

- A round to oval, solid, hypoechoic mass is typical. Refractory acoustic shadowing produced by fibrous elements within the tumor is highly indicative of leiomyoma (Fig. 5.18) [27].
- Inhomogeneous myometrium is produced by numerous small leiomyomas.
- Tumors cause a focal bulge in the uterine contour (intramural leiomyoma), or compress and distort the endometrium (submucosal leiomyoma).
- Necrosis, hemorrhage, and cystic changes are common (Fig. 5.19). Irregular, coarse calcifications are characteristic (Fig. 5.20).
- Isoechoic tumors may be undetectable or cause only uterine enlargement.
- Subserosal fibroids may become pedunculated and present as an adnexal mass. Diagnosis is made by color flow US demonstration of a vascular pedicle continuous with the myometrium (Fig. 5.21).
- Lipomatous leiomyomas contain benign fat cells. With high fat content, the tumors are intensely echogenic.
- Pedunculated serosal leiomyomas on a narrow stalk may parasitize blood supply from adjacent structures and detach from the uterus [28]. These are called *parasitic leiomyomas.*

Leiomyomas are common and so variable in appearance they may be included in nearly every differential diagnosis of pelvic abnormality.

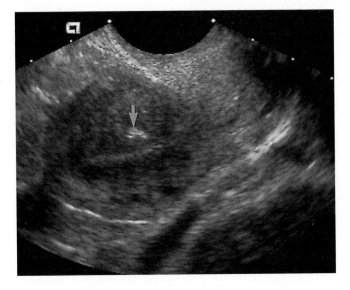

Figure 5.20 *Calcification in Leiomyoma.* A characteristic coarse calcification (*arrow*) is seen within an intramural leiomyoma that causes a focal bulge in the contour of the uterus.

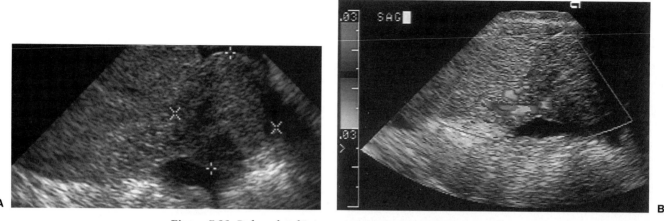

Figure 5.21 *Pedunculated Leiomyoma. A.* Transvaginal US image shows a hypoechoic mass (*outlined by cursors, x, +*) adjacent to the uterus. *B.* Color Doppler image in the same location shows contiguous blood flow from the uterus into the mass, confirming a pedunculated leiomyoma (see Color Figure 5.21A, B).

Leiomyosarcoma

Leiomyosarcoma of the uterus is a rare lesion accounting for approximately 1% of uterine malignancy. Accurate diagnosis by US or other imaging is difficult. Most patients are asymptomatic, although some present with abnormal uterine bleeding.

■ The most suspicious finding is documented rapid enlargement of a solid uterine mass that otherwise has the appearance of a benign leiomyoma. Local invasion, regional adenopathy, and distant metastases are signs of advanced malignancy.

■ Many leiomyosarcomas resemble degenerated leiomyomas in appearance with marked heterogeneity and areas of necrosis and hemorrhage. Some are indistinguishable from benign leiomyomas (Fig. 5.22).

Adenomyosis

Adenomyosis is a common condition with subtle and non-specific US findings. Patients with suspicious findings should be referred for MR to provide a more specific diagnosis.

The presence of endometrial glands and stroma within the myometrium is termed *adenomyosis* [29–31]. Adenomyosis is a major cause of dysmenorrhea, menorrhagia, and uterine enlargement that affects 15–20% of women, especially in their perimenopausal years.

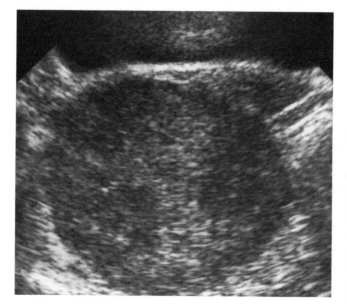

Figure 5.22 *Leiomyosarcoma.* Homogeneous solid mass near the uterine fundus proved to be a leiomyosarcoma. The patient presented with symptoms of partial small bowel obstruction. Computed tomography (not shown) revealed invasion of adjacent small bowel. The echotexture of this leiomyosarcoma is indistinguishable from a benign leiomyoma.

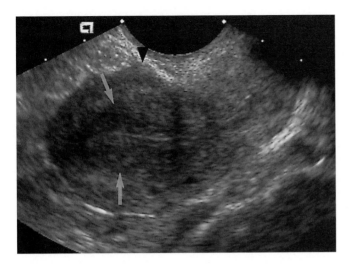

Figure 5.23 *Adenomyosis.* The US findings of adenomyosis are commonly subtle. This image illustrates widening and irregularity of the junctional zone myometrium (*arrows*). A small leiomyoma (*black arrowhead*) causes a focal bulge in the uterine contour.

Dense, tightly packed, myometrial cells surround the ectopic endometrial glands. MR is the most sensitive method for imaging diagnosis. US findings are subtle and non-specific [32].

- US shows areas of decreased echogenicity or heterogeneous myometrium (~75% of cases). The foci of decreased echogenicity correspond to smooth muscle hyperplasia. The heterogeneous foci correspond to the endometrial implants (Fig. 5.23) [32].
- Tiny cysts in the junctional myometrium result from dilated cystic endometrial glands or from foci of hemorrhage.
- Echogenic linear striations extend from the endometrium into the myometrium.
- The junction between endometrium and myometrium is poorly defined.
- Diffuse uterine enlargement with normal-appearing myometrium and endometrium may be the only finding.
- The hypoechoic junctional zone myometrium shows focal or diffuse thickening (Fig. 5.23).

Uterine Arteriovenous Malformations
Arteriovenous malformations (AVMs) of the uterus are a rare cause of uterine bleeding [33]. Most AVMs are isolated and congenital but some occur as a result of curettage or other uterine surgery, pelvic trauma, pregnancy, or uterine cancer. AVMs are a tangle of abnormal vessels without a capillary network.

- On gray-scale US, AVMs appear as tubular spaces in the myometrium, or as an ill-defined mass in the myometrium, endometrium, or cervix [33].
- Parauterine vessels may be prominent.
- Color Doppler shows an intensely colorful, tangled network of vessels with prominent turbulence and aliasing.
- Spectral Doppler shows high systolic velocities (>96 cm/sec) and low resistance spectra (Resistive Index [RI] = 0.25–0.55).

Arcuate Artery Calcification
Arteries that course between the intermediate and outer layers of the myometrium commonly develop atherosclerotic calcification in elderly, diabetic, or hypertensive women.

- Multiple small echogenic foci in the boundary zone between intermediate and outer layer myometrium (Fig. 5.4).
- Doppler confirms arterial flow if the vessels are patent.

Junctional Zone Calcification
Dystrophic calcifications in the junctional zone myometrium are caused by injury from prior instrumentation or biopsy.

■ Punctate echodensities are seen in the junctional zone. Acoustic shadowing may be present.

CERVICAL ABNORMALITIES

Abnormalities of the cervix are best evaluated by clinical examination. TV US demonstrates the cervix well if the transducer is withdrawn slightly and angled toward the cervix. Installation of water into the vagina improves visualization of the cervix [34].

Cervical Stump

Supracervical hysterectomy was formerly a common procedure, leaving behind a stump of cervix that may be mistaken for a mass at the apex of the vaginal vault.

■ Remnant of normal cervix appears as a solid tubular structure with cervical muscle appearing identical to myometrium and the endocervical mucosa forming a thin bright central linear echo.

Nabothian Cysts

Nabothian cysts are common benign inclusion cysts of the cervical mucosa. They are of no clinical significance.

■ Simple cysts are seen within or projecting from the cervix. They vary in size from 1–2 mm up to 4 cm and are commonly multiple (Fig. 5.24).
■ Internal fluid is anechoic except in rare instances when traumatic hemorrhage or infection results in internal debris.

Cervical Polyp

Polyps arise from the endocervical mucosa and are a common cause of abnormal bleeding.

■ Well-defined oval or round masses are seen in the endocervical canal or protruding from the cervix. Polyps are isoechoic with the endocervical mucosa [35].

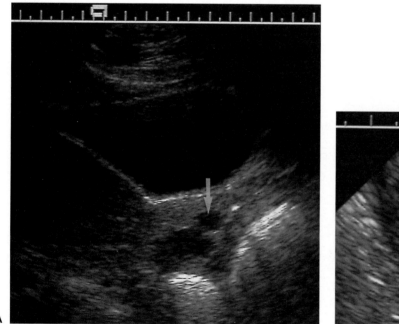
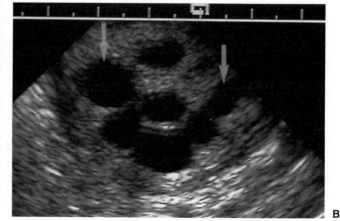

Figure 5.24 *Nabothian Cysts.* Transabdominal longitudinal (*A*) and transvaginal transverse (*B*) images of the cervix illustrate the characteristic appearance of nabothian cysts (*arrows*).

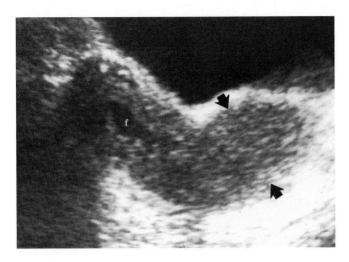

Figure 5.25 *Cervical Carcinoma.* The cervix (*between arrows*) is bulbous and somewhat ill defined on this transabdominal image. A small volume of fluid (f) is present in the uterine cavity. Cervical leiomyoma may have a similar appearance. Carcinoma was confined to the cervix on pathological examination.

Cervical Leiomyoma

Leiomyomas arising in the cervix account for 8% of uterine leiomyomas.

- Solid nodules are seen within or extending from the cervix. Prolapse into the vagina is common.
- Echogenicity is heterogeneous but lesions are hypoechoic compared to endocervical mucosa and usually isoechoic to cervical muscle [35].

Cervical Carcinoma

Cancers of the cervix are primarily diagnosed clinically.

- Inhomogeneous enlarged cervix (Fig. 5.25). Invasion and fixation of paracervical tissues and the upper vagina are common (Fig. 5.26).
- The appearance of early cervical cancer overlaps the appearance of cervical leiomyoma (Fig. 5.25).

DEVELOPMENTAL ABNORMALITIES

Developmental anomalies of the uterus are commonly detected with US but are more completely characterized by MR [36]. Uterine anomalies occur in 5–6% of women and are associated with an increased rate of infertility, spontaneous abortion, and other obstetric complications. The uterus, cervix, fallopian tubes, and upper vagina arise embryologically from paired müllerian ducts, which must migrate caudally and fuse with each other as well as with the distal wolffian ducts to result in normal development. Anomalies result from arrested development of the müllerian ducts, failure of fusion of the müllerian ducts, or fail-

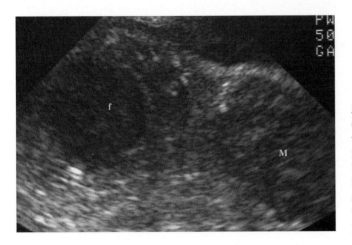

Figure 5.26 *Advanced Cervical Carcinoma.* The cervix and upper vaginal region are replaced by an ill-defined soft tissue mass (M). Echogenic fluid (f) fills the uterine cavity. This cervical cancer, stage IIIB, invaded the anterior vaginal wall and extended to the pelvic side wall.

ure of resorption of the midline uterine septum. Renal anomalies occur in 30% of women with müllerian defects. Unilateral renal agenesis is the most common associated anomaly. US examination must be careful, detailed, and correlated with physical examination to arrive at an accurate diagnosis. Questionable cases should be referred for MR examination.

Uterine Aplasia and Uterus Unicornis Unicollis

These anomalies result from arrested development of the müllerian ducts. If both müllerian ducts are aplastic, the uterus is congenitally absent. If one müllerian duct is aplastic, the uterus develops with only one uterine horn but has a normal single cervix (uterus unicornis unicollis). Hypoplasia of one müllerian duct results in hypoplasia of one uterine horn.

- **Congenital absence of the uterus** is exceedingly rare. The uterus, cervix, fallopian tubes, and upper four-fifths of the vagina are absent in a female of normal genotype. The vagina may be only a shallow external dimple.
- **Unicornate uterus** may be difficult to recognize by US. The uterus appears small and is usually positioned to one side of the pelvis [37]. Hypoplasia of one horn is far more common than aplasia. The hypoplastic horn may contain fluid if endometrium is present within the horn.
- The hypoplastic uterine horn may be mistaken for an adnexal mass.

Duplication Anomalies

Complete failure of fusion of the two müllerian ducts results in complete duplication (uterus didelphys). Greater degrees of müllerian duct fusion result in lesser degrees of duplication.

- The key to US recognition of these anomalies is to recognize a deep external concave fundal cleft that defines the abnormal separation of the two uterine horns. The normal fundus is smoothly contoured and is convex externally.
- **Uterus didelphys** describes the presence of two vaginas, two cervices and two separated uterine horns.
- **Uterus bicornis bicollis** describes two separate uterine horns with two cervices and one vagina.
- **Uterus bicornis unicollis** describes two separate uterine horns with a single cervix and vagina.

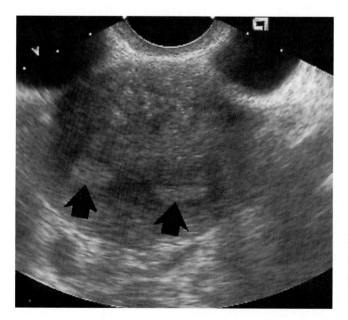

Figure 5.27 *Septate Uterus.* Transvaginal image shows two endometrial complexes (*arrows*) separated by a muscular septum. The uterine fundus was convex externally.

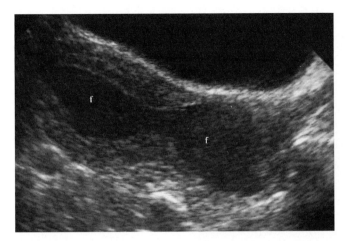

Figure 5.28 *Hematometra.* The endometrial and endocervical canals (f) are distended with bloody echogenic fluid in this patient with cervical stenosis.

- **Arcuate uterus** (uterus arcuatus) describes a partial indentation of the uterine fundus with minimal alteration of the uterine cavity.
- Any uterine anomaly may be associated with a transverse septum that obstructs menstrual outflow and results in hematometra and hematocolpos.
- Uterine anomalies commonly are discovered in early pregnancy when fluid outlines the uterine cavity and reveals the separated uterine horns.
- Careful attention to the endometrial echo, especially in transverse plane, also documents the separated uterine cavity by showing two endometrial complexes (Fig. 5.27).
- Be sure to examine the kidneys for associated anomalies in all cases. Renal agenesis is most commonly associated with uterus bicornis bicollis with a partial uterine septum resulting in unilateral hematometrocolpos.

Septate Uterus

A midline uterine septum may partially or completely divide the uterus into two cavities without duplication of the uterine horns [38]. This anomaly results from failure of resorption of the septum following normal fusion of the müllerian ducts.

- The fundus is convex externally indicating the absence of duplicated uterine horns.
- The uterine cavity is divided completely or partially by midline fibrous or muscular tissue (Fig. 5.27). Two separate endometrial complexes are visualized. Color Doppler may confirm vascularization of the septum and aid in its recognition [38].

Hematometra and Hematocolpos

Obstruction of the genital tract results in the accumulation of menstrual blood in the uterus (hematometra), the vagina (hematocolpos), or both (hematometrocolpos). Congenital obstructions are caused by imperforate hymen, vaginal septum, vaginal atresia, or obstructed, hypoplastic uterine horn. Acquired obstructions result from inflammatory conditions, tumors, radiation treatments, or cervical stenosis [39].

- Echogenic fluid distends the uterus (Fig. 5.28) and/or the vagina (see Fig. 5.62). Anechoic fluid suggests non-hemorrhagic secretions (hydrometrocolpos). Pyometra is suggested by the presence of clinical signs of infection.

OVARIES AND ADNEXA

FOLLICLES

Normal physiologic cysts seen on the ovaries include normal follicles, the developing dominant follicle, and the corpus luteum.

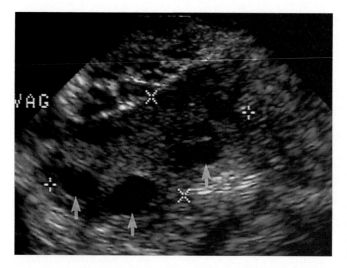

Figure 5.29 *Normal Follicles.* Transvaginal image shows several normal follicles (*arrows*) on the ovary (*between calipers, +, x*). Normal follicles have thin walls, are anechoic, and are <25 mm in size.

- **Normal follicles** are smooth, round, echo-free, thin-walled cysts on the ovary <25 mm in diameter (Fig. 5.29). As the **dominant follicle** enlarges (up to 25 mm) prior to ovulation, the other follicles atrophy. These follicles are normal physiologic structures and must be recognized as such.
- The **corpus luteum** has a varying appearance [6]. It develops at the site of ovulation and is initially a solid structure with blood clot occupying the site of the collapsed dominant follicle. The corpus luteum quickly becomes cystic, enlarges to 15–25-mm size, and persists through menstruation [40]. Thus, a unilocular cyst 25 mm or less in size is normal in the second half of the menstrual cycle as well. The corpus luteum has a slightly thicker wall and more echogenic contents than a follicle. Blood flow to the corpus luteum is low resistance on spectral Doppler (RI <0.4) mimicking the blood flow pattern associated with malignancy [4].

FUNCTIONING CYSTS

Follicles or the corpus luteum may fail to involute and become *functioning cysts* with continued hormone production. These larger cysts have a tendency to hemorrhage internally and become *hemorrhagic cysts*.

- Smooth, round, echo-free, thin-walled ovarian cysts larger than 2.5 cm (up to 8–10 cm) (Fig. 5.30). Cysts larger than 5 cm are less likely to spontaneously regress [41].

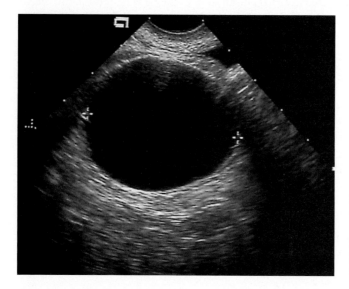

Figure 5.30 *Functioning Ovarian Cyst.* A thin-walled cyst (*between cursors, +*) with anechoic internal fluid and size larger than 2.5 cm meets the definition of a functioning ovarian cyst.

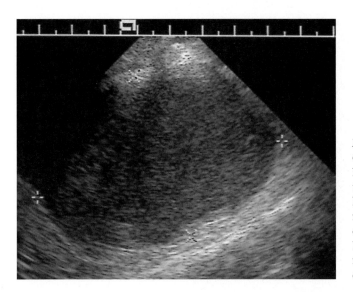

Figure 5.31 *Hemorrhagic Cyst—Homogeneous Echoes.* Mass (*between cursors, +, x*) on the ovary shows a pattern of fine, homogeneous, low-level, internal echoes characteristic of hemorrhage within an ovarian cyst. Doppler is used to verify its cystic nature by confirming the absence of internal blood vessels.

- Doppler shows peripheral blood flow with relatively high resistance (mean RI = 0.65) in the wall of functional cysts. Doppler cannot discriminate between functional cysts and benign ovarian neoplasms [42].
- Because these larger functioning cysts have an appearance identical to early ovarian carcinoma, a follow-up US examination should be performed after one or two menstrual cycles to ensure that resolution of the functioning cyst has occurred. A 6- or 10-week follow-up interval is usually recommended to ensure that the patient is examined in a different phase of her menstrual cycle.

A 10-week follow-up interval is suggested for most patients with benign-appearing ovarian cysts. Ten weeks provides a longer time for resolution of a functional cyst and usually avoids repeating the follow-up examination.

HEMORRHAGIC CYSTS

Hemorrhagic cysts result from bleeding into functioning cysts. Pain and expansion of the cyst may accompany bleeding. Most hemorrhagic cysts resolve in 2–8 weeks [43].

- Homogeneous, low-level, internal echoes are seen in an ovarian cyst with enhanced through-transmission (Fig. 5.31). This appearance is identical to endometrioma.
- A network of fine interdigitating, avascular, fibrous strands (fishnet appearance) is characteristic (Fig. 5.32).
- Retracting clots and fibrous strands are evidence of acute hemorrhage (Fig. 5.33).
- Fluid-fluid levels are common (Fig. 5.34).
- Doppler confirms the absence of internal blood flow. Blood flow may be seen in the wall of the cyst.
- Hemorrhage in a cyst is strong evidence of benignancy [44].

POSTMENOPAUSAL CYSTS

Benign ovarian cysts are found in 3–17% of postmenopausal women [45,46]. Most of these cysts are serous inclusion cysts that arise on the surface of the involuting ovary. Their occurrence is independent of hormone replacement therapy or the time interval since menopause [45].

- Smooth, thin-walled, unilocular, anechoic ovarian cyst in a postmenopausal woman is typical. Most cysts are <5 cm in size. With extended follow-up (2.5 years), the cysts remain stable in appearance and gradually decrease in size [47].
- Normal postmenopausal ovaries are avascular. Doppler US reveals blood flow only in the ovarian artery. Increased blood flow is evidence of neoplasia [4].
- Cysts >5 cm in size or with atypical features should probably be removed because the risk of tumor is increased.

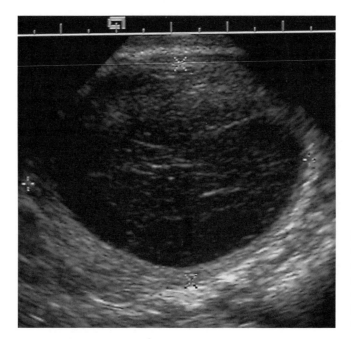

Figure 5.32 *Hemorrhagic Cyst—Fishnet Appearance.* Cyst (*between cursors, +, x*) on the left ovary shows fine internal echoes with a fishnet appearance of thin, linear, fibrous strands characteristic of hemorrhage.

THECA LUTEIN CYSTS

Theca lutein cysts develop on ovaries that are overstimulated by human chorionic gonadotropin (hCG). These cysts occur in patients with gestational trophoblastic disease, in pregnant women with a multiple gestation, and in infertile women receiving hCG for ovulation induction.

- Bilateral, multiseptated ovarian cysts with anechoic contents and thin smooth walls is a typical appearance (Fig. 5.35).
- Cysts commonly persist for weeks after hCG levels return to normal.

OVARIAN HYPERSTIMULATION SYNDROME

Ovulation may be induced in infertile women by treatment with clomiphene citrate, hCG, or gonadotropin releasing factor. Overstimulation of the ovaries results in induction of

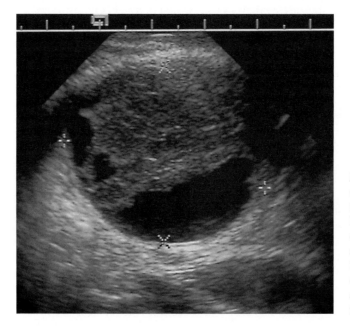

Figure 5.33 *Hemorrhagic Cyst—Retracting Clots.* Retraction of blood clots following hemorrhage within an ovarian cyst (*between cursors, +, x*) forms an irregular echogenic mass. Doppler confirmed the absence of internal vessels. This appearance is characteristic of shrinking blood clots in an ovarian cyst.

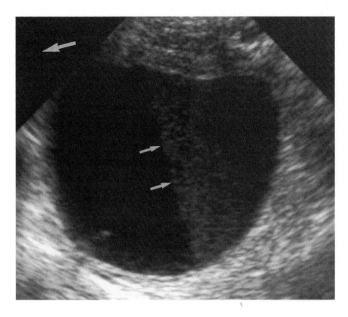

Figure 5.34 *Hemorrhagic Cyst—Layering Blood.* Settling blood products produce a fluid-fluid layer (*small arrows*) within this hemorrhagic ovarian cyst shown on TV US. Large arrow indicates the direction of "up" during transvaginal scanning.

multiple follicles and multiple corpus luteum cysts following multiple ovulations [6]. Very high levels of estrogen are associated with abdominal pain, weight gain, development of ascites and pleural effusions, hemoconcentration, hypotension, and oliguria. Marked ovarian enlargement (>10 cm) is associated with risk of ovarian torsion and rupture.

- Large ovaries (>5–10 cm diameter) with multiple large thin-walled cysts.
- Fluid exudes from the enlarged ovaries. Look for ascites and pleural effusions.

POLYCYSTIC OVARY SYNDROME

A complex endocrine disorder of chronic anovulation, androgen excess, infertility, hirsutism, and obesity is associated with enlarged ovaries with multiple cysts. This disorder is also called the *Stein-Leventhal syndrome.*

- Bilateral large ovaries (>15 cc) with multiple (>11) peripheral follicles (5–8 mm in diameter) (Fig. 5.36).
- The normal shape of the ovary is maintained.

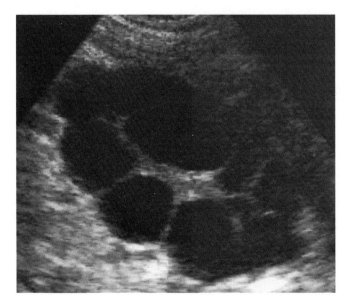

Figure 5.35 *Theca Lutein Cysts.* Multiple thin-walled cysts enlarge the ovary in this patient with gestational trophoblastic disease.

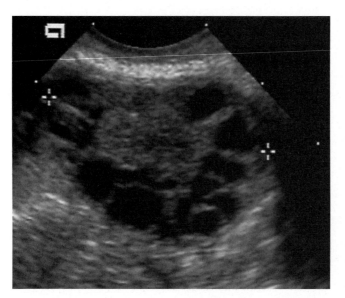

Figure 5.36 *Polycystic Ovary Syndrome.* The ovary (*between cursors,* +) is mildly enlarged and has a large number of follicles arranged around its periphery.

- The ovarian stroma is thickened and significantly increased in echogenicity [48].
- Vascularity of the ovarian stroma is increased. Spectral Doppler shows a low resistance pattern [49].
- The ovaries are normal in size in 30% of cases. The diagnosis is made by biochemical analysis.

OVARIAN CANCER

Ovarian cancer accounts for 4% of all cancer in women and is the leading cause of death from gynecologic malignancy. Although the cancer is usually curable in its early stages, two-thirds of all patients have tumor spread beyond the pelvis when the diagnosis is made.

Epithelial tumors account for 85% of ovarian cancers. These tumors arise from the surface epithelium and the mesothelium of the outer ovarian cortex. Tumors are classified as benign (cystadenoma), borderline malignant (formally called *tumors of low malignant potential*), and malignant (cystadenocarcinoma) [50].

- *Serous* neoplasms account for 60–80% of epithelial tumors and are the most common lesions in both benign and malignant categories. Approximately 50% of tumors are frankly malignant or of low malignant potential. Tumors are bilateral in 20% of benign cases and in 50% of malignant cases. Most tumors are predominantly cystic and contain anechoic fluid. The cysts may be unilocular or multilocular.
- *Mucinous* tumors are approximately 90% benign and are less commonly bilateral (5% of benign tumors and 25% of malignant tumors). Most tumors are predominantly cystic, typically multilocular, and contain fluid of variable echogenicity caused by mucoid material, hemorrhage, and cellular debris. Tumors are often huge (up to 30 cm).
- *Endometrioid* tumors are nearly always malignant with 25% being bilateral. Approximately 20–30% are associated with hyperplasia or carcinoma of the uterine endometrium. Most lesions are mixed cystic and solid, although some are entirely solid.
- *Clear cell* neoplasms are nearly all invasive carcinomas, accounting for 10% of ovarian malignancies. Lesions are most commonly unilocular cysts with mural nodules.
- *Brenner* tumors are uncommon (3% of ovarian tumors) and always benign. The tumors are homogeneously solid, usually small (1–2 cm), and commonly extensively calcified.

Germ cell tumors arise from primitive ovarian germ cells and account for 7% of ovarian malignancy. Benign cystic teratomas (dermoid cysts) are most common (30% of all primary ovarian neoplasms). Malignant lesions are of mixed histology and include immature teratomas, dysgerminomas, yolk sac and endodermal sinus tumors, and choriocarcinoma. Malignant tumors are usually found in girls and young women. Most tumors are large, predominantly solid, heterogeneous, and commonly contain calcifications [51]. Serum α-fetoprotein or hCG may be elevated.

Gonadal stromal (sex-cord stromal) tumors arise from the mesenchymal cells of the embryonic ovaries. Tumors include granulosa cell tumors, thecomas, fibromas, Sertoli and Leydig cell tumors, and steroid cell tumors. This group accounts for 7–8% of ovarian neoplasms. Granulosa cell tumors may produce estrogens and Sertoli-Leydig cell tumors may produce androgens resulting in conspicuous endocrine syndromes. Granulosa cell tumors are typically large and multilocular cystic with solid components. The other tumors are predominantly solid and may be homogeneous or heterogeneous with areas of fibrosis, necrosis, and hemorrhage [52].

Metastases to the ovary most commonly arise from the breast and gastrointestinal tract. Krukenberg tumors are metastatic mucin-producing adenocarcinomas with specific histologic characteristics. Lesions are bilateral, solid, and usually heterogeneous in echogenicity with poorly defined cystic areas commonly present [53].

SIGNS INDICATIVE OF OVARIAN MALIGNANCY

Differentiating benign from potentially malignant ovarian lesions is a primary goal of US examination. Unfortunately, no single gray-scale or Doppler US finding reliably provides this differentiation.

- A solid component (Fig. 5.37) to an ovarian lesion is the most significant predictor of malignancy [44].
- Irregular thick wall (Fig. 5.38) and septa (>3 mm) (Fig. 5.39).
- Solid mural nodules and (Fig. 5.40) papillary projections.
- Doppler demonstration of central blood flow within a solid component correlates well with malignancy (Figs. 5.39, 5.40) [44]. Color flow in septations within an ovarian cyst (Fig. 5.39) is a reliable sign of neoplasm but does not differentiate benign from malignant lesions [54,55]. Spectral Doppler of arterial blood flow usually demonstrates a lower resistance flow pattern (RI < 0.4, pulsatility index < 1.0) in malignant lesions; however, neither RI nor pulsatility index can be used to reliably differentiate benign from malignant [54,56]. Many benign lesions (corpus luteum, hemorrhagic cyst, tuboovarian abscess) will have low RI arterial signals and not all malignancies will have low RI arterial signals.

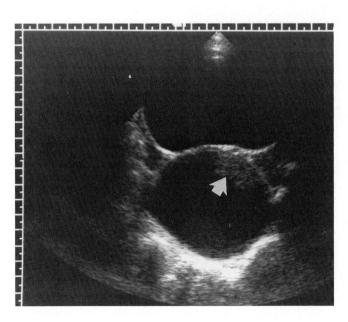

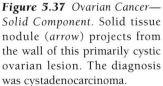

Figure 5.37 *Ovarian Cancer—Solid Component.* Solid tissue nodule (*arrow*) projects from the wall of this primarily cystic ovarian lesion. The diagnosis was cystadenocarcinoma.

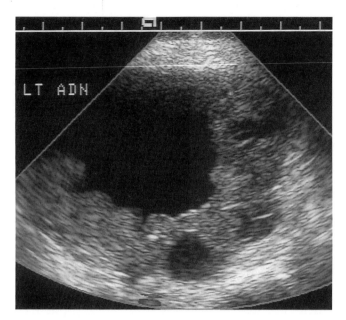

Figure 5.38 *Ovarian Cancer—Irregular Thick Wall.* Cystic ovarian lesion has an irregular nodular thick wall. The diagnosis was endometrioid carcinoma.

- Elevated serum CA-125 [57]. This screening blood test is elevated in only 50% of women with early ovarian cancer [58]. In addition, false-positive rate may exceed 90% in premenopausal women.
- Ovarian lesions larger than 4 cm have a higher incidence of malignancy (Fig. 5.39), but the size of benign and malignant lesions overlaps greatly [59].

Screening for ovarian cancer remains a popular but controversial subject. Because the prevalence of ovarian cancer is relatively low (compared to breast cancer) and the findings associated with malignancy are non-specific, it has been difficult to demonstrate cost-effectiveness or reduced cancer mortality.

SPREAD OF OVARIAN MALIGNANCY

US documentation of tumor spread is obviously evidence of malignancy.

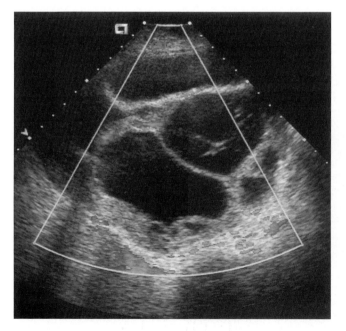

Figure 5.39 *Ovarian Cancer—Blood Flow in Septations.* Power Doppler color flow image confirms blood flow within irregularly thickened septa within this ovarian lesion. Blood flow in septations is highly indicative of the lesion being a neoplasm. In this case, the irregular thickening of the walls and septa and the large size of the tumor (>13 cm) are evidence of malignancy (see Color Figure 5.39).

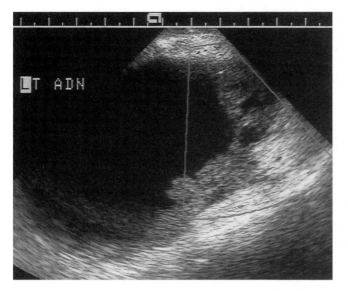

Figure 5.40 *Ovarian Cancer— Blood Flow in Wall.* Color Doppler image reveals blood vessels within the irregular solid thickening of the wall of this cystic ovarian lesion. This finding confirms that the solid-appearing tissue is neoplasm and is not just clotted blood adherent to the cyst wall (see Color Figure 5.40).

- Local extension of tumor beyond the ovarian capsule is manifest by irregular indistinct boundaries with the uterus, localized distortion of uterine contour, encasement of small or large bowel, and displacement or invasion of blood vessels [60]. Tumors with local extension are usually large (>4–5 cm).

- Intraperitoneal spread is a prominent and early feature of metastatic disease. The presence of ascites is non-specific, but is highly suspicious for peritoneal spread in the presence of an ovarian lesion. Loculation of ascites, ascites in the lesser sac, septations, fibrous strands, and echogenic fluid provides further evidence of malignancy. Peritoneal implants are typically tiny and often not visualized by US. Key areas to examine include the posterior cul-de-sac, paracolic gutters, undersurface of the diaphragm, and surfaces of the liver and spleen. Implants appear as nodules or plaque-like lesions (Fig. 5.41). *Omental cake* refers to tumor implantation on the greater omentum. Ill-defined, cake-like mass of cystic and solid tumor (Fig. 5.42) displaces bowel away from the anterior abdominal wall. Bowel involvement is manifest as plaque-like or nodular thickening of the bowel wall, fixation or distortion of bowel, and bowel obstruction.

- Lymphatic spread of tumor occurs along the gonadal lymphatics that parallel the ovarian vein. Lymph nodes larger than 10 mm in short axis are considered involved by metastatic disease. Nodal involvement includes the hypogastric, obturator, external iliac lymph nodes, and nodes adjacent to and between the aorta and inferior vena cava.

- Hydronephrosis is caused by direct tumor invasion of the ureter or by compression of retroperitoneal adenopathy.

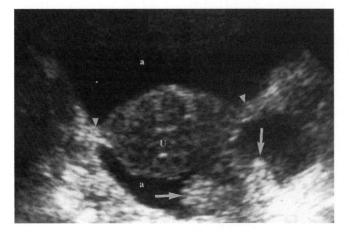

Figure 5.41 *Peritoneal Implants.* Tumor nodules (*arrows*) implanted on peritoneal surfaces in the cul-de-sac are well outlined by ascites (a). The uterus (U) and broad ligaments (*arrowheads*) are also clearly shown. The abrupt onset of ascites in a middle-aged woman without history of liver disease should stimulate a careful examination of the ovaries and a detailed search for peritoneal implants.

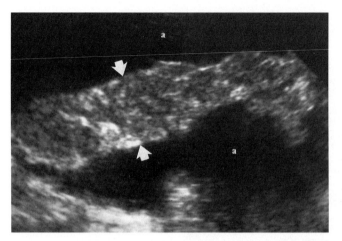

Figure 5.42 *Omental Cake.* Ovarian cancer metastatic implants on the greater omentum (*between arrows*) have caused "cake-like," irregular thickening of the omentum. The omentum is suspended in ascites (a) and floats between bowel and the anterior abdominal wall.

- Hematogenous spread occurs earlier and is more common than previously believed. Intraparenchymal metastases may be seen in the liver, spleen, pancreas, and kidneys. Malignant pleural effusions are associated with lung and pleural metastases.

SIGNS OF A BENIGN OVARIAN MASS

- Purely cystic masses with no visible solid component are nearly always benign and usually represent functioning ovarian cysts (Fig. 5.30) [44,61].
- A markedly hyperechoic solid component (Fig. 5.43) is indicative of cystic teratoma and is always benign [44]. See description of cystic teratoma.
- Absence of color Doppler signal in the mass is reliable evidence of benign lesion (Fig. 5.44) [55].
- Hemorrhage within a unilocular cyst (Fig. 5.44) is statistically strongly associated with non-neoplastic cysts. Most are hemorrhagic functional cysts.

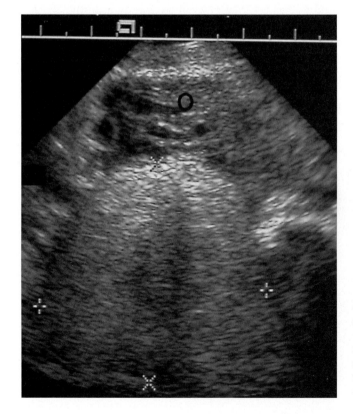

Figure 5.43 *Cystic Teratoma.* A solid markedly hyperechoic mass (*marked by cursors, +, x*) arises from the right ovary (O). This appearance is highly indicative of benign cystic teratoma and effectively excludes malignancy.

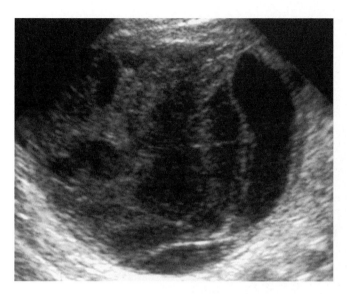

Figure 5.44 *Hemorrhagic Cyst.* Color and spectral Doppler examination showed no internal flow within this complex, solid-appearing, ovarian lesion. The absence of blood vessels indicates the complex, solid-appearing tissue is blood clot within an ovarian cyst. Internal hemorrhage is rarely seen within ovarian cancers.

- Uniform thin septations are common with benign ovarian tumors such as serous or mucinous cystadenomas (Fig. 5.45). Demonstration of blood flow within septations confirms the lesion is a neoplasm but does not differentiate benign from malignant.
- Mucinous tumors commonly secrete mucin, which produces fine low-level echoes within the cyst fluid (Figs. 5.45, 5.46). The presence of this echogenic material suggests a mucinous lesion but is not helpful in differentiating benign from malignant tumors.

CYSTIC TERATOMA

Cystic teratoma is the most common ovarian neoplasm. Most are discovered as asymptomatic adnexal masses. The risk of torsion is significant, as high as 16% in some series. Rarely, the tumor may rupture and produce acute peritonitis. Malignancy occurs in less than 2%. The tumors are cystic but may contain hair, sebum, teeth, or bone that produce a wide variety of US appearances. However, findings are often distinctive enough to provide a specific diagnosis [62,63].

- A characteristic structural feature of most cystic teratomas is the **dermoid plug.** The dermoid plug consists of a mixture of sebaceous material, fat, hair, and soft tissue that

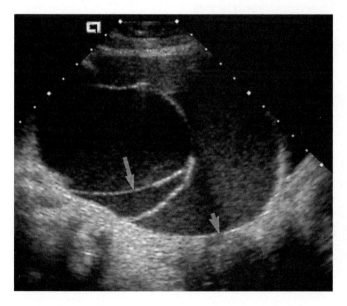

Figure 5.45 *Thin Septations in Benign Neoplasm.* Uniformly thin septations (*long arrow*) and thin wall (*short arrow*) are evident in this benign mucinous cystadenoma. Note the fine low-level echoes within the cyst fluid caused by mucinous fluid.

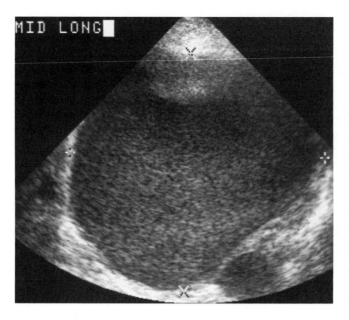

Figure 5.46 *Internal Echoes Caused by Mucin.* A homogeneous pattern of fine, low-level echoes suggests the presence of mucin within this cystic ovarian neoplasm (*between cursors, +, x*). Real-time, US observation of shifting internal echoes with patient movement and Doppler demonstration of the absence of internal vascularity confirm that this is a cystic lesion containing echogenic fluid. The diagnosis was mucinous cystadenocarcinoma.

produces a highly echogenic, amorphous, nodular focus with dirty acoustic shadowing. This appearance is called the *tip of the iceberg* sign (Fig. 5.47) and is considered diagnostic of cystic teratoma. The plug may occupy only a small portion of the mass or may fill the entire mass.

■ Formation of teeth and bone fragments is another highly specific but less common feature of cystic teratoma. These structures produce discrete bright echogenic foci with dense, dark acoustic shadows (Fig. 5.48). Radiographs confirm the presence of ectopic teeth and bone.

■ Hair floating in fluid produces bright linear strands and punctate echoes. The hyperechoic lines and dots pattern is highly predictive of hair within a cystic teratoma [63].

■ Fluid-fluid levels are common and caused by sebum layering on serous fluid in cystic teratomas. This finding is seen in other conditions (such as hemorrhagic cysts and tubo-ovarian abscess) and is not specific for cystic teratoma.

■ Because of the heterogeneous tissues they contain, cystic teratomas commonly appear solid rather than cystic [64]. Because of their high echogenicity, they blend in with pelvic fat and other structures (Fig. 5.49).

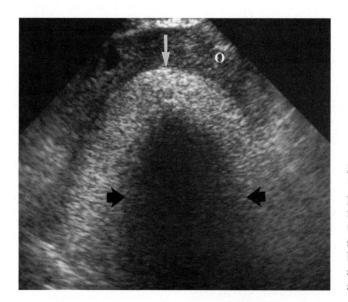

Figure 5.47 *Cystic Teratoma— "Tip of the Iceberg."* The dermoid plug is seen as a highly echogenic mass (*white arrow*) arising from the ovary (O). A dark acoustic shadow (*black arrows*) is produced by sound absorption. This appearance is characteristic of cystic teratoma.

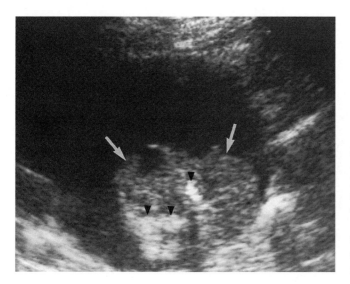

Figure 5.48 *Cystic Teratoma—Bone and Teeth Formation.* A prominent dermoid plug (*white arrows*) within a cystic mass contains coarse echogenic foci (*black arrowheads*) that had the appearance of a primitive teeth and bone on plain film radiographs.

- Approximately three-fourths of cystic teratomas show at least two of the features previously listed. If two of these features are present, the diagnosis can be made with a high degree of confidence [63].
- The cyst may be well defined and anechoic (Fig. 5.50). Sebum is highly echogenic at room temperature (in a specimen bottle) but is anechoic at body temperature within the patient. In the absence of additional findings previously listed, a specific diagnosis of cystic teratoma cannot be made.
- Doppler evaluation demonstrates most cystic teratomas to be devoid of blood flow. Low-to-moderate-impedance blood flow (RI = 0.42–0.72) is found in a few cystic teratomas that histologically demonstrate areas of actively dividing cells [65].

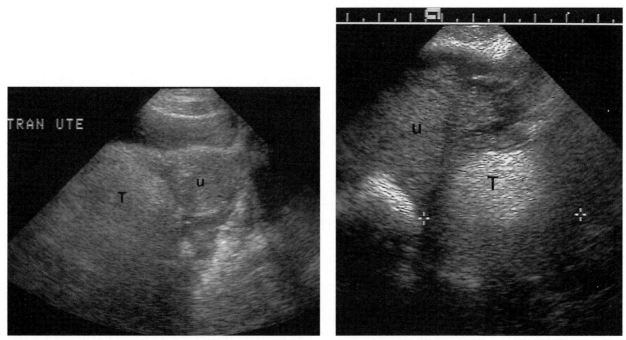

Figure 5.49 *Cystic Teratoma—Easy to Overlook.* A, B. Two large cystic teratomas (T) were easily palpable but difficult to define with US. u, uterus. Cursors (+) show size of the teratoma in B.

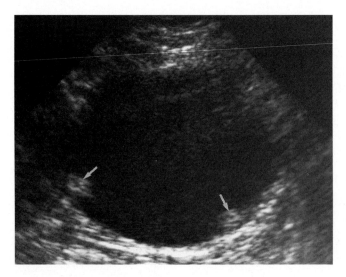

Figure 5.50 *Cystic Teratoma— The Great Mimicker.* This cystic teratoma contains sebum, which is near anechoic. Two small papillary projections (*arrows*) suggest ovarian carcinoma but were proven to be dermoid plugs.

ADNEXAL TORSION

In adnexal torsion, the ovary and/or fallopian tube twist around their vascular pedicle resulting in compromised blood flow. Patients present with intense pelvic pain that is commonly intermittent and mimics many other conditions. Torsion is most common in prepubertal girls and adolescents. Differential diagnosis includes renal stone causing ureteral obstruction, appendicitis, endometriosis, inflammatory bowel disease, and urinary tract infection. Doppler evaluation is essential in the diagnosis. Doppler findings depend upon the completeness and chronicity of torsion. Prompt diagnosis and surgical intervention is required to save the ovary from necrosis. Isolated torsion of the fallopian tube is rare and usually seen in women with a history of tubal ligation.

- The ovary is enlarged, sometimes massively, by edema and interstitial hemorrhage caused by venous obstruction. Central ovarian echogenicity is increased with multiple immature follicles seen in the periphery. Focal hemorrhage produces homogeneous hypoechoic zones in the ovary.
- In some cases an ovarian cyst or tumor is present and is probably responsible for precipitating the torsion. Torsion is extremely rare with malignant ovarian tumors because of adherence to adjacent structures.
- With partial torsion, venous flow is reduced whereas arterial flow is maintained. Spectral Doppler of arterial flow shows high resistance and occasionally reversal of flow in diastole.
- Complete absence of arterial and venous flow is indicative of a non-viable torsed ovary [66].
- The twisted vascular pedicle produces a "whirlpool sign" of concentric tubes in a swirling pattern [67]. Absence of flow in the vascular pedicle is predictive of necrosis of the ovary.
- Isolated tubal torsion is suggested by finding a dilated tube with thickened wall and echogenic contents. Doppler shows absent or high resistance arterial flow [68].
- Fluid is commonly present around the torsed structures.

ENDOMETRIOMA

Endometriosis is the presence of functioning endometrial tissue outside of the uterus. It is seen most commonly in infertile women between the ages of 30 and 40. Implantation of the endometrial tissue may occur anywhere, but implantation on the ovaries is particularly common. Symptoms include pelvic pain and dysmenorrhea. The deposits induce fibrous adhesions that fixate involved structures. Most deposits of endometrial tissue are small and not detectable by US. Larger deposits form hemorrhagic cysts called endometriomas (chocolate cysts). The US appearance of endometriomas is exceptionally diverse [69].

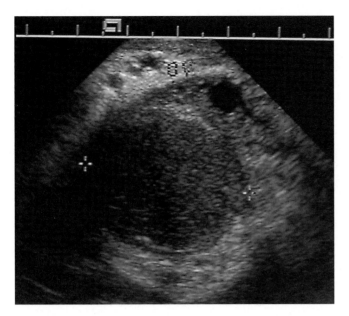

Figure 5.51 *Endometrioma— The Echogenic Cyst.* A 3-cm endometrioma (*between cursors,* +) implanted on the right ovary (OV) has homogeneous, low internal echoes. This appearance is classic for endometrioma, but may also be seen with a hemorrhagic ovarian cyst.

- Adnexal cystic mass with diffuse, low-level internal echoes is highly characteristic of endometrioma (Fig. 5.51).
- The presence of hyperechoic foci in the wall increases the likelihood of endometrioma (Fig. 5.52). These foci may represent cholesterol crystals resulting from cell breakdown in chronic hemorrhage.
- Cyst wall may be thick or thin. Thickness has no diagnostic value [69].
- Wall nodularity may be present and is indistinguishable from the wall nodularity of a neoplasm.
- The ovary is involved in 80% of cases of endometriosis (Fig. 5.51).

Peritoneal Inclusion Cysts

Peritoneal inclusion cysts are benign collections of fluid in the peritoneal cavity confined by adhesions. Patients have a history of multiple prior surgical procedures, endometriosis, or PID. The collections are commonly mistaken for ovarian cancer. No epithelial lining is present [70,71].

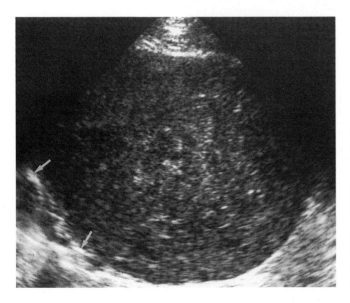

Figure 5.52 *Endometrioma.* This endometrioma contains blood that is higher in echogenicity and more heterogeneous in echotexture. It was initially mistaken for a solid lesion. Subsequently, Doppler demonstrated no internal blood vessels. Echogenic foci in the wall (*arrows*) are a subtle but characteristic sign of endometrioma.

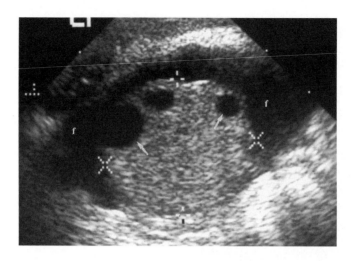

Figure 5.53 *Peritoneal Inclusion Cyst.* The ovary (*between cursors, +, x*), recognized by its follicles (*arrows*), is seen within a loculated fluid collection (f). This finding is characteristic of peritoneal inclusion cyst.

■ The fluid collections may be of any size but are frequently large.
■ Normal-appearing ovaries are frequently seen within the fluid collection. This finding confirms the diagnosis (Fig. 5.53).
■ The fluid collection may be septated and the fluid may contain particulate matter.
■ The fluid is loculated and conforms to peritoneal recesses in the pelvis.

PARAOVARIAN CYSTS

Paraovarian cysts arise between the leaves of the broad ligaments from mesothelial, wolffian duct, or müllerian duct remnants. Most are discovered incidentally in asymptomatic patients. Rare complications include hemorrhage, torsion, and malignant change (2%) [72,73].

■ Cystic mass up to 28-mm size is seen in the adnexa.
■ Cysts are thin walled and unilocular with anechoic internal fluid (Fig. 5.54).
■ Mass is separate from the ovary.

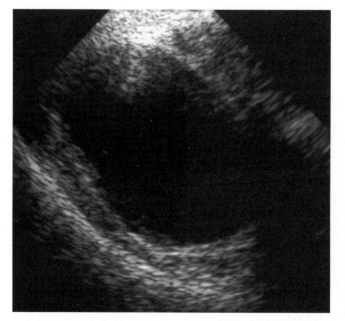

Figure 5.54 *Paraovarian Cyst.* This extra-ovarian cyst in the broad ligament proved to be a wolffian duct remnant cyst. The appearance is non-specific. The diagnosis may be suggested by recognizing that the cyst does not arise from the ovary.

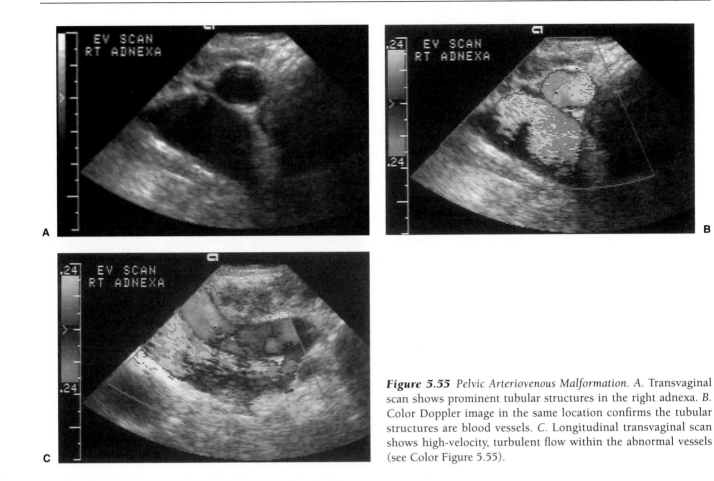

Figure 5.55 *Pelvic Arteriovenous Malformation. A.* Transvaginal scan shows prominent tubular structures in the right adnexa. *B.* Color Doppler image in the same location confirms the tubular structures are blood vessels. *C.* Longitudinal transvaginal scan shows high-velocity, turbulent flow within the abnormal vessels (see Color Figure 5.55).

PELVIC VARICES AND ARTERIOVENOUS MALFORMATIONS

Pelvic varices are associated with pelvic congestion syndrome, which is a common cause of chronic pelvic pain, dysmenorrhea, and dyspareunia [74]. Pelvic varices occur as isolated abnormalities or as a result of portal hypertension. Pelvic AVMs may also cause pelvic pain, back pain, or sciatica [74]. They occur congenitally or as a result of trauma.

- Varices appear as prominent tortuous vessels in the adnexal regions. Doppler confirms venous flow within the vessels. A large varix may be mistaken for hydrosalpinx if Doppler is not utilized.
- AVMs appear as pulsatile tubular structures in the adnexa (Fig. 5.55). They may be mistaken for cysts, fluid collections, or hydrosalpinx. Doppler shows high-velocity, low-resistance arterial flow and pulsatile venous flow.

OVARIAN REMNANTS

Ovarian remnants are fragments of functioning ovarian tissue unintentionally left behind following difficult oophorectomy. Ovarian remnants occur most commonly in patients with adhesions from endometriosis, PID, or previous surgery. The retained ovarian tissue responds to systemic hormonal stimulation and may form cysts and tumors [75]. The enlarging mass may cause pelvic pain or envelop and obstruct a ureter.

- Pelvic mass in a woman with history of bilateral oophorectomy.
- Most ovarian remnants produce simple or hemorrhagic ovarian cysts.
- Remnant ovarian tissue has the potential to produce any ovarian neoplasm.

FOCAL OVARIAN CALCIFICATIONS

Multiple discrete echogenic foci are commonly visualized on the ovary during TV US examination [76]. Histologic data indicate these are psammomatous calcifications associated with tiny superficial epithelial inclusion cysts.

■ Punctate, linear, or globular calcifications in peripheral ovarian tissue appear as discrete echodensities with or without acoustic shadowing. These occur in the absence of a visible ovarian mass. These are incidental findings without documented clinical significance [76].

FALLOPIAN TUBES

Cystic dilatation of the fallopian tubes, hydrosalpinx, hematosalpinx, and pyosalpinx commonly mimic the appearance of ovarian tumors. PID mimics metastatic pelvic tumor and endometriosis. Recognition of the characteristic findings of these conditions prevents misdiagnosis.

PELVIC INFLAMMATORY DISEASE

PID is usually caused by sexually transmitted infection, most commonly chlamydia or gonorrhea. PID also occurs as a complication of appendicitis, diverticulitis, pelvic abscess, and post-abortion or post-delivery infection. Acutely, patients present with fever, pelvic tenderness, and vaginal discharge. The inflammation commonly becomes chronic and patients present with pelvic mass and dyspareunia. Most cases occur in young, sexually active women, although 1–2% of tubo-ovarian abscesses are reported in postmenopausal women [77].

■ **Endometritis** is seen on US as thickening of the endometrium (>14 mm in menstruating women) commonly with fluid in the uterine cavity and echogenic layering fluid

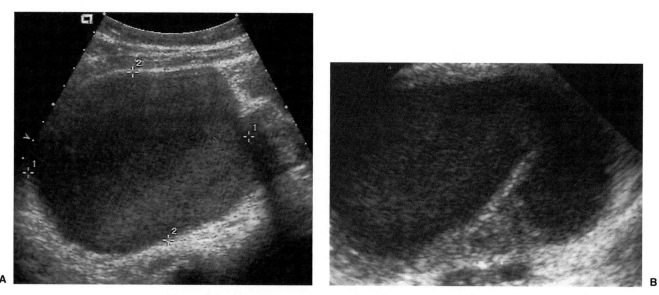

Figure 5.56 *Pyosalpinx. A.* Cystic adnexal mass (*between cursors,* +) contains layering echogenic fluid. The tube is so dilated that it shows no features that identify its etiology. *B.* Transvaginal image in another patient shows a characteristic appearance of a folded dilated tube containing echogenic fluid. Pyosalpinx was confirmed at surgery in both patients.

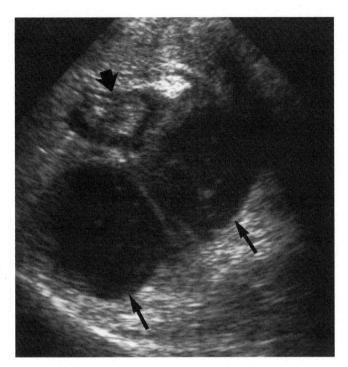

Figure 5.57 *Tubo-Ovarian Complex.* A markedly dilated fallopian tube (*long arrows*) partially envelopes the ovary (*short arrow*) in a patient with pelvic infection.

(pus) in the cul-de-sac. Air produced by bacterial activity produces punctate echodensities. The margin of the inflamed uterus is ill defined [78].

- **Pyosalpinx** is a pus-filled, dilated, fallopian tube and is recognized by the echogenic particulate matter that fills or layers within the tube (Fig. 5.56). Patients are acutely symptomatic. The wall of the dilated tube thickens as the inflammation becomes chronic.

- **Tubo-ovarian complex** results from incorporation of the dilated fallopian tube and inflamed ovary within a mass formed by adhesions (Fig. 5.57). Pus within the mass and surrounding the ovary and tube creates a **tubo-ovarian abscess** (Fig. 5.58). Pus appears as layering echogenic fluid and gas within the mass. Doppler demonstrates increased vascularity with a low resistance pattern (RI <0.5) in the periphery of the abscess. As the process becomes chronic, the RI increases [79,80]. TV US-guided aspiration confirms the diagnosis, obtains fluid for culture, and can be followed by catheter placement for TV drainage.

- **Chronic PID** results in pelvic adhesions that can be a cause of infertility and peritoneal inclusion cysts. Walled-off regions of peritoneum may secrete fluid and may incorporate the ovary and tube in an ill-defined mass that mimics endometriosis and pelvic malignancy.

TUBAL OBSTRUCTION/HYDROSALPINX

Distal obstruction of the fallopian tube causes infertility and may lead to *hydrosalpinx*, the term applied to dilatation of the tube by chronic accumulation of serous secretions. Causes of hydrosalpinx include PID (which may be subclinical), endometriosis, adhesions, surgery involving the tube, and fallopian tube carcinoma. The sensitivity of TV US for detection of a blocked tube has been reported to be as low as 34%. Sonographic diagnosis is dependent upon the blocked tube being dilated with fluid and many are not [81]. Multihormone stimulation during ovulation induction therapy for infertility may dilate a previously unrecognized blocked tube by increasing tubular secretions [82]. SHG and hysterosalpingography are more sensitive than TV US for diagnosis of tubal obstruction because the force of contrast injection dilates the blocked tube. Differential diagnosis of hydrosalpinx includes prominent pelvic blood vessels (Doppler shows blood flow), loops of bowel and dilated distal ureter (look for peristalsis), and cystic ovarian masses (arise from the ovary).

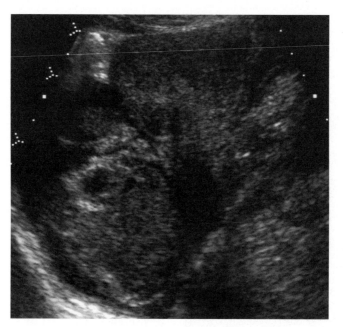

Figure 5.58 *Tubo-Ovarian Abscess.* A dilated tube, a distorted ovary, pus, and marked inflammation cause a complex amorphous adnexal mass in a febrile patient with severe pelvic pain. En bloc resection at surgery confirmed a tubo-ovarian abscess.

- Hydrosalpinx appears as an undulating or folded fluid-filled extraovarian tubular mass (Fig. 5.59).
- Short linear echoes protrude into lumen ("cogwheel pattern"). These represent the longitudinal folds of the tubular mucosa in the ampullary portion of the tube. This finding is characteristic, when present, but is absent in approximately half the cases of hydrosalpinx.
- Well-defined walls are echogenic and 1–2 mm thick.
- Fluid in the tube is anechoic in uncomplicated hydrosalpinx. Echogenic fluid in the tube suggests infection or hemorrhage.
- Doppler demonstrates vascularity in the walls of the dilated tube.
- Hydrosalpinx is most evident during the proliferative phase of the menstrual cycle when tubular secretions are greatest. The dilated tube may empty into the uterine cavity during the secretory phase, making the blocked tube inapparent on US.

CARCINOMA OF THE FALLOPIAN TUBE

This is the rarest (0.3%) of all gynecologic malignancies. Most patients are postmenopausal and older than age 50. A variety of US appearances of an extraovarian mass have been described [83,84].

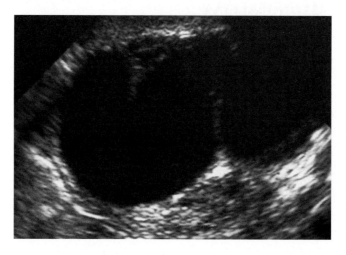

Figure 5.59 *Hydrosalpinx.* Transvaginal image shows the characteristic undulating pattern of a dilated fallopian tube. Careful examination is needed to show the tube in optimal projection. Random cross-sections may show only the non-specific appearance of an adnexal cyst.

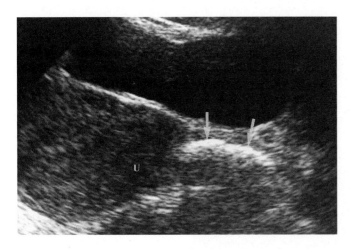

Figure 5.60 *Tampon in Vagina.* An air-filled tampon in the vagina causes a bright linear echo (*arrows*) with acoustic shadowing. U, uterus.

- Sausage-shaped solid mass.
- Dilated tube with multiple solid nodules.
- Multiloculated cystic mass.

VAGINA

The vagina is commonly inspected cursively or is overlooked during pelvic US examination. Because diseases of the vagina are uncommon, they may be unfamiliar or misinterpreted. Examination techniques include TA US with full bladder, translabial US with empty bladder, and TV US with attention to the vaginal wall.

Posthysterectomy, the **vaginal cuff** is usually bulbous at its distal end. During hysterectomy the vaginal wall is folded back on itself and closed, creating a double layer of tissue, more bulbous than the remainder of the vagina. It is important that the bulbous cuff not be mistaken for a mass and that a mass in the cul-de-sac not be mistaken for a bulbous vaginal cuff. A vaginal cuff size larger than 2 cm suggests a mass [85]. The patient should be queried as to the reason for hysterectomy. A history of malignant pelvic tumor reinforces the importance of careful examination of the vaginal cuff. A cervical remnant from a supracervical hysterectomy may be mistaken for a tumor.

Tampons in the vagina trap air and produce a bright linear echo with shadowing and ring down (Fig. 5.60). **Foley catheters** may be misplaced in the vagina and the vagina may

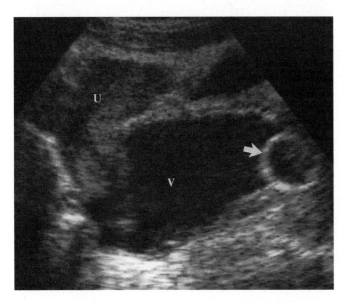

Figure 5.61 *Foley Catheter in Vagina.* In a "misguided" attempt to fill the bladder with saline for pelvic US examination, a Foley catheter (*arrow*) was placed in the vagina and the vagina (V) was filled with fluid. U, uterus.

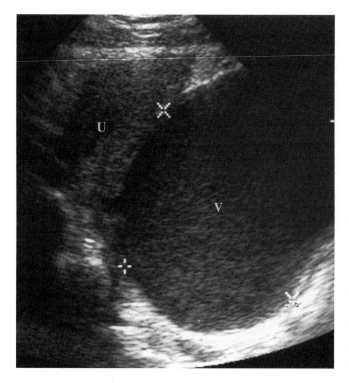

Figure 5.62 *Acquired Hematocolpos.* The vagina (V, *between cursors, +, x*) is markedly distended by menstrual blood. The vagina opening had been sealed shut by healing of mucosal ulcers occurring as a result of Stevens-Johnson syndrome. The patient had been amenorrheic for 3 months following her acute illness. U, uterus.

be filled with fluid meant for the bladder (Fig. 5.61). Blood in the vagina (**hematocolpos**) may be congenital, caused by developmental obstruction of the genital tract, or acquired, caused by inflammatory disease that seals the vagina closed (Fig. 5.62) [39]. Copious bleeding from the uterus may fill the vagina with echogenic material and outline the cervix by blood in the fornices (Fig. 5.63).

SOLID VAGINAL MASSES

Cervical carcinoma and uterine malignancies may protrude into the vagina, appearing as heterogeneous solid masses that obliterate vaginal sonographic landmarks. Primary vaginal

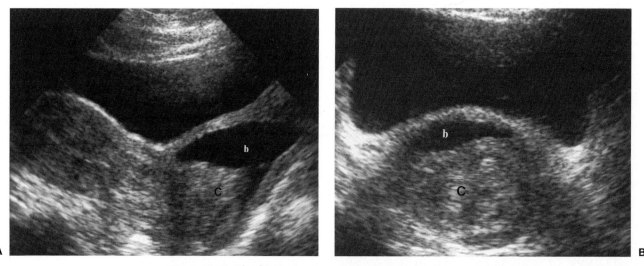

Figure 5.63 *Blood in Vagina.* Longitudinal (*A*) and transverse (*B*) US images of a patient with copious vaginal bleeding shows blood (b) in the vagina filling the fornices and outlining the cervix (C).

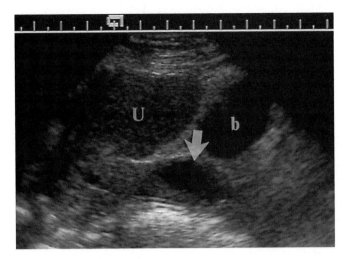

Figure 5.64 *Gartner's Duct Cyst.* Longitudinal image shows an oblong cystic mass (*arrow*) in the anterolateral wall of the vagina. The bladder (b) is only slightly filled. U, uterus.

cancers, clear cell adenocarcinoma, and rhabdomyosarcoma are heterogeneous solid masses that commonly show areas of necrosis.

CYSTIC VAGINAL MASSES

The following cystic lesions may be characterized by US or discovered incidentally during pelvic US examination.

- **Gartner's duct cysts** arise from remnants of the embryologic mesonephric ducts (that form the ductus deferens and ejaculatory ducts in the male). Cysts may form anywhere along the course of the mesonephric duct in the broad ligament and along the lateral wall of the uterus and vagina as far as the hymen. Most cysts are small, but some become large enough to obstruct the vagina. Characteristic location is anterolateral (Fig. 5.64). They may be single or multiple.
- **Inclusion cysts** are common and usually occur near the vaginal outlet. They result from tears or episiotomy incisions that heal with tags of mucosa buried beneath the mucosal surface. The cysts fill with desquamated epithelium.
- **Mucous cysts** (retention cysts) contain mucoid material and result from obstruction of the duct of mucous glands. They may occur anywhere along the vaginal wall.
- **Endometriosis** may occur in the vagina as a result of penetration of disease through the cul-de-sac.
- **Bartholin cysts** present as vulvar masses. Bartholin glands (the greater vestibular glands) lie on the superficial fascia of the urogenital diaphragm on either side of the vagina. Each gland drains into the vestibule through a duct that opens just outside the hymenal ring. The glands secrete a lubricating mucus during sexual arousal. Obstruction of the duct, caused by inflammation and scarring, results in a Bartholin cyst that is a tubular dilatation of the duct to Bartholin's gland. Infected glands or obstructed glands may enlarge to 5–6 cm and obstruct the rectum.
- **Nabothian cysts** arising in the cervix are common and, when large, must be differentiated from a vaginal cyst. Chronic inflammation results in squamous epithelium plugging the ducts of mucous glands of the cervix. The resulting cysts are anechoic, often multiple, and vary in size from 2–3 mm up to 4 cm.

REFERENCES

1. American Institute of Ultrasound in Medicine. Guidelines for performance of the female pelvic examination. Rockville, Maryland: AIUM, 1991.
2. Martensson O, Duchek M. Translabial sonography in evaluating the lower female urogenital tract. AJR Am J Roentgenol 1996;166:1327–1331.

3. Dubinsky TJ, Parvey HR, Maklad N. The role of transvaginal sonography and endometrial biopsy in the evaluation of peri- and postmenopausal bleeding. AJR Am J Roentgenol 1997; 169:145–149.

4. Cullinan JA, Fleischer AC, Kepple DM, et al. Sonohysterography: a technique for endometrial evaluation. Radiographics 1995;15:501–514.

5. Dubinsky TJ, Parvey HR, Gormaz G, et al. Transvaginal hysterosonography in the evaluation of small endoluminal masses. J Ultrasound Med 1995;14:1–6.

6. Ritchie WG. Sonographic evaluation of normal and induced ovulation. Radiology 1986;161:1–10.

7. Surratt JT, Siegel MJ. Imaging of pediatric ovarian masses. Radiographics 1991;11:533–548.

8. Cohen H, Shapiro M, Mandel F, et al. Normal ovaries in neonates and infants: a sonographic study of 77 patients 1 day to 24 months old. AJR Am J Roentgenol 1993;160:583–586.

9. Cohen H, Tive H, Mandel F. Ovarian volumes measured by US: bigger than we think. Radiology 1990;177:189–192.

10. Tepper R, Zalel Y, Markov S, et al. Ovarian volume in postmenopausal women—suggestions to an ovarian size nomogram for menopausal age. Acta Obstet Gynecol Scand 1993;74:208–211.

11. Jorizzo J, Riccio G, Chen M, et al. Sonohysterography: the next step in the evaluation of the abnormal endometrium. Radiographics 1999;19:S117–S130.

12. Dubinsky TJ, Stroehlein K, Abu-Ghazzeh Y, et al. Prediction of benign and malignant endometrial disease: hysterosonographic-pathologic correlation. Radiology 1999;210:393–397.

13. Karlsson B, Granberg S, Wikland M, et al. Transvaginal ultrasonography of the endometrium in women with postmenopausal bleeding: a Nordic multicenter study. Am J Obstet Gynecol 1995;172:1488–1494.

14. Dorum A, Kristensen B, Langebrekke A, et al. Evaluation of endometrial thickness measured by endovaginal ultrasound in women with postmenopausal bleeding. Acta Obstet Gynecol Scand 1993;72:116–119.

15. Levine D, Gosink BB, Johnson LA. Change in endometrial thickness in postmenopausal women undergoing hormone replacement therapy. Radiology 1995;197:603–608.

16. Kupfer MC, Schiller VL, Hansen GC, et al. Transvaginal sonographic evaluation of endometrial polyps. J Ultrasound Med 1994;13:535–539.

17. Laifer-Narin SL, Ragavendra N, Lu DSK, et al. Transvaginal saline hysterosonography: characteristics distinguishing malignant and various benign conditions. AJR Am J Roentgenol 1999;172:1513–1520.

18. Atri M, Nazarnia S, Aldis AE, et al. Transvaginal US appearance of endometrial abnormalities. Radiographics 1994;14:483–492.

19. Ascher S, Imaoka I, Lage J. Tamoxifen-induced uterine abnormalities: the role of imaging. Radiology 2000;214:29–38.

20. Hann LE, Giess CS, Bach AM, et al. Endometrial thickness in tamoxifen-treated patients: correlation with clinical and pathologic findings. AJR Am J Roentgenol 1997;168:657–661.

21. Hulka CA, Hall DA. Endometrial abnormalities associated with tamoxifen therapy for breast cancer: sonographic and pathologic correlation. AJR Am J Roentgenol 1993;160:809–812.

22. Vuento MH, Pirhonen JP, Mäkinen JI, et al. Endometrial fluid accumulation in asymptomatic postmenopausal women. Ultrasound Obstet Gynecol 1996;8:37–41.

23. Goldstein SR. Postmenopausal endometrial fluid collections revisited: look at the doughnut rather than the hole. Obstet Gynecol 1994;83:738–740.

24. Fedele L, Bianchi S, Dorta M, et al. Intrauterine adhesions: detection with transvaginal US. Radiology 1996;199:757–759.

25. Wachsberg RH, Kurtz AB. Gas within the endometrial cavity at postpartum US: a normal finding after spontaneous vaginal delivery. Radiology 1992;183:431–433.

26. Karasick S, Lev-Toaff AS, Toaff MEA. Imaging of uterine leiomyomas. AJR Am J Roentgenol 1992;158:799–805.

27. Caoili E, Hertzberg B, Kliewer M, et al. Refractory shadowing from pelvic masses on sonography: a useful diagnostic sign for uterine leiomyomas. AJR Am J Roentgenol 2000;174:97–101.

28. Yeh H-C, Kaplan M, Deligdisch L. Parasitic and pedunculated leiomyomas: ultrasonographic features. J Ultrasound Med 1999;18:789–794.

29. Outwater EK, Siegelman ES, VanDeerlin V. Adenomyosis: current concepts and imaging considerations. AJR Am J Roentgenol 1998;170:437–441.

30. Reinhold C, McCarthy S, Bret PM, et al. Diffuse adenomyosis: comparison of endovaginal US and MR imaging with histopathologic correlation. Radiology 1996;199:151–158.

31. Reinhold C, Atri M, Mehio A, et al. Diffuse uterine adenomyosis: morphologic criteria and diagnostic accuracy of endovaginal sonography. Radiology 1995;197:609–614.

32. Reinhold C, Tafazoli F, Mehio A, et al. Uterine adenomyosis: endovaginal US and MR imaging features with histopathologic correlation. Radiographics 1999;19:S147–S160.

33. Huang M, Muradali D, Thurston W, et al. Uterine arteriovenous malformations: gray-scale and Doppler US features with MR imaging correlation. Radiology 1998;206:115–123.

34. Schiller V, Sarti D, Reynolds D. Transvaginal water instillation during endovaginal sonography: a new method to visualize the cervix. J Ultrasound Med 1995;14:73–75.

35. Bajo J, Moreno-Calvo F, Uguet-de-Resayre C, et al. Contribution of transvaginal sonography to the evaluation of benign cervical conditions. J Clin Ultrasound 1999;27:61–64.

36. O'Neill M, Yoder I, Connolly S, et al. Imaging evaluation and classification of developmental anomalies of the female reproductive system with emphasis on MR imaging. AJR Am J Roentgenol 1999;173:407–416.

37. Brody J, Koelliker S, Frishman G. Unicornuate uterus: imaging appearance, associated anomalies, and clinical implications. AJR Am J Roentgenol 1998;171:1341–1347.

38. Kupesic S, Kurjak A. Septate uterus: detection and prediction of obstetrical complications by different forms of ultrasonography. J Ultrasound Med 1998;17:631–636.

39. Murphy MI, Brant WE. Hematocolpos caused by genital bullous lesions in a patient with Stevens-Johnson syndrome. J Clin Ultrasound 1998;26:52–54.

40. Lenz S, Lindenberg S. Is the corpus luteum normal after ovulation induction? J Clin Ultrasound 1990;18:155–159.

41. Fried AM, Kenney CM, III, Stigers KB, et al. Benign pelvic masses: sonographic spectrum. Radiographics 1996;16:321–334.

42. Alcázar J, Errasti T, Jarado M. Blood flow in functional cysts and benign ovarian neoplasms in premenopausal women. J Ultrasound Med 1997;16:819–824.

43. Okai T, Kobayashi K, Ryo E, et al. Transvaginal sonographic appearance of hemorrhagic functional ovarian cysts and their spontaneous regression. Int J Gynaecol Obstet 1994;44:47–52.

44. Brown D, Doubilet P, Miller G, et al. Benign and malignant ovarian masses: selection of the most discriminating gray-scale and Doppler sonographic features. Radiology 1998;208:103–110.

45. Levine D, Gosink BB, Wolf SI, et al. Simple adnexal cysts: the natural history in postmenopausal women. Radiology 1992;184:653–659.

46. Wolf S, Gosink B, Feldsman M, et al. Prevalence of simple adnexal cysts in postmenopausal women. Radiology 1991;180:65–71.

47. Auslender R, Atlas I, Lissak A, et al. Follow-up of small, postmenopausal ovarian cysts using vaginal ultrasound and CA-125 antigen. J Clin Ultrasound 1996;24:175–178.

48. Pache TD, Wladimiroff JW, Hop WCJ, et al. How to discriminate between normal and polycystic ovaries: transvaginal US study. Radiology 1992;183:421–423.

49. Dolz M, Osborne N, Blanes L, et al. Polycystic ovarian syndrome: assessment with color Doppler angiography and three-dimensional ultrasonography. J Ultrasound Med 1999;18:303–313.

50. Wagner BJ, Buck JL, Seidman JD, et al. Ovarian epithelial neoplasms: radiologic-pathologic correlation. Radiographics 1994;14:1351–1374.

51. Brammer HM, III, Buck JL, Hayes WS, et al. Malignant germ cell tumors of the ovary: radiologic-pathologic correlation. Radiographics 1990;10:715–724.

52. Outwater E, Bagner B, Mannion C, et al. Sex-cord stromal and steroid cell tumors of the ovary. Radiographics 1998;18:1523–1546.

53. Shimizu H, Yamasaki M, Ohama K, et al. Characteristic ultrasonographic appearance of the Krukenberg tumor. J Clin Ultrasound 1990;18:697–703.

54. Jain KA. Prospective evaluation of adnexal masses with endovaginal gray-scale and duplex and color Doppler US: correlation with pathologic findings. Radiology 1994;191:63–67.

55. Stein SM, Laifer-Narin S, Johnson MB, et al. Differentiation of benign and malignant adnexal masses: relative value of gray-scale, color Doppler, and spectral Doppler sonography. AJR Am J Roentgenol 1995;164:381–386.

56. Brown D, Frates M, Laing F, et al. Ovarian masses: can benign and malignant lesions be differentiated with color and pulsed Doppler US? Radiology 1994;190:333–336.

57. Bourne T, Campbell S, Reynolds K, et al. The potential role of serum CA-125 in an ultrasound-based screening program for familial ovarian cancer. Gynecol Oncol 1994;52:379–385.

58. Jacobs I, Bast RJ. The CA-125 tumor-associated antigen: a review of the literature. Human Reprod 1989;4:1–12.

59. Rulin M, Preston A. Adnexal masses in postmenopausal women. Obstet Gynecol 1987;70:578–582.

60. Kawamoto S, Urban B, Fishman E. CT of epithelial ovarian tumors. Radiographics 1999;19:S85–S102.

61. Buy J-N, Ghossain MA, Hugol D, et al. Characterization of adnexal masses: combination of color Doppler and conventional sonography compared with spectral Doppler analysis alone and conventional sonography alone. AJR Am J Roentgenol 1996;166:385–393.
62. Hertzberg BS, Kliewer MA. Sonography of benign cystic teratoma of the ovary: pitfalls in diagnosis. AJR Am J Roentgenol 1996;167:1127–1133.
63. Patel M, Feldstein V, Lipson S, et al. Cystic teratomas of the ovary: diagnostic value of sonography. AJR Am J Roentgenol 1998;171:1061–1065.
64. Lee D, Kim S, Cho J, et al. Ovarian teratomas appearing as solid masses on ultrasonography. J Ultrasound Med 1999;18:141–145.
65. Kurjak A, Kupesic S, Babic M, et al. Preoperative evaluation of cystic teratoma: what does color Doppler add? J Clin Ultrasound 1997;25:309–316.
66. Fleischer AC, Stein SM, Cullinan JA, et al. Color Doppler sonography of adnexal torsion. J Ultrasound Med 1995;14:523–528.
67. Lee E, Kwon H, Joo H, et al. Diagnosis of ovarian torsion with color Doppler sonography: depiction of twisted vascular pedicle. J Ultrasound Med 1998;17:83–89.
68. Richard HI, Parsons R, Broadman K, et al. Torsion of the fallopian tube: progression of sonographic features. J Clin Ultrasound 1998;26:374–376.
69. Patel M, Feldstein V, Chen D, et al. Endometriomas: diagnostic performance of US. Radiology 1999;210:739–745.
70. Sohaey R, Gardner T, Woodward P, et al. Sonographic diagnosis of peritoneal inclusion cysts. J Ultrasound Med 1995;14:913–917.
71. Kim J, Lee H, Woo S, et al. Peritoneal inclusion cysts and their relationship to the ovaries: evaluation with sonography. Radiology 1997;204:481–484.
72. Kim JS, Woo SK, Suh SJ, et al. Sonographic diagnosis of paraovarian cysts: value of detecting a separate ipsilateral ovary. AJR Am J Roentgenol 1995;164:1441–1444.
73. Stein A, Kooning P, Schlaerth J, et al. Relative frequency of malignant paraovarian tumors: should paraovarian tumors be aspirated. Obstet Gynecol 1990;75:1029–1031.
74. Jain K, Gerscovich E. Sonographic spectrum of pelvic vascular malformations in women. J Clin Ultrasound 1999;27:523–530.
75. Fleischer AC, Tait D, Mayo J, et al. Sonographic features of ovarian remnants. J Ultrasound Med 1998;17:551–555.
76. Kupfer M, Ralls P, Fu Y. Transvaginal sonographic evaluation of multiple peripherally distributed echogenic foci of the ovary: prevalence and histologic correlation. AJR Am J Roentgenol 1998;171:483–486.
77. Kremer S, Kutcher R, Rosenblatt R, et al. Postmenopausal tubo-ovarian abscess: sonographic considerations and clinical significance. J Ultrasound Med 1992;11:613–616.
78. Patten R, Vincent L, Wolner-Hanssen P, et al. Pelvic inflammatory disease: endovaginal sonography with laparoscopic correlation. J Ultrasound Med 1990;9:681–689.
79. Tepper R, Aviram R, Cohen N, et al. Doppler flow characteristics in patients with pelvic inflammatory disease: responders versus nonresponders. J Clin Ultrasound 1998;26:247–249.
80. Tinkanen H, Kujansuu E. Doppler ultrasound findings in tubo-ovarian infectious complex. J Clin Ultrasound 1993;21:175–178.
81. Atri M, Tran CN, Bret PM, et al. Accuracy of endovaginal sonography for the detection of fallopian tube blockage. J Ultrasound Med 1994;13:429–434.
82. Schiller VL, Tsuchiyama K. Development of hydrosalpinx during ovulation induction. J Ultrasound Med 1995;14:799–803.
83. Ong CL. Fallopian tube carcinoma with multiple tumor nodules seen on transvaginal sonography. J Ultrasound Med 1998;17:71–73.
84. Slanetz PJ, Whitman GJ, Halpern EF, et al. Imaging of fallopian tube tumors. AJR Am J Roentgenol 1997;169:1321–1324.
85. Schoenfeld A, Levavi H, Hirsch M, et al. Transvaginal sonography in postmenopausal women. J Clin Ultrasound 1990;18:350–358.

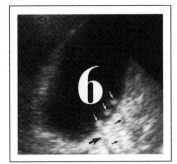

OBSTETRIC ULTRASOUND— FIRST TRIMESTER

- Imaging Technique
- Normal First Trimester Pregnancy
- Abnormal First Trimester Pregnancy
- Normal Developmental Anatomy of the Embryo

The first trimester covers the period from conception to the end of the 13th menstrual week. This is a time of dynamic growth and the differentiation and development of most organ systems. The embryo has the greatest risk of maldevelopment, injury, and death during this period because of external factors (infection, drugs, radiation) or chromosome abnormalities. Approximately 40% of implanted zygotes are lost as a result of unrecognized abortion with menstruation, whereas another 25–35% of the surviving embryos will threaten to abort during the first trimester. Approximately 1–2% of pregnancies will be ectopic, and these pregnancies are a major cause of pregnancy-related morbidity and mortality. Patients presenting with vaginal bleeding or pelvic pain in early pregnancy require urgent and accurate diagnosis (Box 6.1).

IMAGING TECHNIQUE

US remains the imaging method of first choice for diagnostic evaluations in obstetrics. Transvaginal (TV) US is particularly valuable in the first trimester because of its capability to demonstrate in high resolution the detailed anatomic changes of early pregnancy.

Examinations are usually begun using a transabdominal (TA) approach scanning the pelvis through a full bladder with a 3.5–5.0-MHz sector transducer. In our practice, if this examination demonstrates a normal-appearing intrauterine pregnancy with no adnexal abnormalities, the examination is considered satisfactory and is terminated. If the TA examination yields any other result, then TV examination is performed whenever possible. The patient is asked to empty her bladder and the examination continues utilizing a condom-covered 5.0–7.5-MHz intravaginal transducer.

Guidelines for first trimester sonography are provided by the American Institute of Ultrasound in Medicine and endorsed by the American College of Radiology [1]. The location of the gestational sac (GS) is documented. The embryo is identified and its crown-

> **Box 6.1: Differential Diagnosis of Vaginal Bleeding in the First Trimester**
>
> Spontaneous abortion   Ectopic pregnancy
> Anembryonic pregnancy   Subchorionic hemorrhage
> Embryonic demise   Implantation bleed
> Demise of a twin   Gestational trophoblastic disease

Examination of pregnancy in the first trimester should always include evaluation of the adnexa.

rump length (CRL) measured. If no embryo is present the mean diameter of the GS is measured. Gestational age (GA) is estimated by reference of the measurements made to appropriate tables. The presence or absence of embryonic life is determined by real-time observation. M-mode US is utilized to document cardiac activity and to measure cardiac rate. Doppler confirmation of embryonic cardiac activity is not recommended because of the higher US energy involved. Fetal number is documented. The uterus, cervix, and adnexa are carefully examined for any abnormalities.

NORMAL FIRST TRIMESTER PREGNANCY

GESTATIONAL DATING

In clinical obstetrics GA is determined from the first day of the mother's last menstrual period, assuming a regular menstrual cycle of 28 days. In embryology, GA is dated from conception providing a 2-week difference in embryologic dating compared with menstrual dating. In clinical practice and in this text all dating parameters will refer to menstrual dating. For example, 13 weeks GA means that 13 weeks have elapsed since the first day of the mother's last menstrual period. Technically, the developing human is considered an embryo up to 10 weeks menstrual age and a fetus thereafter until birth. Normal pregnancies last 40 weeks with a range of 37–42 weeks.

In the first trimester, GA is determined by measurement of mean sac diameter (MSD) before the embryo is visualized and by measurement of CRL from when the embryo is apparent to 12 weeks GA. MSD is determined by measuring the length (L), width (W), and height (H) of the GS in perpendicular planes, adding the results together and dividing by 3 (MSD = [L + W + H]/3). Measurements of MSD are made from the fluid/tissue interface of the sac and do not include any portion of the wall of the sac (Fig. 6.1). CRL is determined by measuring the maximum length of the visualized embryo (Fig. 6.2). No portion of the yolk sac, umbilical cord, or limbs is included in the measurement. A straight-line measurement is always used even if the torso of the embryo is flexed. Appropriate charts relate the measurements to menstrual age (Table 6.1) [2,3]. Both MSD and CRL measurements are accurate to ±1 week. These early pregnancy charts are acceptably accurate in the first trimester without correction for race, parental size, altitude, or other parameters known to affect birth weight.

NORMAL GESTATION

Understanding the physiology and detailed anatomy of early gestation as shown by TV US is essential to understanding the pathologic changes that occur in early pregnancy.

Ovulation and Fertilization

In a "normal" menstrual cycle of 28 days, days 1–14 are the follicular phase during which the ovary responds to follicle stimulating hormone (FSH) secreted by the pituitary gland [4]. FSH promotes development of a group of follicles that enlarge and produce and release estro-

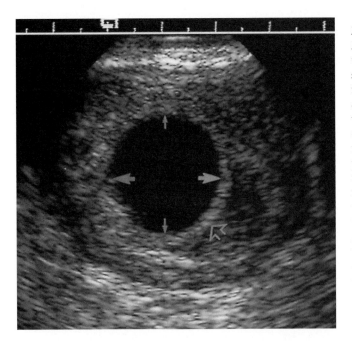

Figure 6.1 *Measurement of Mean Sac Diameter.* The diameter of the gestational sac is measured between fluid-soft tissue interfaces (*between pairs of closed arrows*). No portion of the wall of the sac is included. Three orthogonal measurements are made in perpendicular imaging planes. These three measurements are averaged to calculate mean sac diameter. Standardized tables (Table 6.1) are consulted to relate mean sac diameter to gestational age. Most US scanners provide these tables in the computer memory. The choriodecidual reaction (*open arrow*) that defines the wall of the gestational sac is well defined and uniformly echogenic.

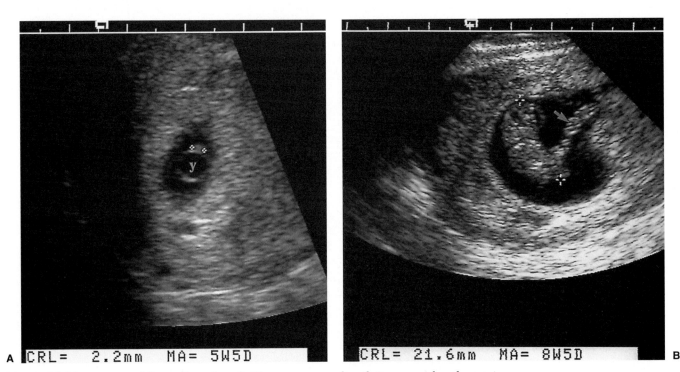

Figure 6.2 *Measurement of Crown-Rump Length.* The crown-rump length is measured as the maximum length of the visualized embryo (*between cursors, +*) when the embryo is small (*A*). When the embryo is larger (*B*), crown-rump length is measured as the straight-line distance from the top of the cranium to the end of the torso (*between cursors, +*) of the embryo. No compensation is made for curvature of the embryo. Care must be taken to avoid including limbs or cord in the measurement. Standardized tables (Table 6.1) relate the crown-rump length measurement to gestational age. The umbilical cord (*arrow*) is visualized. y, yolk sac.

Table 6.1: Gestational Age Estimation

Gestational Sac Size Mean Sac Diameter (mm)	Crown-Rump Length (mm) [3]	Gestational Age Menstrual Dating (weeks) [2]
3	—	4.6
4	—	4.7
5	—	4.9
5.5	—	5.0
6	—	5.1
7	—	5.3
8	—	5.4
9	—	5.6
10	2	5.7
11	3	5.9
12	3.5	6.0
13	4	6.1
14	5	6.3
15	6	6.4
16	7	6.6
17	8	6.7
18	9	6.9
19	9.5	7.0
20	10	7.1
21	11	7.3
22	12	7.4
23	13	7.6
24	14	7.7
25	15	7.9
26	16	8.0
26.5	17	8.1
27	18	8.3
28	19	8.4
29	20	8.6
30	21	8.7
31	22	8.9
32	23	9.0
33	24	9.1
34	25	9.3
35	26	9.4
36	28	9.6
37	29	9.7
38	30	9.9
39	31	10.0
40	32	10.1
41	34	10.3
42	35	10.4
43	37	10.6
44	38	10.7
45	40	10.9
46	40	11.0
47	42	11.1
48	44	11.3
49	46	11.4
50	48	11.6
51	50	11.7
52	52	11.9
53	54	12.0

Adapted from: Robinson H. "Gestational sac" volumes as determined by sonar in the first trimester of pregnancy. Br J Obstet Gynaecol 1975;82:100–107; Hadlock F, Shah Y, Kanon D, et al. Fetal crown rump length: reevaluation of relation to menstrual age (5–18 weeks) with high resolution real time US. Radiology 1992;182:501–505.

gen. Rising estrogen levels suppress secretion of FSH, resulting in atresia of all but one of the stimulated follicles. This **dominant follicle** (graafian follicle) continues to mature and enlarge and will be the source of ovulation. Ovulation occurs around day 14 (range, day 10–18) when the dominant follicle ruptures, releasing the ovum and a small amount of fluid into the peritoneal cavity. The **corpus luteum** develops at the site of the dominant follicle, forming a highly vascular mass that often becomes cystic as it fills with blood and lymph. The corpus luteum produces progesterone that maintains the secretory phase endometrium for successful implantation during the second half of the menstrual cycle. If fertilization of the ovum fails to occur, the corpus luteum will degenerate within 14 days. If fertilization occurs, human chorionic gonadotropin (hCG) from the fertilized ovum stimulates the corpus luteum to continue hormone secretion to support the developing pregnancy. The corpus luteum continues to function through the tenth week of gestation when the placenta replaces its hormone production. The corpus luteum may persist as a visible structure throughout pregnancy and must be recognized and differentiated from pathologic structures.

- **Primordial follicles** are too small to see with US [4].
- **Developing follicles** appear as thin-walled, anechoic cysts that may enlarge up to 14 mm. These follicles are randomly distributed over the surface of the ovary (see Figs. 5.6 and 5.29). They are seen most prominently during cycle days 5–7.
- A follicle larger than 14 mm is likely to be the **dominant follicle**, which continues to enlarge up to 25–30 mm prior to ovulation. In 5–11% of menstrual cycles, dominant follicles develop on each ovary.
- Rupture of the dominant follicle with ovulation results in partial or complete collapse of its cystic structure (Fig. 6.3). Clotted blood and invading fibroblasts occupy the site, which appears as a partially collapsed cyst with wrinkled walls or as an echogenic mass. Fluid volume in the cul-de-sac averages 15–25 mL following ovulation [4].
- The **corpus luteum** initially appears as small irregular cyst containing echogenic blood products (the corpus hemorrhagicum). In most patients the corpus luteum disappears with menstruation. In some patients it continues to enlarge through menstruation up to approximately 40-mm size. This persistent corpus luteum appears as a cystic structure containing anechoic fluid or fluid with particulate matter. It usually disappears within 1 or 2 subsequent menstrual cycles.
- The **corpus luteum of pregnancy** is nearly always identified (98%) with TV US but has a variety of appearances [5,6]:

Recognition of the many appearances of the corpus luteum is essential to correct interpretation of first trimester US examination.

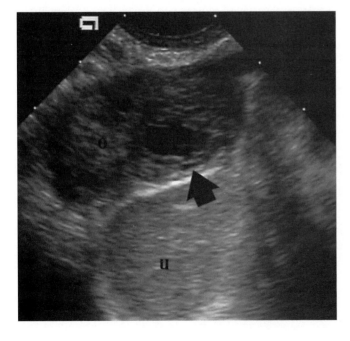

Figure 6.3 *Early Corpus Luteum.* The site of rupture of the dominant follicle soon after ovulation appears as a collapsed cystic structure (*arrow*) on the ovary (o). u, uterus.

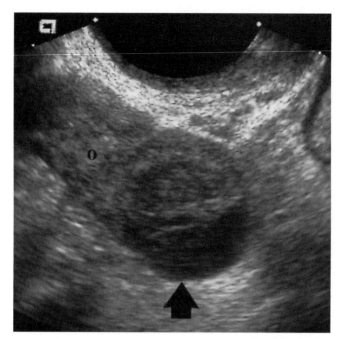

Figure 6.4 *Corpus Luteum—Hypoechoic Solid Appearance.* The corpus luteum appears as a hypoechoic solid mass (*arrow*) on the right ovary (o) on this transvaginal image.

- Identification of origin of the corpus luteum on the ovary is key to its recognition and differentiation from other similar appearing structures.
- Size of the corpus luteum averages 2 cm and varies up to 5–6 cm.
- A solid-appearing hypoechoic structure on the ovary is most common (34%) (Fig. 6.4).
- A cyst containing anechoic fluid and having a thick wall is seen in 27% (Fig. 6.5).
- A cyst with floating debris and particulate matter is present in 23%.
- A thin-walled cyst with anechoic fluid is seen in 15% (Fig. 6.6).
- Intense blood flow surrounds the corpus luteum on color Doppler and may resemble the intense trophoblastic flow surrounding a GS (see Fig. 6.22). Spectral Doppler shows a low-resistance, spectral pattern with mean resistance index of 0.50.

Implantation and Early Appearance of the Gestational Sac

A **zygote** is formed when a sperm fertilizes the ovum, usually in the ampullary portion of the fallopian tube. Cell division occurs as the zygote migrates to the endometrial cavity. A

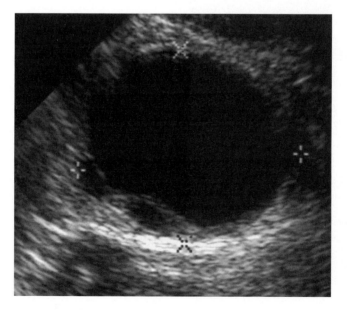

Figure 6.5 *Corpus Luteum—Thick-Walled Cyst Appearance.* Transvaginal scan shows an anechoic ovarian cyst (*between calipers, +, x*) with moderately thick walls.

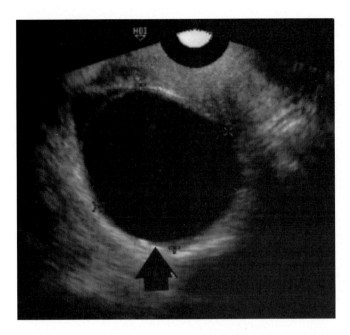

Figure 6.6 *Corpus Luteum—Thin-Walled Cyst Appearance.* This corpus luteum (*arrow, between cursors, +, x*) has a thin wall and contains anechoic fluid.

cystic structure called the **blastocyst** is formed with two cell layers present. The outer cell layer is the **trophoblast** that forms the chorion and the fetal components of the placenta. The inner cell layer forms the embryo, umbilical cord, amnion and secondary yolk sac. The blastocyst implants 7–10 days after fertilization (around menstrual day 23) by burrowing into the endometrium. The thickened, secretory-phase endometrium, characteristic of the second half of the menstrual cycle, begins to secrete glycogen rich in mucin to support the pregnancy. The thickening and functional change of the endometrium in response to pregnancy is called *decidual reaction*, and the endometrium is now called **decidua**. The blastocyst continues to develop forming a recognizable GS completely covered by decidua.

- The early GS is first visible by TV US at approximately 4.5 weeks menstrual age. A small cystic structure 2–3 mm in size is seen burrowed into and completely covered by echogenic decidua, giving it the appearance of a thick-walled cyst (Fig. 6.7). The appearance of this very early GS is called the **intradecidual sign** [7]. This appearance is highly characteristic of early intrauterine pregnancy, although care must be taken to avoid mistaking fluid in the uterine cavity or an endometrial cyst for an early GS [8]. The thin

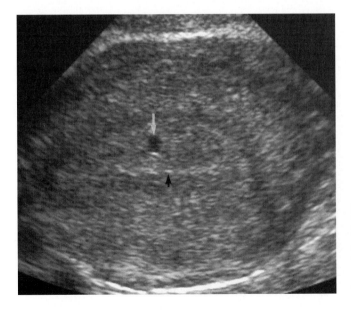

Figure 6.7 *Intradecidual Sign.* A 3-mm gestational sign (*white arrow*) is seen burrowed within the decidua. An echogenic line (*black arrow*) represents the uterine cavity.

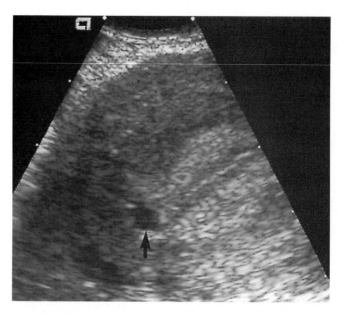

Figure 6.8 *Endometrial Cyst.* An endometrial cyst (*arrow*) in a non-pregnant patient has an appearance very similar to the early gestational sac shown in Figure 6.7. Note the location of the endometrial cyst in the basal layer of the endometrium near the myometrium.

echogenic line of the uterine cavity must be recognized and observed to pass by, rather than meet, the sac burrowed in the decidual lining [9]. A fluid collection that meets or forms a beak with the uterine cavity line represents fluid in the uterine cavity and not an intradecidual GS. Endometrial cysts are found close to the basal layer of the endometrium and have a thin wall (Fig. 6.8), rather than the thick wall characteristic of a GS.

Visualization of the yolk sac confirms that a cystic structure is a GS.

- The secondary **yolk sac** is the first structure visible within the GS and is a finding that unequivocally confirms identification of the GS (Fig. 6.9). The yolk sac is usually visible by TV US at the start of the sixth menstrual week when the GS measures 8–10 mm. It serves a primary source of nutrients for the embryo before placental function is established. The yolk sac should always be visible on TA US when the GS measures 20-mm MSD [10]. It should always be seen with TV US when the GS measures 8-mm diameter [11]. The normal yolk sac is a thin-walled, fluid-filled cyst that does not normally exceed 6 mm in diameter [12]. The yolk sac is located in the chorionic cavity (Fig. 6.10). It is connected to the umbilicus of the embryo by the vitelline duct (omphalomesenteric duct).
- The **double bleb sign** describes the early appearance of the amniotic cavity and the yolk sac seen as early as 5.5 weeks [13]. The yolk sac and amniotic cavity appear as two fluid-filled, thin-walled, spherical structures approximately equal in size within the GS (Fig. 6.11).

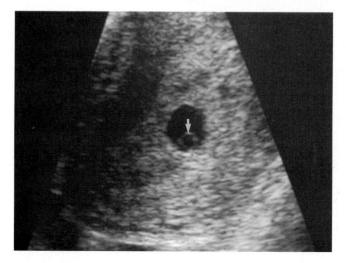

Figure 6.9 *Yolk Sac in Early Pregnancy.* Magnified transvaginal image shows a tiny cystic structure that contains a yolk sac (*white arrow*). Visualization of the yolk sac is diagnostic of this cystic structure being a gestational sac.

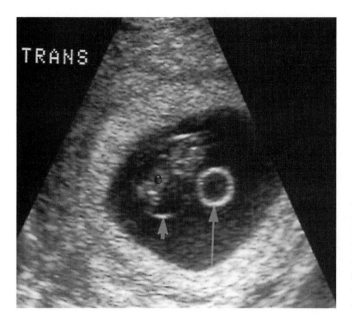

Figure 6.10 *Yolk Sac in Chorionic Cavity.* In a more advanced gestation with an embryo (e) present, the yolk sac (*long arrow*) is a prominent cystic structure in the chorionic cavity outside of the amnion (*short arrow*).

- The **embryo** is first visualized as an echogenic, disk-like structure approximately 2 mm long within the amniotic cavity. The embryo is normally seen by the end of the fifth menstrual week (Figs. 6.2A, 6.11). The normal embryo grows approximately 1 mm per day in length.
- **Embryonic cardiac activity** may be seen with TV US when the embryo is as small as 1–2 mm. All normal embryos should have cardiac activity visible on TV US when the embryo measures 5 mm or more in length [14]. Initial visible embryonic heart rate at 5–6 weeks GA is 100 beats/minute. The rate increases over the next 2–3 weeks to 140 beats/minute [15].

Normal Structure of the Gestational Sac

The normal anatomy of the GS must be recognized to correctly interpret early pregnancy US examinations (Fig. 6.12). The maternal decidua consists of three layers (Fig. 6.13). The **decidua capsularis** covers the surface of the expanding GS as it protrudes into the uterine cavity. The **decidua basalis** combines with **chorion frondosum** to form the placenta at the site of implantation. The **decidua vera** (also called *decidua parietalis*) lines the remainder of the uterine cavity away from the placenta. Because the GS is implanted within and is cov-

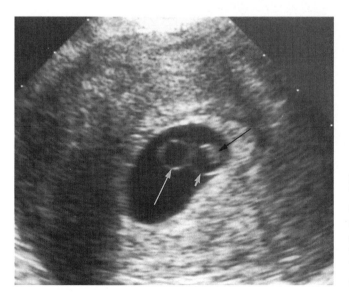

Figure 6.11 *Double Bleb Sign.* The yolk sac (*long white arrow*) and amniotic sac (*short white arrow*) appear as two cystic structures of equal size within the fluid of the chorionic cavity. The embryo (*black arrow*) is seen within the amniotic cavity.

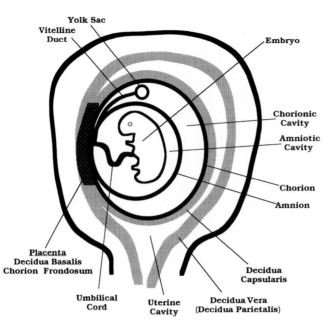

Figure 6.12 *Anatomy of Early Pregnancy.* A line drawing illustrates the anatomic structures of early pregnancy.

ered by decidua, the uterine cavity remains open to the cervix. Bleeding associated with the pregnancy occurs into the uterine cavity and exits the uterus via the cervix. The outer membrane of the GS is the **chorion**. The inner membrane is the **amnion** (Fig. 6.10), which defines the **amniotic cavity** containing the developing embryo. The yolk sac is in the **chorionic cavity**, between amnion and chorion (Fig. 6.10). Low-level echoes are commonly seen within the fluid of the chorionic cavity. As the embryo grows, the amnion expands and becomes adherent to the chorion, obliterating the chorionic cavity at 15–16 weeks. Occasionally the amnion and chorion remain unfused throughout pregnancy. US features of the normal GS are listed below:

- The normal GS is round or oval in shape, smooth in contour, and is positioned in the fundus of the uterus. The choriodecidual reaction produces a smooth echogenic rim >2 mm in thickness around the GS (Fig. 6.1) [10].
- The **double decidual sign** describes the appearance of two echogenic arcs of decidual tissue separated by a hypoechoic arc of fluid in the endometrial cavity (Fig. 6.14) [16].

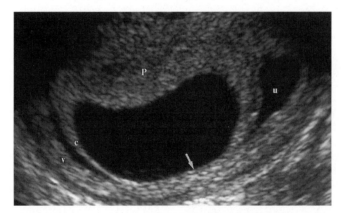

Figure 6.13 *Three Layers of Decidua.* Transvaginal image illustrates the three layers of decidua. The amniotic sac and a normal embryo were visible elsewhere within this gestational sac. The placenta (P) forms from decidua basalis and chorion frondosum at the site of implantation of the blastocyst. Decidua capsularis (c) covers the portion of the gestational sac that protrudes into the uterine cavity (u). Decidua vera (v) lines the remainder of the uterine cavity. This uterine cavity contains a small amount of blood. The chorion is a very thin membrane defined only by the sharp fluid-tissue interface (*arrow*) of the gestational sac.

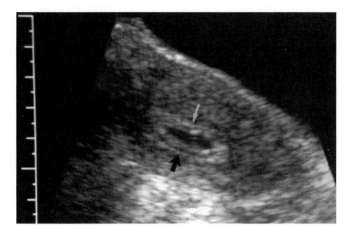

Figure 6.14 *Double Decidual Sign.* Transabdominal image illustrates the two layers of echogenic decidua separated by a thin echolucent line that make up the double decidual sign (*black arrow*). The double decidual appearance extends only part way around the circumference of the sac. It is not present at the site of placental development (*white arrow*).

The visualized decidual arcs consist of decidua vera and decidua capsularis. The double decidual sign partially encircles the GS. The decidual arcs are incomplete because of development of the placenta at the site of implantation.

- Normal growth of the GS is 1.1 mm/day MSD for the first 8 weeks.
- Doppler examination of the trophoblastic tissue that surrounds a pregnancy shows intense vascularity with a high-velocity, low-resistance spectral waveform. This vascular pattern has been characterized as a "ring of fire." The presence of this rim of high vascularity can be used to differentiate intrauterine pregnancy (IUP) from the intrauterine pseudogestational sac of ectopic pregnancy [17]. The use of Doppler is controversial in early pregnancy because of the higher US energies utilized and concern for potential, but unproven, adverse effects on a normal embryo.

Role of Quantitative β-hCG Determinations

Radioimmunoassay (RIA) for the serum beta subunit of human chorionic gonadotropin (β-hCG) provides a specific and sensitive laboratory test for the presence of a fertilized ovum. If the RIA is negative, the patient is not pregnant. If RIA is positive, serial quantitative measurements are useful in diagnosis of normal and abnormal pregnancy. The problem comes in interpretation of results. Numerous papers have been written touting the value of "discriminatory levels" of β-hCG. For example, one study states that if serum β-hCG exceeds 1000 mIU/mL, then an intrauterine GS should always be identified in a normal pregnancy on TV US [18]. To apply this criterion, the first pitfall is to correlate the reporting standard used in the published study with the reporting standard used by the laboratory where you practice. Since the 1960s, a number of reporting standards have been utilized, including the First International Standard, the Second International Standard, the Third International Standard, and the International Reference Preparation. Reported values differ significantly depending on which standard is used. The second pitfall is that different laboratories using the same standard will report different results depending on which laboratory test kit they use. The range of normal values for a given week of pregnancy varies widely from one laboratory to another. These pitfalls make the use of reported discriminatory levels hazardous in any given practice unless specific correlation has been individually studied for a given laboratory and patient population. Further caution is warranted because even if these studies are correlated at each practice location, hospitals commonly change laboratories and test kits for cost considerations without informing practicing physicians.

> The use of "discriminatory levels" of β-hCG in the interpretation of first trimester US has many pitfalls.

In view of these difficulties with using numerical reported values, several uses of β-hCG are unequivocally valuable in any setting. First, if the qualitative β-hCG is positive, a pregnancy "event" has unequivocally occurred. The differential diagnosis may include all of normal and abnormal pregnancy. Second, for a given patient following serial β-hCG is useful in determining normal development. In normal pregnancy, **β-hCG levels double every 48 hours.** Failure to double in value every 48 hours is strong evidence of a nonviable, possibly ectopic, pregnancy.

Box 6.2: US Signs of Failed First Trimester Pregnancy

Empty gestation sac (absent yolk sac)
    At MSD >20 mm on transabdominal US
    At MSD >8 mm on transvaginal US
Absent embryo
    At MSD >25 mm on transabdominal US
    At MSD >16 mm on transvaginal US

Empty amniotic cavity
    Visualization of amnion without visualization of embryo
Absent cardiac activity
    In embryo >4–5 mm in crown-rump length

ABNORMAL FIRST TRIMESTER PREGNANCY

ABNORMAL INTRAUTERINE PREGNANCY

Threatened Abortion

Bleeding and cramping in the first trimester of pregnancy while the cervix is closed is clinically diagnosed as a **threatened abortion**. US is utilized to make a specific and accurate diagnosis on which to base appropriate therapy. Threatened abortion affects 25% of all clinically apparent pregnancies. Up to 50% of these patients will abort their pregnancy. The differential diagnosis of threatened abortion is listed in Box 6.1.

Signs of Failed Pregnancy

Approximately 12% of all clinically apparent pregnancies will fail. These pregnancies develop to an early stage and then become non-viable. The following are diagnostic signs of a failed pregnancy (Box 6.2). Each sign depends upon visualization of a given structure of a minimum "discriminatory size" before the sign can be considered diagnostic. In every instance, TV US allows accurate diagnosis at an earlier stage of pregnancy. When measurements are close to the discriminatory size, follow-up examination should be considered to give the benefit of the doubt to the pregnancy [19]. Failed pregnancies may be classified an **anembryonic pregnancy** if no embryo is visualized, or as **embryonic demise** or **fetal demise** if an embryo or fetus is present.

- **Empty GS.** Visualization of an "empty" GS, exceeding a discriminatory size that contains neither yolk sac nor embryo, is evidence of failed pregnancy (Fig. 6.15). Discriminatory sac size for non-visualization of a yolk sac is 8-mm MSD for TV US and 20-mm MSD for TA US [10,11].
- **Absent embryo.** Discriminatory sac size for non-visualization of an embryo is 16 mm for TV US and 25 mm for TA US [10,11]. A failed pregnancy with absence of a visualized embryo is termed an *anembryonic pregnancy* or *blighted ovum* (Fig. 6.15).

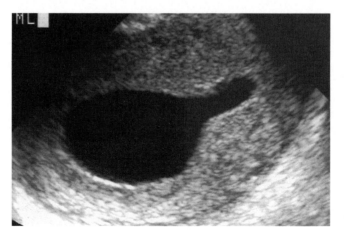

Figure 6.15 *Empty Gestational Sac.* Transvaginal image shows a large, misshapen gestational sac. This sac measured 31 mm mean sac diameter. At this size both a yolk sac and an embryo should be visualized on a transabdominal US examination. The sac is keyhole-shaped rather than round or oval. The choriodecidual reaction is thin and only weakly echogenic. This appearance is diagnostic of an anembryonic pregnancy.

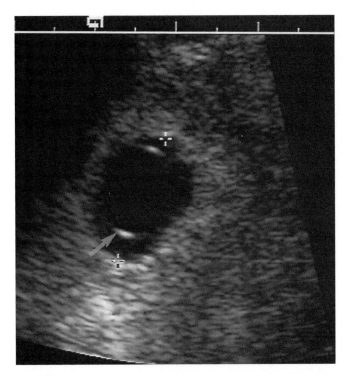

Figure 6.16 *Empty Amnion.* Visualization of the amnion (*arrow*) without the presence of an embryo is evidence of a failed pregnancy. The size of the amniotic sac (~12 mm) far exceeds the normal size of the yolk sac (~6 mm) and confirms identification of this membrane as amnion. Cursors (+) measure the diameter of the gestational sac.

- **Empty amnion.** Visualization of the amnion without visualization of an embryo is a related sign of failed pregnancy (Fig. 6.16). Between 6.5 and 10 weeks gestation (GS-MSD of 14–36 mm), the diameter of the amniotic cavity is normally equal to the CRL of the fetus [20]. An embryo should always be visualized if the amniotic cavity measures 6-mm diameter or above. The amnion is a thin membrane that separates the amniotic cavity from the chorionic cavity. Visualization requires high-quality technique.
- **Dead embryo.** Visualization of an embryo without cardiac activity is proof of a failed pregnancy (Fig. 6.17). The discriminatory embryonic size to unequivocally diagnose absent heartbeat is 4–5-mm CRL for TV US and 9-mm CRL for TA US [21–23]. Absent

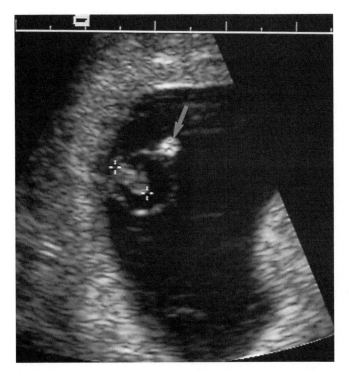

Figure 6.17 *Dead Embryo— Calcified Yolk Sac.* A 6.3-week embryo (*between cursors*, +, crown-rump length = 5.8 mm) without a heartbeat is seen within the amniotic cavity. The yolk sac (*arrow*) is calcified. Calcification of the yolk sac is associated with embryonic demise.

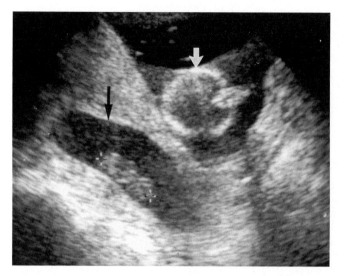

Figure 6.18 *Abortion in Progress*. Transabdominal image shows a gestational sac (*black arrow*) containing a dead embryo (*between cursors, +*) presenting at an open cervical os. Expulsion of the pregnancy is inevitable. The balloon (*white arrow*) of a Foley catheter is evident in the bladder.

heartbeat is distinguished from bradycardia by observing the cardiac area for at least 2 minutes, preferably by two US examiners. Most early embryonic demise is caused by fatal chromosome abnormalities [24].

■ **Abortion in progress.** A distorted GS presenting in the lower uterine segment with an open cervical os is classified as an abortion in progress or inevitable abortion (Fig. 6.18). Complete expulsion of the GS soon follows.

■ **Blighted twin.** Demise of one twin in a twin pregnancy is a relatively common event in the first trimester. The dead embryo will usually be reabsorbed while the live embryo usually develops normally (Fig. 6.19). US reveals no embryo or a dead embryo in a usually smaller or partially collapsed GS. Alternatively, one GS contains an embryo and the second GS is empty. The GS of a blighted twin may be mistaken for a subchorionic hemorrhage.

Signs That Predict a Poor Outcome of Pregnancy
The following US signs are predictive of poor outcome (failure) of a first trimester pregnancy (Box 6.3).

■ **Bradycardia.** An embryonic heart rate below 85 beats per minute is strong evidence of impending embryonic demise [25].

■ **Oligohydramnios** in the first trimester results in small size of the GS relative to the size of the embryo. The MSD of the GS normally exceeds the CRL by 5 mm or more between

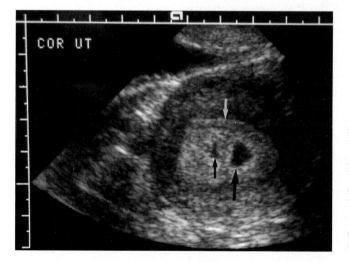

Figure 6.19 *Blighted Twin*. Transvaginal image shows two gestational sacs (*black arrows*). The larger sac (*large black arrow*) contained a live embryo. The smaller, deformed sac (*small black arrow*) contained no embryo. Note the double decidual sign (*white arrow*).

Box 6.3: US Signs of Poor Prognosis for First Trimester Pregnancy

· ·

Abnormal yolk sac   **Abnormal appearance of gestational sac**

    Large yolk sac (>6 mm)   Irregular margin of gestational sac
    Thick wall, irregular, or calcified yolk sac   Abnormal pointed, flattened, or
Bradycardia   crenated shape of gestational sac
    Heart rate <85 bpm at 5–8 weeks gesta-   **Abnormal location of gestational sac**
    tion age   Low implantation near cervix
Abnormal decidual reaction   Gestational sac protruding into or
    Thin decidua   through open cervix
    Decidua of low echogenicity

5.5 and 9 weeks GA. A small sac (less than 5 mm larger than CRL) is an indicator of incipient spontaneous abortion [26].

- **Subchorionic hemorrhage** is a common cause of vaginal bleeding in the first trimester affecting up to 18% of women who present with bleeding [27]. Subchorionic hemorrhage is believed to be a mild form of placental abruption with venous bleeding arising from the edge of the placenta (Fig. 6.20). Hemorrhage strips chorion from the myometrium and extends into the uterine cavity. US shows the hemorrhage as a crescent-shaped collection of fluid between the GS and the uterine wall. The appearance of hemorrhage depends upon its age. Acute clotted blood is isoechoic or hyperechoic to the placenta. As the clots dissolve the collection becomes progressively hypoechoic to anechoic. Small subchorionic hemorrhages are of no clinical significance. However, large hemorrhages exceeding 40% of the volume of the GS are associated with fetal loss rates of up to 50% [28,29]. Risk of spontaneous abortion increases with the size of the hemorrhage, older age of the mother (>35 years), and with earlier gestations (8 weeks or less) [30].
- **Abnormal yolk sac.** An abnormal appearance of the yolk sac correlates with early pregnancy failure. The yolk sac may be too large (>6 mm) (see Fig. 6.28), irregular in shape, have a thick wall, or be calcified (Fig. 6.17) [12,31,32]. Differentiation of an enlarged yolk sac from the amniotic cavity is difficult but irrelevant because any empty cystic structure within the GS larger than 6-mm diameter predicts a failed pregnancy.
- **Thin (<2 mm), poorly echogenic decidua** is a poor prognostic sign for first trimester pregnancy but is difficult to recognize with certainty (Fig. 6.15). It adds to the evidence of impending failure of pregnancy when other signs are present [10].
- **Abnormal position** of the GS correlates with poor prognosis (Fig. 6.21). Any position of the GS except within the fundus of the uterus is abnormal.
- Uterine anomalies are associated with an increased rate of pregnancy loss (Fig. 6.22).

Retained Products of Conception

Retention of products of conception (POC) within the uterus following spontaneous abortion or delivery is associated with risk of bleeding, uterine infection, and synechiae formation. Following death of the embryo, the pregnancy is usually retained in the uterus for a week or longer until hormone levels decrease and vascular support of the pregnancy atrophies. Decidual necrosis causes uterine irritability that expels the pregnancy. Patients who present with bleeding or signs of infection following spontaneous or assisted abortion are examined for retained POC.

- Thin endometrium (<2 mm) is indicative of the absence of retained POC. The decidua becomes necrotic following demise of the pregnancy and should be completely sloughed with expulsion of the pregnancy [33].
- Any cystic or echogenic space-occupying collection in the uterine cavity should be considered to be POC (Fig. 6.23).

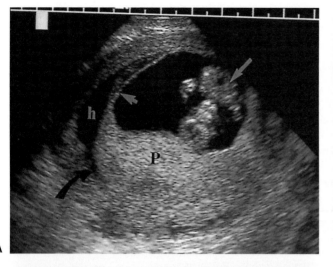

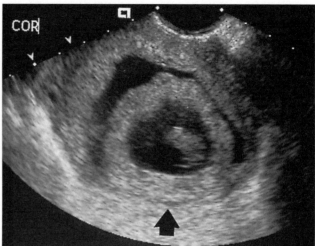

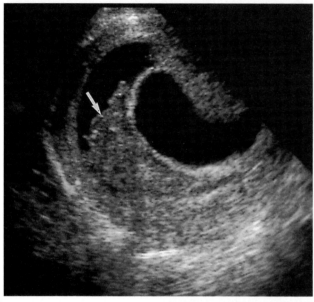

Figure 6.20 *Subchorionic Hemorrhage. A.* A subchorionic hemorrhage results from bleeding from the margin (*curved black arrow*) of the placenta (P) into the uterine cavity (h). The amniotic cavity containing the developing embryo (*long white arrow*) is separated from the hemorrhage by fused amnion/chorion (*short white arrow*) covered by decidua capsularis. *B.* A larger subchorionic hemorrhage is seen in another patient nearly completely encircling the gestational sac. The sac is anchored to the uterine wall at its placental attachment (*arrow*). *C.* Another hemorrhage shows clotted blood (*arrow*) in the uterine cavity.

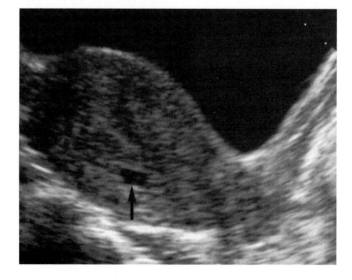

Figure 6.21 *Low Position of Gestational Sac.* This small deformed gestational sac (*arrow*) is positioned low in the uterine body. Implantation of the gestational sac anywhere except in the uterine fundus is a poor prognostic sign.

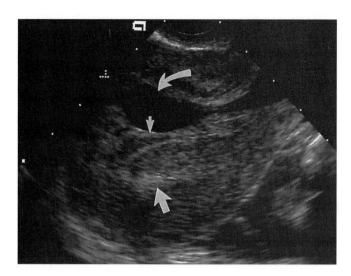

Figure 6.22 *Pregnancy in Septate Uterus.* Transvaginal image shows an empty gestational sac (*curved arrow*) in the left horn of a septate uterus. Echogenic decidual reaction is seen in the right horn (*fat arrow*). A thin muscular septum (*short arrow*) separates the two chambers of the uterus. A small septum, such as this one, can usually be resected hysteroscopically and result in improved prognosis for successful completion of subsequent pregnancies.

- Thickening of the hyperechoic endometrium >5 mm is suggestive of POC [33].
- A thin layer of hypoechoic material in the uterine cavity is more likely to be blood than POC.
- Gas in the endometrial cavity produces focal bright echoes with ring down or acoustic shadowing. Gas is found in the uterine cavity in 15% of normal pregnancies postpartum and cannot by itself be considered evidence of endometritis [34].

ECTOPIC PREGNANCY

An ectopic pregnancy is implantation of a fertilized ovum outside of the fundus or body of the uterine cavity. Any pregnant woman may have an ectopic pregnancy but the risk is increased when there is a past history of pelvic inflammatory disease, tubal surgery, previous ectopic pregnancy, use of intrauterine device, ovulation induction, or *in vitro* fertilization. The ectopic pregnancy is prone to rupture with hemorrhage that may be fatal. Ectopic

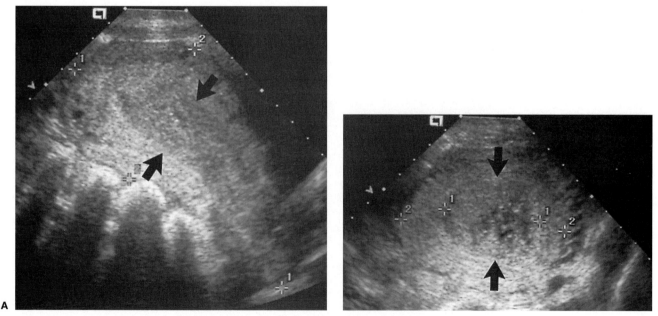

Figure 6.23 *Retained Products of Conception.* Longitudinal (*A*) and transverse (*B*) transabdominal images show an enlarged uterine cavity containing amorphous echogenic material (*between arrows*).

In the setting of "rule out ectopic pregnancy," US examination is most often an exercise in risk assessment.

pregnancy is responsible for approximately 15% of maternal deaths. Patients present with pelvic pain, cramping, or vaginal bleeding.

US currently plays a critical role in the diagnosis or exclusion of ectopic pregnancy. US findings most often provide an assessment of the risk of ectopic pregnancy, rather than a specific diagnosis. The initial goal of US examination is to demonstrate evidence of an IUP. When an IUP is definitely present, the risk of coexisting ectopic pregnancy is small, estimated at 1 in 30,000 for the general population and 1 in 6,000–7,000 for the high-risk population [35]. Patients at higher risk for heterotopic pregnancy (simultaneous intrauterine and ectopic pregnancy) are those who are under treatment for infertility. Detailed evaluation of the adnexa is mandatory even if an IUP is present.

Most (95%) of ectopic pregnancies implant within the ampullary or isthmic portions of the fallopian tube. Approximately 2–4% of ectopics implant within the intramural (interstitial) portion of the tube as it traverses the uterine wall. Cervical, abdominal, and ovarian implantations are rare with each accounting for less than 1% of ectopic pregnancies.

A definitive diagnosis of ectopic pregnancy is made only when a live embryo or GS containing a yolk sac is identified clearly outside of the uterus (Figs. 6.24, 6.25). Unfortunately this result is present in only 20% of ectopic pregnancies.

The following is a list of US findings in ectopic pregnancy. The approximate risk of ectopic pregnancy associated with each finding is stated. This risk is stated with the caveat that no IUP is identified in association with the extrauterine findings.

- IUP is confirmed by demonstration of intrauterine GS containing a yolk sac or living embryo. Risk = 1 in 7,000 to 1 in 30,000 for general population [35]. However, it is reported as high as 1 in 100 for infertility patients treated with ovulation induction or *in vitro* fertilization [36].
- Intradecidual sac. This sign is highly but not perfectly predictive of IUP. Follow-up US to identify a yolk sac or embryo and serial serum β-hCG to confirm appropriately increasing levels are needed to confirm IUP. Risk = very low, follow-up needed [8].
- Extrauterine GS containing yolk sac is diagnostic of ectopic pregnancy (Fig. 6.24). Risk = 100%.
- Extrauterine GS containing living embryo is diagnostic of ectopic pregnancy (Fig. 6.25). Risk = 100%.
- Extrauterine "tubal ring," an echogenic thick-walled, ring-like mass separate from the ovary, represents a GS with surrounding trophoblastic reaction (Figs. 6.24, 6.25A). Risk = ~95% [37].
- Complex cystic or solid adnexal mass without distinguishing features. This finding is consistent with tubal rupture and clotted blood (Fig. 6.26). Risk = ~86% [38].

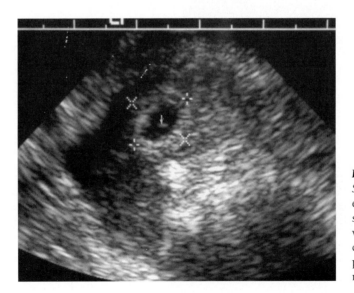

Figure 6.24 *Ectopic Gestational Sac Containing Yolk Sac.* An extrauterine sac (*between cursors, +, x*) shows a tubal ring sign with thick echogenic wall and contains a yolk sac (*arrow*). The presence of the yolk sac is diagnostic of extrauterine gestation.

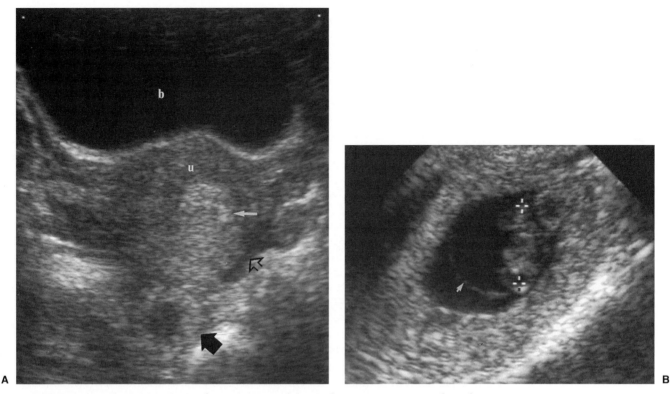

A

B

Figure 6.25 *Ectopic Pregnancy—Live Embryo. **A.** A transabdominal image in transverse plane shows an empty uterus (u) with thickened endometrium (white arrow) representing decidual reaction. Posterior to the uterus is a thick-walled cystic mass (solid black arrow), a "tubal ring sign." Fluid is seen in the cul-de-sac (open black arrow). b, urine-filled bladder. **B.** Transvaginal image in the same patient shows a small living embryo (between cursors, +) with cardiac motion easily visible during real-time US examination. The amnion (arrow) is also seen within this ectopic gestational sac.*

■ Small volume of anechoic-free intraperitoneal pelvic fluid. Risk = normal finding, not predictive of ectopic pregnancy.

■ Moderate or large volume of free intraperitoneal fluid, particularly if the fluid is echogenic (Fig. 6.27). Risk = ~70% [37].

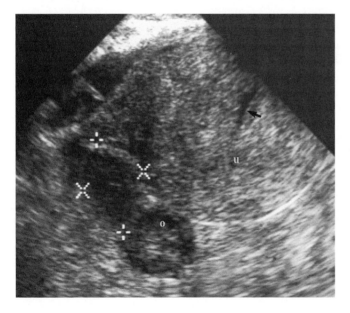

Figure 6.26 *Ectopic Pregnancy—Amorphous Adnexal Mass. Transvaginal image shows a lobulated heterogeneous mass (between cursors, +, x) posterior to the uterus (u). This mass proved to be a tubal ectopic pregnancy adjacent to the right ovary (o). A small volume of fluid is present in the uterine cavity (arrow).*

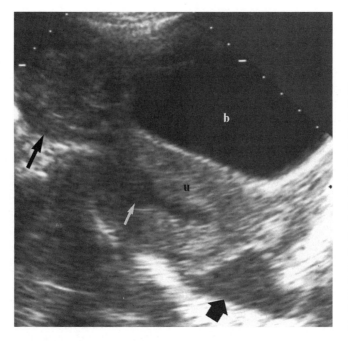

Figure 6.27 *Ectopic Pregnancy—Echogenic Fluid in Cul-de-Sac.* Longitudinal transabdominal image shows a moderate volume of echogenic fluid in the cul-de-sac (*fat black arrow*). A round, amorphous, solid-appearing mass (*long black arrow*) is evident superior to the uterus (u). Within the uterus is an unusually shaped fluid collection (*white arrow*), a "pseudosac" of ectopic pregnancy. The combination of adnexal mass and echogenic cul-de-sac fluid makes this patient very high risk (~98%) for ectopic pregnancy. b, bladder.

- The presence of both complex or solid adnexal mass and echogenic fluid is virtually diagnostic of ectopic pregnancy. Risk = ~98%.
- Ovarian masses are unlikely to represent an ectopic pregnancy. Most ovarian masses are corpus luteum cysts. The wide range of appearance of corpus luteum cysts has been previously described (Figs. 6.3–6.6). Thick-walled cysts may closely resemble the tubal ring of an ectopic pregnancy. Clot within a hemorrhagic cyst may closely resemble a dead embryo. Blood flow within or adjacent to the cyst may resemble the ring of fire on color flow US. Risk = physiologic finding not predictive of ectopic pregnancy.
- Thin-walled ovarian cyst containing anechoic fluid is likely the corpus luteum. Risk = normal finding, not predictive of ectopic pregnancy.
- Double decidual sign (Fig. 6.14) is highly predictive of IUP, although the IUP may not be viable. Risk = very low.
- Intrauterine fluid collection may represent the "pseudogestational sac" seen with ectopic pregnancy or may be retained fluid associated with recent failed pregnancy or spontaneous abortion (Figs. 6.27, 6.28). The intrauterine fluid collection must be differentiated from a true GS by careful attention to detail. Pseudosac fluid is commonly echogenic and may show dependent layering. The shape of the fluid collection is usually non-spherical. No double decidual sign is present. Doppler shows minimal low-velocity flow or no flow. Risk depends upon coexisting findings. An IUP is not confirmed.
- Normal US examination. Because the patient is pregnant an ectopic pregnancy is not excluded. Differential diagnosis includes early normal IUP, early abnormal IUP, completed abortion, and ectopic pregnancy. Risk = ~5% [38].
- Doppler findings on adnexal masses are usually noncontributory. The prominent low-impedance "ring of fire" blood flow (Fig. 6.29) seen in trophoblastic tissue surrounding the GS is also seen with tubo-ovarian abscess, corpus luteum cyst, malignant ovarian tumors, and pedunculated leiomyomas. Risk = not affected.

Interstitial Ectopic Pregnancy

An interstitial ectopic pregnancy implants in the intramural portion of the tube as it traverses the uterine wall. It tends to present clinically later in the course of development with the GS and its blood supply is significantly larger. Rupture then presents a greater risk of massive hemorrhage.

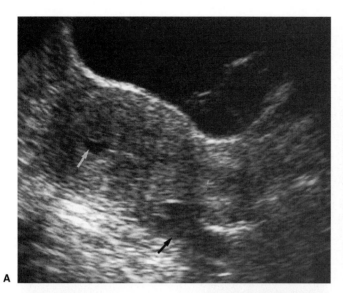

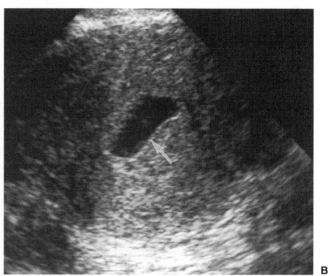

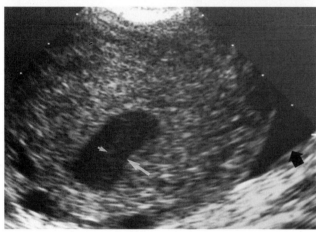

Figure 6.28 *Pseudogestational Sac of Ectopic Pregnancy. A. Trans-abdominal image shows a small fluid collection (white arrow) in the uterine cavity. Transvaginal US is needed to characterize the appearance of the fluid collection. Echogenic fluid is noted in the cul-de-sac (black arrow). B. Transvaginal image in the same patient shows the fluid collection (arrow) is oblong, not round or oval, and lacks the well-defined echogenic rim of choriodecidual reaction. No double decidua sign is present. This patient had a small tubal pregnancy in the right adnexa. C. In another patient, transvaginal US shows a pseudosac (long white arrow) containing layering echogenic fluid (short white arrow). No double decidual sign is present. Fluid is also evident in the cul-de-sac (black arrow).*

- Asymmetric thickness of myometrium around the GS (Fig. 6.30). The myometrial mantle may be partially absent [39].
- GS is eccentric to empty uterine cavity (Fig. 6.30).
- Many cases do not have a recognizable GS. An inhomogeneous mass is seen in the cornual region [40].

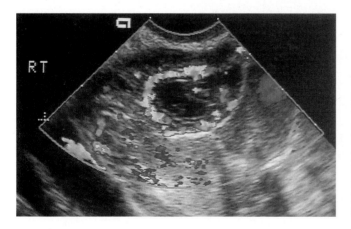

Figure 6.29 *Ring of Fire.* This ring of fire surrounds a corpus luteum. Similar intense color depicting hypervascularity may be seen surrounding a normal pregnancy, ectopic pregnancy, tubo-ovarian abscess, malignant ovarian tumor, or pedunculated leiomyoma (see Color Figure 6.29).

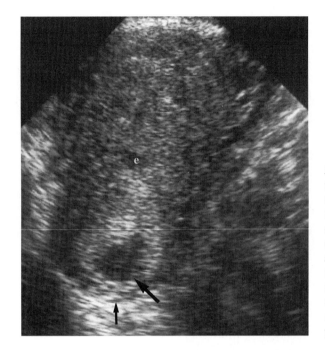

Figure 6.30 *Interstitial Ectopic Pregnancy.* Transvaginal image shows an eccentric intrauterine gestational sac (*long arrow*) with well-defined echogenic rim. The endometrium (e) of the fundal region was ill defined, and the uterine cavity was empty. Note the asymmetric and thin myometrium (*short arrow*) surrounding a portion of the sac. Surgery confirmed a gestational sac implanted in the interstitial portion of the fallopian tube.

- The interstitial line sign has been reported as a reliable sign of interstitial ectopic pregnancy. An echogenic line extends from the uterine cavity to abut the center of the eccentric mass or GS. This line represent the interstitial portion of the fallopian tube [40].
- Leiomyomas may displace the GS and simulate an interstitial ectopic pregnancy (Fig. 6.31).
- Uterine anomalies, such as septate uterus, may also be mistaken for interstitial ectopic pregnancy (Fig. 6.32).

Ovarian Ectopic Pregnancy
Ectopic pregnancy implantation on the ovary is rare. Most ovarian masses discovered in a pregnant woman are corpus luteum cysts or preexisting ovarian lesions such as benign cystic teratoma or cystadenoma.

- A GS is implanted on the ovary.

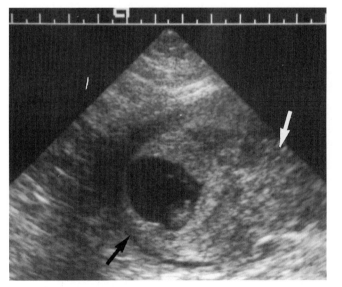

Figure 6.31 *Leiomyoma Simulates Interstitial Pregnancy.* The gestational sac is eccentrically positioned in the uterus and is surrounded by an asymmetrically thinned mantle of myometrium (*black arrow*). An interstitial ectopic pregnancy was suspected. At surgery, a leiomyoma was found to be displacing the gestational sac. The leiomyoma was seen in retrospect as a heterogeneous area of myometrium (*white arrow*).

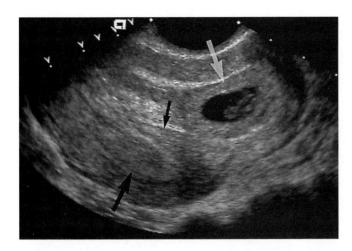

Figure 6.32 *Eccentric Gestational Sac in a Septate Uterus.* An intrauterine pregnancy in a septate uterus also demonstrates an eccentric gestational sac (*white arrow*). An empty smaller horn can be recognized as the cause of the eccentricity. The endometrium of the empty horn (*long black arrow*) is thickened and echogenic, representing decidual reaction. The septum (*short black arrow*) is visualized.

Cervical Ectopic Pregnancy

Patients usually present with painless vaginal bleeding at 6–12 weeks of pregnancy. Implantation in the less vascular cervical tissue provides insufficient blood supply for the pregnancy to progress.

- The GS is implanted abnormally low within or near the cervical canal.
- Differentiation from an aborting GS in the cervix may be difficult. A live embryo within a normal-appearing GS is found with a cervical ectopic pregnancy. An aborting sac appears misshapen and contains an embryo without a heartbeat.
- A large nabothian cyst may simulate a cervical ectopic pregnancy.

Abdominal Pregnancy

Abdominal pregnancies are associated with fetal mortality as high as 90% and maternal mortality of 6–14%. Despite its importance this diagnosis is commonly missed. The pregnancy may implant anywhere in the abdominal cavity but is most common in the pouch of Douglas, the posterior uterine wall, and the anterior abdominal wall.

- No myometrium is present around the fetus or the GS. However, this seemingly obvious finding may be difficult to recognize because trophoblastic tissue and the mother's abdominal wall may simulate the myometrium (Fig. 6.33).
- An empty uterus is identified. The uterus may be squashed deep in the pelvis and is difficult to identify, particularly if the pregnancy is large. The endometrium is thickened due to decidual reaction.
- The location of the fetus is unusual.
- The presentation of the fetus is unusual. Persistent transverse lie is common.
- The lower uterine segment and cervix are not clearly identified.
- Magnetic resonance imaging may be definitive when the US diagnosis is uncertain.

Heterotopic Pregnancy

The simultaneous presence of intrauterine and ectopic pregnancy has become increasingly common with the use of *in vitro* fertilization as treatment for infertility. In some reports, heterotopic pregnancy is as common as 1-in-100 pregnancies in this population [36]. This fact stresses the need for detailed examination of the adnexa, even when an IUP is documented.

- An IUP is present.
- Signs of one or more ectopic pregnancies are also present (Fig. 6.34).

GESTATIONAL TROPHOBLASTIC DISEASE

Gestational trophoblastic disease (GTD) is a proliferative disease of the trophoblast that ranges from benign and highly curable to aggressively malignant [41,42]. The **trophoblast**

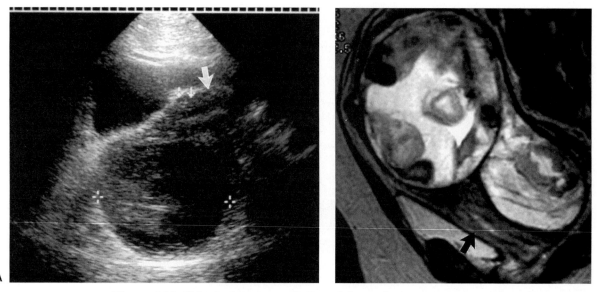

Figure 6.33 *Abdominal Pregnancy. A.* Transabdominal image in transverse plane demonstrates an empty uterus (*arrows*) and a complex cystic mass (*between cursors,* +) in the cul-de-sac. *B.* Sagittal MR image clearly shows the empty uterus (*arrow*) and the advanced pregnancy in the abdominal cavity.

is the functional unit of the placenta, originating as the outer covering of the blastocyst. The normal trophoblast has vigorous invasive and proliferative properties, needed for normal placental development, that are accentuated in this disease. GTD tissue usually has an abnormal karyotype. Patients present in the first trimester with hyperemesis, toxemia, or bleeding. Uterine size is usually larger than expected for gestational age. Serum β-hCG is always substantially elevated. The spectrum of GTD includes hydatidiform mole (complete and partial), invasive mole, and choriocarcinoma.

Complete Hydatidiform Mole

Complete (classic) mole is the benign, non-invasive, most common (80% of cases) type of GTD. Placental villi show excessive proliferation and hydropic swelling. Karyotype is dip-

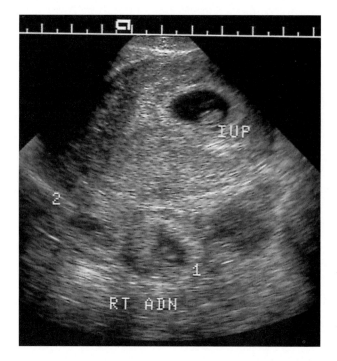

Figure 6.34 *Heterotopic Pregnancy.* Transabdominal image documents a live intrauterine pregnancy (IUP) and two ectopic pregnancies (1, 2) in this patient who had recently undergone *in vitro* fertilization.

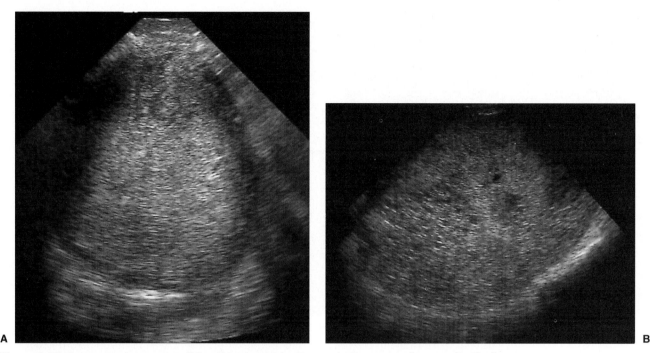

A   B

Figure 6.35 *Snowstorm Appearance of First Trimester Molar Pregnancy.* Transvaginal images (*A, B*) of two patients show the echogenic "snowstorm" appearance characteristic of molar pregnancy in the first trimester. In *B*, tiny cysts are barely visualized.

loid (46, XX) with all chromosomes of paternal origin. The ovum is believed to lose its haploid (23, X) chromosomes. Fertilization by a 23, X sperm follows and these paternal chromosomes are duplicated. US is usually diagnostic. Treatment is dilatation and suction curettage with evacuation of all POC [41,42].

- The uterus is larger than expected for dates.
- In the first trimester, the US appearance is more variable. A "snowstorm" appearance of a coarse granular echogenic mass without discrete cysts filling the uterine cavity is often seen (Fig. 6.35). A variant appearance seen in early gestation is a large central fluid collection indistinguishable from anembryonic pregnancy. Theca lutein ovarian cysts are rarely present in first trimester molar pregnancy [43].
- In the second trimester, the US appearance is usually classic and diagnostic. The uterine cavity is distended and filled with a moderately echogenic heterogeneous mass. TV US resolves innumerable small cystic spaces within the heterogeneous mass (Fig. 6.36). These small cysts correspond to the hydropic chorionic villi seen pathologically. The vesicles increase in size up to 30 mm with increasing gestational age [41,42].
- In the second trimester the ovaries commonly (40% of cases) demonstrate enlargement with multiple bilateral theca lutein cysts (Fig. 6.37). These result from ovarian hyperstimulation caused by high circulating levels of β-hCG. Hemorrhage or rupture occasionally complicates these cysts. They resolve within a few months of effective treatment of the mole. Persistence or enlargement of the cysts post-treatment is evidence of continued disease.
- Coexistence of a fetus with a complete mole is rare (1–2% of cases) and occurs only with dizygotic twinning. The karyotype of the fetus is normal while that of the mole is abnormal. The fetus is supplied by a normal placenta. The "twin" is a complete mole. Survival of the fetus is unlikely because of complications of treatment of the molar twin [44].
- Interpretation must be made in coordination with complete clinical evaluation. The differential diagnosis of cystic mass in the uterus of a pregnant patient is given in Box 6.4.

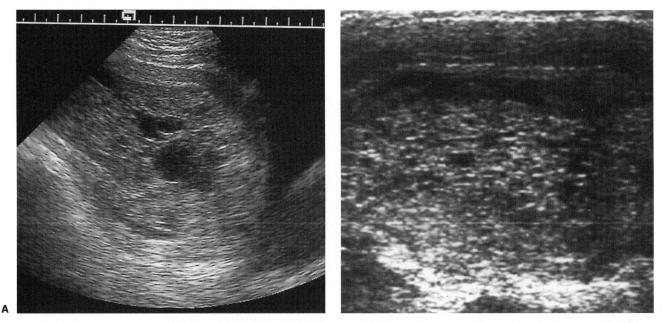

Figure 6.36 *Classic Molar Pregnancy in Second Trimester.* Transabdominal images (*A, B*) in two patients demonstrate the classic appearance of molar pregnancy seen in the second trimester. The uterine cavity is expanded and filled with an echogenic mass with innumerable cysts of varying size. No embryo is present.

Partial Hydatidiform Mole

In distinction from complete mole in which all placental villi are hydropic, in partial mole normal villi are mixed in with hydropic villi and trophoblastic proliferation is much less pronounced. The karyotype is triploid with fertilization of an ovum by two sperm (69, XXX; 69, XXY; or 69, XYY). Partial moles have an abnormal fetus present. The fetus is trip-

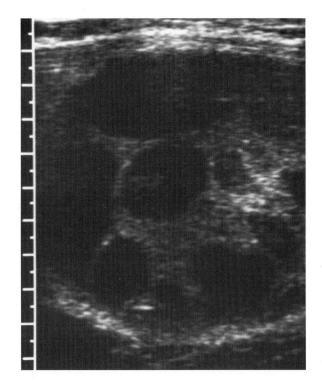

Figure 6.37 *Theca Lutein Cysts.* The ovary is massively enlarged by the presence of numerous cysts. In this patient, the enlargement of the ovary with theca lutein cysts 7 weeks after evacuation of the uterus for molar pregnancy was evidence of persistent gestational trophoblastic disease.

Box 6.4: Differential Diagnosis of Cystic Uterine Mass in Pregnancy

Molar pregnancy   Hydropic degeneration of the placenta
   Complete mole   Retained products of conception
   Partial mole   Degenerating leiomyoma

---

loid with the same karyotype as the molar tissue and does not survive. Partial moles commonly present with spontaneous abortion or fetal demise.

- The placental changes of mole are less pronounced and may be focal with areas of more normal-appearing placenta (Fig. 6.38) [42].
- The fetus is usually grossly abnormal with multiple anomalies and growth retardation. Fetal demise is frequent.

Invasive Mole

Invasive mole is a form of persistent GTD that occurs in approximately 10% of patients with complete mole and less frequently in patients with partial mole. Patients present with bleeding and persistent elevation of β-hCG after treatment for molar pregnancy. In invasive mole the trophoblasts invade the myometrium and blood vessels and may metastasize to the lungs and other tissue. The diagnosis is made by clinical findings and elevated β-hCG levels. US is used primarily to exclude pregnancy as a cause of elevated β-hCG [41,42]. Treatment is chemotherapy.

- US shows the findings of complete mole. Invasion of the myometrium by the echogenic mass is sometimes evident. MR is more sensitive in demonstrating invasion of the junctional zone myometrium but has little impact on therapy.

Choriocarcinoma

Choriocarcinoma is a malignant neoplasm of the chorionic epithelium that complicates 2–5% of molar pregnancy, but may also occur following normal pregnancy, ectopic pregnancy, or spontaneous abortion. Prognosis is best when choriocarcinoma follows molar pregnancy

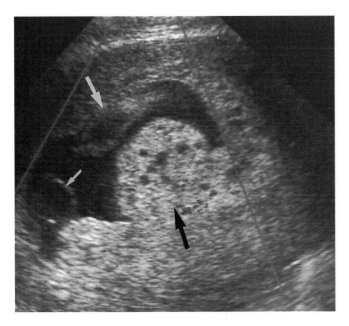

Figure 6.38 *Partial Molar Pregnancy.* The placenta (*black arrow*) is enlarged, misshapen, and contains small cysts throughout. A yolk sac (*small white arrow*) and portion of a dead embryo (*large white arrow*) are visualized. The yolk sac is abnormally large, measuring 11 mm. The patient's serum β-hCG was elevated well above normal for gestational age.

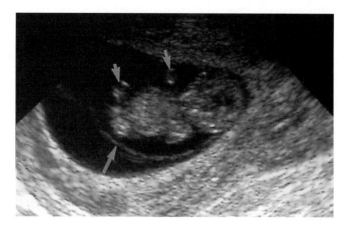

Figure 6.39 *Embryonic Limb Buds.* Primitive limb buds (*short arrows*) are seen in this 9.5-week embryo. The amnion (*long arrow*) is also visible.

with nearly all cases curable. Pathology shows invasive trophoblasts without formation of villi. Extensive necrosis and hemorrhage are usually present. As with invasive mole, patients present with bleeding and persistent elevation of β-hCG. Treatment is chemotherapy [41,42].

- US shows a heterogeneous, necrotic, hemorrhagic, infiltrative mass enlarging the uterus. The mass may extend through the uterine wall into the parametrium [41,42].
- Large, frequently hemorrhagic metastases may be found in the lungs (75%), brain, vagina, kidneys, bowel, and liver. Metastases to lymph nodes and bone are uncommon.

NORMAL DEVELOPMENTAL ANATOMY OF THE EMBRYO

Normal embryologic structures developing in the first trimester must be recognized to avoid mistaking them for anomalies.

- Primitive limb buds are visible by 8 weeks menstrual age (Fig. 6.39).
- The rhombencephalon is seen as a normal but prominent cystic structure in the posterior cranial fossa at 6–8 weeks (Fig. 6.40). This structure must not be mistaken for Dandy-Walker or other cranial anomaly. The rhombencephalon will form the fourth ventricle [45].

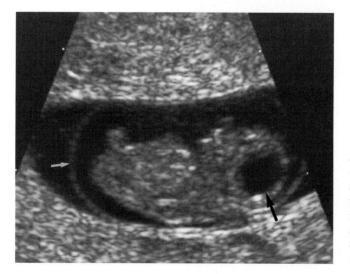

Figure 6.40 *Normal Rhombencephalon.* Transvaginal image of an 8-week embryo shows a prominent, but normal, cystic rhombencephalon (*black arrow*) as the dominant structure in the cranium. The amnion is evident (*white arrow*).

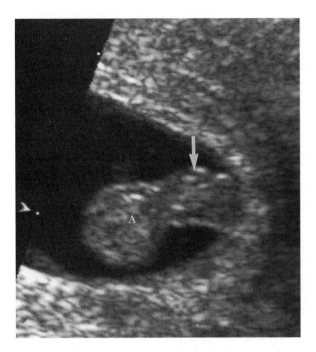

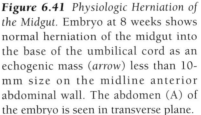

Figure 6.41 *Physiologic Herniation of the Midgut.* Embryo at 8 weeks shows normal herniation of the midgut into the base of the umbilical cord as an echogenic mass (*arrow*) less than 10-mm size on the midline anterior abdominal wall. The abdomen (A) of the embryo is seen in transverse plane.

- The midgut herniates into the base of the umbilical cord between 9 and 11 weeks. This physiological event must not be mistaken for omphalocele. Normal herniated bowel forms a small echogenic mass 6–9 mm in size on the midline anterior abdominal wall (Fig. 6.41) [46].
- The choroid plexus becomes visible as prominent bilateral echogenic structures in the brain by 9–10 weeks. The choroid is normally very large compared to the size of the cranial fossa (Fig. 6.42). As the brain and cranium grow, the choroid changes little in size and appears relatively smaller later in pregnancy.
- Nuchal lucency. Between 9 and 12 weeks, an anechoic area between the neck or occiput and the skin of the embryo that measures 3 mm or greater in thickness is indicative of increased risk of the fetus having trisomy 21 (Down's syndrome) or other chromosome anomaly (Fig. 6.43A) [47]. The risk is approximately 7% in women over age 35. Amnio-

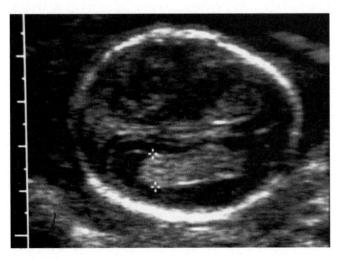

Figure 6.42 *Normal Choroid Plexus.* The normal choroid plexus is seen as a prominent echogenic structure in the brain of the embryo. The choroid plexus fills the lateral ventricle (*between cursors, +*). Note that brain anatomy is usually obscured by reverberation artifact in the portion of the cranium nearest the transducer.

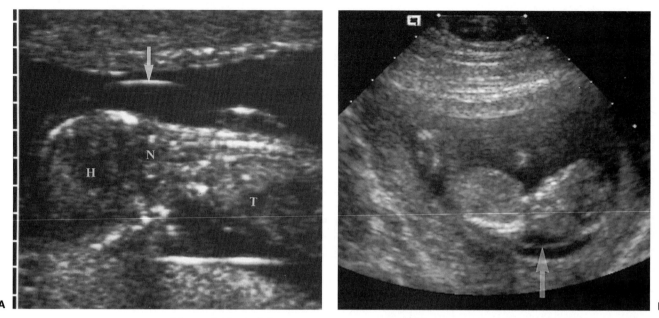

Figure 6.43 *Nuchal Lucency. A.* Prominent nuchal lucency extends over the head (H), neck (N), and thorax (T) of this 11.5-week fetus. In the neck region, the nuchal lucency (*arrow*) measured 7 mm, exceeding the normal upper limit of 3 mm in the first trimester. Amniocentesis confirmed the presence of trisomy 21. *B.* Apparent nuchal lucency (*arrow*) was confirmed by careful examination to be caused by the amnion lying in close proximity to the neck of the embryo. This is the major pitfall in recognizing abnormal nuchal lucency in the first trimester.

centesis or chorionic villus sampling for karyotype is usually recommended. Care must be taken to ensure the nuchal lucency is not caused by covering amnion (Fig. 6.43B).

REFERENCES

1. American Institute of Ultrasound in Medicine. Guidelines for performance of the antepartum obstetrical ultrasound examination. Rockville: American Institute of Ultrasound in Medicine, 1991.
2. Robinson H. "Gestational sac" volumes as determined by sonar in the first trimester of pregnancy. Br J Obstet Gynaecol 1975;82:100–107.
3. Hadlock F, Shah Y, Kanon D, et al. Fetal crown rump length: reevaluation of relation to menstrual age (5–18 weeks) with high resolution real time US. Radiology 1992;182:501–505.
4. Ritchie W. Sonographic evaluation of normal and induced ovulation. Radiology 1986;161:1–10.
5. Durfee S, Frates M. Sonographic spectrum of the corpus luteum in early pregnancy: gray-scale, color, and pulsed Doppler appearance. J Clin Ultrasound 1999;27:55–59.
6. Salim A, Zalud I, Farmakides G, et al. Corpus luteum blood flow in normal and abnormal early pregnancy: evaluation with transvaginal color and pulsed Doppler sonography. J Ultrasound Med 1994;13:971–975.
7. Yeh H, Goodman J, Carr L, et al. Intradecidual sign: a US criterion of early intrauterine pregnancy. Radiology 1986;161:463–467.
8. Laing FC, Brown DL, Price JF, et al. Intradecidual sign: is it effective in diagnosis of an early intrauterine pregnancy? Radiology 1997;204:655–660.
9. Yeh H-C. Efficacy of intradecidual sign and fallacy of double decidual sac sign in the diagnosis of early pregnancy (Letter). AJR Am J Roentgenol 1999;210:579–582.
10. Nyberg DA, Laing FC, Filly RA. Threatened abortion: sonographic distinction of normal and abnormal gestation sacs. Radiology 1986;158:397–400.
11. Levi CS, Lyons EA, Lindsay DJ. Early diagnosis of nonviable pregnancy with endovaginal US. Radiology 1988;167:383–385.
12. Lindsay D, Lovett I, Lyons E, et al. Yolk sac diameter and shape at endovaginal US: predictors of pregnancy outcome in the first trimester. Radiology 1992;183:115–118.

13. Yeh H-C, Rabinowitz J. Amniotic sac development: ultrasound features of early pregnancy—the double bleb sign. Radiology 1988;166:97–103.
14. Goldstein S, Snyder J, Watson C, et al. Very early pregnancy detection with endovaginal ultrasound. Obstet Gynecol 1988;72:200–204.
15. Doubilet P, Benson C. Embryonic heart rate in early first trimester: what rate is normal? J Ultrasound Med 1995;14:431–434.
16. Nyberg DA, Laing FC, Filly RA, et al. Ultrasonographic differentiation of the gestational sac of early intrauterine pregnancy from the pseudogestational sac of ectopic pregnancy. Radiology 1983;146:755–759.
17. Parvey H, Dubinsky T, Johnston D, et al. The chorionic rim and low-impedance intrauterine arterial flow in the diagnosis of early intrauterine pregnancy: evaluation of efficacy. AJR Am J Roentgenol 1996;167:1479–1485.
18. Nyberg D, Mack L, Laing F, et al. Early pregnancy complications: endovaginal sonographic findings correlated with human chorionic gonadotropin levels. Radiology 1988;167:619–622.
19. Rowling SE, Coleman BG, Langer JE, et al. First-trimester US parameters of failed pregnancy. Radiology 1997;203:211–217.
20. McKenna K, Feldstein V, Goldstein R, et al. The "empty amnion": a sign of early pregnancy failure. J Ultrasound Med 1995;14:117–121.
21. Levi C, Lyons E, Zheng X, et al. Endovaginal US: demonstration of cardiac activity in embryos of less than 5.0 mm in crown-rump length. Radiology 1990;176:71–74.
22. Brown DL, Emerson DS, Felker RE, et al. Diagnosis of early embryonic demise by endovaginal sonography. J Ultrasound Med 1990;9:631–636.
23. Pennell R, Needleman L, Pajak T, et al. Prospective comparison of vaginal and abdominal sonography in normal early pregnancy. J Ultrasound Med 1991;10:63–67.
24. Byrne J, Warburton D, Kline J, et al. Morphology of early fetal deaths and their chromosome characteristics. Teratology 1985;32:297–315.
25. Laboda L, Estroff J, Benacerraf B. First trimester bradycardia: a sign of impending fetal loss. J Ultrasound Med 1989;8:561–563.
26. Bromley B, Harlow B, Laboda L, et al. Small sac size in the first trimester: a predictor of poor fetal outcome. Radiology 1991;178:375–377.
27. Pederson J, Mantoni M. Prevalence and significance of subchorionic hemorrhage in threatened abortion: a sonographic study. AJR Am J Roentgenol 1990;154:535–537.
28. Stabile I, Campbell S, Grudzinskas J. Threatened miscarriage and intrauterine hematomas: sonographic and biochemical studies. J Ultrasound Med 1989;8:289–292.
29. Sauerbrei E, Pham D. Placental abruption and subchorionic hemorrhage in the first half of pregnancy: US appearance and clinical outcome. Radiology 1986;160:109–112.
30. Bennett GL, Bromley B, Lieberman E, et al. Subchorionic hemorrhage in first-trimester pregnancies: prediction of pregnancy outcome with sonography. Radiology 1996;200:803–806.
31. Stampone C, Nicotra M, Muttinelli C, et al. Transvaginal sonography of the yolk sac in normal and abnormal pregnancy. J Clin Ultrasound 1996;24:3–9.
32. Harris R, Vinclent L, Askin F. Yolk sac calcification: a sonographic finding associated with intrauterine embryonic demise in the first trimester. Radiology 1988;166:109–110.
33. Kurtz A, Shlansky-Goldberg R, Choi H, et al. Detection of retained products of conception following spontaneous abortion in the first trimester. J Ultrasound Med 1991;10:387–395.
34. Wachsberg R, Kurtz A. Gas within the endometrial cavity at postpartum US: a normal finding after spontaneous vaginal delivery. Radiology 1992;183:431–434.
35. Hann L, Bachman D, McArdle C. Coexistent intrauterine and ectopic pregnancy: a reevaluation. Radiology 1984;152:151–154.
36. Tal J, Haddad S, Gordon N, et al. Heterotopic pregnancy after ovulation induction and assisted reproductive technologies: a literature review from 1971 to 1993. Fertil Steril 1996;66:1–12.
37. Nyberg DA, Hughes MP, Mack LA, et al. Extrauterine findings of ectopic pregnancy at transvaginal US: importance of echogenic fluid. Radiology 1991;178:823–826.
38. Brown DL, Doubilet PM. Transvaginal sonography for diagnosing ectopic pregnancy: positivity criteria and performance characteristics. J Ultrasound Med 1994;13:259–266.
39. Chen G-D, Lin M-T, Lee M-S. Diagnosis of interstitial pregnancy with sonography. J Clin Ultrasound 1994;22:439–442.
40. Ackerman T, Levi C, Dashevsky S, et al. The interstitial line: a new sonographic finding in interstitial (cornual) ectopic pregnancy. Radiology 1993;189:83–87.
41. Wagner BJ, Woodward PJ, Dickey GE. Gestational trophoblastic disease: radiologic-pathologic correlation. Radiographics 1996;16:131–148.

42. Green CL, Angtuaco TL, Shah HR, et al. Gestational trophoblastic disease: a spectrum of radiologic diagnosis. Radiographics 1996;16:1371–1384.

43. Lazarus E, Hulka C, Siewert B, et al. Sonographic appearance of early complete molar pregnancies. J Ultrasound Med 1999;18:589–593.

44. Winter TI, Brock B, Fligner C, et al. Coexistent surviving neonate twin and complete hydatidiform mole. AJR Am J Roentgenol 1999;172:451–453.

45. Cyr D, Mack L, Nyberg D, et al. Fetal rhombencephalon: normal US findings. Radiology 1988;166:691–692.

46. Schmidt W, Yarkoni S, Crelin E, et al. Sonographic visualization of physiologic anterior abdominal wall hernia in the first trimester. Obstet Gynecol 1987;69:911–915.

47. van Vugt J, van Zalen-Sprock R, Kostense P. First trimester nuchal translucency: a risk analysis on fetal chromosome abnormality. Radiology 1996;200:537–540.

OBSTETRIC ULTRASOUND—SECOND AND THIRD TRIMESTER

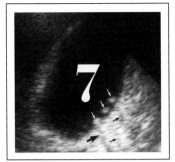

US is widely used in the evaluation of pregnancy with more than 70% of all pregnancies in the United States undergoing sonographic evaluation [1]. Indications for US examination are expansive and include estimation of gestational age (GA), evaluation of fetal growth, determination of fetal position, detection of multiple gestations, evaluation of fetal well-being, and detection of fetal anomalies. The American Institute of Ultrasound in Medicine provides well-accepted guidelines for the performance of obstetric ultrasound examination [2].

GUIDELINES FOR OBSTETRIC ULTRASOUND EXAMINATION

Obstetric US examination in the second and third trimester should include the following standards [2], which are endorsed by the American College of Radiology [3]:

- Documentation of fetal life, number, and presentation.
- An estimate of the amount of amniotic fluid.
- The location and appearance of the placenta and its relationship to the internal cervical os.
- Assessment of GA using a combination of biparietal diameter (BPD), head circumference (HC), abdominal circumference (AC), and femur length (FL).
- Evaluation of the uterus and adnexa. The presence, location, and size of myomas and adnexal masses should be reported.
- The study should encompass evaluation of fetal anatomy including, but not limited to, the cerebral ventricles, four-chamber view of the fetal heart, spine, stomach, urinary bladder, umbilical cord insertion site, and renal region.

Many obstetric US practices expand the evaluation to include the fetal neck, posterior fossa, extremities, ventricular outflow tracts, fetal bowel, and Doppler evaluation of the umbilical artery.

Fetal Measurements and Growth

Determination of gestational age is a primary goal of obstetric US.

Some of the most important aspects of obstetric care are the determination of GA and the assessment of fetal growth. By convention, clinical gestational dating is based on the first day of the last menstrual period (LMP). Conception is assumed to occur on day 14 of the menstrual cycle. A normal, full-term pregnancy is 40 weeks with a range of 37–42 weeks. Clinical dating, based on the mother's history of LMP, is notoriously inaccurate. Sonographic dating is based on measurement of fetal parameters. Standardized charts correlate GA with measurements of fetal parameters. Serial measurements are used to document fetal growth. In the second and third trimesters, four fetal measurements are routinely used.

Biparietal Diameter

The BPD measurement is greatly affected by shape of the fetal head.

- The BPD is determined on an axial image of the fetal head at the level of the thalamus (Fig. 7.1). The measurement is taken from the outer edge of the near cranium to the inner edge of the far cranium.
- The BPD may be low for GA if the head is unusually long and narrow in shape (dolichocephaly) (Fig. 7.2A) [4].
- The BPD may be high for GA if the head is unusually round (brachycephaly) (Fig. 7.2B) [4].
- The fetal head may be compressed by excessive transducer pressure or the molding that occurs with oligohydramnios.

Head Circumference

The HC measurement is independent of head shape. The BPD and HC reflect growth of the fetal brain.

- The HC is measured on the same axial image as the BPD. The HC is a perimeter measurement of the fetal cranium excluding subcutaneous soft tissues (Fig. 7.3).

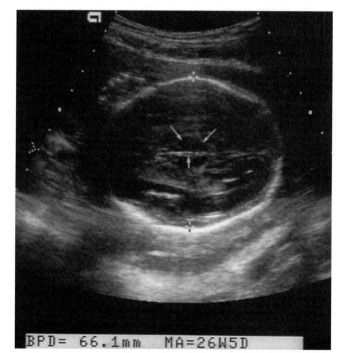

BPD= 66.1mm   MA=26W5D

Figure 7.1 *Biparietal Diameter.* The biparietal diameter is measured from the outer edge of the near skull to the inner edge of the far skull (*between cursors*, +) on an image plane through the thalamus (*long arrows*) and third ventricle (*short arrow*).

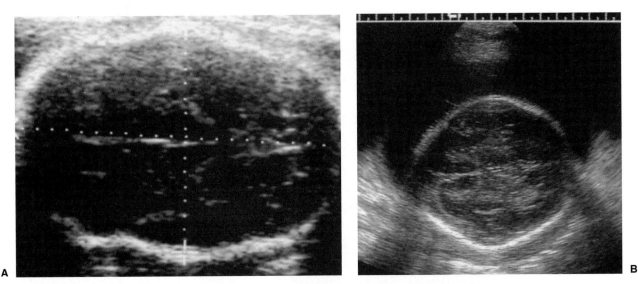

A   B

Figure 7.2 *Dolichocephaly and Brachycephaly. A.* This fetal head is exceptionally elongated in shape (dolichocephaly), disproportionally reducing the biparietal diameter measurement. *B.* This fetal head is exceptionally round in shape (brachycephaly), disproportionally increasing the biparietal diameter measurement.

ABDOMINAL CIRCUMFERENCE

The AC reflects the growth of intraabdominal organs.

■ The AC is measured in axial plane at the level of the junction of the umbilical vein with the left portal vein (Fig. 7.4). The abdomen should appear round, not oval, when a true axial section is obtained. The fluid-filled stomach is routinely seen on this plane. The AC is measured as the length of the peripheral circumference of the fetal abdomen including subcutaneous soft tissues.

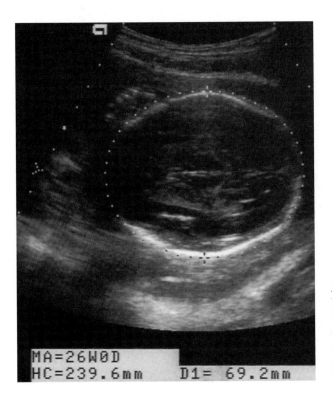

MA=26W0D
HC=239.6mm   D1= 69.2mm

Figure 7.3 *Head Circumference.* The head circumference is measured on the same image plane as the biparietal diameter. The measurement is the circumference of the fetal cranium with no soft tissues of the scalp included.

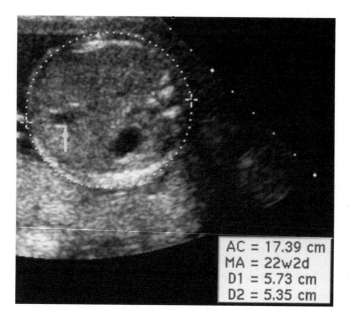

AC = 17.39 cm
MA = 22w2d
D1 = 5.73 cm
D2 = 5.35 cm

Figure 7.4 Abdominal Circumference. The abdominal circumference is measured on a transverse image of the abdomen obtained at the level where the umbilical vein (*arrow*) is in the substance of the liver. The outer circumference is measured to include all soft tissues.

FEMUR LENGTH

The FL serves as a monitor for growth of the long bones.

■ The femoral shaft is seen as a slightly curved, echogenic structure that produces an acoustic shadow. The longest dimension of the femoral shaft is measured for the FL (Fig. 7.5). The femoral epiphysis, seen as a spike on one end of the femoral shaft, is not included in the measurement. The measurement is most accurate when the femur is perpendicular to the US beam.

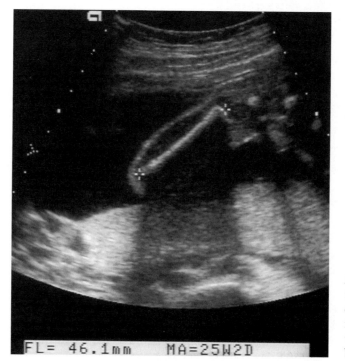

FL= 46.1mm   MA=25W2D

Figure 7.5 Femur Length. The femur length is the longest dimension of the shaft of the femur (*between cursors, +*). Note the acoustic shadow cast by the bone.

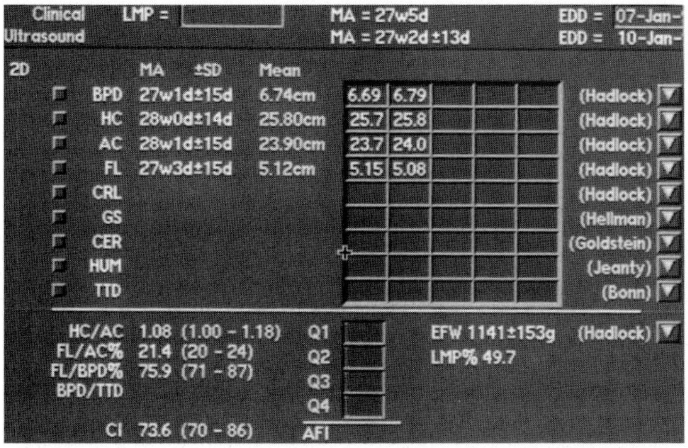

Figure 7.6 *Composite Age—Fetal Biometry Report.* Most US units provide a data page that summarizes fetal measurements and calculations. This report (top) compares clinical dating by last menstrual period (LMP) to US dating by fetal measurements. The US estimate of menstrual age (MA) is the composite age based on an average of the four measurements listed. Mean fetal measurements are listed, along with the gestational age (GA) predicted by each measurement. The right hand column indicates the measurement chart used for the computer determination of GA. Measurement ratios and estimated fetal weight (EFW) calculation is provided at the bottom. The LMP% notation provides the EFW percentile for GA based on LMP.

ESTIMATED FETAL WEIGHT

Estimated fetal weight (EFW) is used to identify fetuses that are small for GA and potentially growth retarded, and fetuses that are large for GA and may be difficult to deliver.

- EFW may be determined by measurement of BPD and AC [5] or by measurement of AC and FL [6]. Many computer programs include an automatic printout of the EFW with weight percentile compared to GA determined by LMP (Fig. 7.6).

Assignment of GA is an *interpretation* based on clinical history, physical examination, and sonographic assessment. It is not just a value taken from a chart. GA is routinely determined at the time of the first US examination and is not changed thereafter. Measurements made on subsequent US examinations are compared to the GA determined on the first US examination to determine if interval growth is normal. Sonographic estimates of GA are most accurate in early pregnancy and become progressively less accurate as the pregnancy advances. Sonographic GA in the second and third trimesters is routinely based on composite age, which is the average GA determined by measurement of multiple parameters, usually BPD, HC, AC, and FL (Fig. 7.6). Fetal anomalies may make individual measurements invalid. If so, the affected measurement is excluded and composite age is determined from the remaining measurements. GA based on crown rump length in the first trimester is accurate to approximately 0.5 week. Composite GA based on the four routine measurements is accurate to 1.2 week between 12 and 18 weeks, but is accurate to only 3.1 weeks at 36–42 weeks. Measurement charts are included within the calculation packages in computer software on most US units. The range of error of each measurement is routinely listed. In the United States, most physicians use the Hadlock charts as the standards of reference, although a variety of measurement charts and formulas are available [7–12].

> Gestational age is determined at the time of the first US examination and is not changed on subsequent US examinations.

INTRAUTERINE GROWTH RETARDATION

Intrauterine growth retardation (IUGR) is associated with high perinatal morbidity and mortality and an increased risk of impaired neurodevelopment. Infant mortality rate is 4–8 times greater than non-IUGR infants [13]. The diagnostic challenge is to differentiate fetuses that are pathologically small from those that are normal, but constitutionally small. Causes of IUGR are listed in Box 7.1. The approach to diagnosis of IUGR is as follows:

Box 7.1: Causes of Intrauterine Growth Retardation

Chromosome abnormality
  Trisomy 13, 18, 21
  Triploidy
Major congenital anomalies
Congenital infections
  Rubella
  Cytomegalovirus
  Toxoplasmosis
Teratogen exposure
  Drugs

Maternal hypertension
Diabetes
Smoking
Alcohol
Cocaine
Poor maternal nutrition
Maternal chronic diseases
Placental infarction
Placental abruption
Placental insufficiency

- Estimate the GA. Make the best estimate possible based on early US, clinical history, and physical assessment.
- Compare the AC measurement to the expected AC value based on GA. An AC below the tenth percentile for GA suggests IUGR.
- Compare the EFW to the expected EFW for GA. An EFW below the tenth percentile for GA suggests IUGR. If EFW is below the fifth percentile for GA, the risk of IUGR is very high.
- An FL-to-AC ratio (FL/AC) >23.5 suggests IUGR.
- Obtain an umbilical artery spectral Doppler tracing (Fig. 7.7) [14]. A systolic-to-diastolic (S/D) velocity ratio >4 suggests IUGR [15]. Absent or reversed flow in diastolic is a highly specific sign of fetal distress, often indicative of imminent fetal death [16]. Normally the umbilical artery shows a low-resistance Doppler spectral pattern [S/D <3, resistance index (RI) <0.70]. A high resistance pattern indicates high vascular resistance within the placenta and impaired blood flow to the placenta.
- Fetuses that measure small for GA but have normal Doppler studies (Fig. 7.7A) are likely to have a normal outcome [17].
- Check for oligohydramnios. Low amniotic fluid volume [amniotic fluid index (AFI) <5] is found with severe IUGR [15].

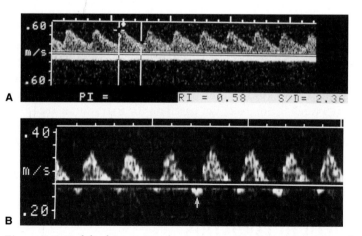

Figure 7.7 *Umbilical Artery Doppler. A.* A normal umbilical artery Doppler spectrum is displayed above the baseline, whereas the umbilical vein spectrum is displayed below the baseline indicating normal blood flow in opposite directions. Distinct, moderately high-velocity blood flow is seen in the umbilical artery throughout diastole, resulting in a resistance index (RI) of 0.58 and a systole/diastole (S/D) ratio of 2.36. *B.* Doppler spectrum from the umbilical artery of a growth-retarded fetus shows reversal of blood flow direction in diastole (*arrow*). This is a highly specific finding of severe fetal distress.

- The combination of IUGR with polyhydramnios is also ominous and is associated with a high incidence of chromosome abnormality (38%), major congenital anomalies, and high mortality (59%) [18].
- Fetuses that are determined by these criteria to be "at risk" for IUGR are routinely followed on a weekly basis with reassessment of the listed parameters. Surveillance of fetal well-being often includes serial biophysical profiles.

BIOPHYSICAL PROFILE

The biophysical profile is a commonly performed test used to identify fetuses that are compromised and may require expedited delivery [19]. Four "neurologic" tests are used to assess for acute hypoxia and one test (amniotic fluid) is used to check for chronic hypoxia. A score of 2 is given if the test is normal and a score of 0 is given if the test is abnormal. A total score of 8 or 10 is considered normal. Lower scores correlate with increased risk to the fetus. Abnormal results are reported only after a minimum observation period of 30 minutes.

- *Amniotic fluid.* At least one pocket of fluid that measures 2 cm or more in a vertical plane yields a score of 2. No pockets of fluid measuring 2 cm or more in a vertical plane equals a score of 0.
- *Fetal movement.* At least three discrete body movements of the limbs or trunk equals a score of 2. Less than three distinct body movements equals a score of 0.
- *Fetal tone.* At least one episode of limb extension from a flexed position with return to a flexed position equals a score of 2. No extension or sluggish limb extension with failure of return to full flexion equals a score of 0.
- *Fetal breathing.* At least one episode of breathing motion lasting at least 30 seconds equals a score of 2. No breathing motion, or breathing lasting less than 30 seconds, equals a score of 0.
- *Nonstress test.* A normal (reactive) stress test is the observation of two or more fetal heart rate accelerations of at least 15 beats per minute (bpm) and of 30 seconds or longer duration equals a score of 2. Anything less constitutes an abnormal (nonreactive) stress test with a score of 0.

MACROSOMIA

Macrosomia describes babies who are large for GA. For these babies life *in utero* is usually uncomplicated but they are at high risk for complications during and after delivery. Many large babies are found in mothers who have gestational diabetes. Complications of macrosomia include shoulder dystocia, neurologic damage to the brachial plexus (Erb's palsy), fractures, perinatal asphyxia, neonatal hypoglycemia, and meconium aspiration.

- Macrosomia is defined as EFW above the ninetieth percentile for GA or greater than 4,000 grams.

PLACENTA

NORMAL PLACENTA

Normal growth and development of the fetus are critically dependent upon the normal function and integrity of the placenta. The union of chorionic villi, arising from the fertilized ovum, with maternal decidual basalis forms the normal placenta. Spiral arteries carry maternal blood to intervillous spaces between branching chorionic villi. Extensive branching provides a large surface area for exchange of metabolites [20].

- The placenta is first visualized by US at 8 weeks as a focal thickening along the periphery of the gestational sac at the site of implantation.

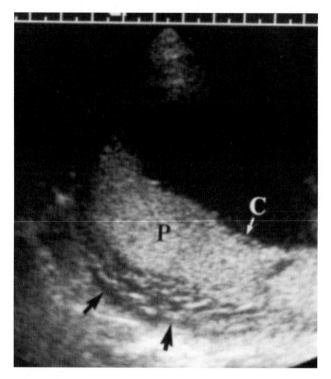

Figure 7.8 *Normal Placenta.* The normal placenta (P) has a granular appearance with a smooth surface defined by its covering chorionic membrane (C, *arrow*). The retroplacental complex of blood vessels (*black arrows*) is an important sonographic landmark in the diagnosis of placental abruption.

The retroplacental complex of blood vessels serves as an important sonographic landmark in the diagnosis of previa, abruption, and accreta.

- By 12 weeks GA, the disc shape of the placenta is evident. Its substance appears finely granular and its surface is smooth and sharply defined by the covering chorion (Fig. 7.6).
- A retroplacental complex of decidual and myometrial veins creates a network of tubular sonolucent channels along the basal aspect of the placenta (Fig. 7.8). Doppler clearly defines these channels as blood vessels. Excessive transducer pressure may obliterate visualization of these normal vessels.
- Normal placenta aging is manifest by the appearance of hypoechoic areas, septations, and calcifications (Fig. 7.9). Calcifications occur randomly throughout the substance of

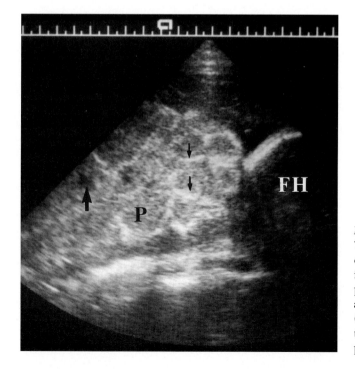

Figure 7.9 *Placental Aging.* This placenta (P) shows normal changes associated with advancing gestational age. The aging placenta develops hypoechoic areas (*large arrow*), septations (*small arrows*), and calcifications along the septations and placental surface. FH, fetal head.

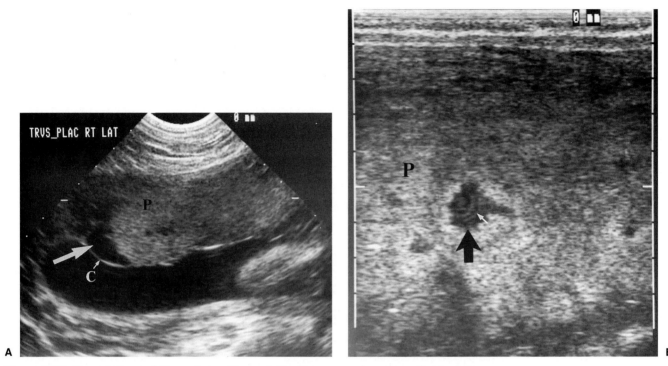

Figure 7.10 *Normal Placental Venous Lakes.* Venous lakes (*large arrows*) appear as focal echolucent areas just beneath the chorionic membrane (*C, small arrow*), *A*, or within the substance of the placenta (*P*), *B*. Note the swirling blood flow (*small arrow*) in *B*. Venous lakes are incidental finding of no clinical significance.

the placenta and prominently along placental septations. Acoustic shadowing may or may not be evident. Attempts to correlate the appearance of the placenta with fetal lung maturity have been unsuccessful.

■ Echolucencies within the placenta commonly represent venous lakes (Fig. 7.10). Slow swirling flow may be visualized with real-time US. Flow is often too slow to demonstrate with Doppler. These venous lakes may thrombose and remain as echolucent fibrin deposits [21].

■ Placental thickening normally does not exceed 4 cm. Causes of an abnormally thick placenta are listed in Box 7.2 [22].

■ An abnormally thin placenta (<1 cm) is associated with placental insufficiency (Box 7.3).

PLACENTA PREVIA

Placenta previa describes low implantation of the placenta that covers all, or a portion of, the internal os of the cervix. Placenta previa is present at term in only 0.3–0.6% of all pregnancies, but may be suggested by US in 45% of pregnancies in the first and second trimesters. Risk factors for placenta previa include previous caesarian section, previous placenta previa, multiparity, and maternal age >35 years. Complications of placenta previa are

---

Box 7.2: Causes of a Thickened Placenta (>4 cm)

Maternal diabetes mellitus	Congenital fetal neoplasm
Fetal hydrops	Congenital infection
Maternal anemia (severe)	Placental abruption
Triploidy	

Box 7.3: Causes of a Thinned Placenta (<1 cm)

Placental insufficiency   Toxemia of pregnancy
Maternal hypertension   Trisomy 13, 18
Maternal diabetes mellitus

---

maternal hemorrhage, premature delivery, IUGR, and perinatal death. Patients present with painless vaginal bleeding in the third trimester caused by dilatation of the cervical os, which disrupts placental blood vessels.

- **Marginal previa** is present when the edge of the placenta reaches or partially covers the dilating cervical os.
- **Complete previa** is present when the os is completely covered by placenta (Fig. 7.11).
- Taipale reported the risk of placenta previa at term is 5.1% when placenta previa is present on US performed at 12–16 weeks [23]. Follow-up of these patients is controversial. Some suggest that all be re-examined for placenta previa in the third trimester, whereas others recommend follow-up on only patients with risk factors or third trimester bleeding [24]. Rosati suggests following only those patients with a placenta that extends 14 mm or more beyond the internal os [25].
- US diagnosis of placenta previa should always be made with the bladder empty. A full bladder distorts the appearance of the lower uterine segment and commonly creates a false appearance of previa. The cervix and placenta are easily examined with the bladder empty by a translabial approach (Fig. 7.9) [26]. Transvaginal examination is an alternative. The probe must be inserted cautiously and with direct visualization to stop at the cervix.
- **Vasa previa** describes a membranous insertion of the cord that crosses the internal cervical os. The insertion of the cord into the placenta is velamentous. That is, the cord inserts into the peripheral membranes of the placenta rather than into the bulk of the placenta near its center. An accessory lobe of the placenta (a **succenturiate lobe**) may be connected to the main body of the placenta only by membranous vessels that may cross

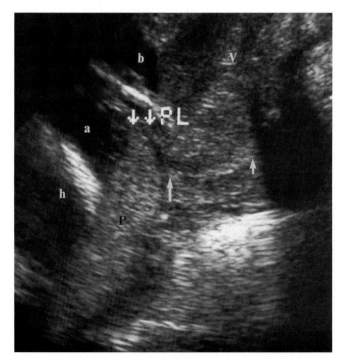

Figure 7.11 *Placenta Previa.* A translabial image down the "tube" of the vagina (V) shows the internal (*long arrow*) and external (*short arrow*) os of the cervix. The internal os is covered by placenta (P, PL, *dual arrows*). Also seen are a portion of the near-empty bladder (b), a bit of amniotic fluid (a), and a portion of the fetal head (h). The translabial view allows optimal visualization of the cervix with the bladder empty.

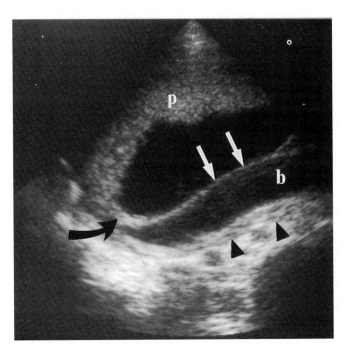

Figure 7.12 *Subchorionic Hemorrhage—Marginal Placental Abruption.* Subchorionic hemorrhage results from venous bleeding caused by detachment of the margin (*curved arrow*) of the placenta (p). Low pressure bleeding (b) dissects beneath the chorion (*white arrows*) separating it from the myometrium (*black arrowheads*).

the os. Disruption of these vessels with cervical dilatation results in rapid exsanguination of the fetus. Doppler shows blood vessels adherent to and crossing the internal os [27].

PLACENTAL ABRUPTION

Abruption is defined as the premature separation of a normally positioned placenta from its myometrial attachment. Hemorrhage occurs from disrupted maternal vessels. Risk factors for placental abruption include maternal hypertension, toxemia, cocaine abuse, smoking, and previous placental abruption. Complications include precipitous delivery, prematurity, coagulopathy, and fetal death.

- US diagnosis of abruption depends upon visualization of the resulting hematoma [28].
- **Subchorionic hemorrhage** represents separation of the placenta at its margin (a "marginal" abruption). Bleeding is primarily venous and extends beneath the chorionic membrane (Fig. 7.12) (see Fig. 6.20). Large hematomas are associated with high risk of early pregnancy loss. Most subchorionic hemorrhages occur before 20 weeks gestation [29–31].
- **Retroplacental abruption** is much more serious because the associated bleeding is arterial (Fig. 7.13). Extensive placental detachment disrupts placental function, causes placental infarctions, and may result in fetal hypoxia and death. Tears in the amnion allow blood to enter the gestational sac. Amniotic fluid leakage into the maternal bloodstream may cause consumption coagulopathy.
- The hematoma appears as an anechoic or mixed echogenicity mass beneath the placenta and commonly extending beneath the chorion (Figs. 7.12, 7.13). The appearance of the hematoma varies with its age and physical state. The hematoma is anechoic before clot forms, isoechoic to placenta with clot formation, and becomes hypoechoic to anechoic with hemolysis 1–2 weeks after hemorrhage. When the clot is isoechoic, the placenta may appear only diffusely thickened.
- Disruption of the retroplacental complex of blood vessels is an important confirmatory finding with abruption (Fig. 7.13A). Myometrial contractions and leiomyomas beneath the placenta simulate the US appearance of abruption but displace rather than disrupt the placental blood vessels.

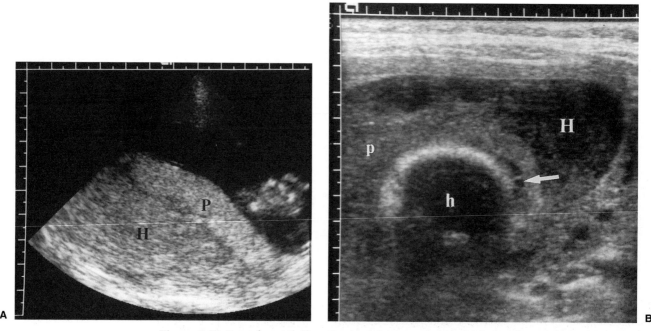

Figure 7.13 *Retroplacental Abruption. A.* A large retroplacental hemorrhage (H) displaces the placenta (P) away from the myometrium and disrupts the retroplacental complex of blood vessels. *B.* A large retroplacental hematoma (H) compresses the umbilical cord (*arrow*) against the fetal head (h), causing marked fetal distress. This mother was a frequent user of cocaine. p, placenta.

PLACENTA CRETA

Placenta creta describes abnormal placental invasion of the myometrium with complete or partial absence of the decidua basalis. Severity is graded as **accreta** with chorionic villi directly contacting the myometrium, **increta** with chorionic villi invading the myometrium, and **percreta** with chorionic villi penetrating the myometrium and invading the bladder wall. Risk factors are similar to those for placenta previa and include previous cae-

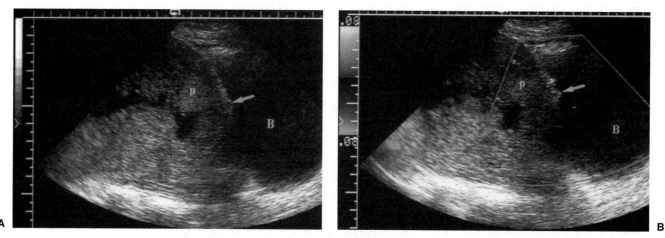

Figure 7.14 *Placenta Percreta. A.* Gray scale image shows a lumped-up placenta (p) with complete placenta previa. The placenta is in close proximity to the wall of the bladder (B). Note the absence of a normal retroplacental complex of blood vessels and the thin, difficult-to-visualize myometrium. The inner surface of the bladder wall has a lobulated appearance (*arrow*). *B.* Color Doppler image shows abnormal placental blood vessels (*arrow*) penetrating the wall of the bladder and protruding into the bladder lumen. This patient had a previous history of two cesarean sections and previous placenta previa. (See Color Figure 7.14B).

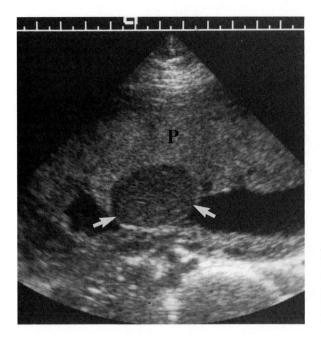

Figure 7.15 *Placental Chorioangioma. The tumor (arrows) appears as a well-defined hypoechoic mass within the placenta (P) and bulging from its surface. Spectral Doppler shows blood flow within the mass at fetal heart rate.*

sarian section, increased parity, and previous uterine infection. Definitive US diagnosis may be difficult, but the diagnosis should be suggested when these findings are present [32,33].

■ The placenta is low lying and anterior with placenta previa often present (Fig. 7.14).
■ The retroplacental complex of vessels is partially or completely absent. Care must be taken to avoid compression of these vessels by excessive transducer pressure or bladder overdistention.
■ The myometrium underlying the placenta appears thinned (<1 mm) or absent.
■ The bright reflection of the serosa separating the uterus from the bladder is absent.
■ Color Doppler may show contiguous blood vessels extending from the myometrium into the bladder wall (Fig. 7.14B). The abnormal blood vessels may cause focal elevations of the bladder mucosa.

PLACENTAL CHORIOANGIOMA

Chorioangioma is a benign tumor of the placenta sometimes classified as a *hamartoma*. They are found in 1% of placentas pathologically but most are small and not clinically significant [21]. US detects only the larger lesions which are associated with elevation of maternal serum alpha-fetoprotein (MS-AFP).

■ Chorioangiomas appear as well-defined, hypoechoic, or mixed echogenicity masses within the placenta, often near the cord insertion site (Fig. 7.15) [34]. Detected chorioangiomas are usually 1–5 cm in size.
■ Spectral Doppler is diagnostic with demonstration of vessels within the tumor with blood flow pulsating at fetal heart rate.
■ Placental hematomas may have a similar appearance but have no blood flow on Doppler US.

UMBILICAL CORD

NORMAL UMBILICAL CORD

■ The normal umbilical cord contains two arteries and a single vein (Fig. 7.16A, C). The cord is easily visualized in amniotic fluid. Color Doppler shows its spiraling configuration.

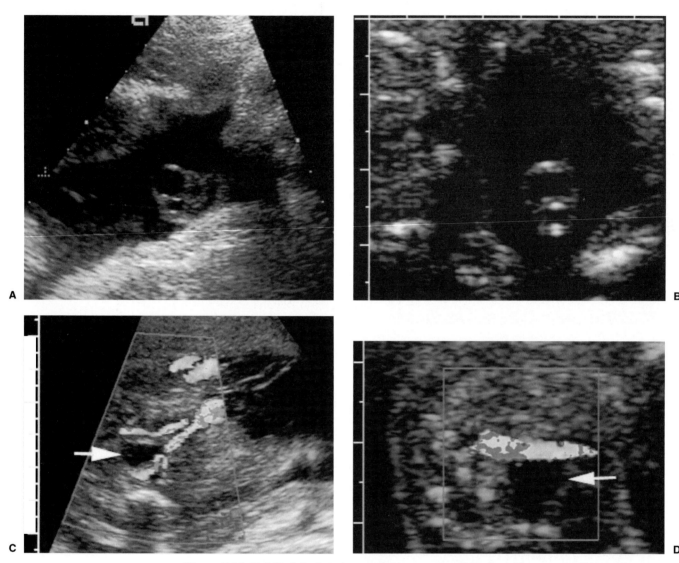

Figure 7.16 *Umbilical Cord. A.* A normal three-vessel umbilical cord has two smaller arteries carrying blood from the fetus to the placenta and one larger vein carrying oxygenated blood and nutrients from the placenta to the fetus. *B.* A two-vessel umbilical cord has a single artery and a single vein. Color flow images of the bladder (*arrow*) confirms the presence of two, *C,* or one, *D,* umbilical arteries coursing adjacent to the bladder from the fetal hypogastric arteries to the umbilicus. Imaging the bladder is useful when optimal cross sectional images of the cord cannot be obtained. (See Color Figures 7.16C, D).

■ Confirmation of one or two umbilical arteries is easily made by examining the fetus and demonstrating the umbilical arteries coursing on both sides of the bladder (Fig. 7.16C, D) [35].

TWO-VESSEL UMBILICAL CORD

A single umbilical artery is found in up to 1% of pregnancies. A two-vessel cord is associated with chromosome anomalies and a variety of fetal malformations [36].

■ The cord contains one artery and one vein. Only a single umbilical artery is seen adjacent to the bladder in the fetus (Fig. 7.16B, D).
■ A careful and complete anatomic survey of the fetus is indicated to detect developmental anomalies. Most centers do not perform amniocentesis if no anomalies are found [37].

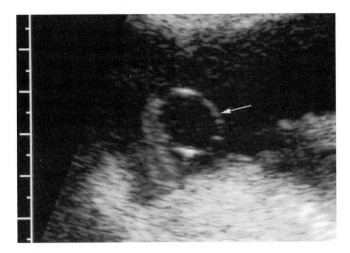

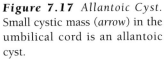
Figure 7.17 *Allantoic Cyst.* Small cystic mass (*arrow*) in the umbilical cord is an allantoic cyst.

NUCHAL CORD

The cord encircles the fetal neck in up to 25% of pregnancies. Multiple encircling loops and a tight nuchal cord put the fetus at risk for fetal distress especially during labor [35].

- Color Doppler provides a high sensitivity for detecting nuchal cord.

MASSES IN THE UMBILICAL CORD

- Umbilical cord cysts arise from remnants of the omphalomesenteric duct (vitelline duct) or allantoic duct (Fig. 7.17). Fetal anomalies are commonly associated. Cysts are usually small (4–6 mm).
- Tumors of the umbilical cord are exceedingly rare and include hemangiomas and teratomas [35].
- Hematomas of the cord usually occur only with manipulation or puncture of the cord (percutaneous umbilical cord sampling).

UTERUS AND CERVIX

LEIOMYOMAS IN PREGNANCY

Leiomyomas are the most common pregnancy-associated pelvic tumor present in up to 3% of pregnant women. Myomas are associated with bleeding, premature uterine contractions, malpresentation, and obstruction during labor. Approximately 15% of myomas will increase in size during pregnancy. The remainder remain stable in size or disappear because of progressive stretching of the myometrium [38,39].

- Leiomyomas appear as spherical masses that distort the contour of the myometrium, and have heterogeneous, usually decreased, echogenicity compared to myometrium. Calcifications may be present. Color Doppler shows myometrial vessels displaced around the myoma [40].
- Uterine contractions must be differentiated from myomas. Contractions are transient, although they may persist for 1 hour. Contractions are homogeneous and isoechoic to myometrium. They bulge the inner, but usually not the outer, uterine wall. Color Doppler shows no vessel displacement in the area of a contraction [40].
- Myomas with a volume >200 cm³ show a higher rate of complications than smaller myomas [39].

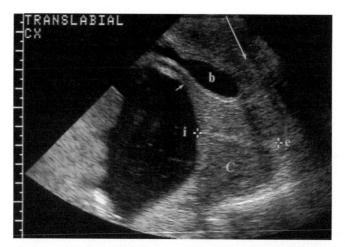

Figure 7.18 *Normal Translabial View of the Cervix.* Positioning the US transducer on the labia directs the US beam down the long axis (*long arrow*) of the vagina and perpendicular to the cervix (C). The cervix is seen as a muscular cylinder contiguous with the myometrium (*tiny arrow*). The endocervical canal (*between cursors, +*) appears as an echogenic line in the middle of the cervix. The internal os (i) is outlined by amniotic fluid. The external os (e) in indicated by the end of the endocervical canal. The bladder (b) contains a small volume of urine on this image. Imaging the cervix with the bladder empty allows an accurate measurement of the length of the cervix. This cervix measured 4.2 cm.

NORMAL CERVIX

The normal cervix remains closed during pregnancy to physically retain the fetus *in utero* and to prevent ascending infection of the uterus [24].

Translabial US with the bladder empty provides excellent visualization of cervical abnormalities.

- A translabial approach is optimal to evaluate the cervix with the bladder empty (Fig. 7.18) [41]. A 3.5–4.0-MHz sector transducer is routinely utilized. The transducer is covered by a sterile glove or condom and is placed directly on the patient's labia. The US beam is directed down the long axis of the vagina and is perpendicular to the cervix.
- The normal cervix is seen as a hypoechoic cylinder contiguous with the myometrium (Fig. 7.18). The cervical canal is seen as an echogenic line commonly surrounded by a hypoechoic zone. The internal os is defined by the point at which the amniotic sac meets the cervical canal. The external os is interpreted as the point at which echogenic cervical canal is no longer visible [41].

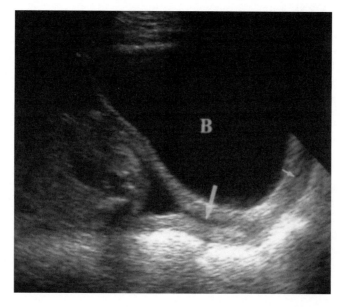

Figure 7.19 *Elongated Cervix.* A transabdominal view of the cervix (*large arrow*) with bladder (B) overdistended falsely elongates the apparent cervix by coapting the myometrium of the lower uterine segment. This cervix measured 5.8 cm. The vagina (*tiny arrow*) appears as a hypoechoic muscular tube.

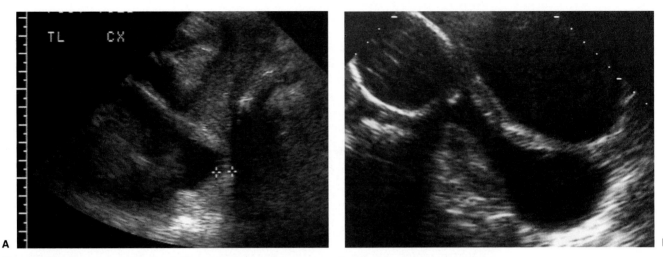

Figure 7.20 *Incompetent Cervix. A.* Translabial view shows a very short cervix (*between cursors, +*) measuring less than 1 cm in length. *B.* Transabdominal view in another patient shows a completely dilated cervix distended by amniotic fluid with membranes presenting at the external os.

- The length of the cervix is measured along the endocervical canal from internal to external os. The normal cervix has a mean length of 3.4–3.7 cm and a minimum length of 2.5 cm [42]. A full bladder compresses the lower uterine segment and falsely elongates the cervix (Fig. 7.19). Cervical length is most accurately measured with the bladder empty (Fig. 7.18).

INCOMPETENT CERVIX

A shortened cervix is predictive of cervical incompetence with its associated high risk of premature delivery. Cervical incompetence is responsible for approximately 16% of premature deliveries [24].

- The cervix is considered abnormally short when the closed endocervical canal is <2.5 cm in length (Fig. 7.20A) [42]. Cervical length >3.0 cm effectively excludes pre-term delivery.
- Fluid within the cervical canal indicates dilatation of the cervix. Measurement of the distance between the anterior and posterior wall of the cervix indicates the degree of dilatation. The closed portion of the endocervical canal, measured between the dilated portion of the cervix and the external os, is considered the functional cervical length.
- Membranes may bulge into or through the cervical canal. When membranes bulge into the vagina, delivery is inevitable (Fig. 7.20B).

AMNIOTIC FLUID

NORMAL AMNIOTIC FLUID

Amniotic fluid protects the fetus from injury, allows growth and fetal movement, and is essential for normal lung maturation. In early pregnancy, fluid in the amnion and chorionic spaces is a filtrate of the membranes. After 16 weeks GA, nearly all of the amniotic fluid originates from fetal urination. Fetuses with bilaterally impaired renal function have profound oligohydramnios by 18 weeks. Amniotic fluid is removed from the amniotic cavity primarily by fetal swallowing.

- The volume of amniotic fluid rises steadily to a maximum at 22 weeks GA and stays at that level until delivery [43]. Accurate measurement of amniotic fluid volume by US is difficult and most sonographers rely on estimating fluid volume subjectively based on their experience [44].

■ Normal fluid volume allows free but not unlimited movement of fetal limbs. Fluid is seen around the fetus but both the anterior and posterior uterine walls are in contact with the fetus.

■ The amniotic fluid index (AFI) is widely utilized in an attempt to be more objective. The index is determined by measuring the vertical height of the deepest fluid pocket in each quadrant of the uterus and summing the 4 measurements. Umbilical cord and fetal parts are excluded from any measurement. The normal range of the AFI is 5–20 cm.

■ Fine particulate matter suspended in the amniotic fluid is usually a normal finding. It usually represents vernix in the third trimester, but may also result from blood or meconium [45].

OLIGOHYDRAMNIOS

Oligohydramnios indicates abnormally low volume of amniotic fluid. Oligohydramnios is associated with increased perinatal morbidity. Causes include reduced urine output (renal agenesis, bilateral renal dysplasia, and urinary tract obstruction), IUGR, premature rupture of membranes, and post-term pregnancy.

■ AFI below 5 cm is indicative of oligohydramnios (Fig. 7.21A).

POLYHYDRAMNIOS

Polyhydramnios is an excessive volume of amniotic fluid. Polyhydramnios is associated with maternal diabetes under poor control, gastrointestinal and central nervous system anomalies, lethal skeletal dysplasias, and chromosome anomalies. Severe polyhydramnios may cause abdominal pain, breathing difficulty, premature rupture of membranes and pre-

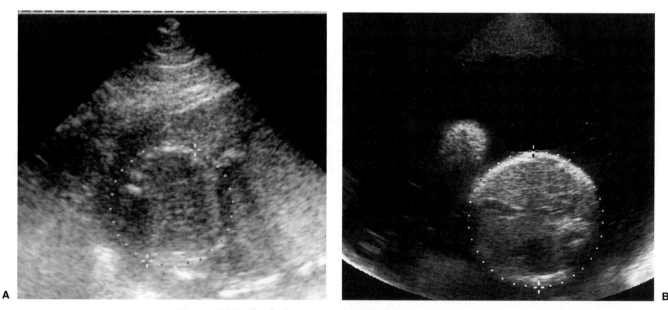

A B

Figure 7.21 *Oligohydramnios and Polyhydramnios. A. Oligohydramnios. The abdominal circumference is measured on a fetus with renal agenesis. No amniotic fluid was seen in the uterine cavity. Visualization of fetal anatomy is very difficult when severe oligohydramnios is present. B. Polyhydramnios. A huge volume of fluid surrounds the fetus. At least 8 cm of amniotic fluid separates the abdomen from the anterior wall of the uterus. This fetus had esophageal atresia.*

mature delivery. Polyhydramnios is commonly idiopathic and many fetuses with mild poly-hydramnios will have a normal outcome.

- AFI above 20 cm is indicative of polyhydramnios.
- A single fluid pocket >8 cm in vertical height indicates polyhydramnios.
- The fetus is observed to float in the excessive fluid (Fig. 7.21B).
- Fluid is seen anteriorly between the fetus and the anterior uterine wall.

MEMBRANES

CHORIOAMNIOTIC SEPARATION

The amnion is seen separately from the chorion until 16 weeks GA when the two membranes normally fuse (see Chapter 6). Persistent separation of chorion and amnion is a normal variant but may also result from amniocentesis. No morbidity is associated with persistent separation [46].

- The amnion appears as a thin, undulating membrane suspended in fluid (Fig. 7.22). While the chorion is tightly adherent to the surface of the placenta, the amnion is commonly seen separately over the placenta.

AMNIOTIC SHEETS

Amniotic sheets develop over uterine synechiae that cross the uterine cavity. Synechiae result from previous uterine surgery or infection. Membranes drape over the synechiae as the pregnancy develops and the sac enlarges [47,48].

- Visualized membranes are thick because they consist of two layers of chorion and two layers of amnion. The membrane forms a shelf-like structure about which the fetus moves freely (Fig. 7.23).
- Visualization of a free edge is diagnostic. The edge is usually rounded and is thicker than the membrane because it includes the synechiae.
- A Y-shaped splitting of the membrane is seen at the attachment to the uterine wall as the double layers of chorion and amnion separate [47,48].
- No fetal anomalies are associated with amniotic sheets. The risk of malpresentation or poor pregnancy outcome is not increased [49].

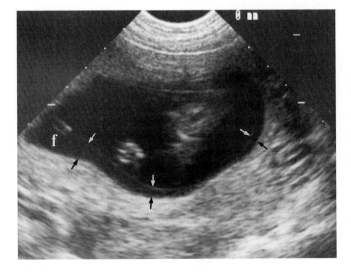

Figure 7.22 *Normal Chorioamniotic Separation.* The amnion (*white arrows*) is a delicate membrane, uniform in thickness that floats in fluid. The amnion may separate from the surface of the placenta, whereas the chorion is fixed to the placenta. The chorion (*black arrows*) defines the limit of the fluid-filled gestation sac. The chorionic cavity is between the amnion and chorion. f, fluid in the chorionic cavity.

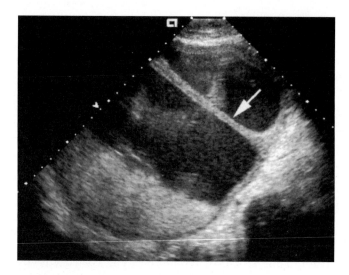

Figure 7.23 *Amniotic Sheet.* Amniotic sheets are caused by layers of amnion and chorion folding over a uterine synechiae to form a thick membranous shelf (*arrow*). The folded membrane always has a thickened free edge. The fetus moves freely on both sides of the shelf.

AMNIOTIC BAND SYNDROME

Amniotic band syndrome is a common cause of fetal malformations present in 1 in 1200 births [50]. Disruption of the amnion allows the fetus to enter the chorionic cavity where it becomes entangled by sticky fibrous septa. Entrapment of random fetal parts results in amputations and slash defects that are nonembryological in distribution.

- Amniotic bands appear as septa of varying thickness that may produce a spider web appearance (Fig. 7.24). Extension of bands to entangled limbs may be visualized. Absence of US visualization of amniotic bands does not exclude the diagnosis of amniotic band syndrome.
- Extremities are most frequently involved with asymmetric amputations that involve only one digit or the entire limb. Focal constriction may result in marked lymphedema of the peripheral limb.
- Head defects include asymmetric anencephaly, encephaloceles away from the midline, and facial clefts that extend beyond normal boundaries.
- Truncal deformities may include the chest and abdomen and resemble gastroschisis with associated angulation deformities of the spine. The distal spine may be amputated.

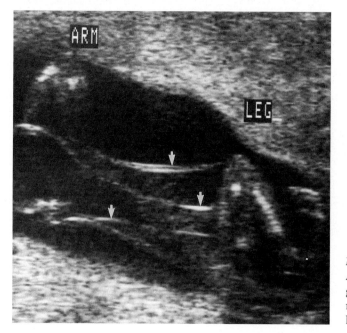

Figure 7.24 *Amniotic Bands.* Amniotic bands (*arrows*) entangle the arm and leg of this fetus, restricting both movement and limb growth.

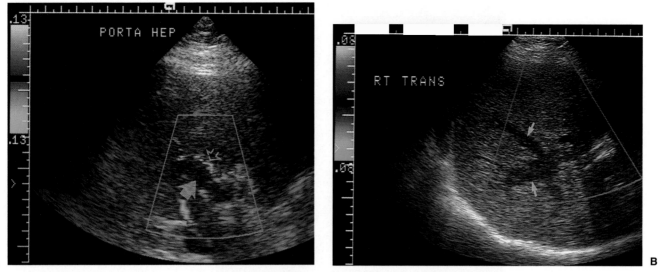

Color Figure 2.32 *Thrombosed Portal Vein. A.* Color Doppler image through the porta hepatis shows absence of blood flow in the dilated portal vein (*fat arrow*). High-velocity turbulent blood flow (mixed colors) is evident in the adjacent hepatic artery (*open arrow*). *B.* Transverse color Doppler image of the right lobe reveals extension of blood clot into intrahepatic branches (*arrows*) of the portal vein.

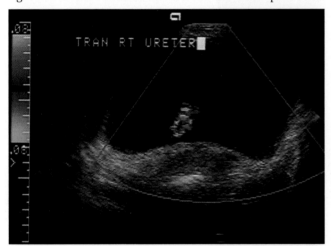

Color Figure 3.4 *Normal Ureteral Jet.* Ureteral peristalsis produces a flash of color as urine squirts into the bladder lumen.

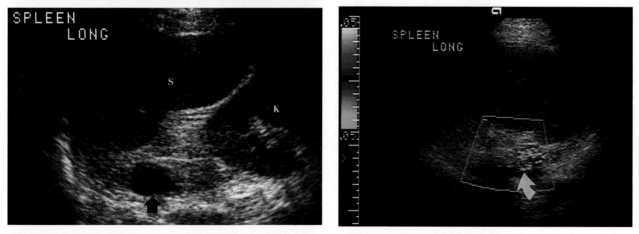

Color Figure 3.59 *Varix Mimics an Adrenal Mass.* This patient was referred for biopsy of a left adrenal mass seen on a CT of the abdomen performed without contrast because the patient had impaired renal function. *A.* US revealed a homogeneous, hypoechoic, left suprarenal mass (*arrow*). K, left kidney; S, spleen. *B.* Color Doppler confirmed the "mass" was a varix (*arrow*) formed because of the patient's portal hypertension.

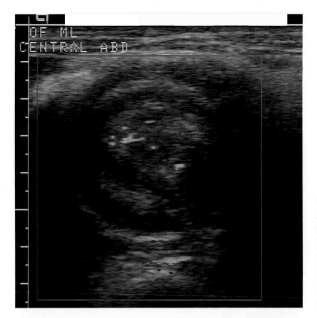

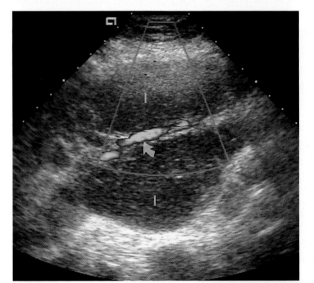

Color Figure 4.23 *Intussusception—Potentially Reducible.* Color Doppler image confirms blood flow within the loops of bowel involved in the intussusception. The presence of blood flow is excellent evidence that the intussusception will be successfully reduced by enema.

Color Figure 4.25 *Sandwich Sign of Mesenteric Lymphoma.* A mesenteric artery (*arrow*) is sandwiched between two homogeneous hypoechoic masses of lymphoma (l).

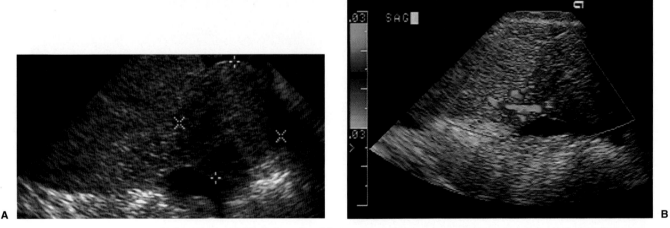

A

B

Color Figure 5.21 *Pedunculated Leiomyoma.* A. Transvaginal US image shows a hypoechoic mass (*outlined by cursors, x, +*) adjacent to the uterus. B. Color Doppler image in the same location shows contiguous blood flow from the uterus into the mass, confirming a pedunculated leiomyoma.

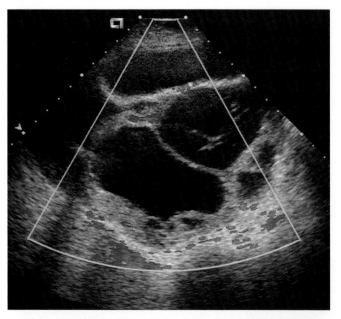

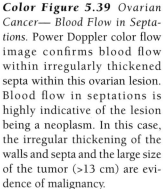

Color Figure 5.39 *Ovarian Cancer— Blood Flow in Septations.* Power Doppler color flow image confirms blood flow within irregularly thickened septa within this ovarian lesion. Blood flow in septations is highly indicative of the lesion being a neoplasm. In this case, the irregular thickening of the walls and septa and the large size of the tumor (>13 cm) are evidence of malignancy.

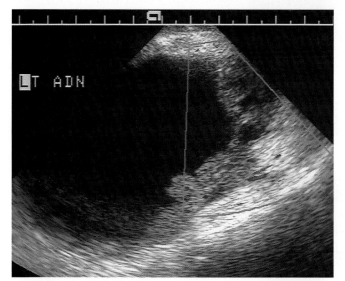

Color Figure 5.40 *Ovarian Cancer—Blood Flow in Wall.* Color Doppler image reveals blood vessels within the irregular solid thickening of the wall of this cystic ovarian lesion. This finding confirms that the solid-appearing tissue is neoplasm and is not just clotted blood adherent to the cyst wall.

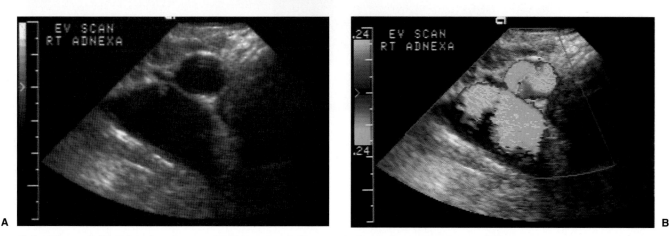

A B

Color Figure 5.55 *Pelvic Arteriovenous Malformation.* A. Transvaginal scan shows prominent tubular structures in the right adnexa. B. Color Doppler image in the same location confirms the tubular structures are blood vessels (*continued*).

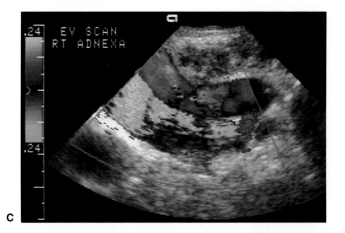

Color Figure 5.55 *(continued)* *C.* Longitudinal transvaginal scan shows high-velocity, turbulent flow within the abnormal vessels.

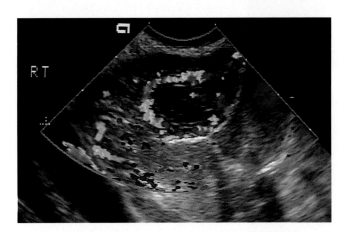

Color Figure 6.29 *Ring of Fire.* This ring of fire surrounds a corpus luteum. Similar intense color depicting hypervascularity may be seen surrounding a normal pregnancy, ectopic pregnancy, tubo-ovarian abscess, malignant ovarian tumor, or pedunculated leiomyoma.

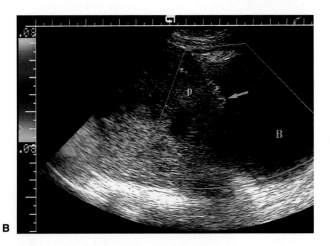

Color Figure 7.14 *Placenta Percreta. B.* Color Doppler image shows abnormal placental blood vessels (*arrow*) penetrating the wall of the bladder (B) and protruding into the bladder lumen. This patient had a previous history of two cesarean sections and previous placenta (p) previa.

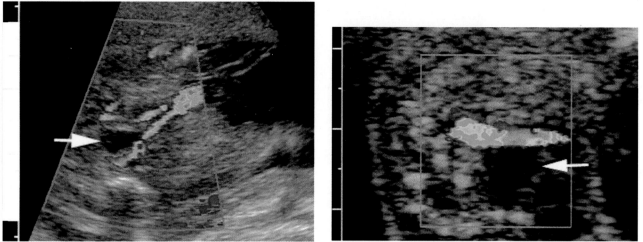

C   D

Color Figure 7.16 *Umbilical Cord.* Color flow images of the bladder (*arrow*) confirms the presence of two, *C*, or one, *D*, umbilical arteries coursing adjacent to bladder from fetal hypogastric arteries to umbilicus. Imaging the bladder is useful when optimal cross-sectional images of the cord cannot be obtained.

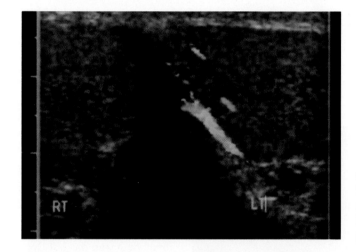

Color Figure 8.4 *Testicular Torsion.* Color Doppler image demonstrates normal flow to the left testis (LT) and no flow to the painful right testis (RT).

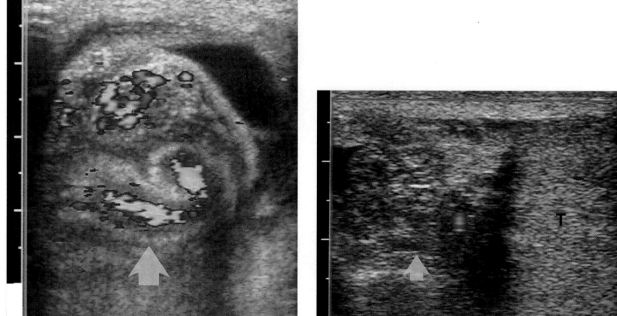

C   D

Color Figure 8.5 *Acute Epididymitis.* Color Doppler images show a marked increase in vascularity in the right (*C*) epididymis (*arrow*) compared to the left (*D*) epididymis (*arrow*). T, left testis.

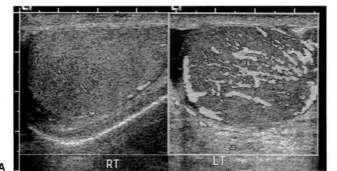

Color Figure 8.6 *Acute Orchitis. A.* Color flow images of both testes in a patient with a painful left testis demonstrate marked hypervascularity on the left compared to the right.

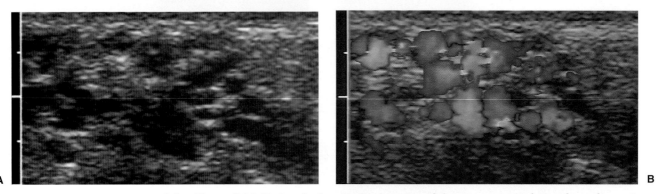

Color Figure 8.11 *Varicocele.* Longitudinal images of the spermatic cord just above the testis demonstrates a serpiginous network of tubular lucencies (*A*) that are confirmed to be dilated veins by color Doppler (*B*).

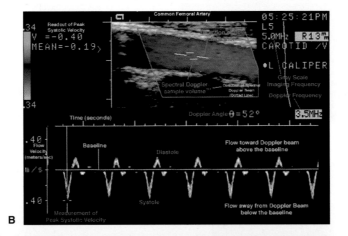

Color Figure 11.2 *Spectral Doppler Display. B.* In this illustration, color Doppler and gray-scale US are used to locate and display the vessel being interrogated in the box at the top of the image. The spectral Doppler sample volume, the direction of the spectral Doppler US beam, and the Doppler angle indicator are shown. The Doppler spectrum is shown at the bottom of the image. See text for explanation of the spectral Doppler display.

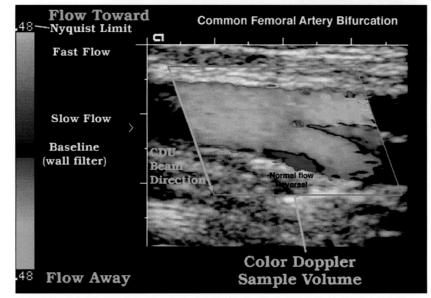

Color Figure 11.3 *Color Doppler Imaging Display.* The color map is shown on the left side of this image. See text for detailed explanation of the color Doppler display.

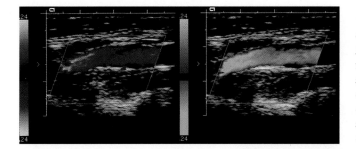

Color Figure 11.4 *Color Maps.* Inversion of the color map radically changes the appearance of the color image of a carotid artery. Choice and orientation of the color map are at the option of the US operator.

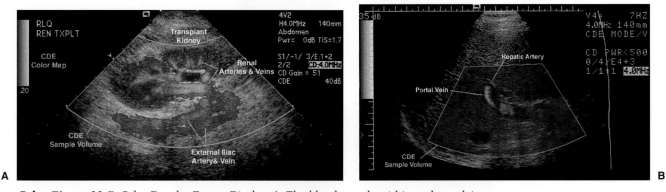

A

B

Color Figure 11.5 *Color Doppler Energy Display. A.* The blood vessels within and supplying a renal transplant are displayed on this color Doppler energy (CDE) (power Doppler) image. CDE shows the presence of blood flow with high sensitivity. However, direction of blood flow is not determined, and adjacent arteries and veins with blood flow in opposite directions are shown in the same color. The CDE sample volume is adjusted by the operator to include the tissues of interest. *B.* CDE image of the liver shows flow in the portal vein and hepatic artery. In this example the Doppler sample volume is shaded in color.

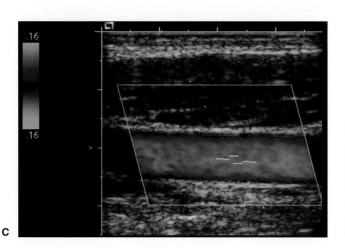

C

Color Figure 11.6 *Normal Laminar Blood Flow. C.* Color Doppler image of the common carotid artery at mid-systole shows bright color in midstream, indicating faster flow, and darker color near the vessel wall, indicating slower flow.

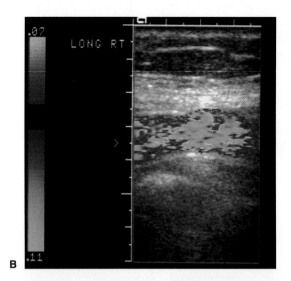

B

Color Figure 11.8 Turbulence. B. Severe turbulence within a venous shunt is seen on color Doppler.

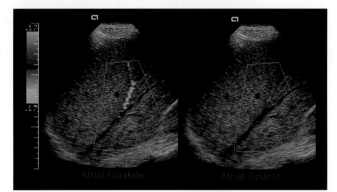

Color Figure 11.15 Normal Hepatic Vein Flow. Blood flow in the hepatic veins is normally toward the heart during atrial filling and away from the heart during atrial contraction. Note that a static color Doppler image represents only an instant in time during the cardiac cycle. Compare to the hepatic vein waveform in Figure 11.14.

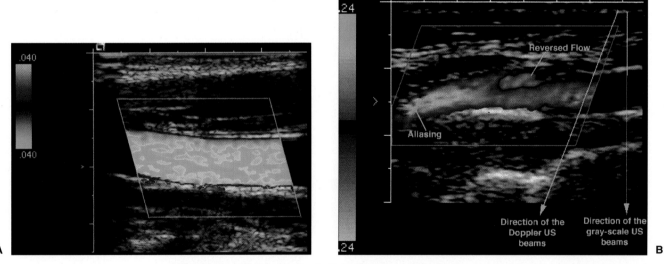

A

B

Color Figure 11.18 Aliasing in Color Doppler. A. The dominant color displayed within this vessel is yellow from the top side of the color map. Yellow indicates flow toward the Doppler beams, or in this case, from right to left. The splotches of green color are areas of aliasing. Note the absence of a black border. The color velocity scale is set low with a Nyquist limit of 0.040 m/sec. When the detected mean blood flow velocity exceeds this limit, aliasing occurs, and color from the bottom portion of the color map is displayed. Aliasing must be recognized, but in this case may be useful by providing identification of highest velocity flow. B. This color Doppler image of the internal carotid artery demonstrates the appearance of true reversal of blood flow direction as indicated by the black border around the region of color shift. A small area of flow reversal is a normal finding opposite the flow divider at the bifurcation of the common carotid artery. Note that the direction of the Doppler beams is different than the direction of the gray-scale image beams.

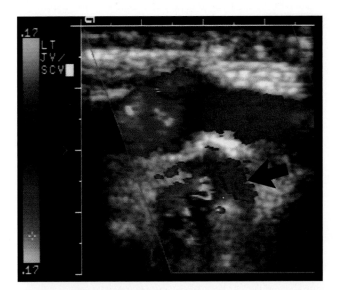

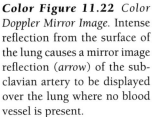

Color Figure 11.22 Color *Doppler Mirror Image.* Intense reflection from the surface of the lung causes a mirror image reflection (*arrow*) of the subclavian artery to be displayed over the lung where no blood vessel is present.

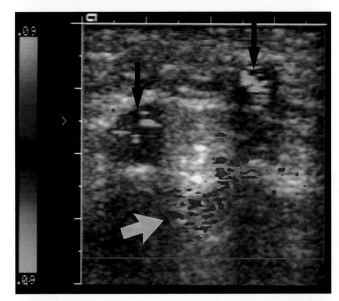

Color Figure 11.23 Tissue *Vibration Artifact.* Turbulent blood flow in a hemodialysis shunt produces a "visible bruit" of tissue vibration artifact seen as a random pattern (*white arrow*) of red and blue color displayed over the soft tissues adjacent to the shunt. The random color pattern within the two limbs of the shunt (*black arrows*) are indicative of turbulent blood flow.

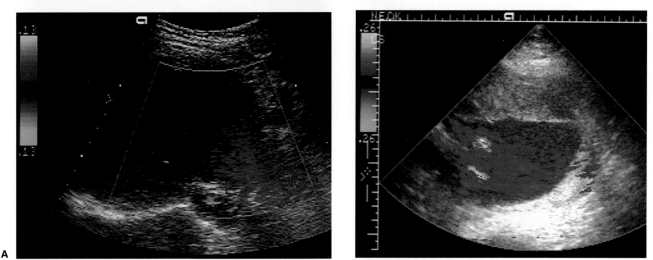

A   B

Color Figure 11.26 Color *Flash—Fluid Motion. A.* Cardiac motion causes color flash artifact and obscures the junction of hepatic veins and inferior vena cava. *B.* A kicking motion by a baby *in utero* moves the amniotic fluid to produce a prominent color flash artifact.

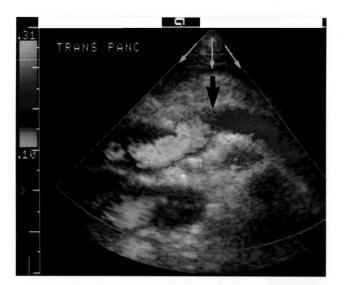

Color Figure 11.27 *Color Change Caused by Changing Doppler Angle.* A sector transducer is used to produce a color image of the splenic vein as it curves through the pancreas (PANC). The sector transducer sends diverging Doppler beams (*tiny white arrows*) through the pancreas. On the right side of the image, the red color in the splenic vein indicates flow toward the Doppler beams. In the mid-portion of the image (*black arrow*), the Doppler beams intersect the moving blood at a 90-degree angle; therefore, no color is displayed in this portion of the vein. On the left side of the image, the blue color indicates blood flow away from the Doppler beams. The yellow color without a black border indicates aliasing caused by an unbalanced velocity scale as shown on the color map. In summary, the color changes indicate normal flow in the splenic vein toward the portal confluence and the liver.

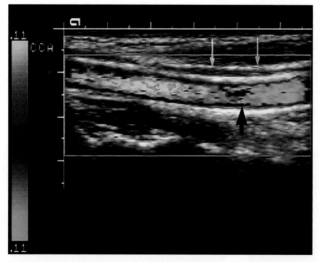

Color Figure 11.28 *Linear Array—Vertical Doppler Beams.* In this color image, the Doppler beams are vertical (*tiny white arrows*) and parallel to the gray-scale US beams. The common carotid artery (CCA) has a gently curving course through the color field-of-view. On the right side of the image, the blue color indicates flow relatively away from the Doppler beams. On the left side of the image, the red/yellow color indicates flow relatively toward the Doppler beams. In summary, blood flow is from left to right, indicating normal flow direction toward the brain. Note the black border of transition between the red and blue colors (*black arrow*) where the color changes because of change in Doppler angle. Aliasing is indicated by patches of green without a black border in the yellow colored flow.

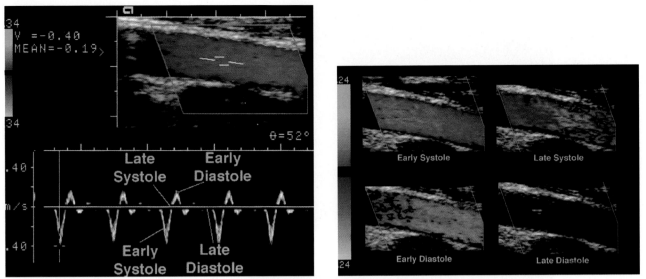

A

B

Color Figure 11.29 *Color Changes in the Cardiac Cycle. A.* Spectral Doppler shows the characteristic changes of the Doppler spectrum of the common femoral artery during the cardiac cycle. *B.* Color Doppler images show the corresponding changes in color images that correspond to phases of the cardiac cycle.

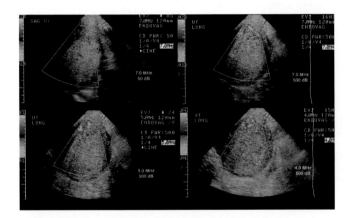

Color Figure 11.30 *Effect of Transducer Frequency and Doppler Power Settings.* This series of transvaginal images of a uterus containing a first trimester molar pregnancy provides graphic example of the effect of transducer frequency and power settings on the color Doppler image. The best color image is obtained using the lowest transducer frequency (4 MHz) with the highest power setting (500 dB).

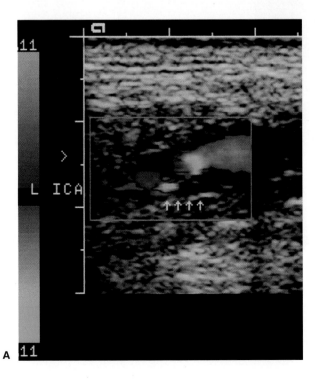

A

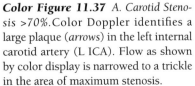

Color Figure 11.37 *A. Carotid Stenosis >70%.* Color Doppler identifies a large plaque (*arrows*) in the left internal carotid artery (L ICA). Flow as shown by color display is narrowed to a trickle in the area of maximum stenosis.

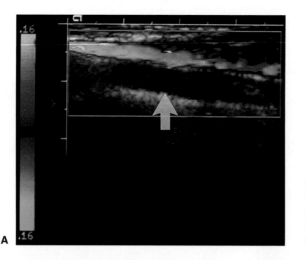

A

Color Figure 11.39 A. Occlusion of the Internal Carotid Artery. Color Doppler image shows no flow in the internal carotid artery (*arrow*). The lumen is filled with hypoechoic thrombus.

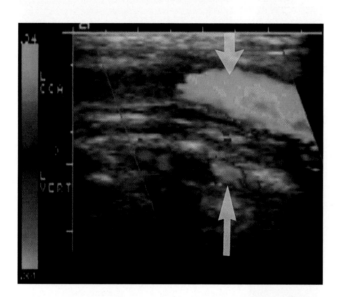

Color Figure 11.40 Subclavian Steal. Color Doppler image of the common carotid artery (CCA) (*short arrow*) and the vertebral artery (*long arrow*) shows colors on opposite sides of the color map, indicating blood flow in different directions. The vertebral artery is flowing away from the brain while the CCA shows normal blood flow direction toward the brain.

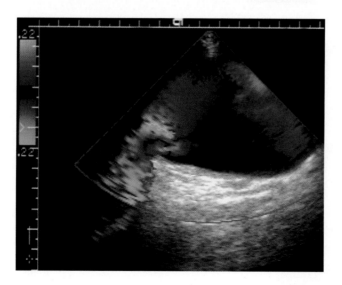

Color Figure 11.42 Aneurysm of the Abdominal Aorta. Longitudinal color Doppler image shows swirling blood flow within a 5-cm diameter aneurysm.

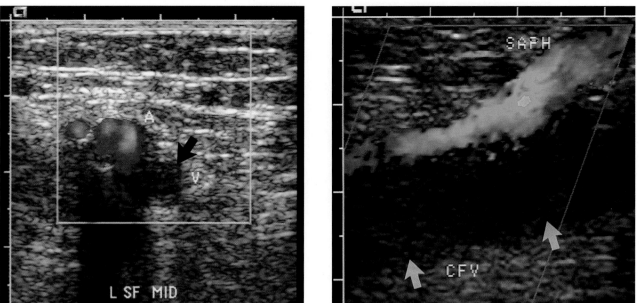

A

B

Color Figure 11.44 *Deep Venous Thrombosis—Lower Extremity. A.* Transverse power Doppler image with transducer compression applied shows flow in the femoral artery (A) and no flow in the femoral vein (V, *arrow*). The vein does not compress with transducer pressure, indicating intraluminal thrombus. *B.* Longitudinal color Doppler image of the junction of the greater saphenous vein (SAPH) with the common femoral vein (CFV, *arrows*) shows enlargement of the CFV with intraluminal thrombus. Note the flow of blood around the thrombus above the venous junction.

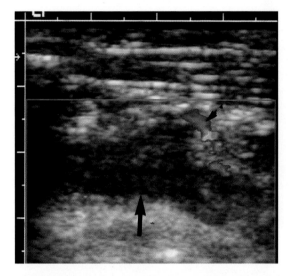

Color Figure 11.46 *Deep Vein Thrombosis—Upper Extremity.* Color Doppler image of the subclavian vein (*long arrow*) shows that the lumen is distended with thrombus. No blood flow in the vein is evident. Flow is present in an adjacent artery (*short arrow*).

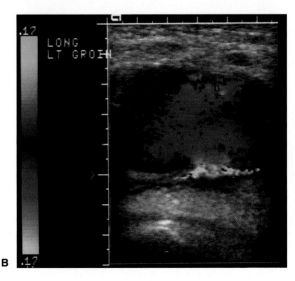

B

Color Figure 11.47 *Pseudoaneurysm. B.* Color Doppler shows blood flow that enters a pseudoaneurysm via a large neck connecting to the parent artery.

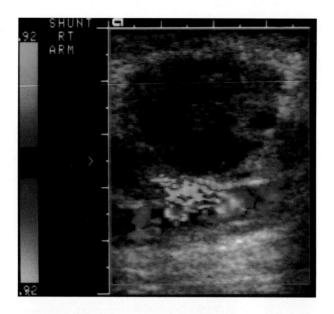

Color Figure 11.48 *Hematoma.* Color Doppler reveals no flow in a hematoma adjacent to a dialysis shunt graft in the arm.

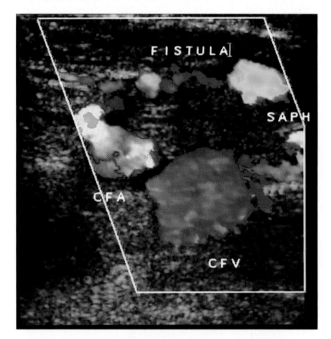

Color Figure 11.49 *Arteriovenous Fistula.* Color Doppler shows a fistula between the greater saphenous vein (SAPH) and the common femoral artery (CFA). The common femoral vein (CFV) is also seen.

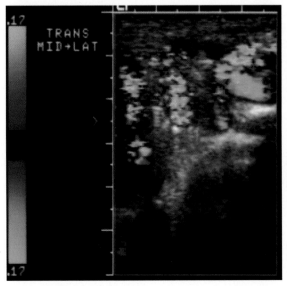

Color Figure 11.50 *Arteriovenous Malformation.* B. Color Doppler confirms blood flow in the tubular structures, representing a complex of vessels of an arteriovenous malformation.

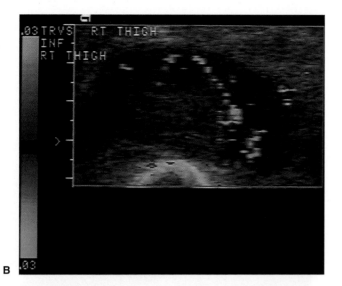

B

Color Figure 13.8 *Soft Tissue Sarcoma. B.* Color Doppler US shows prominent internal vascularity, indicating this mass is a tumor, not a hematoma.

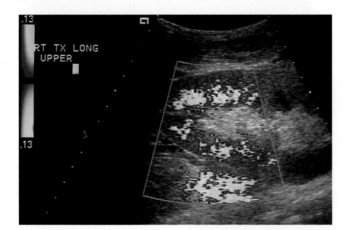

Color Figure 14.2 *Normal Color Doppler of Renal Transplant.* Color Doppler of a normal well-perfused renal transplant shows color signal well into the peripheral parenchyma.

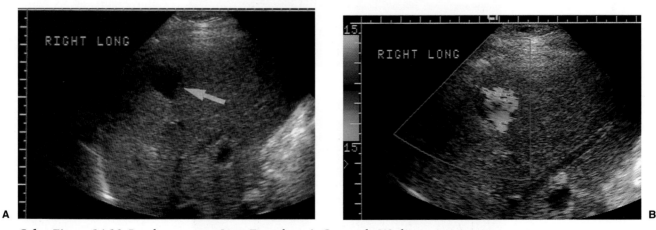

A

B

Color Figure 14.10 *Pseudoaneurysm—Liver Transplant. A.* Gray-scale US shows a cystic mass (*arrow*) in the liver. *B.* Color Doppler confirms swirling blood flow in the cystic mass. The pseudoaneurysm was a complication of biopsy of the liver transplant.

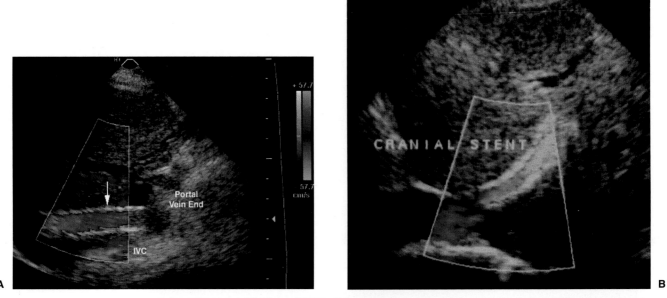

A   B

***Color Figure* 14.12** *Normal TIPS.* Color Doppler images show the portal (*A*) and hepatic (*B*) ends of the shunt. Note the bright wall of the shunt caused by the metallic mesh. IVC, inferior vena cava.

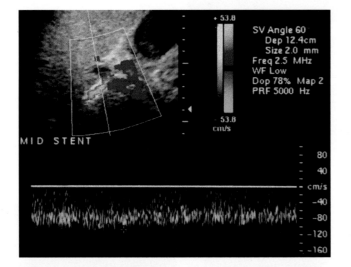

***Color Figure* 14.13** *Normal TIPS Spectral Doppler.* Spectral Doppler tracing obtained in the mid-portion of the shunt shows normal turbulent venous flow.

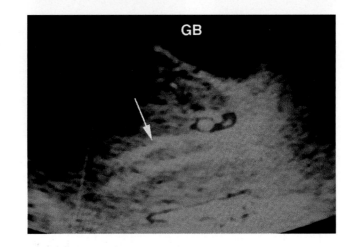

***Color Figure* 14.14** *Occluded TIPS.* Color Doppler image shows echogenic thrombus and no blood flow in the shunt (*arrow*). GB, gallbladder.

CHROMOSOME ANOMALIES AND BIOCHEMICAL SCREENING

Approximately 4 infants per 1000 live births have a significant chromosome abnormality [51]. The incidence of chromosome abnormalities is much higher in spontaneous abortions and stillbirths. **Aneuploidy** is the state of having an abnormal number of chromosomes (more or less than 46). The risk of aneuploidy increases with increasing age. **Triploidy** refers to the presence of a complete extra set of chromosomes (69 chromosomes). Most triploidies result in spontaneous abortions. Triploidy is associated with partial hydatidiform mole. **Trisomy** is the state of having three, instead of the usual pair, of any one chromosome. Trisomy implies aneuploidy with 47 chromosomes. Common trisomies are trisomy 21 (Down's syndrome), trisomy 18 [52], and trisomy 13 [53].

Initial screening for chromosome abnormalities was based on maternal age alone [54]. The risk of Down's syndrome is 1 in 910 at age 30 and progressively increases to 1 in 110 at age 40. At age 37 the risk is 1 in 240, which is approximately equal to the risk of fetal loss associated with amniocentesis, approximately 1 in 200. If amniocentesis is offered to all pregnant women age 35 and older, approximately 40–60% of Down's syndrome fetuses will be detected [54]. Additional efforts at detection of chromosome anomalies are based on biochemical screening of maternal serum and on US examination.

MATERNAL SERUM ALPHA-FETOPROTEIN

Biochemical screening for fetal abnormalities initially focused on alpha-fetoprotein (AFP) as a marker of neural tube and other fetal anatomic defects [55]. AFP is a glycoprotein made initially in the yolk sac and later by the fetal liver. MS-AFP levels vary with GA and peak at 28–32 weeks. Fetal tissue not covered by skin leaks AFP into the amniotic fluid where it is absorbed into the maternal bloodstream. Levels of AFP in maternal blood that exceed 2.5 multiples of the median (MOM) for GA are considered abnormal for singleton pregnancies. Levels >4.5 MOM are abnormal for multiple fetus pregnancies. MS-AFP screening detects 98% of open spina bifida defects and anencephaly. See Box 7.4 for a summary of abnormalities associated with elevated MS-AFP.

Low levels of MS-AFP (0.63–1.0 MOM) are associated with increased risk of Down's syndrome. However the sensitivity of low MS-AFP for Down's is only approximately 21%. This has led to the use of "triple marker" maternal serum screening.

Box 7.4: Causes of Elevated Maternal Serum Alpha-Fetoprotein

Neural tube defect
  Open spina bifida (98% of cases)
  Anencephaly (98%)
  Cephalocele
Abdominal wall defects
  Gastroschisis (77–90%)
  Omphalocele (40%)
  Amniotic band syndrome

Placental abnormalities
  Chorioangioma
  Placental hematoma
  Placental insufficiency
Chromosome abnormalities
  Trisomy 13
  Trisomy 18
  Turner's syndrome (XO)
  Triploidy
Incorrect menstrual dating
Multiple fetus gestation
Fetal demise

Box 7.5: US Markers of Down's Syndrome

. . . .

"Soft" Markers

Short femur length—Also seen with skeletal dysplasias [135].

Echogenic bowel (≥bone)—Also seen with bowel obstruction, intrauterine infection, cystic fibrosis, and bowel ischemia. Finding implies a risk of adverse outcome of the pregnancy [114].

Choroid plexus cyst—Has a higher association with trisomy 18. The presence of a choroid plexus cyst is an indication for detailed fetal anatomic survey for additional anomalies (Fig. 7.47) [54,56].

Nuchal fold—Nuchal translucency ≥3 mm in the first trimester, or nuchal skin thickness ≥6 mm in the second trimester is highly associated with the presence of Down's syndrome [60,61]. Increased nuchal fold thickness in the second trimester is also associated with Turner's syndrome (XO).

Echogenic focus in cardiac ventricle—Associated risk of Down's syndrome is increased by as much as fourfold [101,136,137].

Mild renal pyelectasis—(≥4 mm at 15–20 weeks) Is seen in 17–25% of fetuses with Down's syndrome [138].

"Hard" Markers

Duodenal atresia—Is the most common intraabdominal abnormality associated with Down's syndrome. However, US can rarely make the diagnosis before 22 weeks GA.

Congenital heart disease—Up to 50% of fetuses with Down's syndrome have congenital heart disease, most commonly complete atrioventricular canal or ventricular septal defect.

TRIPLE MARKER SCREENING

Expanded AFP, or triple marker, screening measures the levels of AFP, human chorionic gonadotropin, and unconjugated estriol in maternal serum. Race, ethnicity, maternal age, and accurate determination of GA are used to determine the risk level for chromosome abnormality.

SONOGRAPHIC SCREENING FOR DOWN'S SYNDROME

US findings associated with Down's syndrome are summarized in Box 7.5. The presence of an abnormal nuchal fold, a "hard" marker, or two soft markers is considered an indication for parental counseling and consideration of amniocentesis for chromosome analysis [56,57]. Use of sonographic markers in a high-risk population can identify up to 75% of fetuses with Down's syndrome [58]. A number of centers recommend against counseling if only one "soft" marker is present because of the high price of parental anxiety for what is most likely to be an insignificant problem [54,59].

■ Nuchal thickening is one of the strongest predictive signs of chromosome abnormality. Nuchal thickness is measured on the transcerebellar view. Nuchal thickness >3 mm in the first trimester [60] or >6 mm in the second trimester is associated with the presence of chromosome anomalies (Fig. 7.25) [61].

MULTIPLE PREGNANCY

Multiple pregnancies carry an increased risk of nearly every complication of pregnancy.

Mortality of twins is 15% higher than mortality of singleton pregnancies. The incidence of congenital anomalies is increased 4-fold in twin pregnancies. In addition, twins may experience a variety of disorders that are unique to twinning.

Approximately 1 in 80–90 deliveries involves twins. Triplets are much less common, approximately 1 in 6400 births. Quadruplets occur in 1 in 512,000 births.

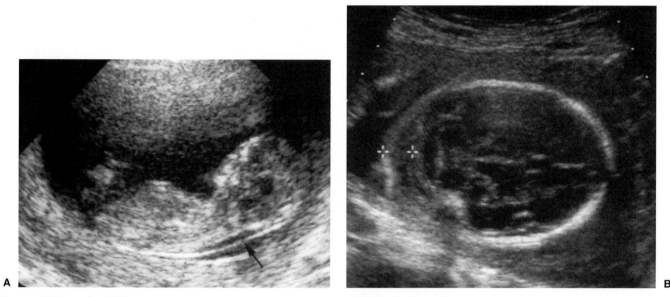

Figure 7.25 *Nuchal Thickening. A.* On this 9-week fetus, the nuchal lucency (*arrow*) measures 4 mm. This fetus was proven to have Down's syndrome on amniocentesis. *B.* On this 20-week fetus, the nuchal thickness (*between cursors,* +) measures 9 mm. This fetus has Turner's syndrome (XO).

PLACENTATION

The risks of twin pregnancies are related to the type of twinning [62]. Dizygotic twins are always dichorionic, diamniotic. The placentation of monozygotic twins depends upon the timing of the division of the fertilized ovum that results in twinning. When division is early (first 3–4 days), the twins are dichorionic, diamniotic (1/3). When division occurs at 4–7 days, the twins are monochorionic, diamniotic (2/3). When division occurs after 8 days, the twins are monoamniotic (<1%) and at highest risk for adverse outcome. Division later than 13 days results in conjoined twins.

- In the first trimester, the presence of a thick membrane separating the two sacs indicates dichorionic twins. If the membrane is thin or not seen, the pregnancy is monochorionic. Because the amnion membrane separating the twins may not be evident, amnionicity cannot be reliably determined until the second trimester. The presence of two yolk sacs indicates diamniotic twins. If only one yolk sac is present, the pregnancy is monoamniotic [63].
- In the second trimester the pregnancy is dichorionic if the twins are of different gender or if two separate placentas are clearly visualized.
- A single placental mass may consist of two abutting placentas or a single placenta that supplies both twins. A thick membrane, consisting of two chorions and two amnions, separating the twins indicates dichorionic twinning. A thin membrane, consisting of two layers of amnion, separating the twins indicates monochorionic, diamniotic twins. An easy-to-see membrane of 1–2 mm is considered "thick." A difficult-to-see membrane is "thin." Differentiation of thin and thick is obviously subjective and not very accurate (Fig. 7.26).
- The "twin-peak sign" is more definitive [64]. A beak-like tongue of placenta protrudes between the two double-membranes of dichorionic diamniotic twins (Fig. 7.26A). The single chorion of a monochorionic pregnancy prevents this protrusion of placenta between membranes.
- Visualization of an amnion in the second trimester is definitive for diamniotic pregnancy. However, when the amnion is not visualized it still may be present. Diagnosis of monoamniotic twinning requires additional findings such as entangled umbilical cords or fetal parts (Fig. 7.26C).

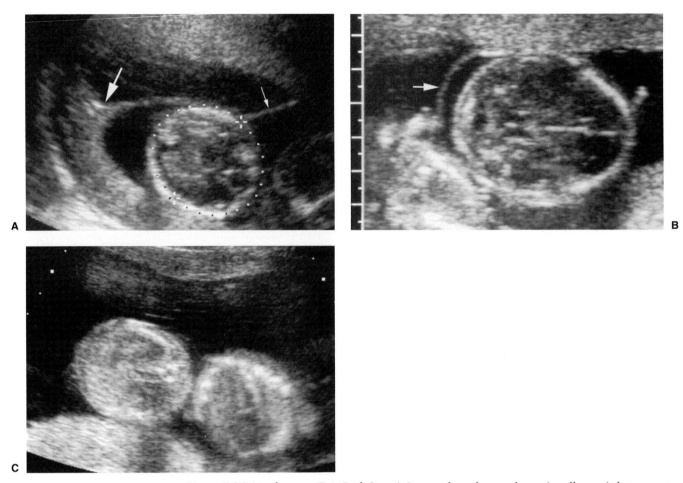

Figure 7.26 *Membranes—Twin Peak Sign. A.* Image where the membrane (*small arrow*) that separates twins joins the placenta shows the "peak" of placental tissue (*large arrow*) that protrudes between the membrane layers. This is, therefore, a "thick" membrane of two layers of chorion and two layers of amnion in a dichorionic diamniotic twin pregnancy. Compare to the "thin" membrane (*arrow*) in *B* and note the minimal difference in apparent thickness. The apparent thickness of the membrane is determined more by US physics and angle of the US beam than by the physical thickness of the membrane. *B.* This membrane (*arrow*) of a monochorionic diamniotic twin pregnancy varies little in apparent thickness compared to *A.* Note that the membrane is fairly closely applied to the head of one twin, simulating a cystic hygroma; however, the characteristic midline septum is not present. Membranes may simulate nuchal lucencies and cystic hygroma. *C.* Monoamniotic twins have no separating membrane and demonstrate intermingling of fetal parts and umbilical cords. Monoamniotic twins have the highest rate of complications.

GROWTH OF TWINS

Twins closely parallel the growth of singletons in the first and second trimesters, so the same growth charts can be used [65,66]. In the third trimester, the weight gain of normal twins slows and charts specific to twins may be used for more accurate assessment. IUGR affects approximately 25% of twin pregnancies.

- GA is determined at the first US examination by averaging the composite GA of the twins, provided they are not grossly discordant. Subsequent US examinations are compared to the first examination for growth. Once established, the GA of the twins is not changed [62]. If the first US examination is performed late in pregnancy, FL measurements appear to be most reliable for determining GA.
- A 15% difference in EFW or AC between the twins is considered evidence of significant growth discordance.

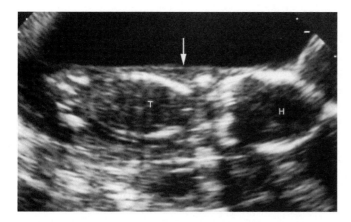

Figure 7.27 *Twin-Twin Transfusion Syndrome—Stuck Twin.* The donor twin suffering from twin-twin transfusion syndrome is trapped in a small sac with almost no amniotic fluid by a tightly adherent membrane (*arrow*). The recipient twin floated in a huge volume of amniotic fluid. H, head; T, trunk of the donor twin.

TWIN-TWIN TRANSFUSION SYNDROME

In monoamniotic twin pregnancies, vascular communications exist in the placenta between the two twins. If a large arterial to venous shunt exists, blood and nutrients are progressively transfused between a donor twin and a recipient twin. The donor twin becomes anemic and growth restricted. The recipient twin becomes hypervolemic and hydropic [67]. This condition affects 15–30% of monochorionic pregnancies and is commonly fatal to both twins (40–87%) [62].

- Significant (>20%) difference in EFW between the twins is caused by growth restriction of the donor twin.
- The size and amniotic fluid volume of the two sacs are greatly different. In some cases the donor twin appears "stuck" to the wall of the uterus (Fig. 7.27). This twin experiences severe oligohydramnios caused by diminished urine output and its movement is greatly restricted by adherent amnion. The stuck twin is commonly fixed in position in a nondependent portion of the uterus. The recipient twin floats freely in polyhydramnios.
- The recipient twin commonly shows evidence of congestive heart failure or hydrops.
- Doppler shows a marked difference in the umbilical artery spectrum of the twins with the growth-restricted donor twin showing high resistance [68].

INTRAUTERINE DEMISE OF ONE TWIN

Death of one twin may occur at any time during gestation. Death late in gestation carries increased risk to the surviving fetus.

- Loss of one twin early in pregnancy is very common, affecting as many as 50% of early twins. Often one twin will "vanish" with no residual evidence of its presence. A blighted twin is evidenced by the presence of a recognizable second fetus without a heartbeat. The non-viable twin may persist in the uterus throughout gestation as a flattened fetal remnant (fetus papyraceous).
- The live twin may lose blood to the dead twin resulting in hypovolemic shock and death.
- The dead twin may embolize necrotic tissue to the live twin resulting in disseminated intravascular coagulation, tissue ischemia, and infarction. This is called *twin-twin embolization syndrome.* This syndrome occurs only in monochorionic twins with significant vascular intercommunications in the placenta.

TWIN REVERSED ARTERIAL PERFUSION SEQUENCE

Intraplacental shunts result in pairing of arteries of one twin to the arteries of the other twin and vein-to-vein pairing between the twins. Preferential perfusion to the lower body of one twin results in absence of development of the upper body and absence of the heart (acardiac

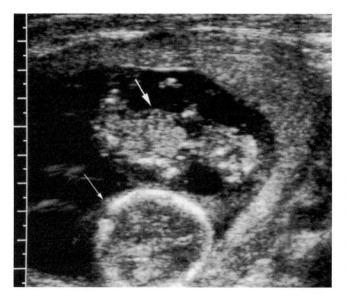

Figure 7.28 *Acardiac Twin.* The acardiac twin (*larger arrow*) is grossly deformed with no identifiable head or heart. The normal twin (*smaller arrow*) shows no evidence of hydrops or cardiac decompensation at this stage of pregnancy.

twin). Blood flow is reversed in the acardiac twin while the "pump" twin experiences high output cardiac failure. If the acardiac twin is large (>70% EFW of the co-twin), the co-twin will usually die.

■ No beating heart is present in the severely deformed acardiac twin (Fig. 7.28).
■ Doppler shows umbilical artery flow *toward* and umbilical vein flow *away from* the acardiac twin. The blood flow to the acardiac twin is deoxygenated by flow through the pump twin. In most cases only a single umbilical artery perfuses the acardiac twin.
■ The head and upper body of the acardiac twin is either absent or shows major anomalies of development.
■ The pump twin is usually anatomically normal and will survive if the strain on its heart is not excessive.

NORMAL FETAL ANATOMY

BRAIN

Three image planes provide effective US screening of the brain for anomalies [69].

■ The **transthalamic plane** is used to measure the BPD and HC (Figs. 7.1, 7.3). Anomalies of head shape and head size are evident on this image plane. The third ventricle is routinely identified on this image plane [70].
■ The **transventricular plane** is used to assess the size and appearance of the lateral ventricles (Fig. 7.29). It is an axial plane through the fetal cranium at the level of the atria of the lateral ventricles. The diameter of each atrium is measured on this plane and remains unchanged throughout the second and third trimesters. Normal atria measure 7–8 mm in diameter and do not exceed 10 mm throughout pregnancy. The echogenic choroid plexus nearly completely fills the atria. More than 3 mm of separation of the choroid plexus from the medial wall of the lateral ventricle is a sign of ventriculomegaly.
■ The **transcerebellar plane** provides a standardized image for assessment of the posterior fossa (Fig. 7.30). This plane is an axial plane obtained by angling the transducer 10–15 degrees posteriorly and inferiorly from the transthalamic plane. The anatomic landmarks of this plane are the posterior aspect of the third ventricle and the prominent cerebellar hemispheres and vermis outlined by fluid in the cisterna magna. Demonstration of normal size and appearance of the cisterna magna virtually excludes the presence of lumbosacral meningomyelocele. The width of the cisterna magna is measured in the

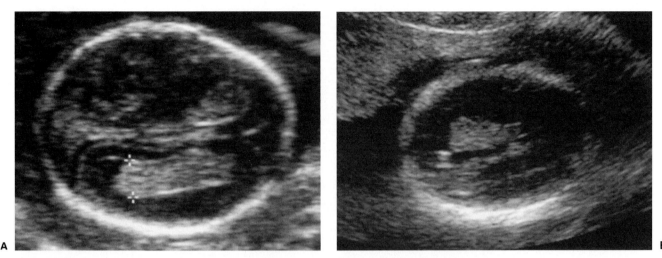

Figure 7.29 *Normal Transventricular Plane. A.* The echogenic choroid plexus nearly completely fills the lateral ventricle at the atrium (*between cursors, +*). Note that only the downside ventricle can be visualized. The upside ventricle is obscured by shadowing and reverberation artifact from the near skull. *B.* The upside ventricle can be imaged by angling the transducer slightly from a direct axial plane.

midline from the inner table of the occiput to the posterior aspect of the vermis. The normal cisterna magna measures 2–11 mm in diameter. A small cisterna magna (<2 mm) suggests a Chiari II malformation. A large cisterna magna (>11 mm) suggests Dandy-Walker malformation, cerebellar hypoplasia, arachnoid cyst, or maybe a normal variant "mega-cisterna magna." Echogenic lines that cross the cisterna magna have been shown to represent bridging arachnoid septations. A cyst-like configuration of these septa is a normal variant of no significance [71].

FACE AND NECK

- By 13–14 weeks GA, a sagittal profile view (Fig. 7.31A) will show normal features of the fetal face including nose, maxilla, mandible, and orbits [72].
- A coronal view shows the lips and mouth (Fig. 7.31B). The normal depression, called the *fulcrum*, in the upper lip beneath the nose should not be mistaken for a facial cleft. Tooth buds are seen as echogenic structures within the maxilla and mandible. The tongue is seen to move within the open mouth.

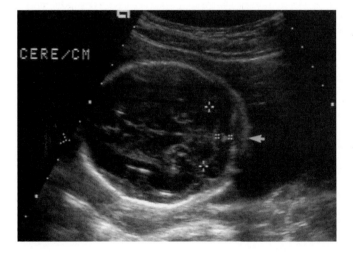

Figure 7.30 *Normal Transcerebellar Plane.* By angling the transducer posteriorly from the transthalamic plane, the posterior fossa, cerebellum (*between cursors, +*), and cisterna magna (*between cursors, x*) can be visualized and measured. This same plane is used to measure nuchal thickness from the outer aspect of the cranium to the surface of the skin (*arrow*). The width of the cerebellum in millimeters is approximately equal to gestational age in weeks.

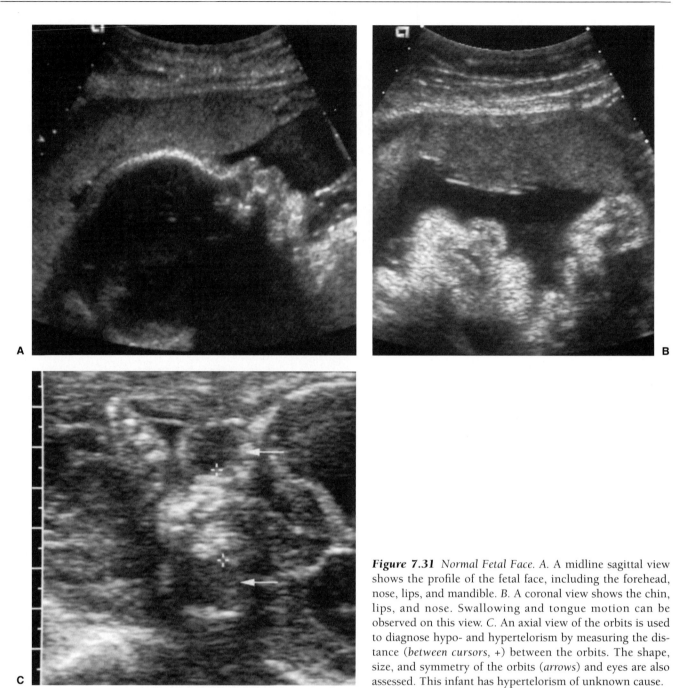

Figure 7.31 *Normal Fetal Face. A.* A midline sagittal view shows the profile of the fetal face, including the forehead, nose, lips, and mandible. *B.* A coronal view shows the chin, lips, and nose. Swallowing and tongue motion can be observed on this view. *C.* An axial view of the orbits is used to diagnose hypo- and hypertelorism by measuring the distance (*between cursors,* +) between the orbits. The shape, size, and symmetry of the orbits (*arrows*) and eyes are also assessed. This infant has hypertelorism of unknown cause.

■ Axial views show the orbits (Fig. 7.31C). The distance between the medial and lateral walls of the orbits can be measured and compared to charts related to GA to diagnose hypo- and hypertelorism.

■ The neck is well seen on axial (Fig. 7.32) and longitudinal views [73]. Landmarks are the larynx, thyroid gland, and pulsating carotid arteries.

SPINE

■ Ossification of the fetal spine occurs in three prominent ossification centers; paired dorsal centers that will become the lateral masses and posterior arch and a single central ventral center that will become the vertebral body (Fig. 7.33) [74].

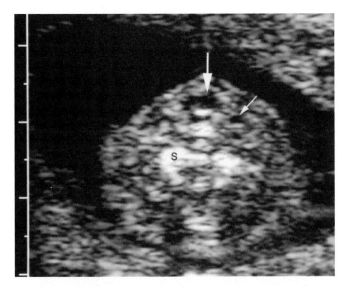

Figure 7.32 *Normal Neck.* Axial view of the fetal neck shows the centrally positioned spine (S), the fluid-filled trachea (*large arrow*), and the carotid artery (*small arrow*). Vascular pulsations in the carotid arteries are prominent on real-time imaging.

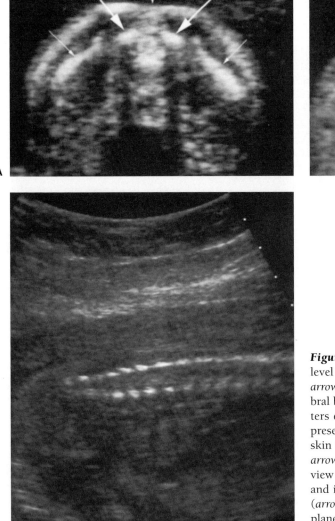

Figure 7.33 *Normal Spine. A.* Transverse view of the spine at the level of L5 vertebra shows the three ossification centers, two (*large arrows*) for the posterior elements and one anteriorly for the vertebral body. With advancing GA, the two posterior ossification centers elongate and converge on each other. When spina bifida is present, the posterior ossification centers diverge. Note that the skin (*arrowhead*) is intact over the spine. The iliac wings (*skinny arrows*) are prominent landmarks of the bony pelvis. *B.* Transverse view of L4 vertebra shows converging posterior ossification centers and intact skin (*arrowhead*). The hypoechoic paraspinal muscles (*arrows*) are well seen. *C.* Longitudinal view of the spine in coronal plane shows normal tapering of the distance between posterior elements toward the sacrum.

■ Transverse views allow simultaneous imaging of all three ossification centers, whereas sagittal and coronal views provide images of only two centers at a time but allow visualization of many vertebral segments (Fig. 7.33). Transverse images are best for detection of subtle spina bifida anomalies whereas sagittal and coronal images are best for demonstration of scoliosis, hemivertebrae, and disorganized vertebral development. Normal dorsal ossification centers converge toward each other on transverse views. Divergence is evidence of spina bifida. Longitudinal views are inspected for normal thoracic kyphosis and lumbar lordosis [74].

CHEST

The chest cavity is defined by the shadowing ribs and the dome-shaped, thin, hypoechoic muscle of the diaphragm.

■ On axial view the heart occupies approximately one-third of the cross-sectional area of the thorax (Fig. 7.34A).
■ Normal fetal lungs surround the heart and have homogeneous echogenicity approximately equal to the liver. Color Doppler will show the vascularity of the lungs.
■ The normal esophagus may be seen in the lower neck and posterior thorax as a multi-layered tubular structure [75].

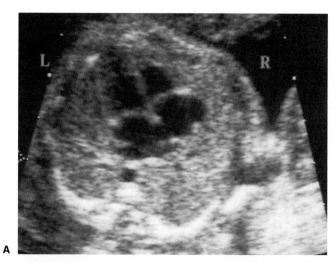

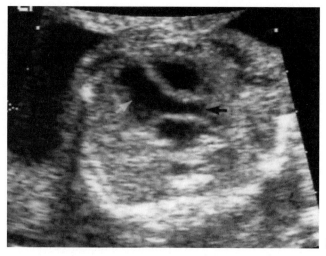

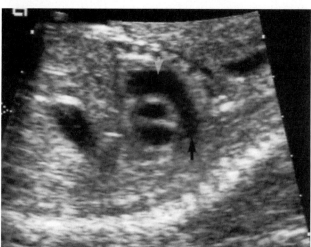

Figure 7.34 *Normal Chest and Heart. A.* Axial 4-chamber view of the heart clearly shows both cardiac atria and ventricles, interventricular and interatrial septa, and the atrioventricular valves. See Box 7.6 for a description of normal features of this view. R, fetal right side. L, fetal left side. *B.* The left ventricular outflow tract view shows the left ventricle (*white arrow*) and root of the aorta (*black arrow*). *C.* The right ventricular outflow tract view shows the right ventricle (*white arrow*) and the main pulmonary artery (*black arrow*).

HEART

Routine screening of the fetal heart for anomalies of the cardiovascular system and thorax includes the 4-chamber view and views of the right and left ventricular outflow tracts (RVOT and LVOT) [76,77]. These three views will identify the majority (83%) of cardiac anomalies [78].

- The 4-chamber view is an axial section through the lower thorax and heart (Fig. 7.34A) [77,79]. The cross-sectional area of the normal heart occupies approximately one-third of the cross-sectional area of the thorax on this view. The cardiac axis is evaluated by drawing one line to connect the spine and sternum and a second line through the interventricular septum. The normal cardiac axis is 45 degrees to the left (normal range = 22–75 degrees). Situs is determined by evaluating fetal position and confirming that both the cardiac apex and the stomach are on the left. The right and left ventricles are equal in size in the fetus and are separated by a muscular septum of uniform thickness. The ventricular septum has a normal thin membranous portion near the atrio-ventricular valves that should not be mistaken for a ventricular septal defect. The moderator band of muscle near the apex of the right ventricle is commonly prominent. The papillary muscles are occasionally brightly echogenic. Echogenic foci in the ventricular chambers may be associated with chromosome anomalies as previously discussed. The atrioventricular valves are inspected for symmetry of size and motion. Normal features of the 4-chamber view are listed in Box 7.6 [77,79,80].
- The LVOT view (Fig. 7.34B) is obtained by rotating the transducer approximately 90 degrees from the 4-chamber view to visualize the aorta exiting from the *center* of the heart. The left ventricle, aortic valve, and ascending aorta are well visualized on this view [77].
- The RVOT view (Fig. 7.34C) is obtained by rotating the transducer approximately 90 degrees from the 4-chamber view in the opposite direction from that used to obtain the LVOT view. At the same time that the transducer is rotated, it is also angled cephalad. The pulmonary artery exits the heart anterior to the aorta. The RVOT view shows the right ventricle, pulmonic valve, and main pulmonary artery [77].
- The size of the pulmonary artery should be approximately equal to the size of the aorta. Distinct differences in size of the great vessels suggests atresia or cardiac shunts with asymmetric volumes of blood passing out of each side of the heart.

Box 7.6: Features of a Normal 4-Chamber View of the Fetal Heart

Cardiac size is approximately equal to one-third of the thorax.
Cardiac axis is directed 45 degrees to the left.
Heart and stomach are both on the left side of the fetus.
Right ventricle is substernal and contains the muscular moderator band near the apex.
Left ventricle borders the left lung.
Right and left ventricular walls are equal in thickness.
Right and left ventricular chambers are equal in size.
Right and left atrial chambers are equal in size.
Ventricular septum is uniform in thickness and has no defects.
The foramen ovale is a normal defect in the atrial septum.
The flap covering the foramen ovale opens on the left.
The tricuspid valve is positioned slightly closer to the cardiac apex than the mitral valve.
The tricuspid and mitral valves are equal in thickness and move symmetrically.
A thin hypoechoic rim of outer myocardium should not be mistaken for a pericardial effusion.
A thin sliver of pericardial fluid (<2 mm at its thickest point) is a normal finding.

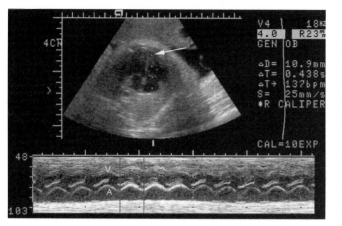

Figure 7.35 *M-Mode Documentation of Fetal Heart Rate.* The direction of the M-mode US beam can be steered by the operator and is indicated by the dotted line (*arrow*). In this case, the beam is directed through both the right ventricle and the right atrium of this fetal heart seen in 4-chamber view. The M-mode tracing shows an identical heart rate for the atrium and the ventricle at 137 beats per minute.

- If the pulmonary artery is not clearly anterior to the aorta, transposition of the great vessels must be suspected.
- M-mode US is used to document fetal heart rate and rhythm (Fig. 7.35). If the fetal heart rate is below 100 bpm, above 180 bpm, or is irregular, M-mode tracings should be obtained and compared to both the atrial rate and the ventricular rate. Doppler is not recommended for this indication because of the high-energy settings required for Doppler US.

ABDOMINAL WALL

- The umbilical cord enters the fetus at the umbilicus and diverges immediately into the two umbilical arteries, which extend caudally, and the umbilical vein, which courses superiorly and dorsally.
- The umbilical arteries course from their origin on the internal iliac arteries around both sides of the bladder and along the anterior abdominal wall to the umbilicus. A single umbilical artery (two-vessel cord) is easily confirmed by observing that only one umbilical artery is seen adjacent to the bladder.
- The umbilical vein crosses the peritoneal cavity in the free edge of the falciform ligament to enter the liver and join the left portal vein. Oxygenated blood is divided equally between liver via the portal circulation and the IVC via the ductus venosus.
- Midgut herniation into the base of the umbilical cord is normal between 8 and 12 weeks GA. US shows a round or oval echogenic mass 4–10 mm in size in the base of the umbilical cord.
- The cord insertion site should be inspected on every second and third trimester examination (Fig. 7.36).
- The abdominal wall musculature may be mistaken for ascites [81]. Abdominal wall muscles create a sonolucent band of uniform thickness that merges with the rib ends. No fluid is seen within the peritoneal recesses.

ABDOMEN—GASTROINTESTINAL

- The fetal stomach is visualized as a fluid-filled structure (Fig. 7.37) in the left upper quadrant as early as 11 weeks and in 98% of normal fetuses after 12 weeks.
- The liver occupies most of the upper abdomen. In the fetus the left lobe is larger than the right lobe and commonly extends to the left flank.
- The gallbladder is seen as an ovoid cystic structure to the right of the intrahepatic umbilical vein.
- The spleen is seen as a solid organ posterior and to the left of the stomach.
- In the first and second trimester, bowel is ill defined, somewhat heterogeneous, and moderately echogenic in mid- to lower abdomen.

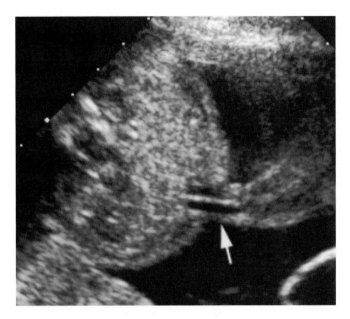

Figure 7.36 *Normal Umbilical Cord Insertion.* Axial view through the fetal abdomen at the level of the umbilicus shows the normal appearance of the umbilical cord insertion (*arrow*).

- After 20 weeks, large bowel is seen as a continuous hypoechoic tubular structure in the periphery of the abdomen. Normal size is 3–5 mm at 20 weeks, increasing to a maximum of 23 mm at term [82]. Liquid meconium in the colon may be mistaken for a cystic mass near term.
- Small bowel is seen more centrally in the abdomen. Meconium becomes increasingly echogenic with advancing GA. Normal loops are <6 mm diameter [82]. Active peristalsis is evident in the third trimester and helps to differentiate small from large bowel.
- Compared to adults, the fetal abdomen is relatively large and the fetal pelvis is relatively small resulting in the bladder, uterus, and ovaries lying mainly in the abdomen.

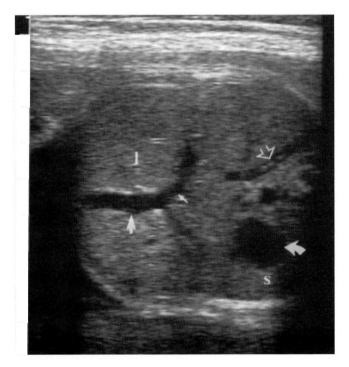

Figure 7.37 *Normal Fetal Abdomen.* Axial view of the abdomen in a 30-week fetus shows the umbilical vein (*short arrow*) passing through the liver (l) to enter the left portal vein (*tiny arrow*). A normal, prominent fetal adrenal gland (*open arrow*) is apparent. The fetal stomach (*curved arrow*) is fluid filled. The spleen (S) occupies the left upper quadrant posterior and lateral to the stomach.

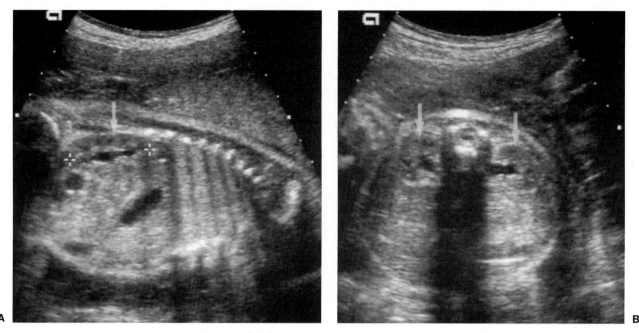

Figure 7.38 *Normal Kidneys.* Long axis, *A*, and transverse, *B*, views of the fetal kidneys (*arrows*) show prominent corticomedullary differentiation and mild pelviectasis. Mild dilatation of the fetal renal pelvis is a common normal finding. The dilatation will commonly disappear when the fetus empties its bladder. Note the prominent shadow of the spine on the transverse view. Abnormal structures that touch the fetal spine are likely renal in origin.

ABDOMEN—GENITOURINARY TRACT

- The fetal adrenal glands are 20 times their relative size in the adult and form prominent masses above the kidneys. The inner medulla is echogenic and the thick outer cortex is hypoechoic (Fig. 7.37).
- Kidneys are seen as distinct structures at 14 weeks and show characteristic internal morphology by 18–20 weeks. The kidneys are identified by their characteristic shape and their position adjacent to the spine (Fig. 7.38). Fetal lobulation becomes more prominent with advancing GA. The pyramids are lucent and may be mistaken for hydronephrosis. The kidneys grow throughout gestation with normal fetal renal length in mm being approximately equal to GA in weeks.
- Ureters are not seen unless they are dilated. Visualization of a fetal ureter indicates the ureter is dilated.
- The urinary bladder may be observed to fill and empty every 30–45 minutes. When distended, its wall is very thin.
- Amniotic fluid volume beyond 16 weeks reflects the volume of urine production and excretion.

GENDER DETERMINATION

Although fetal gender is probably the most common question asked by prospective parents, answering the question correctly may be difficult [83].

- In approximately 30% of cases, the perineum is not adequately visualized.
- Seeing the testes in the scrotum is reliable in confirming a male fetus; however, the testes do not descend to the scrotum until 28–34 weeks (Fig. 7.39).
- The labia may be enlarged by circulating maternal hormones and may closely resemble the scrotum (Fig. 7.39). A hypertrophied clitoris may mimic the penis.

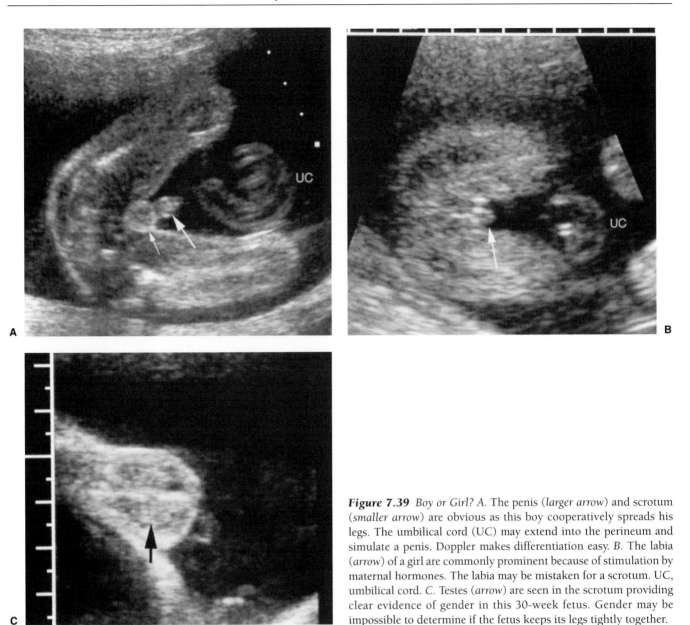

Figure 7.39 *Boy or Girl? A.* The penis (*larger arrow*) and scrotum (*smaller arrow*) are obvious as this boy cooperatively spreads his legs. The umbilical cord (UC) may extend into the perineum and simulate a penis. Doppler makes differentiation easy. *B.* The labia (*arrow*) of a girl are commonly prominent because of stimulation by maternal hormones. The labia may be mistaken for a scrotum. UC, umbilical cord. *C.* Testes (*arrow*) are seen in the scrotum providing clear evidence of gender in this 30-week fetus. Gender may be impossible to determine if the fetus keeps its legs tightly together.

SKELETAL SYSTEM

The high reflectivity of bone makes the skeletal system easy to visualize with US. However, complete examination is difficult because of wide variations in fetal position and orientation of the limbs. The sonographer is completely at the mercy of the fetus. However, with experience the skeletal system can usually be comprehensively evaluated.

- Identify individual bones by anatomic continuity, not just by position. A limb adjacent to the fetal head may be either an arm or a leg.
- Image the short axis of a limb to confirm whether one or two bones are present. The presence of two bones differentiates the forearm and leg from the upper arm and thigh. Bones that begin and end at the same level are the tibia and fibula. The ulna is longer than the radius and extends more proximally than the radius at the elbow.
- Make sure that *both* upper and lower extremities are examined and that the same extremity is not examined twice because the fetus has moved.

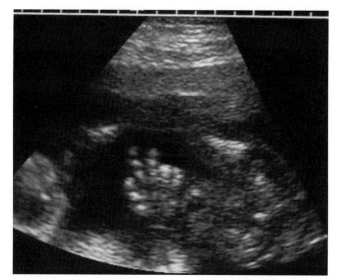

Figure 7.40 *Normal Hand.* Bones, even tiny ones like the phalanges, are highly echogenic and easy to visualize. This baby is celebrating its peaceful life *in utero.*

- Measure the greatest length of the echogenic surface of each long bone and refer to appropriate charts that relate bone length to GA to determine if measurements are within normal range.
- Documentation of normal opening and closing of the fetal hand is more important than counting the number of phalanges (Fig. 7.40).

FETAL ANOMALIES

HYDROPS

Fetal Hydrops

Fetal hydrops is defined as the abnormal accumulation of serous fluid in at least two body cavities or tissues. Causes of hydrops are usually classified as immune and nonimmune. Immune hydrops is caused by maternal antibodies that cross the placenta to attack and hemolyze fetal red blood cells, resulting in severe fetal anemia, tissue hypoxia, and eventually fetal death (erythroblastosis fetalis). The majority of cases are associated with maternal sensitization to Rh factor from previous pregnancy. Nonimmune hydrops is the terminal stage of many severe fetal anomalies. Most cases in the United States are caused by severe congenital heart disease, congenital infections, and chromosome abnormalities.

- US diagnosis is based on the presence of two or more of the following abnormalities: ascites, pleural effusion, pericardial effusion, and subcutaneous edema.
- Placental edema may be present late in the course of hydrops. The placenta is thickened (>4–5 cm) and diffusely decreased in echogenicity.
- Additional signs of fetal distress include abnormal biophysical profile and abnormal umbilical artery Doppler.

BRAIN

Anencephaly

Anencephaly is the most common of the neural tube defects reported in 1 in 1000 births. Anencephaly is uniformly fatal, although some infants may survive several months [84].

- Absence of the cranium and cerebral hemispheres above the orbits is the characteristic finding of anencephaly (Fig. 7.41).

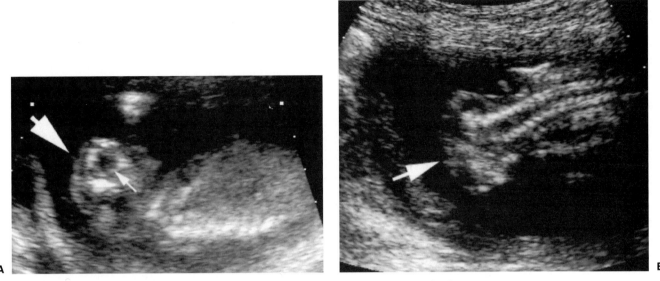

Figure 7.41 *Anencephaly. A.* The cranium and cerebral cortex (*large arrow*) are obviously absent on this sagittal view of the fetus. Small arrow indicates the orbit. *B.* Coronal view of the same fetus shows the spine ending abruptly at the flattened cranium. Disorganized brain tissue (*arrow*) floats freely not covered by bone.

- The brainstem, midbrain (mesencephalon), and base of the cranium are typically present.
- A variable amount of disorganized soft tissue commonly protrudes from the cranial defect. This vascular (angiomatous) stroma is called *area cerebrovasculosa.*
- Polyhydramnios is present in most cases after 25 weeks GA.

Cephalocele

The term *cephalocele* describes herniation of brain, meninges, or cerebrospinal fluid (CSF) through defects in the cranium. Prognosis depends on the size of the defect and the presence of brain in the herniated tissue [85].

- Encephalocele describes herniation of brain and meninges through a cranial defect (Fig. 7.42). The herniated mass is solid and shows a gyral pattern contiguous with intracranial brain.

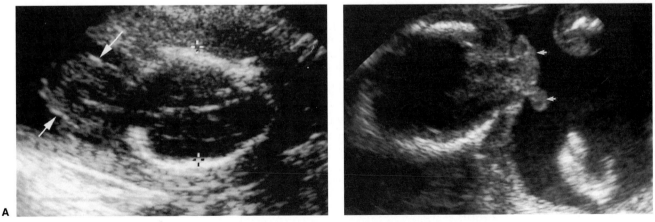

Figure 7.42 *Encephalocele. A.* Occipital encephalocele. Axial image shows a large posterior protrusion of brain tissue (*arrows*) through a defect in the occiput. The biparietal diameter (*between cursors,* +) is smaller than normal for gestational age. *B.* Frontoethmoid encephalocele. Polypoid masses of brain tissue (*arrows*) protrude through a frontoethmoid cranial defect seen on this axial image.

> **Box 7.7: Causes of Ventriculomegaly in the Fetus**
>
> Hydrocephalus (obstruction to flow of cerebrospinal fluid)
>   Neural tube defects (Chiari II malformation)
>   Congenital aqueductal stenosis
>   Dandy-Walker malformation
>
> Anomalous brain development
>   Holoprosencephaly
>   Agenesis of the corpus callosum
>   Idiopathic
>   Chromosome anomaly
> Brain atrophy—brain tissue destruction
>   Congenital infection
>   Brain infarction (porencephaly)

- Meningoencephaloceles involve herniation of brain tissue, CSF, and meninges. The mass has cystic and solid elements.
- Meningocele is less common (10%) and describes herniation of meninges and CSF without brain tissue. The herniated mass is purely cystic and is defined by its covering of meninges.
- The cranial defect is characteristically midline and may be occipital (75%), frontoethmoid (13%), or parietal (12%).
- Hydrocephalus and microcephaly are usually present.
- Cephaloceles in atypical location, asymmetric and not in the midline, are often caused by amniotic band syndrome.
- Cephaloceles are found in a variety of multiple anomaly syndromes including Meckel-Gruber syndrome.

Ventriculomegaly

Ventriculomegaly is a generic term used to describe abnormal dilatation of the cerebral ventricles. Ventriculomegaly has many causes.

The term *ventriculomegaly* refers to abnormal enlargement of the ventricles. The term *hydrocephalus* should be reserved for cases of ventriculomegaly that are caused by obstruction to the flow of CSF. Non-obstructive causes of ventriculomegaly include brain maldevelopment and diffuse brain atrophy (Box 7.7).

- The lateral ventricles are considered to be enlarged when the width of the ventricular atrium exceeds 10 mm on the standard transventricular plane image (Fig. 7.43A) [86]. Ventriculomegaly is differentiated from hydranencephaly and holoprosencephaly by the presence of the falx and a distinct rim of peripheral cortex (Fig. 7.43B).
- Separation of the choroid plexus from the medial wall of the lateral ventricle ≥3 mm is another widely accepted sign of ventriculomegaly (Fig. 7.43A) [87]. This measurement is also made on the transventricular plane image.
- A choroid angle of >29 degrees is indicative of ventriculomegaly. The choroid angle is measured between the midline and the long axis of the choroid plexus on the transventricular view. The normal choroid angle is between 16 degrees and 22 degrees.
- Aqueduct stenosis is a common cause of hydrocephalus with enlargement of the lateral and third ventricles. Aqueduct stenosis may be inherited (X-linked recessive) or caused by tumor, infection, or hemorrhage. Many cases are not evident until late second or third trimester.
- Ventriculomegaly is commonly associated with additional anomalies. The diagnosis of ventriculomegaly is an indication for careful and detailed fetal survey.

Chiari II Malformation

Chiari II malformation accompanies nearly all cases of lumbosacral myelomeningocele. The posterior fossa is small and the cerebellum is squeezed upward against the tentorium, downward through the foramen magnum, and anteriorly around the brainstem.

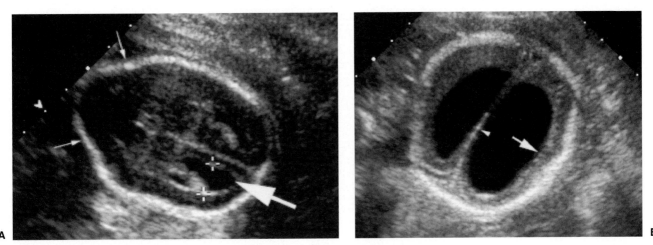

Figure 7.43 *Ventriculomegaly. A.* Axial view of an 18-week fetal head shows dilatation of the ventricular atrium (*between cursors,* +) to 11 mm. Separation (*large arrow*) of the choroid plexus from the medial wall of the ventricle exceeds 4 mm. Flattening of the frontal bones (*small arrows*) creates a lemon-shaped head. This is an example of hydrocephalus associated with Chiari II defect. A myelomeningocele was also present. *B.* Another fetus has more severe ventriculomegaly caused by idiopathic aqueductal stenosis. Note the presence of a thinned rim of peripheral cortex (*arrow*) and the falx (*arrowhead*). These findings differentiate severe hydrocephalus from hydranencephaly and holoprosencephaly.

- The lemon sign is seen as a concave deformity of the frontal bones that results in a lemon-shaped outline of the fetal head on axial section (Figs. 7.43A, 7.44A). The lemon sign usually disappears by 34 weeks gestation.
- The banana sign describes the appearance of the cerebellar hemispheres as they are compressed downward toward the foramen magnum and anteriorly around the brainstem (Fig. 7.44A). Sonographically recognizing obliteration of the cisterna magna is far more important than identifying the banana. Compression of the posterior fossa with absence of fluid in the cisterna magna is a highly specific finding of Chiari II malformation.
- Hydrocephaly is seen in 80–90% of cases of Chiari II (Fig. 7.43A). The degree of ventricular dilatation is mild in the second trimester and increases in the third trimester.
- The corpus callosum is partially or completely absent.

Holoprosencephaly
Holoprosencephaly is a spectrum of disorders resulting from failure of cleavage of the forebrain during early development.

- Alobar holoprosencephaly is the most severe and presents with a large central monoventricle, small brain, fused thalami, and absence of the corpus callosum, cavum septum pellucidum, and falx (Fig. 7.45A).
- Semilobar holoprosencephaly has partial fusion of the hemispheres and formation of a portion of the posterior interhemispheric fissure and falx.
- Lobar holoprosencephaly has partial absence of the anterior interhemispheric fissure and absent cavum septum pellucidum.
- Facial anomalies are commonly associated with alobar and semilobar holoprosencephaly. Abnormalities include midline clefts, cyclopia, cebocephaly, and proboscis (Fig. 7.45B) [88].

Hydranencephaly
Hydranencephaly is believed to result from total cerebral infarction *in utero* caused by bilateral thrombosis of the internal carotid arteries.

- Cerebral hemispheres are completely absent (Fig. 7.46).
- The cranium, falx, skin, meninges, midbrain, and brainstem are present.

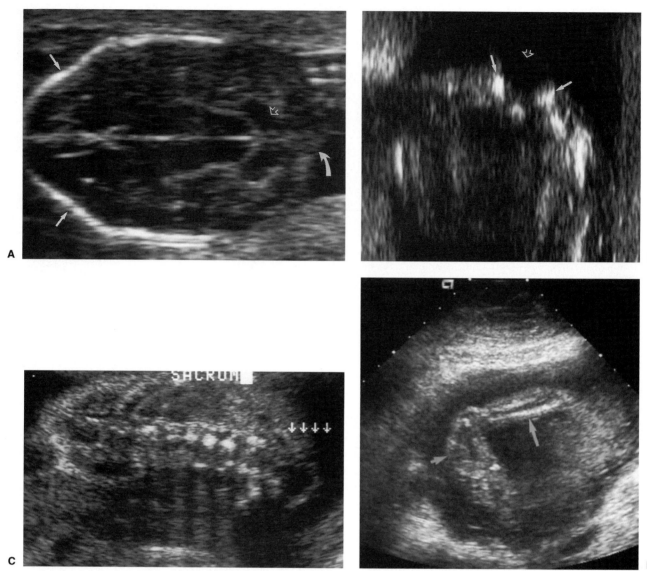

Figure 7.44 *Spina Bifida Defect. A.* Axial transthalamic plane image of the fetal head demonstrates the frontal concavities (*closed arrows*) that cause the lemon sign, and the compression of the cerebral hemispheres that produce the banana sign (*open arrow*). Absence of a visible cisterna magna (*curved arrow*) is indicative of Chiari II defect. *B.* Transverse image of the lumbar spine shows an open spina bifida defect. Note the divergence of the posterior ossification centers (*closed arrows*) and the absence of skin over the defect (*open arrow*). *C.* Longitudinal image of the spine in another fetus shows a myelomeningocele (*arrows*). *D.* Clubfoot deformity is commonly present, reflecting the neurologic deficit caused by the spine defect. A clubfoot deformity is diagnosed by US when the long axis of the foot (*short arrow*) is visible in the same coronal plane that shows the tibia and fibula (*long arrow*).

■ No facial anomalies are associated with hydranencephaly.

Dandy-Walker Malformation

In distinction to the Chiari II malformation, Dandy-Walker syndrome is characterized by a large posterior fossa. Dandy-Walker malformation is a midline posterior fossa cyst associated with absence of the vermis. Dandy-Walker variants are similar but less severe anomalies.

■ The posterior fossa is expanded by cystic dilatation of the fourth ventricle, which exerts mass effect on adjacent structures (Fig. 7.47).

■ The cerebellar hemispheres are hypoplastic and the vermis is hypoplastic or absent.

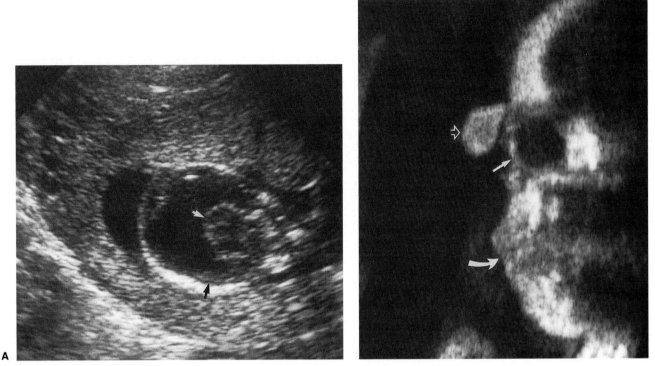

Figure 7.45 *Alobar Holoprosencephaly.* A. Coronal image through the fetal brain shows a large intracranial fluid space representing a monoventricle. The fused thalami (*white arrow*) protrude upward into the fused ventricle. Note the presence of a thin rim of cortex (*black arrow*) peripherally that aids in the differentiation of holoprosencephaly from hydranencephaly. B. Midline sagittal image of the face of another fetus with alobar holoprosencephaly shows absence of the nose, a midline fused eye (*straight arrow*) representing cyclopia, and a proboscis (*open arrow*) protruding from above the fused eye. The curved arrow indicates the mouth. Severe facial anomalies are common with holoprosencephaly.

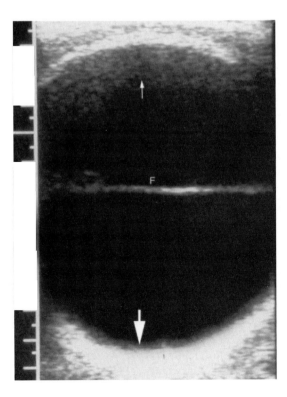

Figure 7.46 *Hydranencephaly.* Axial image of the fetal head shows fluid replacing all visible brain tissue. No rim of cerebral cortex is present (*large arrow*). This finding is best evaluated adjacent to the far cranium because reverberation artifact (*small arrow*) obscures visualization deep to the near cranium. The falx (F) is clearly present.

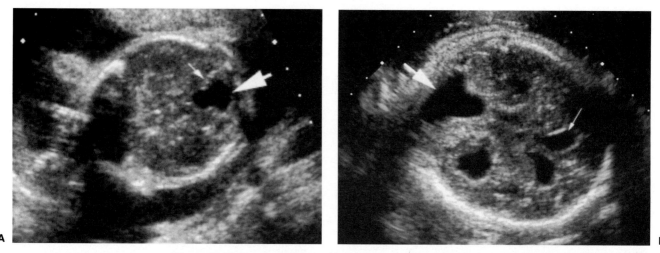

Figure 7.47 *Dandy-Walker Malformation.* A. A large cystic cavity (*large arrow*) fills the posterior fossa. The tentorium is seen as a thin echogenic line (*small arrow*). B. In another fetus, the posterior fossa (*large arrow*) is characteristically expanded by a fluid-filled cavity. Hydrocephaly (*small arrow*) is also present.

- The size of the posterior fossa is usually normal.
- Hydrocephalus and agenesis of the corpus callosum are commonly present.
- Dandy-Walker variant has a normal-sized posterior fossa, lesser dilatation of the fourth ventricle, and lesser degree of cerebellar hypoplasia with no mass effect on adjacent structures.
- Arachnoid cysts are benign developmental cysts of the arachnoid membrane. The cyst does not communicate with the ventricular system. The vermis and remainder of the cerebellum are normally developed but may be compressed.
- Mega cisterna magna has a large (>11 mm) cisterna magna with normal size of the posterior fossa and cerebellum. No mass effect is present.

Vein of Galen Aneurysm

The primary defect is an arteriovenous malformation (AVM) in cerebral tissue. Marked increased blood flow from the AVM causes striking dilatation of the midline vein of Galen that is the major draining vein of both cerebral hemispheres.

- The dilated vein of Galen produces a cystic mass just above the tentorium and just posterior to the corpus callosum.
- Doppler shows turbulent blood flow within the cyst.
- The AVM is occasionally identified as a region of abnormal vascularity in the cerebral hemispheres.

Choroid Plexus Cysts

Choroid plexus cysts are associated with chromosome abnormalities including trisomy 18, trisomy 21, Turner's syndrome (XO), and Klinefelter's syndrome (XXY). Discovery of a choroid plexus cyst is an indication for detailed examination of the fetus to look for additional abnormalities. In the absence of additional findings, trisomy 18 is very unlikely. Genetic counseling and amniocentesis are often offered.

- Choroid plexus cysts appear as round or oval anechoic cystic masses within the echogenic choroid plexus (Fig. 7.48). Most are <10 mm in size. They may be single or multiple, bilateral or unilateral, multiseptated or unilocular. Nearly all disappear before birth regardless of whether they are found in a normal or abnormal fetus.

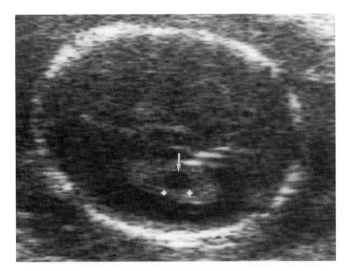

Figure 7.48 *Choroid Plexus Cyst.* Transventricular image shows a 9-mm (*between cursors,* +) cyst (*arrow*) in the echogenic choroid plexus.

SPINE

Spina Bifida

Spina bifida refers to failure of normal fusion of the posterior vertebral elements to complete the bony ring of the spinal canal. Defects may occur at any level but are most common in the lumbosacral region. The defect may involve one or several consecutive vertebrae [74].

- **Open spina bifida** defects refer to defects that are either uncovered or are covered by a very thin translucent membrane (Fig. 7.44B).
- **Closed spina bifida** defects are covered by either skin or a thick opaque membrane.
- **Spina bifida occulta** is a minor internal defect of spine closure seen in 2–3% of the population and not detected prenatally. This condition is nearly always asymptomatic.
- The posterior ossification centers are divergent and often abnormally widely separated (Fig. 7.44).
- The skin is absent over open spina bifida defects.
- A myelomeningocele sac protrudes through the bone and skin defect. A thin membrane defines the sac.
- A myelomeningocele contains both neural elements and CSF.
- A meningocele contains only CSF.
- Chiari II malformations are found in association with nearly all (99%) cases of myelomeningocele.
- Clubfoot deformities and absence of leg movements are commonly associated with large lumbosacral defects (Fig. 7.44D).
- Parallel posterior ossification centers are commonly seen early in the second trimester caused by incomplete ossification. The soft tissues overlying the spine should be carefully inspected for a mass or skin defect. If no defect or mass is present and the cisterna magna is normal, no spina bifida defect is present.

FACE AND NECK

Facial Clefts

Facial clefts are the most common anomaly of the fetal face [72]. Many cases are inherited and up to 30% are associated with chromosome anomalies. Many centers offer amniocentesis [73].

- Lateral facial clefts include isolated cleft lip (25%), isolated cleft palate (25%), and combined cleft lip and cleft palate (50%). The condition may be bilateral (20%).

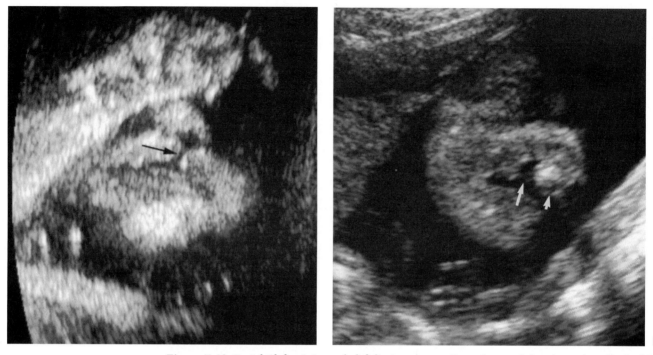

Figure 7.49 *Facial Clefts. A.* Lateral cleft lip is seen as a linear lucent defect (*arrow*) in the fetal lip extending into the left nares. The arm overlies part of the face on this coronal image. *B.* This infant has bilateral cleft lip (*larger arrow*) and palate that has resulted in premaxillary mass (*smaller arrow*) of soft tissue beneath the nose and between the clefts.

- Cleft lip appears as a linear defect extending from either naris through the lip, just lateral of midline (Fig. 7.49). Nearly all of these defects are detected if coronal views of the lips and nose are obtained.
- Cleft palate is much more difficult to detect. Cleft palate without cleft lip is almost never detected prenatally. The major finding is a linear defect through the maxilla with abnormal separation of the tooth buds.
- Median facial clefts are rare and are usually associated with holoprosencephaly. Central facial development is markedly abnormal.
- Amniotic band syndrome causes irregular facial clefting. An amniotic band may be visualized extending through the lip and into the mouth.

Cystic Hygroma

Cystic hygroma results from abnormal connections of the lymphatic system [72]. Most cases are associated with chromosome abnormalities, most commonly Turner's syndrome (XO) and Down's syndrome (trisomy 21). Amniocentesis is indicated [73].

- A complex cystic mass symmetrically surrounds the posterior neck and may extend over the head and upper thorax.
- A midline septum representing the nuchal ligament is always present and helps to differentiate cystic hygroma from occipital meningocele. Additional randomly placed septations are common (Fig. 7.50).
- Fetal hydrops and diffuse cystic lymphangiectasis are commonly present and are usually associated with fetal demise *in utero*.
- Cystic hygromas will commonly be observed to involute with advancing gestation. The residual skin thickening is responsible for the web neck characteristic of Turner's syndrome.

CHEST

Displacement of the fetal heart is a primary US sign of an intrathoracic mass (Boxes 7.8, 7.9) [89].

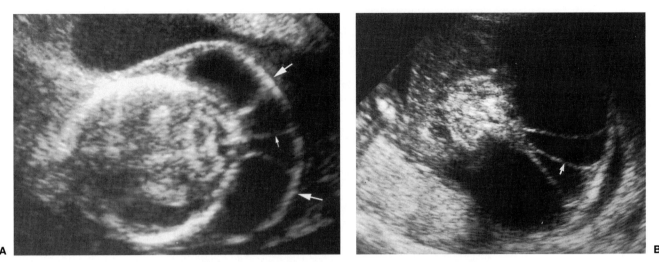

Figure 7.50 *Cystic Hygroma. A.* A cystic mass (*large arrows*) surrounds the posterior neck and occiput. Several septations are evident, one of which (*small arrow*) is the characteristic midline septum that represents the nuchal ligament. *B.* In another fetus, a larger cystic hygroma also has the midline nuchal ligament (*arrow*) and additional septa.

Pleural Effusion

Most pleural effusions in the fetus are associated with hydrops, are bilateral, and consist of serous fluid. Isolated unilateral pleural effusions are most likely chylothorax associated with malformations of the thoracic duct. These are found as isolated abnormalities, or in association with chromosome anomalies, especially trisomy 21 and Turner's syndrome (XO).

- Pleural effusions appear as well-defined anechoic fluid surrounding sharply marginated, triangular-shaped, echogenic lung (Fig. 7.51).
- Isolated unilateral pleural effusions occur most commonly on the right side and usually are chylothorax.

Congenital Diaphragmatic Hernia

Congenital diaphragmatic hernias occur most often at the posterolateral foramen of Bochdalek (90%), predominantly on the left side (85–90%). The remainder are herniations through the anteromedial foramen of Morgagni. Approximately 50% of affected fetuses have chromosome abnormalities or additional structural defects [90].

- Hernias appear as a complex cystic mass of displaced bowel in the chest. Peristalsis in the herniated bowel is often seen (Fig. 7.52).
- The heart is displaced to the right by left-sided hernias.
- No fluid-filled stomach is seen in the abdomen.
- Polyhydramnios is often present.
- The AC is often small for dates. AC below the fifth percentile for GA is associated with large hernias and poor prognosis [91].
- Large hernias compress the ipsilateral lung directly and compress the opposite lung by displacement of the mediastinum. This commonly results in severe pulmonary hypoplasia.

Box 7.8: Causes of Cystic Mass in the Fetal Chest

Diaphragmatic hernia
Cystic adenomatoid malformation, types I and II
Pleural effusion
Pericardial effusion

Duplication cyst
Cystic teratoma
Pericardial cyst

> ## Box 7.9: Causes of Echogenic Mass in the Fetal Chest
>
> Diaphragmatic hernia
> Cystic adenomatoid malformation, type III
> Bronchopulmonary sequestration
>
> Bronchial atresia
> Mediastinal teratoma
> Chest wall hamartoma

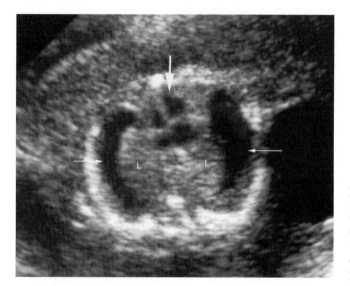

Figure 7.51 *Pleural Effusions.* Bilateral pleural effusions (*small arrows*) are seen as crescentic-shaped fluid spaces compressing the lungs (L). The heart (*large arrow*) is also seen on this axial plane image.

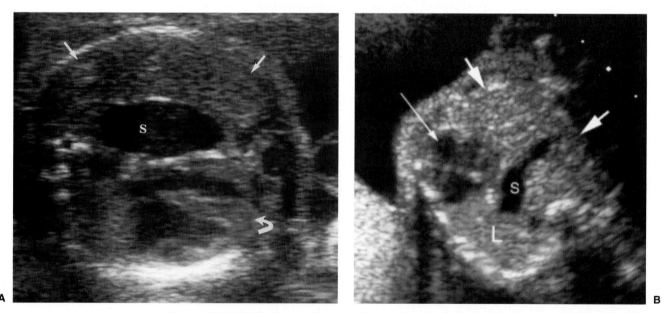

Figure 7.52 *Diaphragmatic Hernia. A.* Transverse image through the chest shows the stomach (S) and a large volume of small bowel (*straight arrows*) occupying the left chest and displacing the heart (*curved arrow*) into the right thorax. No lung is visible, indicating that severe pulmonary hypoplasia is very likely. *B.* In another fetus, a moderate volume of lung (L) is visible in the right thorax even though the heart (*long arrow*) is displaced rightward by the herniation of bowel (*short arrows*) and stomach (S) into the left thorax.

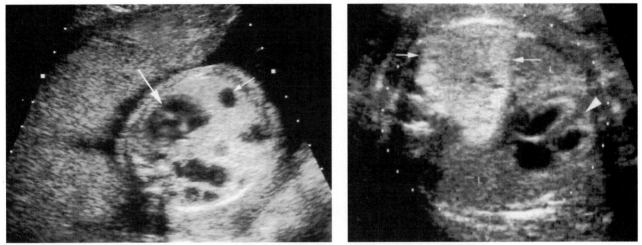

Figure 7.53 *Cystic Adenomatoid Malformation. A.* Type I. Markedly echogenic bilateral cystic adenomatoid malformations replace all visible lung. The heart (*large arrow*) appears compressed by the lung mass. The presence of several large cysts (*small arrow*) indicates a type I malformation. *B.* Type III. The left lower lobe (*small arrows*) is replaced by markedly echogenic cystic adenomatoid malformation. Normal appearing lung (L) is present bilaterally. The heart (*arrowhead*) is seen anteriorly.

Cystic Adenomatoid Malformation

Cystic adenomatoid malformation (CAM) is a hamartoma of the lung. Three pathologic types are described. CAM usually involves only one lobe or a portion of one lobe [92].

- CAM type I consists of one or more large cysts, 2–10 cm in diameter, surrounded by numerous smaller cysts (Fig. 7.53A).
- CAM type II consists of multiple small cysts (<2 cm) of uniform size.
- CAM type III consists of innumerable tiny cysts (<5 mm size) that produce the appearance of a solid echogenic mass (Fig. 7.53B).
- CAM may shrink or disappear *in utero*. However, CT of the neonatal lung will usually reveal a residual pulmonary abnormality.
- Pulmonary hypoplasia is a risk when the CAM is large.
- Hydrops and polyhydramnios may be present.

Pulmonary Sequestration

Pulmonary sequestration is a lung mass separate from the normal bronchial system and supplied by a systemic artery.

- Identification of the systemic artery supply is diagnostic of pulmonary sequestration. Doppler is used to identify the systemic artery that usually arises from the thoracic or upper abdominal aorta.
- Intralobar sequestrations (75%) share the visceral pleura with the normal lung and drain via pulmonary veins into the left atrium [93].
- Extralobar sequestrations (25%) are separated from normal lung by a separate covering of visceral pleura and drain via systemic veins into the azygous or hemiazygous system to the right atrium [94]. Although less common overall, extralobar sequestrations are more likely to present *in utero*.
- Approximately 5% of pulmonary sequestrations are below the diaphragm.
- Sequestrations appear as homogeneous well-defined, usually solid, echogenic masses in the posterior basal thorax, most commonly on the left. Occasionally cystic areas are seen within the mass. The mass is usually triangular in shape.
- Polyhydramnios and hydrops may occur.
- Additional developmental defects occur in 15–60% of fetuses with extralobar sequestrations. Foci of CAM type II are found in 15–25% of extralobar sequestrations [92].

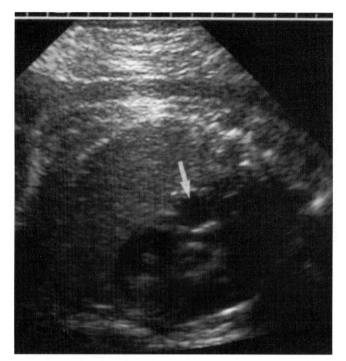

Figure 7.54 *Bronchogenic Cyst.* Transverse scan of the chest shows a well-defined unilocular cystic mass (*arrow*) in the mediastinum. This is a characteristic appearance and location for a bronchogenic cyst.

Foregut Duplication Cysts

Foregut malformations cause cystic masses in the thorax.

- Bronchogenic cysts are unilocular cysts found in the anterior mediastinum or in the lung parenchyma (Fig. 7.54) [95]. They are isolated defects usually not associated with other congenital anomalies. Cysts are sharply marginated and unilocular or multilocular. Echogenic debris may layer within the fluid.
- Enteric cysts in the thorax are duplications of the esophagus and appear as unilocular cysts in the posterior mediastinum.
- Neurenteric cysts are attached to the spine and are associated with spinal dysraphism, absent vertebrae, hemivertebrae, and meningomyelocele.

Pulmonary Hypoplasia

Pulmonary hypoplasia is an absolute decrease in lung volume or lung weight for GA. Any process that interferes with distension of the lung with lung fluid or fetal respiratory movements may result in pulmonary hypoplasia. Etiologic factors include severe or prolonged oligohydramnios (bilateral renal disease), chest mass or fluid that compresses the lung, skeletal dysplasia with small thorax, neurological conditions resulting in decreased breathing movements, and chromosomal abnormalities.

- Determination of lung volume and development is difficult to assess directly.
- Small thoracic circumference (TC) is associated with pulmonary hypoplasia. TC is measured on the axial plane of the chest that shows the 4-chambered heart. Measurements of TC below the fifth percentile for GA predict pulmonary hypoplasia [96].
- The ratio of TC/AC normally exceeds 0.80 beyond 20 weeks GA. Smaller ratios suggest pulmonary hypoplasia [97].
- Shift in cardiac position in the absence of an intrathoracic mass is evidence of unilateral lung hypoplasia (Fig. 7.52) [98].

HEART

The fetal heart is probably the most challenging organ to evaluate with US. Cardiac anomalies are common but quite diverse and complicated. Emphasis should be placed on screen-

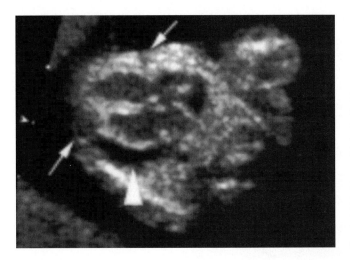

Figure 7.55 *Ectopia Cordis and Cardiomegaly.* Four-chamber view of the chest shows a disproportionately large heart, part of which protrudes out of the chest (*arrows*). A pericardial effusion is also evident (*arrowhead*). This infant had complex congenital heart disease in addition to multiple anomalies caused by trisomy 18.

ing for cardiac anomalies with precise diagnosis often left to tertiary centers with highly experienced pediatric cardiologists. A dedicated fetal cardiac examination can easily take as long to perform as a complete fetal survey. Because the examinations may be long and tedious for the parents, as well as the examining physician, each study should be scheduled on a different day.

Abnormal 4-Chamber View
Approximately 63% of cardiac defects can be detected on the 4-chamber view alone [78].

- When position of the heart is abnormal, consider an extracardiac thoracic mass, unilateral lung hypoplasia, and situs abnormalities (Fig. 7.52).
- When heart size is disproportional to size of the thorax, consider cardiomegaly and skeletal dysplasias (Fig. 7.55).
- When the left ventricle appears small compared to the right ventricle, consider hypoplastic left heart, coarctation of the aorta, and hypoplastic aortic arch [79,99].
- When the right ventricle appears small compared to the left ventricle, consider hypoplastic right heart (pulmonary atresia, tricuspid atresia) or aortic stenosis or insufficiency (large left ventricle) [79,99].
- Abnormal position of the atrioventricular valves is most commonly caused by Ebstein anomaly with downward displacement of the tricuspid valve, a huge right atrium, and a small right ventricle.
- An echogenic focus in the ventricular chamber (Fig. 7.56) is caused by mineralization of the papillary muscle but may be associated with chromosome abnormalities [100,101]. If an echogenic mass is seen within the ventricle consider a rhabdomyoma, which is often associated with tuberous sclerosis (Fig. 7.57) [79].
- If the heart wall is grossly thickened, consider a cardiomyopathy or endocardial fibroelastosis [79].
- A ventricular septal defect appears as an opening in the ventricular septum (Fig. 7.58). The normal, thin, membranous septum near the mitral valve may be mistaken for a septal defect.

Abnormal Views of the Great Vessels
Including images of the RVOT and LVOT adds detection of an additional 25% of congenital heart anomalies compared to obtaining only the 4-chamber view [102].

- When the pulmonary artery is small compared to the aorta, consider tetralogy of Fallot and hypoplastic right heart [76,103].
- When the aorta is small compared to the pulmonary artery, consider hypoplastic left heart or coarctation of the aorta [76,103].

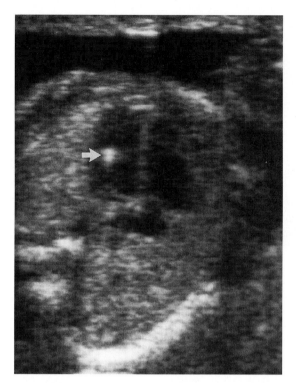

Figure 7.56 *Echogenic Focus in Left Ventricle.* A focus of high echogenicity (*arrow*) corresponds to the location of the papillary muscles in the left ventricle. This finding is not indicative of a congenital heart defect but may be associated with chromosome anomalies.

- When the position of the great vessels appears abnormal, consider transposition of the great vessels and double outlet right ventricle [76,103].
- When only a single, large great vessel is seen, consider truncus arteriosus and tetralogy of Fallot (Fig. 7.59) [76,103].

Pericardial Effusion

Pericardial effusions are seen with hydrops and with cardiac structural anomalies. Isolated pericardial effusions 2–7 mm in thickness are not associated with adverse outcomes [104].

- Pericardial fluid is seen between the thin rim of echogenic pericardium and the thin rim of hypoechoic myocardium (Fig. 7.60). M-mode is useful to confirm the presence of pericardial effusion. Normal pericardial fluid is <2 mm in thickness at its point of maximum width. Pericardial fluid >2 mm is considered a pericardial effusion [104].

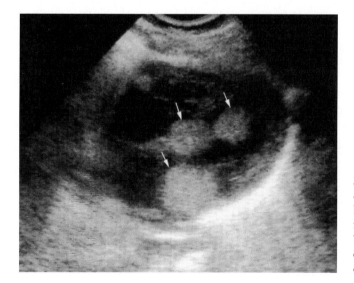

Figure 7.57 *Cardiac Rhabdomyomas.* Axial view of the heart reveals multiple echogenic masses (*arrows*) in the heart. These were proven to be rhabdomyomas in a fetus with tuberous sclerosis.

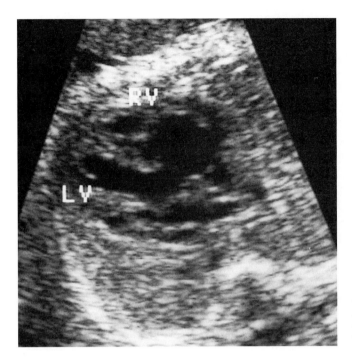

Figure 7.58 *Ventricular Septal Defect.* A large defect is evident in the ventricular septum. LV, left ventricle; RV, right ventricle.

Cardiac Arrhythmias

Arrhythmias are defined as heart rates that are irregular, or too fast, or too slow. Fetuses with arrhythmias deserve complete echocardiography to detect morphological abnormalities. M-mode US is used to determine the atrial and ventricular rates separately [105]. The M-mode cursor must be placed to demonstrate atrial and ventricular motion simultaneously. Ventricular rates are commonly slower than atrial rates because some degree of atrioventricular block is usually present.

■ Irregular rhythms are usually caused by premature atrial or ventricular contractions. Isolated premature ventricular contractions are the most common fetal arrhythmia [105]. Diagnosis is confirmed by an M-mode tracing that shows an early beat followed by a prolonged compensatory pause. Isolated premature contractions are usually innocent. Frequent premature contraction may be induced by maternal smoking, or caffeine or alcohol use. These activities should be discontinued and the fetus rechecked. Premature contractions resulting in tachycardia are treated with digoxin.

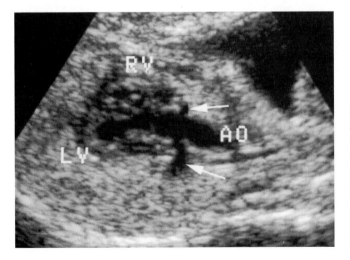

Figure 7.59 *Truncus Arteriosus Anomaly.* Only one great vessel (the truncus arteriosus) was shown to arise from the heart primarily from the left ventricle (LV). This solitary vessel continued as the aorta (AO). Both pulmonary arteries (*arrows*) arose from the truncus arteriosus. RV, right ventricle.

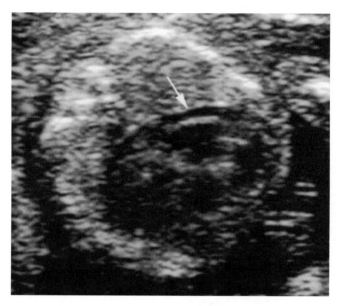

Figure 7.60 *Pericardial Effusion.* A 4-chamber view of the heart shows a small anechoic pericardial effusion (*arrow*). The shape and width of the pericardial effusion change with cardiac motion viewed with real-time imaging.

- Tachycardia is usually defined as fetal heart rate >180 bpm [105]. Causes include supraventricular tachycardia, atrial fibrillation, and atrial flutter. Tachycardia may lead to congestive heart failure, hydrops, and fetal death. Digoxin, administered intravenously through the maternal circulation, is the usual treatment of choice.
- Bradycardia is defined as fetal heart rate <100 bpm [105]. Transient bradycardia is common and is usually caused by vasovagal reaction, sometimes induced by excessive transducer pressure. Scanning should be temporarily stopped. Heart rate usually returns to normal in 15–30 seconds. Complete heart block is the most common cause of sustained bradycardia. Atrial rates are usually 120–140 bpm, while ventricular rates are 40–60 bpm. Sustained bradycardia may result in hydrops. Prognosis is poor if cardiac malformations are also present.

ABDOMINAL WALL

Gastroschisis

Gastroschisis results from a defect in the anterior abdominal wall on the right side of the umbilicus [106]. Bowel and abdominal contents herniate through the defects to float freely in the amniotic cavity [107]. Gastroschisis is nearly always surgically repairable in the postnatal period. Prognosis depends upon presence and severity of other anomalies [108].

- Free-floating bowel loops are seen outside of the abdominal cavity (Fig. 7.61).
- No covering membrane is present.
- The cord insertion is normal. The cord is most easily identified and the insertion site visualized by use of color flow US (Fig. 7.61C). Herniation occurs to the right of the cord insertion site.
- Large defects may contain liver, urinary bladder, uterus, and adnexa.
- Gastroschisis is usually (75%) an isolated defect without associated chromosome abnormality or risk of recurrence. Amniocentesis is usually not indicated.
- Approximately 25% of affected fetuses have other anomalies including cardiac defects, cleft palate, scoliosis, or diaphragmatic hernia.
- Complications include non-rotated bowel (always present), ischemia caused by rotation and kinking of the mesenteric vessels, perforation, obstruction, and bowel atresia.
- US demonstration of bowel wall thickening or intestinal dilatation is not a useful predictor of the presence of complications [109].

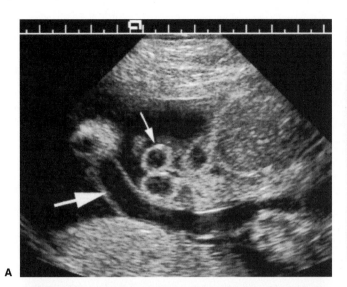

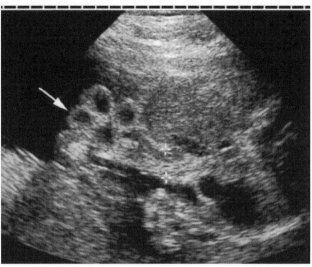

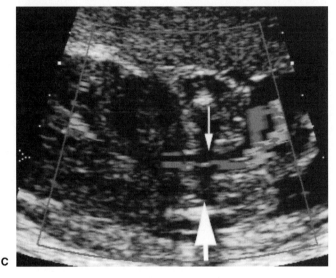

Figure 7.61 *Gastroschisis. A.* Bowel loops (*small arrow*) float freely in amniotic fluid. No covering membrane is present. These are diagnostic findings of gastroschisis. The umbilical vein (*large arrow*) in the cord courses adjacent to the protruding bowel loops. *B.* The abdominal wall defect (*between cursors,* +) is shown on this transverse image. Bowel loops (*arrow*) extend from the abdomen to the amniotic cavity through this defect. *C.* Color Doppler, shown here as a gray scale image, shows a normal insertion (*small arrow*) of the umbilical cord on the abdominal wall. The gastroschisis defect (*large arrow*) is adjacent to the cord insertion site on the right side.

Omphalocele

Omphalocele is a midline defect in the anterior abdominal wall through which abdominal contents herniate into the base of the umbilical cord [106–108].

- US shows a midline mass protruding through the abdominal wall (Fig. 7.62). The mass commonly contains liver, stomach, and bowel.
- A covering membrane produces a smooth, well-defined surface to the mass.
- The umbilical cord inserts into, rather than next to, the mass (Fig. 7.62B, C).
- Ascites is common and helps to define the covering membrane.
- Polyhydramnios is present in one-third of cases.
- Most cases (67–88%) have associated anomalies including cardiac, central nervous system, urinary tract, and gastrointestinal malformations.
- Chromosome anomalies, most commonly trisomy 13 or 18, are found in 30–45% of cases. Amniocentesis is usually performed.
- **Pentalogy of Cantrell** is the association of an ectopic heart (ectopia cordis) with omphalocele. The anterior wall defect includes the thorax as well as the abdomen. The fetal heart is seen outside of the thoracic cavity (Fig. 7.55) [110].

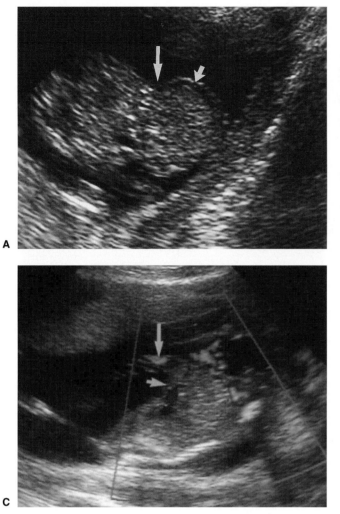

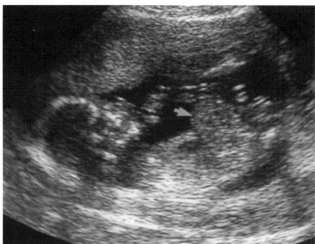

Figure 7.62 *Omphalocele. A.* An omphalocele is seen as a rounded mass protruding from the anterior abdominal wall. A covering membrane (*short arrow*) is clearly visible. Note the characteristic obtuse angle (*long arrow*) that the omphalocele forms with the abdominal wall. This omphalocele contains liver and bowel. *B.* In a 14-week fetus, an omphalocele forms a 20-mm mass (*arrow*) protruding from the anterior abdominal wall. *C.* Color Doppler image (shown in gray scale) of the same fetus as in *B* shows the umbilical cord (*long arrow*) inserting into the mass (*short arrow*) confirming an omphalocele.

Amniotic Band Syndrome

Disruption of the amnion allows the fetus to enter the chorionic cavity where fibrous bands form and entangle the fetus. Entrapment of fetal parts results in amputation deformities that range from partial finger amputations to being incompatible with life [50].

- Amniotic bands trapping the fetus are commonly visualized.
- Extension of bands across the abdomen results in gastroschisis and truncal defects.
- Bands across the cranium may result in anencephaly, encephaloceles, and facial clefts.
- Spine deformities, marked scoliosis, and extremity amputations are common.

ABDOMEN—GASTROINTESTINAL

Esophageal Atresia

Almost two-thirds of cases of esophageal atresia are associated with additional anomalies including chromosome anomalies (20%) [111].

- Association of polyhydramnios with non-visualization of a fluid-filled stomach is strong but not perfect evidence of esophageal atresia (Fig. 7.21B).
- Visualization of a fluid-filled stomach does not exclude esophageal atresia because the stomach may fill with amniotic fluid through a tracheoesophageal fistula.
- Rarely, a blind-ended pouch of proximal esophagus may be visualized [111].

Box 7.10: Causes of Non-Visualization of Fetal Stomach

Transient normal—due to physiologic emptying—reexamine patient
Mechanical obstruction
  Esophageal atresia
  Chest mass
Too little fluid to swallow
  Oligohydramnios

Impaired swallowing
  Central nervous system anomalies
  Neuromuscular disorders
  Cleft lip/palate
  "Sick" fetus
Ectopic stomach
  Congenital diaphragmatic hernia—stomach in chest
  Situs inversus—stomach in right side of abdomen
Chromosome abnormality
  Trisomy 18, trisomy 21

Non-Visualization of Fluid-Filled Stomach

The normal fetal stomach is visualized as a fluid-filled structure in the left upper quadrant of the abdomen in most fetuses by 14–15 weeks GA [112,113].

- Non-visualization of the stomach is indication for follow-up examination. Look for associated abnormalities. Causes are listed in Box 7.10 [114,115].

Duodenal Obstruction—The Double Bubble

The duodenum is not fluid-filled in normal fetuses (Box 7.11) [116]. Approximately one-half of the cases have additional anomalies. Amniocentesis is indicated because of a 30% incidence of Down's syndrome.

- "Double bubble" describes the appearance of a fluid-distended duodenal bulb associated with an overdistended stomach (Fig. 7.63). Careful scanning will usually reveal the pylorus connecting the two structures. This finding confirms a true double bubble and is highly indicative of duodenal obstruction.
- Care must be taken to confirm a true double bubble. Other cystic masses in the upper abdomen include choledochal cyst, renal cyst, bowel duplication, omental or mesenteric cyst, hepatic cyst, and gallbladder.

Echogenic Bowel

Echogenic bowel may be a normal variant or may be associated with significant fetal abnormalities (Box 7.12) [114,115].

- Normal fetal bowel varies from being isoechoic with liver to being moderately echogenic compared to liver.
- Bowel is abnormally echogenic when its echogenicity is equal to or greater than that of bone. Comparison is often made to the echogenicity of the iliac crest (Fig. 7.64).

Box 7.11: Causes of Duodenal Obstruction

Duodenal atresia	Malrotation with Ladd's bands
Duodenal stenosis	Volvulus
Duodenal web	Intestinal obstruction
Annular pancreas	

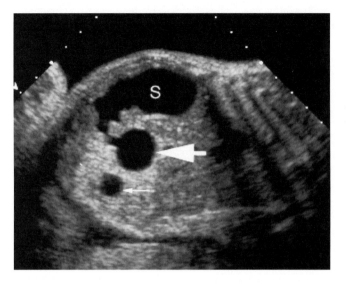

Figure 7.63 *Double Bubble— Duodenal Atresia.* Image of the fetal abdomen shows a distended stomach (S) in contiguity with a dilated duodenal bulb (*large arrow*) making the "double bubble" sign of duodenal obstruction. Care must be taken to not mistake the gallbladder (*small arrow*) for a second "bubble." This fetus had duodenal atresia and Down's syndrome.

- When abnormally echogenic bowel is present, parents are routinely offered genetic counseling and opportunity for amniocentesis.
- High-frequency transducers (8 MHz) increase the apparent echogenicity of bowel compared to lower frequency transducers (5 MHz) [117].

Small Bowel Obstruction

Dilatation of small bowel is indicative of obstruction (Box 7.13).

- Diameter of small bowel >6 mm is considered dilated. Multiple, interconnecting, dilated, small bowel loops indicate small bowel obstruction (Fig. 7.65).
- Small bowel dilatation is generally not seen until after 16–20 weeks because insufficient meconium is present to distend the small bowel.
- Polyhydramnios is commonly present.
- A dilated and tortuous ureter may simulate dilated small bowel loops. Differentiation is made by careful examination of the kidney for hydronephrosis.
- Normal colon is differentiated from dilated small bowel by its normal more peripheral location.

Meconium Ileus

Meconium ileus is small bowel obstruction caused by abnormally thick meconium in the distal ileum. Most cases (90%) are associated with cystic fibrosis. Approximately 10–15% of fetuses with cystic fibrosis present with meconium ileus [118].

Meconium Peritonitis

Perforation of the fetal small bowel *in utero* spills meconium into the peritoneal cavity and incites a chemical peritonitis. Approximately 50% of cases are idiopathic, 15–20% are

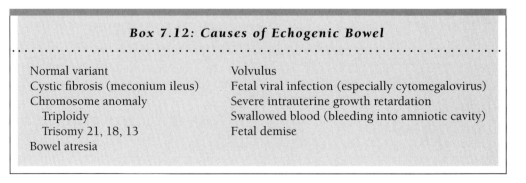

Box 7.12: Causes of Echogenic Bowel

Normal variant
Cystic fibrosis (meconium ileus)
Chromosome anomaly
  Triploidy
  Trisomy 21, 18, 13
Bowel atresia

Volvulus
Fetal viral infection (especially cytomegalovirus)
Severe intrauterine growth retardation
Swallowed blood (bleeding into amniotic cavity)
Fetal demise

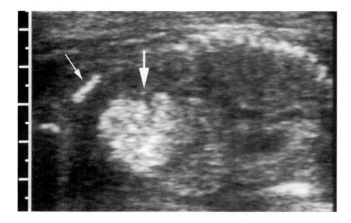

Figure 7.64 *Echogenic Bowel. This bowel (large arrow) is considered to be abnormally echogenic because it is equal in echogenicity to the nearby iliac crest (small arrow).*

caused by small bowel atresia, and 15–40% of cases are associated with cystic fibrosis. Isolated small bowel perforation has a good prognosis [118].

- Calcifications occur on peritoneal surfaces and appear as linear or punctate bright echoes with or without acoustic shadowing (Fig. 7.66).
- Ascites is commonly present (Fig. 7.66).
- Loculations of fluid may form in the peritoneal cavity from the chemical peritonitis. These thick-walled cystic masses are called **meconium pseudocysts** and may have a calcified wall (Fig. 7.66).
- Fetal bowel is commonly dilated.

Large Bowel Obstruction

- Normal colon can be seen as a prominent structure in the periphery of the abdomen as early as 22 weeks. Normal colon can be especially prominent and have echolucent contents in the third trimester [113].
- Colonic dilatation >23 mm is reliable evidence of colon obstruction (Box 7.14).
- Normal meconium-filled rectum may be mistaken for a presacral mass, especially in the third trimester (Box 7.15) [119].
- Anal atresia results in dilatation of the colon apparent only late in the third trimester. **VATER syndrome** refers to the association of vertebral anomalies, anal atresia, tracheoesophageal fistula, radial dysplasia, and renal dysplasia.
- **Meconium plug syndrome** describes transient colonic obstruction caused by inspissated meconium. Approximately 25% of patients have cystic fibrosis.

Ascites

Ascites is always abnormal in the fetus. Most ascites is associated with hydrops. Additional causes include bowel perforation and urine ascites resulting from rupture of an obstructed bladder [120].

- Ascites appears as anechoic fluid surrounding abdominal organs and distending peritoneal recesses. Fluid outlines the falciform ligament and umbilical vein (Fig. 7.67A).

Box 7.13: Causes of Dilatation of Small Bowel (>6 mm)

Jejunal atresia/stenosis (most common)	Meconium ileus
Ileal atresia	Meconium peritonitis
Colonic atresia (rare, but usually proximal)	Enteric duplication

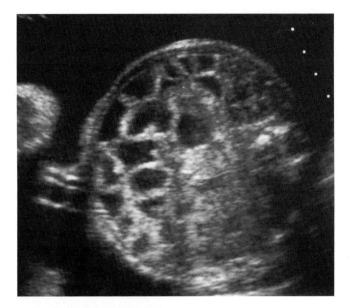

Figure 7.65 *Small Bowel Obstruction.* Transverse image of the fetal abdomen demonstrates multiple dilated loops of small bowel measuring up to 10–11 mm in diameter. This infant had ileal atresia.

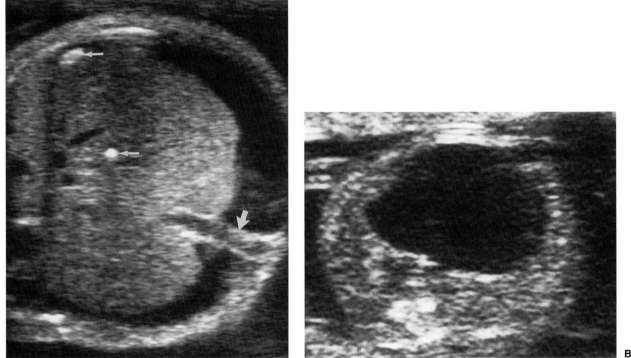

A   B

Figure 7.66 *Meconium Peritonitis.* A. View of the abdomen shows the umbilical vein (*large arrow*) crossing ascites in the peritoneal cavity. Several calcifications (*small arrows*) are present that provide diagnostic evidence of meconium peritonitis. B. Image of another fetus shows a large, cystic, abdominal mass with calcifications in its wall. Calcifications seen elsewhere in the abdominal cavity confirm meconium peritonitis and a diagnosis of meconium pseudocyst.

Box 7.14: Causes of Dilatation of Large Bowel (>23 mm)

Anorectal atresia   Hirschsprung's disease
Meconium plug syndrome

Box 7.15: Causes of Presacral Mass

Normal meconium-filled rectum   Rectal duplication
Sacrococcygeal teratoma   Anorectal atresia
Presacral meningocele

- Fluid may accumulate between the leaves of the unfused greater omentum resulting in a cystic intraperitoneal mass.
- The thin lucent rim of abdominal musculature must not be mistaken for ascites (Fig. 7.67B).

Abdominal Calcifications

Isolated abdominal calcifications without associated abnormality are usually incidental findings associated with a normal fetal outcome (Fig. 7.68) (Box 7.16).

- Calcifications appear as echogenic foci with or without acoustic shadowing.
- Localize the calcifications as being associated with a mass, within an organ, within the bowel lumen, or within the peritoneal cavity (Box 7.16).

Cystic Abdominal Masses

Cystic masses in the fetal abdomen are virtually never malignant (Box 7.17).

- If the cyst touches the spine, renal origin is likely.
- Ovarian cysts may be huge and appear simple, complex, or septated. Simple ovarian cysts result from excessive stimulation of fetal ovaries by maternal and placental hormones. Most disappear spontaneously by 6 months of age.

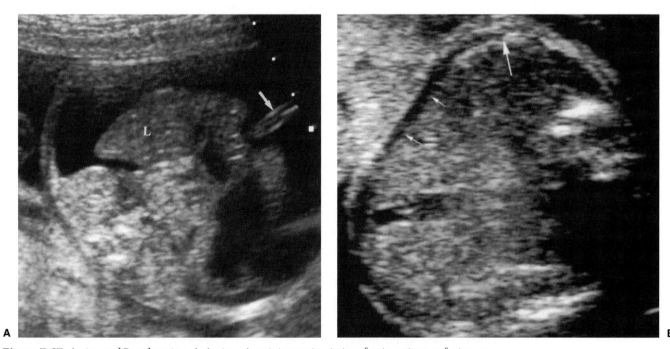

A   **B**

Figure 7.67 *Ascites and Pseudoascites. A. Ascites.* A recipient twin victim of twin-twin transfusion syndrome shows large volume ascites surrounding the liver (L) and outlining the umbilical vein (*arrow*). *B. Pseudoascites.* The abdominal wall muscles (*small arrows*) appear hypoechoic, especially when well seen late in pregnancy. This finding has been mistaken for ascites. Note the thin uniform width of the musculature and the fact that the muscles merge with the ribs (*large arrow*). Use these findings to differentiate musculature from true ascites, which should be seen in numerous peritoneal recesses.

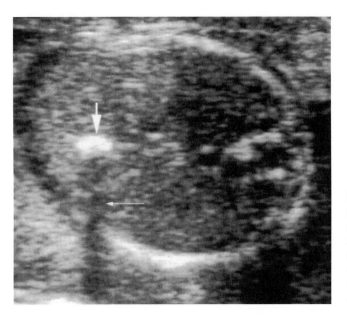

Figure 7.68 Isolated Abdominal Calcification. Image of the abdomen shows a solitary coarse calcification (*large arrow*) with acoustic shadowing (*small arrow*) within the liver. As an isolated finding, this is of no consequence.

- Enteric duplication cysts may occur anywhere in the GI tract. They may appear entirely cystic to solid, commonly have thick walls and contain internal debris [111].
- Mesenteric and omental cysts are solitary, unilocular or multilocular and are generally found as isolated defects.
- Choledochal cysts are found near the porta hepatis. Intrahepatic bile ducts may be dilated [111].
- Meconium pseudocysts have calcification in the walls and usually elsewhere in the abdomen (Fig. 7.66B).

Sacrococcygeal Teratoma

The sacrococcygeal region is the most common location for teratomas in children. Additional anomalies are present in approximately 18% of patients [121]. Tumors may be mature benign (60%), immature benign (18%), or malignant (22%). Differential diagnosis of a sacral region mass is presented in Box 7.18.

- The mass occupies the presacral region and usually extends caudally as an obvious exophytic mass (Fig. 7.69A).
- The most common appearance is a complex mass of approximately equal cystic and solid components. Echogenic areas represent fat. Calcification or ossification is present in 50%.
- Some tumors are predominantly cystic, unilocular, or multilocular, with a small solid nodule often present within the cyst.
- Entirely solid masses are uncommon.
- The tumor may obstruct the urinary tract.
- US does not reliably differentiate benign from malignant teratomas.

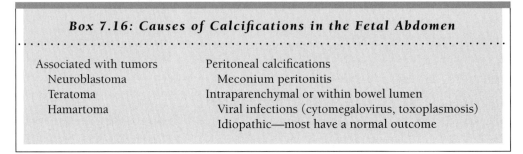

Box 7.16: Causes of Calcifications in the Fetal Abdomen

Associated with tumors
   Neuroblastoma
   Teratoma
   Hamartoma

Peritoneal calcifications
   Meconium peritonitis
Intraparenchymal or within bowel lumen
   Viral infections (cytomegalovirus, toxoplasmosis)
   Idiopathic—most have a normal outcome

Box 7.17: Causes of Cystic Mass in Fetal Abdomen

. . . .

Urinary tract	Ovarian cyst
Renal cyst	Meconium pseudocyst
Hydronephrosis	Omental/mesenteric cyst
Hydroureter	Enteric duplication
Urinoma	Choledochal cyst
Distended bladder	Hepatic cyst
	Hydrometrocolpos

- Polyhydramnios is common. The presence of hydrops caused by arteriovenous shunting within the mass indicates a poor prognosis.
- A normal, fluid-filled rectum may simulate a pelvic teratoma late in pregnancy (Fig. 7.69B).

ABDOMEN—URINARY TRACT

Because nearly all amniotic fluid after 16 weeks GA is fetal urine, evaluation of the urinary tract starts with assessment of amniotic fluid volume as a measure of fetal urine production.

Renal Agenesis

Bilateral renal agenesis (Potter's syndrome) is incompatible with life because of the severe pulmonary hypoplasia that results from the lack of amniotic fluid. Unilateral agenesis is 4–20 times more common than bilateral renal agenesis. It has a good prognosis provided the opposite kidney is normal.

- Severe oligohydramnios is always present with bilateral renal agenesis (Fig. 7.21A).
- The fetal kidneys are not visualized.
- The normally large fetal adrenal gland may "lie down" and mimic the appearance of the missing fetal kidney.
- The bladder is not visualized or is small.
- If one renal fossa is empty, search for an ectopic kidney.

Hydronephrosis

Hydronephrosis is the most common cause of an abdominal mass in a neonate and is readily detected by prenatal US (Box 7.19).

- Significant fetal hydronephrosis is unequivocally present when the anteroposterior (AP) diameter of the renal pelvis is ≥10 mm, or when the ratio of AP diameter of the renal pelvis to AP diameter of the kidney is >0.5 (Fig. 7.70A) [122].
- Calyceal dilatation is a sign of significant hydronephrosis independent of the size of the renal pelvis (7.70B, C).

Box 7.18: Differential Diagnosis of Sacral Region Mass

. . . .

Sacrococcygeal teratoma	Rectal duplication cyst (no solid elements)
Meconium-filled rectum (characteristic tubular shape in third trimester)	Neuroblastoma
	Hemangioma
Sacral meningocele (less septated than teratoma)	Lipoma

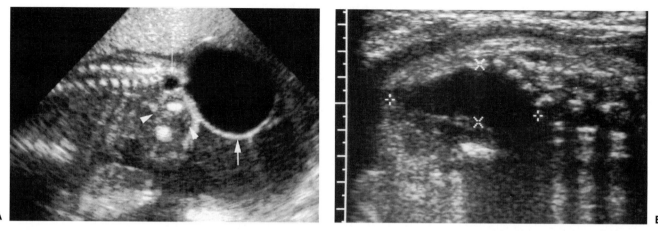

Figure 7.69 *Sacrococcygeal Teratoma.* A. Longitudinal image shows a large cystic mass (*big arrow*) protruding inferiorly from the pelvis. Careful inspection reveals another cystic component of the mass within the sacrum (*small arrow*) and a solid component of the mass filling the pelvis (*arrowheads*). B. A fluid-filled rectum (*between cursors, +, x*) may create a pelvic mass and simulate a sacrococcygeal teratoma. Note the characteristic location anterior to the sacrum and elongated normal shape of the rectum.

- Patients with significant hydronephrosis are usually followed with periodic US *in utero* and undergo postnatal evaluation of the urinary tract with renal US, voiding cystourethrography, and radionuclide renography with diuretic challenge. Postnatal renal US should not be performed until after 48 hours of life to allow for sufficient urine production to dilate the obstructed system.

- Mild pyelectasis in common in normal fetuses. The upper limit of "normal" pyelectasis in a fetus of <20 weeks GA has been defined as 4 mm or 5 mm depending on the publication. This small degree of dilatation is not associated with significant pathology and does not require follow-up [123]. The upper limit of normal pelvis AP diameter is increased to 7 mm after 33 weeks GA [124].

- Dilatation of the renal pelvis between 5 and 10 mm without dilatation of the calyces remains a source of controversy as to proper management. The incidence of significant urinary pathology at birth is low in this group. Some authors recommend aggressive evaluation and others challenge that approach as not being necessary or cost effective [125,126].

- **Ureteropelvic junction obstruction** is the most common cause of fetal hydronephrosis (Fig. 7.70B, C). The renal pelvis and calyces are dilated but the ureter is not. The degree of pelvicalyectasis is dependent upon the degree of obstruction. Polyhydramnios may occur because of increased production of dilute urine by the affected kidney. Oligohydramnios is uncommon unless the opposite kidney is also abnormal. Rarely, obstruction may be severe enough to rupture the collecting system and result in a perinephric urinoma. These severely affected kidneys usually have minimal renal function.

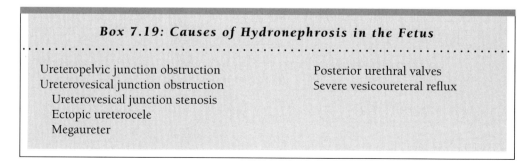

Box 7.19: Causes of Hydronephrosis in the Fetus

Ureteropelvic junction obstruction
Ureterovesical junction obstruction
   Ureterovesical junction stenosis
   Ectopic ureterocele
   Megaureter

Posterior urethral valves
Severe vesicoureteral reflux

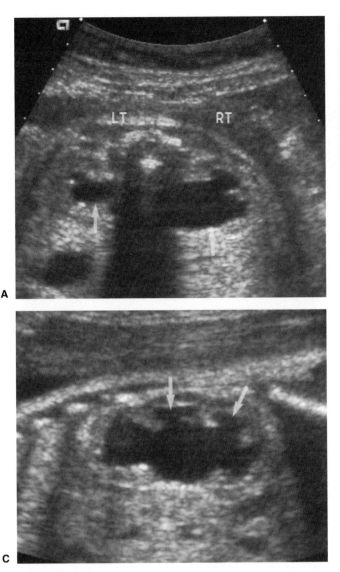

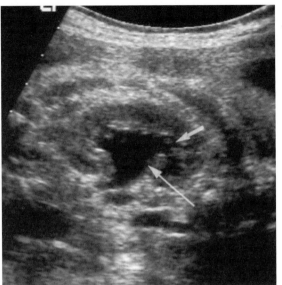

Figure 7.70 *Hydronephrosis. A.* Transverse image shows dilatation of both renal pelvises (*arrows*). The right pelvis (RT) measures 18 mm in anteroposterior diameter, and the left pelvis (LT) measures 8 mm in anteroposterior diameter. *B.* Longitudinal image of the kidney shows pelviectasis (*long arrow*) with mild calyectasis (*short arrow*) caused by mild ureteropelvic junction obstruction. *C.* Longitudinal image of the kidney in another fetus shows a greater degree of hydronephrosis. Note the prominently dilated calyces (*arrows*).

- **Ureterovesical junction (UVJ) obstruction** is the cause of approximately 23% of fetal hydronephrosis.
- **Megaureter** may be caused by distal obstruction (ureterovesical junction), vesicoureteral reflux, or congenital megaureter. These three entities cannot be differentiated by prenatal US. Postnatal testing is required.
- **Complete ureteral duplication** shows characteristic findings. The upper pole ureter is commonly obstructed because of its ectopic insertion inferior and medial to the normal bladder insertion of the lower pole ureter. Severe obstruction may result in dysplasia of the upper pole. Ureteroceles appear as a thin-walled cystic mass in or below the bladder.

Posterior Urethral Valves

A flap-like structure or web blocks the prostatic urethra causing bladder outlet obstruction. This condition is seen only in males. The condition is easily corrected with surgery but irreversible damage may occur *in utero* before the diagnosis is made. Catheter placement to drain the obstructed bladder may be performed *in utero* using US guidance. Females may have similar findings when urethral obstruction is caused by urethral atresia or a cloacal anomaly.

- The bladder is dilated, frequently massively. The wall undergoes smooth muscle hypertrophy and is thickened and trabeculated.

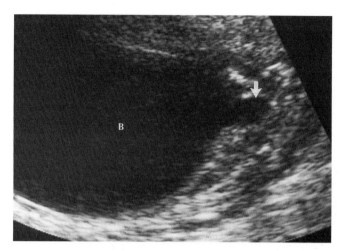

Figure 7.71 *Posterior Urethral Valve.* The fetal bladder (B) is massively distended. The posterior urethra (*arrow*) is dilated to the level of the obstructing valve.

- Ureters are dilated and sometimes thick-walled.
- The kidneys are hydronephrotic and commonly dysplastic with abnormally echogenic parenchyma and cyst formation.
- Oligohydramnios may be profound, depending upon the degree of urethral obstruction.
- Dilatation of the prostatic urethra produces a characteristic "keyhole" appearance to the bladder (Fig. 7.71).

Renal Dysplasia

Renal dysplasia has a spectrum of US appearances from solid renal dysmorphism with a few cysts to total replacement of the kidney with cysts.

Early (before 20 weeks) severe obstruction results in renal dysplasia. Dysplastic kidneys have disorganized parenchymal development and a marked increase in fibrous tissue [127].

- Renal cysts in the setting of renal obstruction indicate renal dysplasia (Fig. 7.72) [128].
- Increased echogenicity of the renal parenchyma indicates dysplasia when the kidney is hydronephrotic.
- Some normal appearing kidneys may be severely dysplastic.

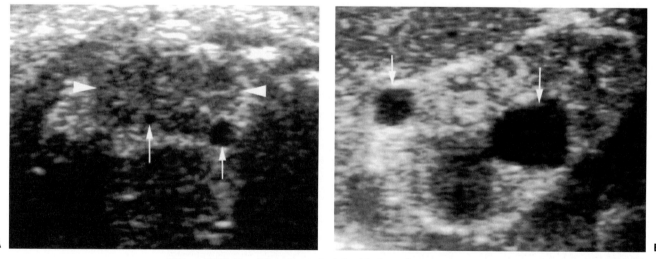

Figure 7.72 *Renal Dysplasia. A.* A fetal kidney (*between arrowheads*) is abnormally small with poor corticomedullary differentiation. Several discrete renal cysts (*arrows*) are evident, providing strong evidence of renal dysplasia. *B.* Similar findings are present in a newborn. The kidney is abnormally echogenic with renal cysts (*arrows*).

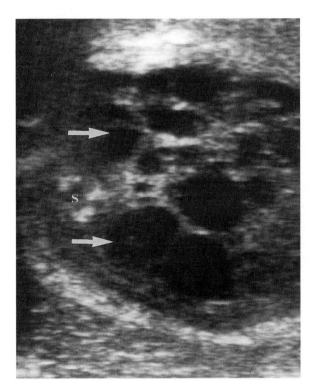

Figure 7.73 *Multicystic Dysplastic Kidney.* Both fetal kidneys (*arrows*) are completely replaced by cysts of varying size. No amniotic fluid was detected. Bilateral multicystic dysplastic kidneys are a fatal condition. Without amniotic fluid, the fetal lungs will not develop properly. S, spine.

Multicystic Dysplastic Kidney

- The kidney is replaced by numerous cysts of varying size that do not communicate (Fig. 7.73).
- Approximately 40% of cases are associated with anomalous development of the opposite kidney. Anomalies include ureteropelvic junction obstruction, agenesis, and bilateral multicystic dysplastic kidney.

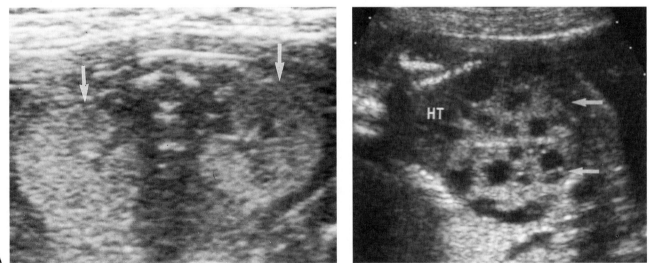

Figure 7.74 *Polycystic Kidney Disease. A.* Bilateral large, diffusely echogenic kidneys (*arrows*) are indicative of autosomal recessive polycystic disease in the fetus. Image is in transverse plane. *B.* Multiple bilateral discrete renal cysts in enlarged kidneys (*arrows*) are indicative of autosomal dominant polycystic disease in the fetus. Image is in coronal plane. HT, heart.

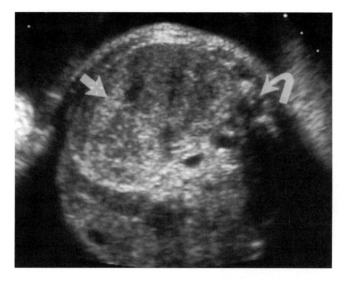

Figure 7.75 *Mesoblastic Nephroma.* Transverse image of the abdomen demonstrates a large solid mass (*straight arrow*) replacing the kidney. Note that the mass touches the spine (*curved arrow*), providing excellent evidence that the mass is renal in origin.

- Bilateral multicystic dysplastic kidneys produce no urine, have severe oligohydramnios, and are always fatal.

Polycystic Kidney Disease

- Autosomal recessive polycystic disease produces large, very echogenic kidneys (Fig. 7.74A). The numerous very tiny cysts are usually too small to see with US. Amniotic fluid is minimal or absent.
- Autosomal dominant polycystic disease may produce large echogenic kidneys with multiple cysts (Fig. 7.74B), but amniotic fluid volume is usually normal.

Solid Renal Mass

Mesoblastic nephroma is the most common solid renal mass seen in the fetus. The tumor is a benign hamartoma.

- A solid heterogeneous infiltrating mass replaces some or the entire affected kidney (Fig. 7.75). When only a portion of the kidney is replaced by tumor, the margin between tumor and normal parenchyma is ill defined.
- Polyhydramnios is usually present.
- Wilms tumor is exceedingly rare in the fetus. The tumor is seen as a solid mass with a discreet capsule separating tumor from normal parenchyma.

SKELETAL SYSTEM

Fetal limb anomalies are associated with skeletal dysplasias, exposure to teratogens, and certain metabolic disorders [129]. More than 200 skeletal dysplasias have been described

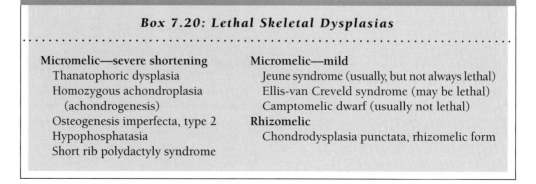

Box 7.20: Lethal Skeletal Dysplasias

Micromelic—severe shortening	Micromelic—mild
Thanatophoric dysplasia	Jeune syndrome (usually, but not always lethal)
Homozygous achondroplasia (achondrogenesis)	Ellis-van Creveld syndrome (may be lethal)
Osteogenesis imperfecta, type 2	Camptomelic dwarf (usually not lethal)
Hypophosphatasia	**Rhizomelic**
Short rib polydactyly syndrome	Chondrodysplasia punctata, rhizomelic form

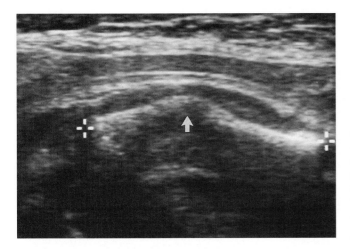

Figure 7.76 *Osteogenesis Imperfecta.* The femur (*between cursors, +*) is abnormally thin and obviously fractured in its mid-portion (*arrow*). Multiple bones were affected in this fetus with a family history of osteogenesis imperfecta.

and differentiating between them is a daunting task. Fortunately, skeletal dysplasias are rare, affecting only 0.03% of births. Unfortunately, approximately half of all skeletal dysplasias are lethal. Keep several features in mind. If a family has a history of skeletal anomalies and a skeletal anomaly is found in the fetus, the anomaly is very likely to be the same one. Extremely short bones (more than 4 standard deviations from the mean for GA) are indicative of a lethal bone dysplasia (Box 7.20) [130,131]. Demonstrating a small fetal thorax is confirmatory of a lethal dysplasia. Precise identification of the lethal syndrome is not necessary for management.

Approach to Skeletal Dysplasias
Spirt and Mahony provide excellent algorithmic approaches to the diagnosis of skeletal dysplasias [130,132].

■ A short femur (below fifth percentile for GA) is a highly sensitive but not specific sign of a skeletal dysplasia [133]. If FL is more than 2 standard deviations below the mean length for GA, measure all the long bones and refer to appropriate tables for normal values. IUGR is another common cause of a short FL.
■ If FL is normal and a skeletal anomaly is suspected on the basis of family history, reexamine the fetus at a later date. Limb shortening may be evident only late in pregnancy (after 25 weeks) [129].
■ Evaluate bones for fractures, bowing, and mineralization (Fig. 7.76). Signs of decreased mineralization are decreased echogenicity of bone, decreased or absent acoustic shadowing, poor visualization of the fetal spine, and increased prominence of the falx [130].

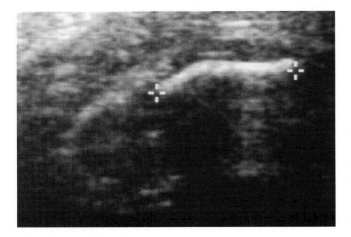

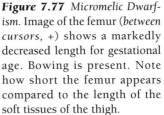

Figure 7.77 *Micromelic Dwarfism.* Image of the femur (*between cursors, +*) shows a markedly decreased length for gestational age. Bowing is present. Note how short the femur appears compared to the length of the soft tissues of the thigh.

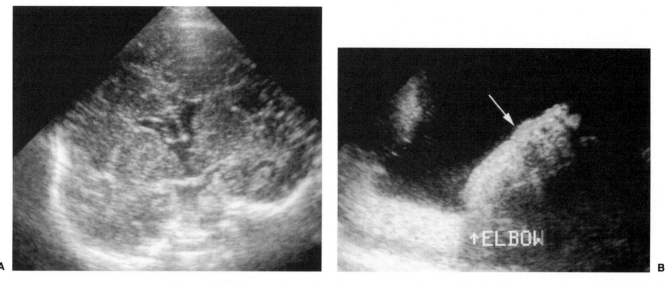

Figure 7.78 *Thanatophoric Dysplasia. A.* Coronal view of the fetal brain reveals remarkable detail. The skull is so thin that the US beams penetrate it easily. Excellent visualization through bone is a sign of poor bone mineralization. *B.* A view of the arm *(arrow)* shows severe deformity. This is a lethal dysplasia.

The brain is seen "too well" (Fig. 7.76). Bones appear abnormally thickened because the US beam is only weakly attenuated.

- Evaluate for evidence of small thorax. Measure TC and compare to tables for GA. Measure cardiothoracic ratio. Cardiac anomalies are associated with increased cardiothoracic ratio with normal TC. Bone dysplasias have increased cardiothoracic ratio and decreased TC.
- Evaluate hands and feet for polydactyly [134].
- **Micromelia** refers to proportional shortening of all long bones (Fig. 7.77).
- **Rhizomelia** refers to shortening of the humerus and/or the femur.
- **Mesomelia** refers to shortening of the radius and ulna and/or tibia and fibula. Mesomelic dysplasias are rare and non-lethal.
- **Acromelia** refers to shortening of the bones of the hands and feet.

Lethal Skeletal Dysplasias

Diagnosis of a lethal, or possibly lethal, skeletal dysplasia is essential to appropriate family counseling and delivery planning. Postnatal evaluation is usually required to confirm a specific diagnosis.

- Severe bone shortening is a hallmark of a lethal skeletal dysplasia (Figs. 7.77, 7.78) [131].
- Small thorax results in pulmonary hypoplasia and respiratory insufficiency.
- Cloverleaf skull deformity is seen with thanatophoric dysplasia.
- Polydactyly is seen with Jeune syndrome, Ellis-van Creveld syndrome, and short rib-polydactyly syndrome.
- Fractures, bowing, and severely deficient mineralization are seen with osteogenesis imperfecta, type 2.

REFERENCES

1. American College of Obstetrics and Gynecology. Ultrasonography in pregnancy. Technical Bulletin 1993;187:1–9.
2. American Institute of Ultrasound in Medicine. Guidelines for performance of the antepartum obstetrical ultrasound examination. Rockville: American Institute of Ultrasound in Medicine, 1991.

3. American College of Radiology. ACR standards for the performance of antepartum obstetrical ultrasound. 1990, revised 1995.

4. Hadlock FP, Deter RL, Carpenter RJ, et al. Estimating fetal age: effect of head shape on BPD. AJR Am J Roentgenol 1981;137:83–85.

5. Shepard MJ, Richards VA, Berkowitz RL, et al. An evaluation of two equations for predicting fetal weight by ultrasound. Am J Obstet Gynecol 1982;142:47–52.

6. Hadlock FP, Harrist RB, Carpenter RJ, et al. Sonographic estimation of fetal weight: the value of the femur in addition to head and abdomen measurements. Radiology 1984;150:535–540.

7. Hadlock FP, Deter RL, Harrist RB, et al. Fetal biparietal diameter: a critical re-evaluation of the relation to menstrual age by means of real-time ultrasound. J Ultrasound Med 1982;1:97–100.

8. Hadlock FP, Deter RL, Harrist RB, et al. Fetal head circumference: relation to menstrual age. AJR Am J Roentgenol 1982;138:649–653.

9. Hadlock FP, Deter RL, Harrist RB, et al. Fetal abdominal circumference as a predictor of menstrual age. AJR Am J Roentgenol 1982;139:367–370.

10. Hadlock FP, Harrist RB, Deter RL, et al. Fetal femur length as a predictor of menstrual age: sonographically measured. AJR Am J Roentgenol 1982;138:875.

11. Hadlock FP, Deter RL, Harrist RB, et al. Estimating fetal age: computer-assisted analysis of multiple growth parameters. Radiology 1984;152:497–501.

12. Lessoway VA, Schlzer M, Wittman BK, et al. Ultrasound fetal biometry charts for a North American Caucasian population. J Clin Ultrasound 1998;26:433–453.

13. Doubilet PM, Benson CB. Sonographic evaluation of intrauterine growth retardation. AJR Am J Roentgenol 1995;164:709–717.

14. Fong DW, Ohlsson A, Hannah ME, et al. Prediction of perinatal outcome in fetuses suspected to have intrauterine growth restriction: Doppler US study of fetal cerebral, renal, and umbilical arteries. Radiology 1999;213:681–689.

15. Dubinsky T, Lau M, Powell F, et al. Predicting poor neonatal outcome: a comparative study of noninvasive antenatal testing methods. AJR Am J Roentgenol 1997;168:827–831.

16. Woo JSK, Liang ST, Lo RLS. Significance of an absent or reversed end diastolic flow in Doppler umbilical artery waveforms. J Ultrasound Med 1987;6:291–297.

17. Ott WJ. Intrauterine growth restriction and Doppler ultrasonography. J Ultrasound Med 2000;19:661–665.

18. Sickler GK, Nyberg DA, Sohaey R, et al. Polyhydramnios and fetal intrauterine growth restriction: ominous combination. J Ultrasound Med 1997;16:609–614.

19. Finberg HJ, Kurtz AB, Johnson RL, et al. The biophysical profile: a literature review and reassessment of its usefulness in the evaluation of fetal well-being. J Ultrasound Med 1990;9:583–591.

20. Brant WE. Ultrasonography of the placenta. Perspectives in Radiology 1989;2:157–170.

21. Harris RD, Cho C, Wells WA. Sonography of the placenta with emphasis on pathological correlation. Semin Ultrasound CT MRI 1996;17:66–89.

22. Spirt BA, Gordon LP. Practical aspects of placental evaluation. Sem Roentgen 1991;26:32–49.

23. Taipale P, Hilesma V, Ylostalo P. Diagnosis of placenta previa by transvaginal sonographic screening at 12–16 weeks in a nonselected population. Obstet Gynecol 1997;89:364–368.

24. Wong G, Levine D. Sonographic assessment of the cervix in pregnancy. Semin Ultrasound CT MRI 1998;19:370–380.

25. Rosati P, Guariglia L. Clinical significance of placenta previa detected at early routine transvaginal scan. J Ultrasound Med 2000;19:581–585.

26. Hertzberg BS, Bowie JD, Carroll BA, et al. Diagnosis of placenta previa during the third trimester: role of transperineal sonography. AJR Am J Roentgenol 1992;159:83–87.

27. Hertzberg BS, Kliewer MA. Vasa previa: prenatal diagnosis by transperineal sonography with Doppler evaluation. J Clin Ultrasound 1998;26:405–408.

28. Kaakaji Y, Nghiem HV, Nodell C, et al. Sonography of obstetric and gynecologic emergencies: Part I, obstetric emergencies. AJR Am J Roentgenol 2000;174:641–649.

29. Pederson JF, Mantoni M. Prevalence and significance of subchorionic hemorrhage in threatened abortion: a sonographic study. AJR Am J Roentgenol 1990;154:535–537.

30. Sauerbrei EE, Pham DH. Placental abruption and subchorionic hemorrhage in the first half of pregnancy: US appearance and clinical outcome. Radiology 1986;160:109–112.

31. Bennett GL, Bromley B, Lieberman E, et al. Subchorionic hemorrhage in first-trimester pregnancies: prediction of pregnancy outcome with sonography. Radiology 1996;200:803–806.

32. Finberg HJ, Williams JW. Placenta accreta: prospective sonographic diagnosis in patients with placenta previa and prior Cesarean section. J Ultrasound Med 1992;11:333–343.

33. Kim H, Hill MC, Winick AB, et al. Prenatal diagnosis of placenta accreta with pathologic correlation. Radiographics 1998;18:237–242.

34. Bromley B, Benacerraf BR. Solid masses on the fetal surface of the placenta: differential diagnosis and clinical outcome. J Ultrasound Med 1994;13:883–886.

35. Dudiak CM, Salomon CG, Posniak HV, et al. Sonography of the umbilical cord. Radiographics 1995;15:1035–1050.

36. Nyberg DA, Mahony BS, Luthy D, et al. Single umbilical artery—prenatal detection of concurrent abnormalities. J Ultrasound Med 1991;10:247–253.

37. Wu M-H, Chang F-M, Shen M-R, et al. Prenatal sonographic diagnosis of single umbilical artery. J Clin Ultrasound 1997;25:425–430.

38. Strobelt N, Ghidini A, Cavallone M, et al. Natural history of uterine leiomyomas in pregnancy. J Ultrasound Medicine 1994;13:399–401.

39. Rosati P, Exacoustos C, Mancuso S. Longitudinal evaluation of uterine myoma growth during pregnancy—a sonographic study. J Ultrasound Med 1992;11:511–515.

40. Kessler A, Mitchell DG, Kuhlman K, et al. Myoma vs. contraction in pregnancy: differentiation with color Doppler imaging. J Clin Ultrasound 1993;21:241–244.

41. Mahony BS, Nyberg DA, Luthy DA, et al. Translabial ultrasound of the third-trimester uterine cervix—correlation with digital examination. J Ultrasound Med 1990;9:717–723.

42. Iams JD, Goldenberg RL, Meis PJ, et al. The length of the cervix and the risk of spontaneous premature delivery. N Engl J Med 1996;334:567–572.

43. Brace RA, Wolf EJ. Normal amniotic fluid volume changes throughout pregnancy. Am J Obstet Gynecol 1989;161:382–388.

44. Magann EF, Perry KG, Jr., Chauhan SP, et al. The accuracy of ultrasound evaluation of amniotic fluid volume in singleton pregnancies: the effect of operator experience and ultrasound interpretative technique. J Clin Ultrasound 1997;25:249–253.

45. Petrikovsky B, Schneider EP, Gross B. Clinical significance of echogenic amniotic fluid. J Clin Ultrasound 1997;26:191–193.

46. Levine D, Callen PW, Pender SG, et al. Chorioamniotic separation after second-trimester genetic amniocentesis: importance and frequency. Radiology 1998;209:175–181.

47. Randel SB, Filly RA, Callen PW, et al. Amniotic sheets. Radiology 1988;166:633–636.

48. Finberg HJ. Uterine synechiae in pregnancy: expanded criteria for recognition and clinical significance in 28 cases. J Ultrasound Med 1991;10:547–555.

49. Ball RH, Buchmeier SE, Longnecker M. Clinical significance of sonographically detected uterine synechiae in pregnant patients. J Ultrasound Med 1997;16:465–469.

50. Burton DJ, Filly RA. Sonographic diagnosis of the amniotic band syndrome. AJR Am J Roentgenol 1991;156:555–558.

51. Evans HJ. Chromosome anomalies among live births. J Med Genet 1977;14:309–312.

52. Nyberg DA, Kramer D, Resta RG, et al. Prenatal sonographic findings of trisomy 18: review of 47 cases. J Ultrasound Med 1993;2:103–113.

53. Lehman CD, Nyberg DA, Winter TC, III, et al. Trisomy 13 syndrome: prenatal US findings in a review of 33 cases. Radiology 1995;194:217–222.

54. Dubbins PA. Screening for chromosome abnormality. Semin Ultrasound CT MRI 1998;19:310–317.

55. Filly RA, Callen PW, Goldstein RB. Alpha-fetoprotein screening programs: what every obstetric sonologist should know. Radiology 1993;188:1–9.

56. Benacerraf BR, Nadel A, Bromley B. Identification of second-trimester fetuses with autosomal trisomy by use of a sonographic scoring index. Radiology 1994;193:135–140.

57. Benacerraf BR. Use of sonographic markers to determine the risk of Down syndrome in second-trimester fetuses. Radiology 1996;201:619–620.

58. Bromley B, Shipp T, Benacerraf BR. Genetic sonogram scoring index: accuracy and clinical utility. J Ultrasound Med 1999;18:523–528.

59. Filly RA. Obstetrical sonography: the best way to terrify a pregnant woman. J Ultrasound Med 2000;19:1–5.

60. Nicolaides KH, Brizot ML, Snijders RJM. Fetal nuchal translucency: ultrasound screening for fetal trisomy in the first trimester of pregnancy. Br J Obstet Gynecol 1994;101:782–786.

61. Watson WJ, Miller RC, Menard MK, et al. Ultrasonographic measurement of fetal nuchal skin to screen for chromosomal abnormalities. Am J Obstet Gynecol 1994;170:583–586.

62. Benson CB, Doubilet PM. Sonography in multiple gestations. Radiologist 1994;1:147–154.

63. Bromley B, Benacerraf BR. Using the number of yolk sacs to determine amnionicity in early first trimester monochorionic twins. J Ultrasound Med 1995;14:415–419.

64. Finberg HJ. The "twin peak" sign: reliable evidence of dichorionic twinning. J Ultrasound Med 1992;11:571–577.

65. Reece EA, Yarkoni S, Abdalla M, et al. A prospective longitudinal study of growth in twin gestations compared to growth in singleton pregnancies: I. The fetal head. J Ultrasound Med 1991;10:439–443.

66. Reece EA, Yarkoni S, Abdalla M, et al. A prospective longitudinal study of growth in twin gestations compared to growth in singleton pregnancies: II. The fetal limbs. J Ultrasound Med 1991;10:445–450.

67. Brown DL, Benson CB, Driscoll SG, et al. Twin-twin transfusion syndrome: sonographic findings. Radiology 1989;170:61–63.

68. Hecher K, Ville Y, Nicolaides KH. Fetal arterial Doppler studies in twin-twin transfusion syndrome. J Ultrasound Med 1995;14:101–108.

69. Filly RA, Cardoza JD, Goldstein RB, et al. Detection of fetal central nervous system anomalies: a practical level of effort for a routine sonogram. Radiology 1989;172:403–408.

70. Hertzberg BS, Kliewer MA, Freed KS, et al. Third ventricle: size and appearance in normal fetuses through gestation. Radiology 1997;203:641–644.

71. Knutson RK, McGahan JP, Salamat MS, et al. Fetal cisterna magna septa: a normal anatomic finding. Radiology 1991;180:799–801.

72. Brant WE. Ultrasound of the fetal face and neck. Radiologist 1994;1:235–244.

73. Mernagh JR, Mohide PT, Lappalainen RE, et al. US assessment of the fetal head and neck: a state-of-the-art pictorial review. Radiographics 1999;19:S229–S241.

74. Budorick NE, Pretorius DH, Nelson TR. Sonography of the fetal spine: technique, imaging findings, and clinical implications. AJR Am J Roentgenol 1995;164:421–428.

75. Avni EF, Rypens R, Milaire J. Fetal esophagus: normal appearance. J Ultrasound Med 1994;13:175–180.

76. Benacerraf BR. Sonographic detection of fetal anomalies of the aortic and pulmonary arteries: value of the four-chamber view vs direct images. AJR Am J Roentgenol 1994;163:1483–1489.

77. Frates MC. Sonography of the normal fetal heart: a practical approach. AJR Am J Roentgenol 1999;173:1363–1370.

78. Bromley B, Estroff JA, Sanders SP. Fetal echocardiography: accuracy and limitations in a population at high and low risk for heart defects. Am J Obstet Gynecol 1992;166:1473–1481.

79. McGahan JP. Sonography of the fetal heart: findings on the four chamber view. AJR Am J Roentgenol 1991;156:547–553.

80. Brown DL, DiSalvo DN, Frates MC, et al. Sonography of the fetal heart: normal variants and pitfalls. AJR Am J Roentgenol 1993;160:1251–1255.

81. Hashimoto BE, Filly RA, Callen PW. Fetal pseudoascites: further anatomic observations. J Ultrasound Med 1986;5:151–152.

82. Parulekar SG. Sonography of normal fetal bowel. J Ultrasound Med 1991;10:211–220.

83. Elejalde B, Elejalde M, Heitman T. Visualization of the fetal genitalia by ultrasonography: a review of the literature and analysis of its accuracy and ethical implications. J Ultrasound Med 1985;4:633–636.

84. Goldstein RB, Filly RA. Prenatal diagnosis of anencephaly: spectrum of sonographic appearances and distinction from the amniotic band syndrome. AJR Am J Roentgenol 1988;151:547–550.

85. Goldstein RB, LaPidus AS, Filly RA. Fetal cephaloceles: diagnosis with US. Radiology 1991;180:803–808.

86. Cardoza JD, Goldstein RB, Filly RA. Exclusion of fetal ventriculomegaly with a single measurement: the width of the lateral ventricular atrium. Radiology 1988;169:711–714.

87. Hertzberg BS, Lile R, Foosaner DE, et al. Choroid plexus-ventricular wall separation in fetuses with normal-sized cerebral ventricles at sonography: postnatal outcome. AJR Am J Roentgenol 1994;163:405–410.

88. McGahan JP, Nyberg DA, Mack LA. Sonography of facial features of alobar and semilobar holoprosencephaly. AJR Am J Roentgenol 1990;154:143–148.

89. Sohaey R, Zwiebel WJ. The fetal thorax: noncardiac chest anomalies. Semin Ultrasound CT MR 1996;17:34–50.

90. Guibaud L, Filiatrault D, Garel L, et al. Fetal congenital diaphragmatic hernia: accuracy of sonography in the diagnosis and prediction of outcome after birth. AJR Am J Roentgenol 1996;166:1195–1202.

91. Teixeira J, Sepulveda W, Hassan J, et al. Abdominal circumference in fetuses with congenital diaphragmatic hernia: correlation with hernia content and pregnancy outcome. J Ultrasound Med 1997;16:407–410.

92. Rosado-de-Christenson ML, Stocker JT. Congenital cystic adenomatoid malformation. Radiographics 1991;11:865–886.
93. Frazier AA, Rosado-de-Christenson ML, Stocker JT, et al. Intralobar sequestration: radiologic-pathologic correlation. Radiographics 1997;17:725–745.
94. Rosado-de-Christenson ML, Frazier AA, Stocker JT, et al. Extralobar sequestration: radiologic-pathologic correlation. Radiographics 1993;13:425–441.
95. McAdams HP, Kirejczyk WM, Rosado-de-Christenson ML, et al. Bronchogenic cyst: imaging features with clinical and histopathologic correlation. Radiology 2000;217:441–446.
96. Ohlsson A, Fong K, Rose T, et al. Prenatal ultrasonic prediction of autopsy proven pulmonary hypoplasia. Am J Perinatol 1992;9:334–337.
97. D'Alton M, Mercer B, Riddick E, et al. Serial thoracic versus abdominal circumference ratios for the prediction of pulmonary hypoplasia in premature rupture of the membranes remote from term. Am J Obstet Gynecol 1992;166:658–662.
98. Abdullah MM, Lacro RV, Smallhorn J, et al. Fetal cardiac dextroposition in the absence of an intrathoracic mass: sign of significant right lung hypoplasia. J Ultrasound Med 2000;19:669–676.
99. McGahan JP, Choy M, Parrish MD, et al. Sonographic spectrum of fetal cardiac hypoplasia. J Ultrasound Med 1991;10:539–546.
100. Brown DL, Roberts DJ, Miller WA. Left ventricular echogenic focus in the fetal heart: pathologic correlation. J Ultrasound Med 1994;13:613–616.
101. Bromley B, Lieberman E, Shipp TD, et al. Significance of an echogenic intracardiac focus in fetuses at high and low risk for aneuploidy. J Ultrasound Med 1998;17:127–131.
102. Wigton TR, Sabbagha RE, Tamura RK, et al. Sonographic diagnosis of congenital heart disease: comparison between the four-chamber view and multiple cardiac views. Obstet Gynecol 1993;82:219–224.
103. Yoo S-J, Lee YH, Cho KS. Abnormal three-vessel view on sonography: a clue to the diagnosis of congenital heart disease in the fetus. AJR Am J Roentgenol 1999;172:825–830.
104. Di Salvo DN, Brown DL, Doubilet PM, et al. Clinical significance of isolated fetal pericardial effusion. J Ultrasound Med 1994;13:291–293.
105. Brown DL. Sonographic assessment of fetal arrhythmias. AJR Am J Roentgenol 1997;169:1029–1033.
106. Emanuel PG, Garcia GI, Angtuaco TL. Prenatal detection of anterior abdominal wall defects with US. Radiographics 1995;15:517–530.
107. Brant WE. Sonographic evaluation of the fetal abdominal wall. Radiologist 1995;2:149–161.
108. Calzolari E, Volpato S, Bianchi F, et al. Omphalocele and gastroschisis: a collaborative study of five Italian congenital malformation registries. Teratology 1993;47:47–55.
109. Babcook CJ, Hedrick MH, Goldstein RB, et al. Gastroschisis: can sonography of the fetal bowel accurately predict postnatal outcome? J Ultrasound Med 1994;13:701–706.
110. Tongsong T, Wanapirak C, Sirivatanapa P, et al. Prenatal sonographic diagnosis of ectopia cordis. J Clin Ultrasound 1999;27:440–445.
111. Robertson FM, Crombleholme TM, Paidas M, et al. Prenatal diagnosis and management of gastrointestinal anomalies. Semin Perinat 1994;18:182–195.
112. McKenna KM, Goldstein RB, Stringer MD. Small or absent fetal stomach: prognostic significance. Radiology 1995;197:729–733.
113. Hertzberg BS. Sonography of the fetal gastrointestinal tract: anatomic variants, diagnostic pitfalls, and abnormalities. AJR Am J Roentgenol 1994;162:1175–1182.
114. Nyberg DA, Dubinsky T, Resta RG, et al. Echogenic fetal bowel during the second trimester: clinical importance. Radiology 1993;188:527–531.
115. Perez CG, Goldstein RB. Sonographic borderlands in the fetal abdomen. Semin Ultrasound CT MR 1998;19:336–346.
116. Levine D, Goldstein RB, Cadrin C. Distention of the fetal duodenum: abnormal finding? J Ultrasound Med 1998;17:213–215.
117. Vincoff NS, Callen PW, Smith-Bindman R, et al. Effect of ultrasound transducer frequency on the appearance of the fetal bowel. J Ultrasound Med 1999;18:799–803.
118. Rypens FF, Avni EF, Abehsera MM, et al. Areas of increased echogenicity in the fetal abdomen: diagnosis and significance. Radiographics 1995;15:1329–1344.
119. Karcnik TJ, Rubenstein JB, Swayne LC. The fetal presacral pseudomass: a normal sonographic variant. J Ultrasound Med 1991;10:579–581.
120. Zelop C, Benacerraf BR. The causes and natural history of fetal ascites. Prenat Diag 1994;14:941–946.

121. Keslar PJ, Buck JL, Suarez ES. Germ cell tumors of the sacrococcygeal region: radiologic-pathologic correlation. Radiographics 1994;14:607–620.

122. Arger PH, Coleman BG, Mintz MC, et al. Routine fetal genitourinary tract screening. Radiology 1985;156:485–489.

123. Bronshtein M, Bar-Hava I, Lightman A. The significance of early second-trimester sonographic detection of minor fetal renal anomalies. Prenat Diagn 1995;15:627–632.

124. Anderson N, Clautice-Engle T, Allan R, et al. Detection of obstructive uropathy in the fetus: predictive value of sonographic measurements of renal pelvic diameter at various gestational ages. AJR Am J Roentgenol 1995;164:719–723.

125. Corteville JE, Gray DL, Crane JP. Congenital hydronephrosis: correlation of fetal ultrasonographic findings with infant outcome. Am J Obstet Gynecol 1991;165:384–388.

126. Filly RA. Fetal hydronephrosis. Annual meeting of American Roentgen Ray Society, 1998.

127. Risdon RA. Renal dysplasia. J Clin Pathol 1971;24:57–71.

128. Zhou Q, Cardoza JD, Barth R. Prenatal sonography of congenital renal malformations. AJR Am J Roentgenol 1999;173:1371–1376.

129. Machado LE, Bonilla-Musoles F, Osborne NG. Fetal limb abnormalities: ultrasound diagnosis. Ultrasound Q 2000;16:203–219.

130. Spirt BA, Oliphant M, Gottlieb RH, et al. Prenatal sonographic evaluation of short limbed dwarfism: an algorithmic approach. Radiographics 1990;10:217–236.

131. Bowerman RA. Anomalies of the fetal skeleton: sonographic findings. AJR Am J Roentgenol 1995;164:973–979.

132. Mahony BS. Ultrasound evaluation of the fetal musculoskeletal system. In: Callen PW, ed. Ultrasonography in Obstetrics and Gynecology. 3rd ed. Philadelphia: WB Saunders and Co., 1994:254–290.

133. Kurtz AB, Needleman L, Wapner RJ. Usefulness of a short femur in the in utero detection of skeletal dysplasias. Radiology 1990;177:197–200.

134. Bromley B, Benacerraf B. Abnormalities of the hands and feet in the fetus: sonographic findings. AJR Am J Roentgenol 1995;165:1239–1243.

135. FitzSimmons J, Droste S, Shepard TH, et al. Long-bone growth in fetuses with Down syndrome. Am J Obstet Gynecol 1989;161:1174–1177.

136. Wax JR, Philput C. Fetal intracardiac echogenic foci: does it matter which ventricle? J Ultrasound Med 1998;17:141–144.

137. Manning JE, Ragavendra N, Sayre J, et al. Significance of fetal intracardiac echogenic foci in relation to trisomy 21: a prospective sonographic study of high-risk pregnant women. AJR Am J Roentgenol 1998;170:1083–1084.

138. Benacerraf BR, Mandell J, Estroff JA, et al. Fetal pyelectasis, a possible association with Down syndrome. Obstet Gynecol 1990;76:58–60.

SCROTAL ULTRASOUND

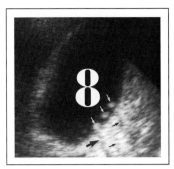

US is the imaging method of first choice for most diseases of the scrotum because of its high accuracy, general availability, and low cost. Indications include acute scrotal pain and scrotal mass [1]. Since most extratesticular masses are benign and most solid intratesticular masses are malignant, making this differentiation is a critical goal and advantage of US imaging.

IMAGING TECHNIQUE

The patient is asked to undress and lie supine on the examination table with his legs together. A folded towel is placed across both legs and beneath the scrotum to support the testes during the examination. The penis is placed on the abdomen and covered with a towel so only the scrotum is exposed. A copious amount of warm gel is placed on the scrotum and examination is performed with a linear array 7.5–10 MHz transducer. Images are obtained of each testis in transverse and longitudinal planes. The epididymides and inguinal canal regions are included in every examination. Color flow imaging and spectral Doppler are used to assess vascularity [2]. At least one image showing both testes on the same image is obtained to compare overall testicular echogenicity (see Fig. 8.16). The use of multiple transmit or focal zones usually improves image quality.

ANATOMY

Normal testes are oval globes approximately equal in size with average dimensions of 3–5 cm in length and 2–4 cm in diameter [3]. The echogenicity of the two testes is identical to each other. Normal echogenicity is medium in intensity with a moderately grainy texture (Fig. 8.1). The **tunica albuginea** is the tough fibrous capsule of the testis, seen as a discrete structure only when a hydrocele is present. The **mediastinum** (Fig. 8.2) is an infolding of the tunica albuginea that marks the entry and exit portal for the testicular arteries, veins, and ducts. The mediastinum appears as a linear bright echo in the long plane of the testes. Normal vascular clefts are seen as linear hypoechoic bands (Fig. 8.3). Their vascular nature is readily confirmed with color flow US. The **epididymis** forms at the mediastinum from anastomosis of the **efferent ductules** [4]. The **head of the epididymis** (globus major) projects cephalad as a moderately echogenic nodule 10–12 mm in size. The markedly con-

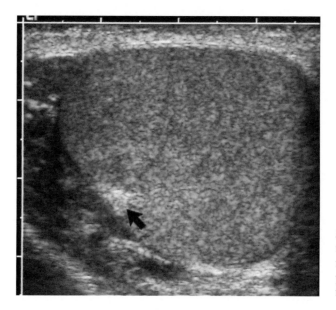

Figure 8.1 *Normal Testis.* The normal testis has a homogeneous, moderately grainy, echotexture. A portion of the mediastinum (*arrow*) is seen on this transverse image.

voluted tube that makes up the **body of the epididymis** courses inferiorly along the posterior aspect of the testis to the lower pole where it turns abruptly cephalad and becomes the **ductus deferens**. The **tail of the epididymis** (globus minor) is seen as a small nodular structure at this abrupt turn in the course of the epididymal tube. The epididymis appears on US to be coarser and more heterogeneous than the testis. The **ductus deferens** is markedly convoluted near its origin but straightens into a thick fibrous tube as it courses superiorly to the spermatic cord. The **appendix epididymis** is a blind-ended efferent tubule sometimes seen as a small tubular or nodular structure near the head of the epididymis. The **appendix testis** is a Müllerian remnant sometimes seen as another small nodule (1–3 mm size) under the epididymal head. These appendages are isoechoic to the epididymis and are usually seen only when a hydrocele is present. Torsion of these appendages clinically mimics torsion of the testis.

Most of the testis and epididymis is covered by the **tunica vaginalis**, a membrane identical to peritoneum that lines the scrotal sac. The tunica vaginalis envelops the head of the epididymis and forms a sinus between the body of the epididymis and testes. The fluid of

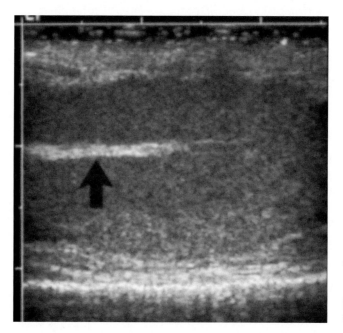

Figure 8.2 *Normal Mediastinum Testis.* The mediastinal portal (*arrow*) to the testis is linear and brightly echogenic on this longitudinal image.

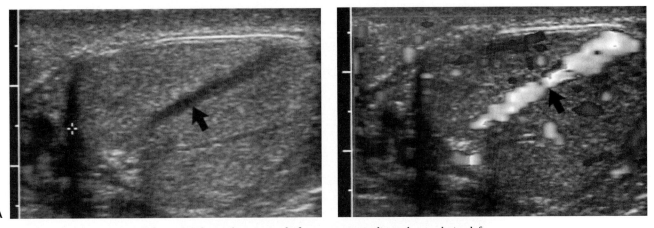

Figure 8.3 *Normal Vascular Cleft. A.* Blood vessels commonly form prominent linear hypoechoic clefts (*arrow*) as they course through the testicular parenchyma. *B.* Color Doppler, shown here in gray scale, readily confirms their vascular nature (*arrow*) and eliminates possible confusion with a testicular fracture.

a hydrocele outlines the epididymal head and fills the epididymal sinus. A "bare area" of the testis is formed posteriorly where the visceral tunica vaginalis reflects to the internal surface of the scrotum isolating the ductus deferens, part of the epididymis and the blood vessels coursing to the mediastinum from the fluid of a hydrocele.

Color flow and spectral Doppler US demonstrate the blood supply of the testis [5,6]. The **spermatic cord** is composed of the **testicular artery**, the **cremasteric artery**, and the **artery of the ductus deferens**; the testicular veins that make up the convoluted **pampiniform plexus**; the ductus deferens (vas deferens); and accompanying lymphatics, nerves, and connective tissue. The testicular artery enters the testes at the mediastinum and arborizes in a subcapsular layer. Redundant branches course through the testes perpendicular to the capsule. The intratesticular arteries normally have a low-resistance spectral waveform with high velocities maintained throughout diastole. The cremasteric and deferential arteries have high-resistance spectral waveforms.

ACUTE SCROTAL PAIN

Acute painful swelling of the scrotum is a common indication for scrotal US. Torsion, infection, or trauma may cause acute pain. Real-time gray scale and Doppler US are needed for complete evaluation [2]. All studies compare the symptomatic side to the asymptomatic side. The asymptomatic side is usually scanned first to provide a baseline for comparison with the symptomatic side. In children, testicular torsion is the most common diagnosis, whereas in adults, infection is most common.

TESTICULAR TORSION

Torsion must be identified and treated within a few hours to prevent infarction of the testis. Patients prone to torsion lack the normal attachment of the testis and epididymis to the posterior scrotal wall. This congenital abnormality is called the *bell-clapper deformity*. The risk of infarction varies with the degree of torsion. Torsion of 90 degrees produces lymphatic and venous obstruction and may not cause infarction for days. Torsion of 720 degrees obstructs arterial flow and may cause infarction within 2 hours.

- Swelling of the testis, epididymis, and spermatic cord below the site of torsion is caused by lymphatic and venous obstruction.
- Echogenicity is decreased with edema, but is heterogeneously increased with superimposed hemorrhage.

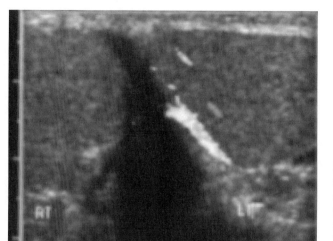

Figure 8.4 *Testicular Torsion.* Color Doppler image demonstrates normal flow to the left testis (LT) and no flow to the painful right testis (RT) (see Color Figure 8.4).

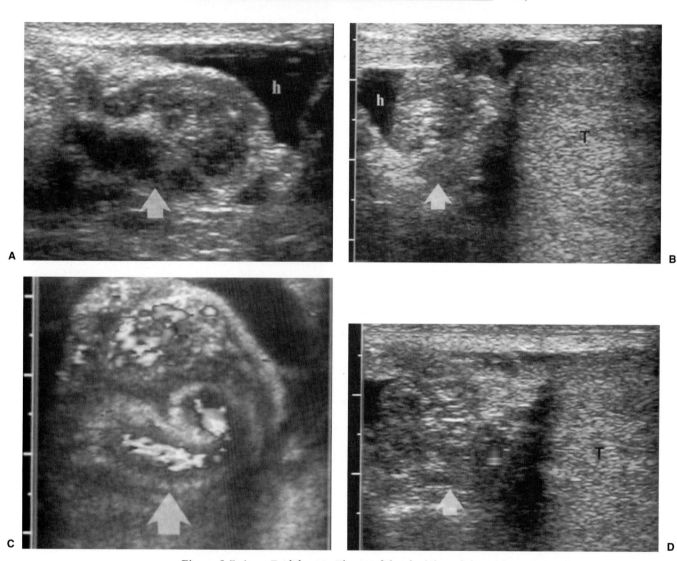

Figure 8.5 *Acute Epididymitis.* The painful right (*A*) epididymis (*arrow*) is enlarged and hypoechoic compared to the asymptomatic left (*B*) epididymis (*arrow*). Small hydroceles (h) are present on both sides. Color Doppler images show a marked increase in vascularity in the right (*C*) epididymis (*arrow*) compared to the left (*D*) epididymis (*arrow*). T, left testis. (See Color Figures 8.5C, D.)

- Venous thrombus may be visible in the spermatic cord as enlarged, clot-filled, occluded veins of the pampiniform plexus.
- Doppler demonstrates absent or decreased flow in the symptomatic testis compared to the opposite testis (Fig. 8.4) [2,7].
- If flow is present, peak systolic velocity is abnormally low.
- With spontaneous detorsion, Doppler findings may be normal or demonstrate reactive hyperemia. The major clue to detorsion is the spontaneous and rapid improvement in pain.

ACUTE EPIDIDYMO-ORCHITIS

Infection ascends in orderly fashion from the prostate or urinary tract through the ductus deferens to the epididymal tail, body, head, and finally into the testis. Patients present with pain and swelling at any time in this progression. Adolescents and adults are most commonly affected. Findings include [8,9]:

- Epididymis is swollen and decreased in echogenicity because of edema (Fig. 8.5A, B).
- Doppler demonstrates asymmetric hypervascularity of the affected epididymis reflecting arterial and venous dilatation (Fig. 8.5C, D). Spectral Doppler shows increased peak systolic and end-diastolic velocities (low-resistance waveform).
- Scrotal skin is often thickened.
- Testicular swelling, heterogeneous decreased echogenicity, and hypervascularity are signs of coexisting orchitis (Fig. 8.6). To exclude the possibility of testicular tumor masquerading as orchitis, all patients with altered testicular echogenicity should be reexamined when symptoms abate.

SCROTAL ABSCESS

Untreated infection can result in abscess formation in the epididymis, testis, or scrotal wall. These abscesses can rupture into the cavity of the tunica vaginalis and cause pyocele.

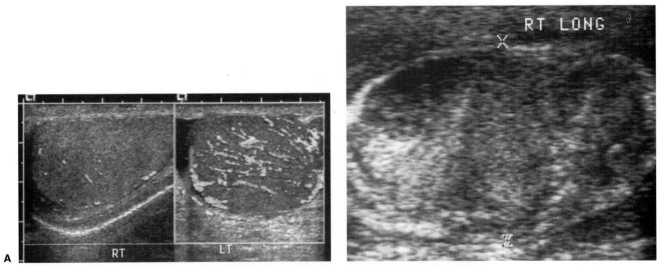

Figure 8.6 *Acute Orchitis. A.* Color flow images of both testes in a patient with a painful left testis demonstrate marked hypervascularity on the left (LT) compared to the right (RT). *B.* Severe orchitis in another patient markedly alters the echotexture of the testes (*between cursors, x*). Differentiation from testicular tumor is difficult (compare to Figure 8.18). Follow-up US examination to ensure complete resolution of orchitis is mandatory (see Color Figure 8.6A).

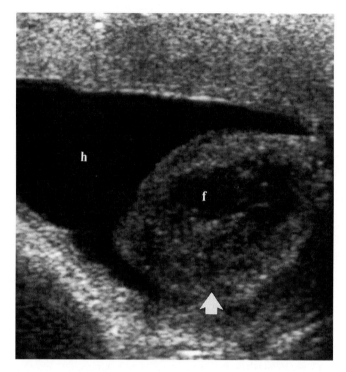

Figure 8.7 *Epididymal Abscess.* The painful epididymis (*arrow*) is markedly enlarged and contains a complex fluid collection (f) that is an abscess. A large reactive hydrocele (h) is present.

- Focal areas of complex echogenicity in epididymis (Fig. 8.7) or testis (Fig. 8.8) suggest abscess formation.
- Surrounding hyperemia on color flow US indicates inflammation. No flow is seen within the complex fluid of the abscess cavity.
- Pyocele appears as echogenic fluid, layering debris, and septations within the cavity of the tunica vaginalis.

TORSION OF TESTICULAR APPENDAGES

Torsion of the appendix testes or appendix epididymis is a common cause of acute scrotal pain in children, mimicking torsion of the testis. In distinction to urgent surgery needed for testicular torsion, torsion of the testicular appendages is self-limited and is treated conservatively with pain management [10,11].

- Enlarged nodule posterior or medial to the head of the epididymis represents the torsed appendage. It may be isoechoic or hypoechoic compared to the epididymal head.

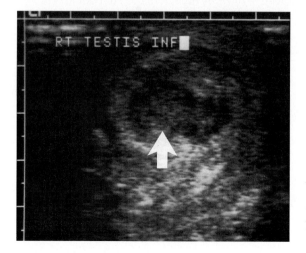

Figure 8.8 *Testicular Abscess.* The right testis is swollen and has markedly heterogeneous echogenicity. A central complex fluid collection (*arrow*) was proven to be an abscess.

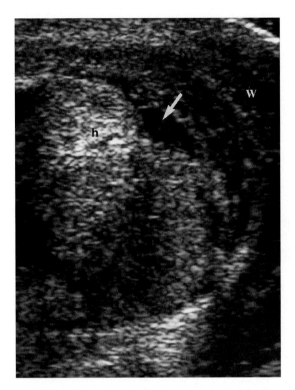

Figure 8.9 *Fractured Testis.* The injured testis is markedly heterogeneous and has a disrupted contour (*arrow*). The area of high echogenicity (h) is caused by hematoma. The scrotal sac is greatly thickened by bleeding into the scrotal wall (W).

- Hydrocele is usually present.
- Scrotal wall is often thickened.
- Increased blood flow is seen in both the epididymal head and the torsed appendage.
- The testis appears normal on gray scale and color flow imaging.

SCROTAL TRAUMA

Trauma is an obvious cause of acute scrotal pain. US is performed to diagnose disruption of the testis that requires surgical repair. A normal intact testis on US excludes significant injury. Rupture is more difficult to diagnose. Fracture planes are uncommonly evident and altered echotexture reflects intratesticular bleeding but not necessarily fracture. Findings include (Fig. 8.9):

- Loss of testicular outline is the most reliable sign of testis rupture.
- Irregular fracture planes extending through the testis are differentiated from vascular clefts by color flow US.
- Altered testis echotexture is usually indicative of testis hematoma or contusion.
- Color flow imaging aids in differentiating hematoma (avascular) from tumor (vascular). Because trauma may cause intratumoral hemorrhage, follow-up US is recommended to insure resolution of hematoma and to exclude tumor.
- Hematocele and scrotal wall hematoma are commonly present.

EXTRATESTICULAR MASS

Extratesticular masses commonly displace or compress the testis but are not encircled by testicular tissue [12,13].

Most extratesticular masses are benign, whereas most intratesticular masses are malignant.

HYDROCELE

Fluid accumulation in the cavity of the tunica vaginalis between its visceral and parietal layers is a common cause of scrotal enlargement. The fluid may be serous (**hydrocele**) (Fig.

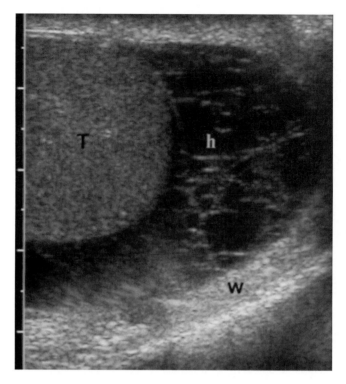

Figure 8.10 *Hematocele.* One week following a direct blow to the scrotum, US reveals complex fluid with septation and debris (h) indicative of hematocele in the cavity of the tunica vaginalis. The scrotal wall (w) is thickened. The testis (T) is intact. Pyocele has a similar appearance.

8.7), blood (**hematocele**), or pus (**pyocele**). Hydroceles may be congenital or result from tumor, inflammation, trauma, or torsion. Hematocele results from trauma, surgery, or rupture of tumor. Pyocele results from infection and rupture of abscess into the cavity of the tunica vaginalis.

- Fluid outlines the anterolateral testis and the head and part of the body of the epididymis. Fluid does not have access to the posterior aspect of the testis where it is anchored to the scrotum, unless the bell clapper anomaly is present.
- Anechoic fluid without septations is characteristic of hydrocele (Fig. 8.7).
- Bloody fluid contains low-intensity echoes that often layer. Septations and loculations are common (Fig. 8.10).
- Purulent fluid appears similar to bloody fluid with heterogeneous layering debris and thick irregular septations.

VARICOCELE

Dilatation of the pampiniform venous plexus in the spermatic cord is termed a *varicocele.* Varicocele is associated with male infertility related to elevated temperature in the testis caused by increased venous flow. They are more common on the left side presumably due to left testicular vein drainage into the left renal vein. Sudden appearance of a varicocele is suspicious for venous obstruction in the retroperitoneum caused by tumor or adenopathy. Findings include (Fig. 8.11):

- Serpiginous network of dilated veins (>3 mm) in the spermatic cord is diagnostic.
- Color flow US confirms venous flow within the tortuous tubes.
- Valsalva maneuver dilates the veins and makes varicocele more obvious.

SPERMATOCELE AND EPIDIDYMAL CYST

These are common and benign causes of a scrotal mass. Spermatoceles result from obstruction of the efferent ductules and contain creamy fluid and sperm. Epididymal cysts occur

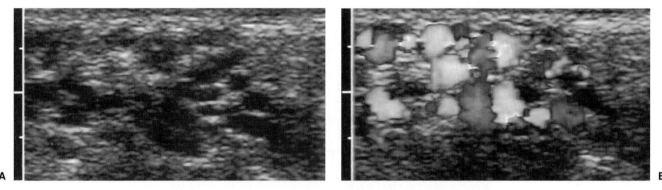

Figure 8.11 *Varicocele.* Longitudinal images of the spermatic cord just above the testis demonstrate a serpiginous network of tubular lucencies (*A*) that are confirmed to be dilated veins by color Doppler (*B*) (see Color Figures 8.11A, B).

anywhere along the course of the epididymis. Both are incidental findings of no clinical significance.

■ **Spermatocele** (Fig. 8.12):
 – Found only at the superior pole of the testis adjacent to the mediastinum.
 – Oval/round cystic mass with echogenic, often layering, fluid.
 – May appear solid if completely filled with echogenic fluid.
 – Septations are common.
 – Solitary, with size up to 2–3-cm diameter.
■ **Epididymal cyst** (Fig. 8.13):
 – Found anywhere along the epididymis.
 – Simple cyst with anechoic fluid.
 – Often multiple with usual size <1 cm.

HERNIA

Inguinal hernias commonly present as a scrotal mass (Fig. 8.14).

■ Heterogeneous mass extends from inguinal canal to scrotum.

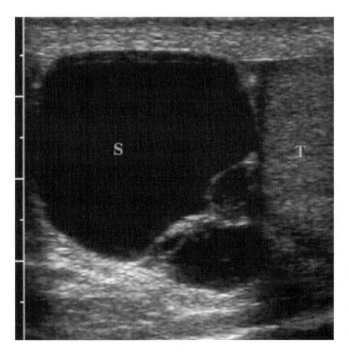

Figure 8.12 *Spermatocele.* Large cystic extratesticular mass (S) with septations and debris above the upper pole of the testis (T) is characteristic for spermatocele.

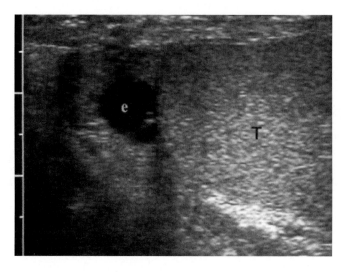

Figure 8.13 *Epididymal Cyst.* A well-defined cystic mass anywhere along the course of the epididymis is characteristic of a benign epididymal cyst. This epididymal cyst (e), above the upper pole of the testis (T), is indistinguishable from spermatocele. Differentiation is not important since both are benign and incidental findings.

- Mass moves and changes size and appearance with Valsalva maneuver.
- Omentum appears as heterogeneous mass with echogenic and hypoechoic components.
- Bowel shows spontaneous peristaltic motion.
- Hydrocele is commonly present.

CHRONIC EPIDIDYMITIS

Chronic inflammation thickens the epididymis and increases its echogenicity. Causative infections include bowel organisms, *Neisseria gonorrhea*, *Chlamydia*, and tuberculosis. Sarcoidosis may produce similar findings (Fig. 8.15) [14].

- Epididymis is enlarged with heterogeneously increased echogenicity.
- Vascularity is normal to slightly increased.
- Scrotal wall may be thickened.

SPERM GRANULOMA

Extravasation of sperm into surrounding tissue results in necrosis and granuloma formation. Sperm granulomas may occur after vasectomy or other forms of obstruction of the epididymis or vas deferens. The masses formed are painful.

- Granulomas appear as a hypoechoic solid mass along the course of epididymis or ductus deferens.
- No increased vascularity is present.
- May calcify in chronic stage.

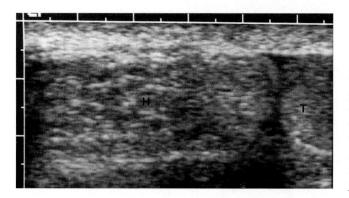

Figure 8.14 *Inguinal Hernia.* Herniation of omental fat into the inguinal canal is seen as a complex echogenic mass that moves within the inguinal canal as the patient strains and relaxes his abdominal muscles. This indirect inguinal hernia (H) extends to just above the testis (T).

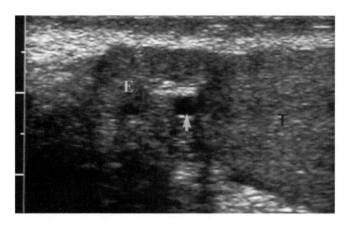

Figure 8.15 *Chronic Epididymitis.* The head of the epididymis (E) is enlarged, heterogeneous, and contains a small epididymal cyst (*arrow*). The patient had noted a mildly painful scrotal mass for more than 1 year. T, testis.

TUMOR OF THE EPIDIDYMIS

All neoplasms of the epididymis are rare and most are benign. Tumor types include adenomatoid tumor (a hamartoma found in adolescents and young adults) [15], papillary cystadenoma, various sarcomas, and metastases.

■ Non-specific solid mass along course of epididymis.

TESTICULAR MASS

Most solid testicular masses are malignant. Differential diagnosis includes orchitis and hematoma. Purely cystic lesions of the testis are benign and require only accurate sonographic characterization.

GERM CELL NEOPLASM

Most malignancies of the testes are germ cell tumors [16]. Peak occurrence is at age 25–35. Seminoma accounts for approximately one-half of the tumors. Non-seminomas include embryonal cell carcinoma, teratoma, yolk sac tumor, and choriocarcinoma. Mixed tumor histology is common. Young men who present with unexplained retroperitoneal adenopathy should be screened sonographically for non-palpable testicular tumor.

■ Homogeneous hypoechoic mass suggests seminoma (Figs. 8.16, 8.17).
■ Irregular heterogeneous mass with cystic, hemorrhagic, and necrotic areas and calcification suggests non-seminoma germ cell tumor (Fig. 8.18).
■ Small masses (<1.5 cm) tend to be hypovascular.

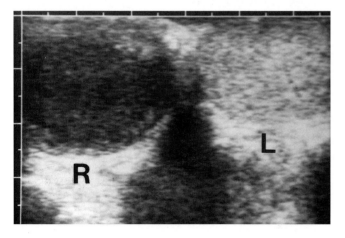

Figure 8.16 *Seminoma.* Transverse image comparing the right (R) and left (L) testis clearly demonstrates the homogeneous tumor replacing the right testis. This image illustrates the value of side-to-side comparison of the testes. The tumor was so homogeneous as to be possibly overlooked on images of the right testis alone.

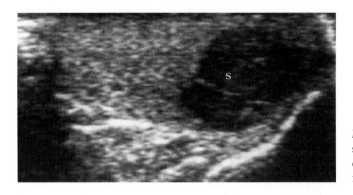

Figure 8.17 *Seminoma.* Another seminoma (S) is seen as a discrete, quite hypoechoic, intratesticular mass with echogenic septations.

- Larger masses (>1.5 cm) tend to be hypervascular with distorted vessels.
- Doppler characteristics are not helpful in differentiating tumor types.

STROMAL TUMORS

Leydig cell and Sertoli cell tumors arise from the supporting stromal tissue of the testis. Most (90%) of these tumors are benign. Leydig tumors secrete androgens and may produce virilizing effects. Sertoli tumors secrete estrogens and may produce feminizing effects. Adrenal rest tumors are often bilateral. These tumors are indistinguishable from germ cell tumors by imaging methods. Diagnosis requires surgical biopsy.

- Well-defined, hypoechoic solid nodule is the usual appearance.

LYMPHOMA AND METASTASES

Solid testicular masses in men older than age 45 are much more likely to be metastases or lymphoma than germ cell tumors.

Solid testicular masses in older men (>45 years) are most likely to be secondary tumors. Metastases originate most commonly from prostate, renal, lung, and gastrointestinal carcinoma and malignant melanoma (Fig. 8.19). The testes are a "safe haven" for lymphoma because systemic chemotherapy does not reach the intratesticular tumor in sufficient concentration to kill the cells [17]. Leukemia in children and adults may spread into and be "protected" in the testis (Fig. 8.20).

- Multiple and bilateral solid masses are seen with metastases, lymphoma, and leukemia. Masses may be well defined or infiltrative.
- Most masses are hypoechoic.
- Diffusely altered echogenicity of testis without discrete mass is common with infiltrative lesions (Fig. 8.21).

ISOLATED TESTICULAR CALCIFICATIONS

These usually reflect previous healed infection, trauma, or ischemia. They are clinically insignificant.

- Most calcifications produce a coarse echogenic focus with acoustic shadowing.
- No adjacent mass is present and parenchymal echogenicity is normal.

TESTICULAR MICROLITHIASIS

Diffuse punctate calcifications in the testicular parenchyma are associated with a variety of conditions including germ cell malignancies, infertility, Klinefelter's syndrome, and cryptorchidism [18]. One study reported the coexistence of germ cell neoplasm in 40% of patients with testicular microlithiasis [19]. Because tumors may develop subsequent to discovery of microlithiasis, follow-up US examination at 6-month intervals has been recommended for early tumor detection [18].

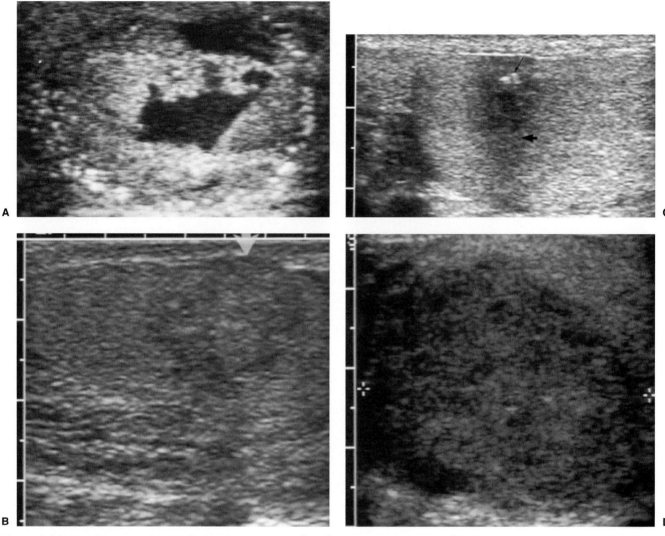

A **C** **B** **D**

Figure 8.18 *Non-Seminoma Germ Cell Tumors.* Four examples of non-seminoma germ cell tumors demonstrate the broad range of appearance. *A.* Choriocarcinoma replaces the testicular parenchyma with heterogeneous tumor. *B.* Embryonal cell carcinoma causes ill-defined disruption of the homogeneous echotexture of the testicular parenchyma. Note the subtle nodular contour change (*arrow*) of the testis. *C.* A teratocarcinoma is seen as small, ill-defined, hypoechoic tumor containing calcifications (*tiny arrow*) and causing a faint acoustic shadow (*arrowhead*). *D.* Mixed histology germ cell tumor is seen as a lobulated, heterogeneous testicular mass (*between cursors,* +).

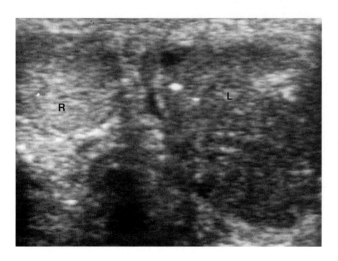

Figure 8.19 *Malignant Melanoma Metastasis.* The left testis (L) of a 55-year-old man is enlarged, heterogeneous, and nodular. The patient had a history of malignant melanoma believed to be in remission until he developed painless testicular enlargement. R, right testis.

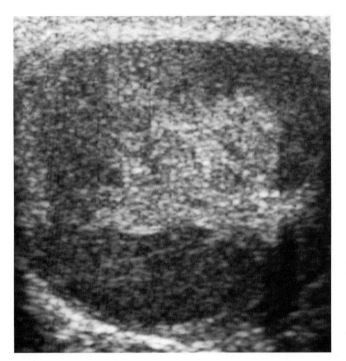

Figure 8.20 Leukemia. A 12-year-old boy with acute lymphocytic leukemia developed tender swelling of both testes. Hypoechoic leukemic infiltrate dramatically alters the echogenicity of the parenchyma of the left testis.

- Tiny (1–3 mm) echodensities scattered diffusely or clustered in the testicular parenchyma (Fig. 8.22).
- Microlithiasis is usually, but not always, bilateral.
- Acoustic shadowing is rare. Comet tail artifacts are occasionally seen.
- Look carefully for testicular mass.

TESTICULAR CYSTS

Benign, simple, intratesticular cysts are found in up to 8% of men and with increased frequency in older men [20].

- Simple, anechoic, well-defined cyst in testicular parenchyma is characteristic (Fig. 8.23).
- Size varies from a few mm to 1–2 cm.
- Cysts may be single or multiple.

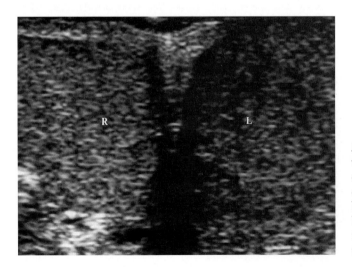

Figure 8.21 Lymphoma. Transverse image of both testes demonstrates the subtle uniform decrease in echogenicity caused by diffuse infiltration of Burkitt's lymphoma into the left testis (L) of a 14-year-old boy. R, right testis.

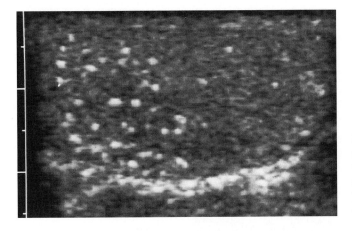

Figure 8.22 *Testicular Microlithiasis.* Punctate echodensities without acoustic shadowing are scattered diffusely but irregularly throughout the testicular parenchyma.

CYSTS OF THE TUNICA ALBUGINEA

Cysts that arise from the tunica albuginea present as a firm, pea-sized, palpable testicular mass. No treatment is needed when accurate diagnosis is made sonographically [21].

- Well-defined, small (2–5 mm) anechoic to hypoechoic cyst in the peripheral testis intimately related to the tunica albuginea is diagnostic (Fig. 8.24).
- Cysts may be single or multiple.
- Most cysts are unilocular, some are septate.

CYSTIC DILATION OF RETE TESTIS

Men with a history of previous vasectomy, recurrent epididymitis, or other obstructions to testicular fluid outflow are prone to develop cystic dilation of the rete testis [22]. The rete testis are irregular anastomosing spaces connecting the seminiferous tubules and the efferent ductules. These may dilate with epididymal obstruction. No treatment is needed.

- Multiple small anechoic cysts and tubes in mediastinum of the testis have a characteristic appearance shown in Fig. 8.25.
- No blood flow is present in these structures.

UNDESCENDED TESTIS

Undescended testis is present at birth in 3–4% of full-term and 30% of preterm boys. In 10–25%, both testes are undescended. Infertility and a 40-to-50–fold increase in risk of cancer

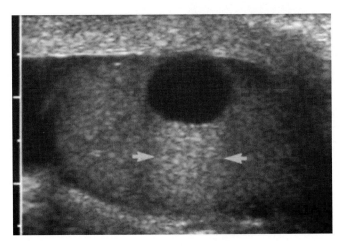

Figure 8.23 *Benign Testicular Cyst.* The cyst is sharply demarcated from the parenchyma and has no discernible wall. The internal fluid is anechoic and causes accentuated through-transmission (*arrows*).

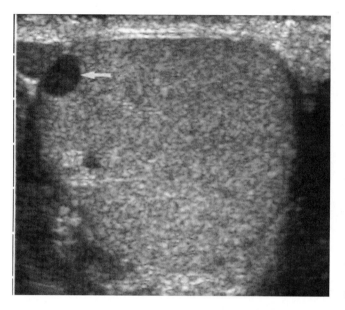

Figure 8.24 *Cyst of the Tunica Albuginea.* This tiny cyst (*arrow*) projects from the fibrous covering of the testis. The fluid has faint internal echoes. No discrete accentuated through-transmission is evident. Although these cysts contain fluid, on palpation, they feel like a hard, pea-sized nodule.

are complications of uncorrected cryptorchidism. Because spontaneous descent is common, surgical correction (orchiopexy) is usually delayed until after the first year of age. In older children and adults, the testis is often surgically removed because of risk of malignancy. US successfully identifies nearly all of the 80% of maldescended testes that are located in the inguinal canal. MR or surgical exploration is indicated in the remaining cases in which the testis is located in the abdomen or is absent.

- The testis is seen as an oval solid mass in the inguinal canal.
  - In infants <1 year, the undescended testis is approximately 1-cm size and is isoechoic to the descended testis.
  - In older children and adults, the testis is often atrophic and appears hypoechoic compared to the descended testis (Fig. 8.26).
- Demonstration of the echogenic mediastinum testis confirms identification of the testis.
  - Lymph nodes may mimic the atrophic undescended testis.

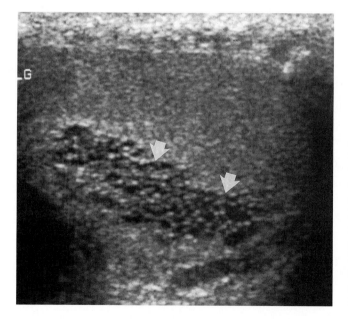

Figure 8.25 *Cystic Dilatation of the Rete Testis.* A network of tiny tubular structures (*arrows*) is evident in the area of the mediastinum of the testis. Color Doppler imaging is used to confirm that these structures are not vascular. The patient had had a vasectomy 5 years previously. This appearance is characteristic of cystic dilatation of the rete testis.

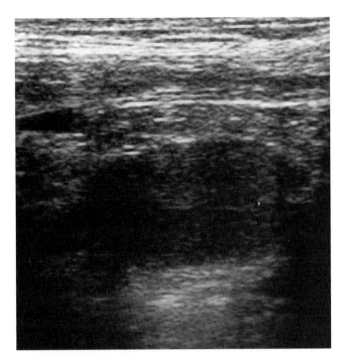

Figure 8.26 *Undescended Testis.* An undescended testis is demonstrated in the upper inguinal canal as an oval hypoechoic mass in this 12-year-old boy. A lymph node may have a very similar appearance. Demonstration of the testicular mediastinum is definitive but only occasionally possible.

- The pars infravaginalis gubernaculi, the bulbous termination of the cordlike gubernaculum that guides descent of the testis, may also be mistaken for the testis [23].
■ Look for testicular tumors in older patients with cryptorchidism.

REFERENCES

1. van Dijk R, Doesburg WH, Verbeek ALM, et al. Ultrasonography versus clinical examination in the evaluation of testicular tumors. J Clin Ultrasound 1994;22:179–182.
2. Herbener TE. Ultrasound in the assessment of the acute scrotum. J Clin Ultrasound 1996;24:405–421.
3. Gerscovich EO. High-resolution ultrasonography in the diagnosis of scrotal pathology: I. normal scrotum and benign disease. J Clin Ultrasound 1993;21:355–373.
4. Black JAR, Patel A. Sonography of the normal extratesticular space. AJR Am J Roentgenol 1996;167:503–506.
5. Middleton WD, Thorne DA, Melson GL. Color Doppler ultrasound of the normal testis. AJR Am J Roentgenol 1989;152:293–297.
6. Horstman WG, Middleton WD, Melson GL, et al. Color Doppler US of the scrotum. Radiographics 1991;11:941–957.
7. Burks DD, Markey BJ, Burkhard TK, et al. Suspected testicular torsion and ischemia: evaluation with color Doppler sonography. Radiology 1990;175:815–821.
8. Keener TS, Winter TC, Nghiem HV, et al. Normal adult epididymis: evaluation with color Doppler US. Radiology 1997;202:712–714.
9. Berman JM, Beidle TR, Kunberger LE, et al. Sonographic evaluation of acute intrascrotal pathology. AJR Am J Roentgenol 1996;166:857–861.
10. Cohen HL, Shapiro MA, Haller JO, et al. Torsion of the testicular appendage—sonographic diagnosis. J Ultrasound Med 1992;11:81–83.
11. Strauss S, Faingold R, Manor H. Torsion of the testicular appendages: sonographic appearance. J Ultrasound Med 1997;16:189–192.
12. Frates MC, Benson CB, DiSalvo DN, et al. Solid extratesticular masses evaluated with sonography: pathologic correlation. Radiology 1997;204:43–46.
13. Black JAR, Patel A. Sonography of the abnormal extratesticular space. AJR Am J Roentgenol 1996;167:507–511.
14. Forte MD, Brant WE. Ultrasonographic detection of epididymal sarcoidosis. J Clin Ultrasound 1988;16:191–194.

15. Mäkäräinen HP, Tammela TLJ, Karttunen TJ, et al. Intrascrotal adenomatoid tumors and their ultrasound findings. J Clin Ultrasound 1993;21:33–37.

16. Gerscovich EO. High-resolution ultrasonography in the diagnosis of scrotal pathology: II. tumors. J Clin Ultrasound 1993;21:375–386.

17. Mazzu D, Jeffrey RB, Jr., Ralls PW. Lymphoma and leukemia involving the testicles: findings on gray-scale and color Doppler sonography. AJR Am J Roentgenol 1995;164:645–647.

18. Miller RL, Wissman R, White S, et al. Testicular microlithiasis: a benign condition with a malignant association. J Clin Ultrasound 1996;24:197–202.

19. Backus ML, Mack LA, Middleton WD, et al. Testicular microlithiasis: imaging appearances and pathologic correlation. Radiology 1994;192:781–785.

20. Gooding GAW, Leonhardt W, Stein R. Testicular cysts: US findings. Radiology 1987;163:537–538.

21. Martinez-Berganza MT, Sarria L, Cozcolluela R, et al. Cysts of the tunica albuginea: sonographic appearance. AJR Am J Roentgenol 1998;170:183–185.

22. Brown D, Benson CB, Doherty FJ, et al. Cystic testicular mass caused by dilated rete testis: sonographic findings in 31 cases. AJR Am J Roentgenol 1992;158:1257–1259.

23. Rosenfield AT, Blair DN, McCarthy S, et al. The pars infravaginalis gubernaculi: importance in identification of the undescended testis. AJR Am J Roentgenol 1989;153:775–778.

THYROID, PARATHYROID, AND NECK ULTRASOUND

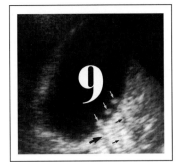

- Imaging Technique
- Anatomy
- Thyroid
- Parathyroid
- Neck

Sonography of the thyroid gland is one of the more frustrating areas of US imaging. Expectations are high because sonography is exquisitely sensitive to thyroid abnormalities. Unfortunately, US findings are rarely specific for any disease. Evaluation of thyroid nodules is particularly annoying because thyroid nodules are exceedingly common and US detects most of them, even as small as 1–2 mm, but can rarely unequivocally differentiate benign from malignant nodules. Most of the nodules detected by US are not clinically significant. Fortunately, thyroid cancer is relatively rare; so criteria can be selected to limit the number of biopsies performed and still diagnose the majority of clinically significant cancers. Sonographic guidance is used to direct aspiration biopsy of nonpalpable thyroid nodules and to guide procedures such as alcohol ablation of thyroid lesions [1–3].

US is utilized to detect parathyroid adenomas in patients with clinical hyperparathyroidism. These adenomas can then be removed surgically or ablated with US-guided, alcohol injection. Preoperative localization of adenomas decreases operative time and surgical morbidity. Sonography is limited by its inability to detect ectopic parathyroid adenomas in the mediastinum. These lesions may be demonstrated by Tc-99m sestamibi scans, CT or MR [4–6].

Masses and adenopathy can be accurately characterized by US, which can also be used to guide aspiration or biopsy.

IMAGING TECHNIQUE

US of the neck is performed with the patient in supine position. The neck is hyperextended by placement of a pillow or folded towels under the patient's shoulders. A linear array transducer with frequency of 5–10 MHz is utilized. Occasionally, when the thyroid is greatly enlarged, curved-array or sector transducers are used to provide the "big picture." Images are obtained in transverse and longitudinal planes. The lobes of the thyroid gland and any

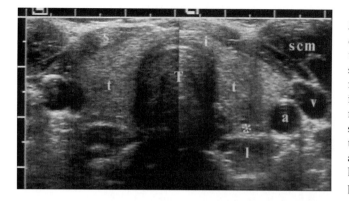

Figure 9.1 *Normal Thyroid Anatomy.* A transverse image through the mid–thyroid gland demonstrates normal sonographic landmarks. a, common carotid artery; i, thyroid isthmus; l, longus colli muscle; s, strap muscles; scm, sternocleidomastoid muscle; t, thyroid lobes; T, trachea (note the acoustic shadow); v, internal jugular vein; *, normal location of the parathyroid glands.

focal lesions are measured in three dimensions. Volumes are calculated using the standard formula for volume of an ellipsoid (length × width × height × 0.52). The neck is thoroughly examined for adenopathy. Intrathoracic extension of thyroid disease can be demonstrated by angling the US transducer downward into the mediastinum from a supra-manubrial position. Spectral, color, and power Doppler are utilized to demonstrate the vascularity of the thyroid gland and any focal lesions.

ANATOMY

The thyroid gland consists of two ellipsoid lobes connected by an isthmus that extends across the lower cervical trachea (Figs. 9.1, 9.2). Normal thyroid parenchyma is homogeneous and hyperechoic relative to the muscles of the neck. Anatomic landmarks include the common carotid artery (CCA), internal jugular vein (IJV), trachea, and neck muscles. The sternocleidomastoid is seen as an oval muscle mass superficial and lateral to the thyroid. The strap muscles, the sternohyoid, sternothyroid, and omohyoid, appear as thinner muscle bands just superficial to the thyroid. The thyroid extends over the midline trachea between the CCA/IJV vascular bundles. It rests on the prevertebral longus colli muscles. The trachea, being air-filled, causes a bright reflection at its surface and a prominent acoustic shadow. The esophagus commonly extends from behind the tracheal shadow between the left thyroid lobe and the longus colli muscle. The esophagus has a target appearance that must not be mistaken for a thyroid or parathyroid nodule (Fig. 9.3). Identification of the esophagus is confirmed by observing the patient swallow, and observing air or fluid move through the esophagus.

The CCA courses along the lateral aspect of the thyroid lobe, which may partially envelop the CCA when the thyroid is enlarged. The IJV are seen lateral to the CCA.

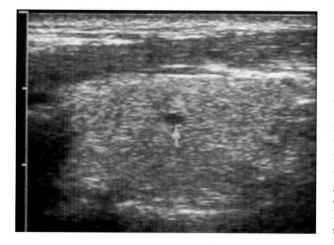

Figure 9.2 *Normal Thyroid Echogenicity.* Longitudinal image demonstrates the normal homogeneous mid-level echogenicity of the thyroid gland. Tiny cysts (*arrow*) are commonly seen in normal thyroid glands. These are large thyroid follicles and are commonly called colloid cysts. They are of no clinical significance.

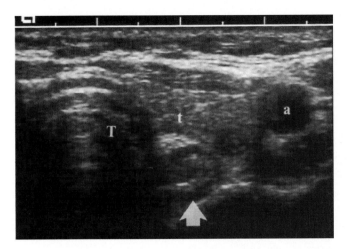

Figure 9.3 *Esophagus.* The esophagus (*arrow*) commonly protrudes from behind the trachea (T) to the area between the thyroid gland and the longus colli muscle on the left, mimicking a thyroid or parathyroid mass. a, common carotid artery; t, left thyroid lobe.

Enlarged lymph nodes may be detected along the vascular sheath of the CCA/IJV. The thyroid and parathyroid glands are supplied by the superior thyroid artery, a branch of the external carotid artery, and the inferior thyroid artery, a branch of the thyrocervical trunk from the subclavian artery. These arteries (1–2 mm diameter) and their accompanying veins (6–8 mm diameter) course between the thyroid lobes and the longus colli muscles. Spectral Doppler of the thyroidal arteries shows a high systolic velocity (20–40 cm/sec), low resistance (high diastolic velocity) pattern. The thyroid parenchyma shows a richly vascular pattern with power Doppler.

Normal parathyroid glands are thin wafers 5 mm in diameter, but only 1 mm in thickness. Normal glands are not visualized by US. US reliably demonstrates adenomas and enlarged glands when they are in the neck. Most patients have four parathyroid glands, although 3% of patients have three glands and 13% have five or more. The paired superior and inferior glands are located deep to the lobes of the thyroid gland and superficial to the longus colli muscle. The inferior glands are ectopically located in the mediastinum in 3% of cases.

THYROID

THYROID NODULES

Most thyroid US is requested to evaluate suspected thyroid nodules. Nodules are exceedingly common, with nodules present in 50% of glands normal to palpation on autopsy series and in 18–36% of palpably normal glands on US studies [7–9]. Although thyroid cancer is the most common malignancy of the endocrine glands, it remains a rare disease accounting for less than 1% of all malignancy, and is the cause of death in only 0.005% of the United States population [10]. Most thyroid cancers are relatively non-aggressive and have a good prognosis with 90% 10-year survival for early disease. The challenge of US is to differentiate benign from malignant nodules. At this task, US fails because no sonographic finding is pathognomonic. To deal with this dilemma and to avoid a huge number of unproductive biopsies, criteria have been developed to select for biopsy only those patients who are at highest risk for carcinoma.

Benign thyroid nodules outnumber malignant thyroid nodules approximately 500 to 1.

Malignant Thyroid Nodules
Thyroid carcinoma is 3 times more common in women with median age of 45–50 years at diagnosis. Radiation to the neck, especially in childhood, is a major risk factor, greatest at 20 years after the radiation [11].

Papillary carcinoma is most common (60–70%), is multifocal in 20–80% of cases, and spreads early to regional lymph nodes. The tumor is commonly at least partially cystic and

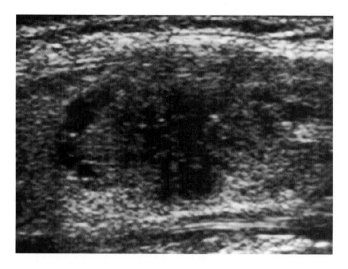

Figure 9.4 *Dominant Nodule.* Longitudinal image shows an ill-defined dominant nodule measuring 42 mm × 30 mm. The remainder of the thyroid gland was normal. This nodule was "cold" on radionuclide imaging. Biopsy is indicated.

the lymph node metastases are cystic in 25%. Punctate psammomatous calcifications are a strong sign of malignancy (see Fig. 9.5).

Follicular carcinoma (15%) is invasive and spreads more commonly hematogenously to bones and lungs. It is uncommonly multifocal and less frequently spreads to cervical lymph nodes.

Medullary carcinoma (5–10%) may be familial (10% of cases) or associated with multiple endocrine neoplasia. Serum calcitonin is elevated and is a marker of disease.

Anaplastic carcinoma (5%) is exceptionally aggressive with average survival time of 6–12 months. The tumor is locally invasive and spreads rapidly to adjacent structures, nodes (which are commonly necrotic), lungs, and bone.

Metastases to the thyroid (from breast, lung, and renal cell carcinoma and melanoma) may be infiltrative masses or well-defined focal nodules.

Lymphoma accounts for approximately 4% of thyroid malignancy [12]. Older women are most commonly affected. The disease is usually non-Hodgkin's lymphoma. Hypoechoic nodules grow rapidly and cause dysphagia or dyspnea. Enlarged lymph nodes are seen elsewhere. Cystic change in the enlarged nodes is common.

Benign Thyroid Nodules

Benign thyroid nodules are most commonly adenomatous nodules (adenomatous hyperplasia) or follicular adenomas. True thyroid cysts are exceedingly rare lesions. Most cystic

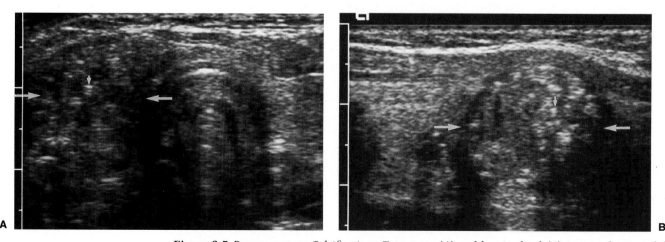

Figure 9.5 *Psammomatous Calcifications.* Transverse (*A*) and longitudinal (*B*) images show a solid thyroid nodule (*between large arrows*) with punctate calcifications (*small arrows*). These calcifications are highly predictive of malignancy. Biopsy was indicated and confirmed a papillary carcinoma.

nodules are cystic degeneration of hyperplastic nodules or adenomas. At least 15–25% of all thyroid nodules have cystic areas within them.

Adenomatous nodules are nodules caused by hyperplasia of benign follicular cells. Most often the nodules are multiple. Cystic degeneration, hemorrhage, and calcification are common.

Follicular adenomas are benign neoplasms arising from follicular epithelium. Most are solitary with a well-developed fibrous capsule. Occasionally, adenomas are hyperfunctioning and result in hyperthyroidism with suppression of function of the remainder of the gland. These hyperfunctioning adenomas are "hot" on radionuclide scans.

Biopsy should be considered with the following findings that are associated with increased risk of malignancy:

- Size >4–5 cm. Large dominant nodules are more likely to be malignant (Fig. 9.4). Few, however, reach size larger than 4 cm before coming to medical attention. Many physicians recommend biopsy of predominantly solid nodules larger than 15 mm.
- Psammomatous calcifications. Microcalcifications <1 mm size (Fig. 9.5) scattered throughout a solid nodule are strong evidence of malignancy (70% positive predictive value) [13,14]. The calcifications appear as punctate echodensities. Many are too small to produce acoustic shadows. Psammomatous microcalcifications are strongly associated with papillary carcinoma. The microcalcifications may also be present in lymph node metastases.
- Solitary cold nodule on radionuclide scan (Fig. 9.4). The risk of malignancy is approximately 15%.
- History of neck irradiation, especially in childhood. The risk is highest at 20 years after radiation exposure and remains high for an additional 20 years [15].
- Family history of thyroid malignancy, especially medullary carcinoma.
- Age <20 years or male patient with solitary nodule. Benign thyroid nodules are uncommon in children and less common in males.
- Irregular contour and poor margination (Fig. 9.4) suggest malignancy but may also be seen with benign nodules.

The following findings are most indicative of a benign lesion that can be followed conservatively or ignored:

- Extensive cystic component is strongly indicative of benignancy (Fig. 9.6). Nearly all of these cystic lesions are the result of cystic degeneration in benign hyperplastic nodules or benign adenomas.

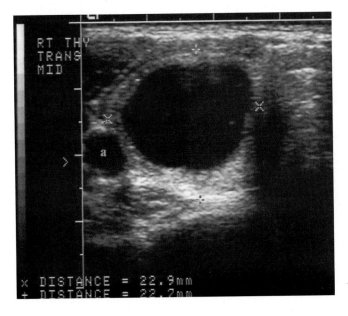

Figure 9.6 *Cystic Thyroid Nodule.* Calipers (+, x) measure a predominantly cystic nodule in the right thyroid lobe, This is a benign thyroid nodule. Biopsy is not indicated. a, common carotid artery.

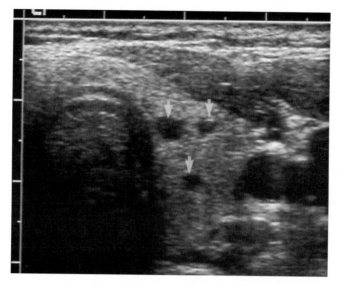

Figure 9.7 *Colloid Cysts.* Three tiny cysts (*arrows*) are seen in the left thyroid lobe. The largest of these measures 3 mm. These tiny cysts are normal findings. Biopsy is not indicated.

- Tiny cysts <5 mm size without an associated solid component are collections of colloid in macrofollicles (Fig. 9.7). These are benign and can be considered a normal finding.
- Comet tail artifacts are produced by inspissated colloid [16]. Their presence is indicative of a benign lesion containing abundant colloid.
- Homogeneous hyperechoic lesions are rarely malignant. Nearly all malignancies (and most benign nodules) are hypoechoic or isoechoic compared to thyroid parenchyma.
- Peripheral rim-like, "eggshell" calcifications (Fig. 9.8) are indicative of a benign lesion.
- Increased radionuclide activity, "hot" nodules with suppression of the remainder of the gland are nearly always benign.

The following findings are indeterminate and are found with benign and malignant nodules:

- Solid, hypoechoic or isoechoic, nodule (Fig. 9.9).
- Amorphous dense calcification.
- Complex nodule with irregular areas of cystic degeneration and hemorrhage (Figs. 9.10, 9.11).
- Increased flow within a nodule on Doppler US (Fig. 9.11) [17,18].
- Multiple nodules on US examination.

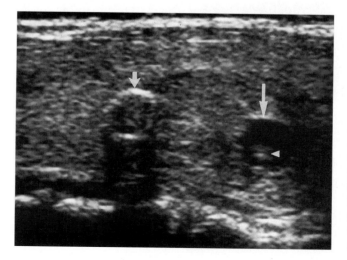

Figure 9.8 *Peripheral Rim-like Calcification.* Longitudinal image reveals two nodules in the thyroid. One nodule appears solid but has a calcified peripheral rim (*short arrow*). The second nodule (*long arrow*) is predominantly cystic but has a solid component projecting from its wall (*arrowhead*). The appearance of each is consistent with a benign adenomatous nodule. Biopsy is not indicated.

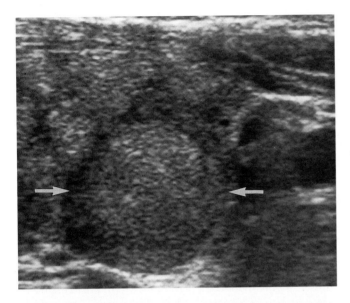

Figure 9.9 *Solid Nodule.* US confirms a homogeneous solid thyroid nodule (*between arrows*) that corresponded to a palpable abnormality. Its benign or malignant nature cannot be determined by further imaging. US-guided biopsy revealed benign lymphocytic thyroiditis (Hashimoto's thyroiditis).

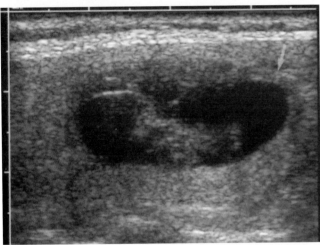

Figure 9.10 *Complex Nodule.* This nodule is predominantly cystic but has a thick wall (*arrow*) and a prominent internal solid component. The appearance is indeterminate. A clinical decision must be made whether to biopsy or follow this nodule. This decision is based on integrating the size and appearance of a given nodule with the clinical information regarding the patient's risk factors, laboratory evaluation, and medical history.

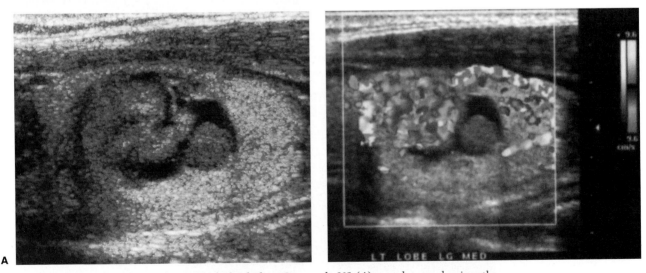

Figure 9.11 *Complex Nodule with Increased Blood Flow.* Gray-scale US (*A*) reveals a predominantly solid nodule with cystic components. The corresponding color Doppler image (*shown here in gray scale*) (*B*) reveals marked increased blood flow within most, but not all, of the solid tissue. Both the gray-scale and the color Doppler appearance are indeterminate. US-guided biopsy of the solid tissue confirmed a benign adenomatous nodule with degeneration.

DIFFUSE THYROID DISEASE

Goiter

The word **goiter** refers to generalized enlargement of the thyroid gland. Goiter is not a specific diagnosis because thyroid enlargement has many causes, including iodine deficiency, Graves' disease, adenomatous goiter, and thyroiditis. The size of the normal thyroid gland increases with body weight, decreases with age, and is larger in men than in women. Normal values are 19.6 ± 4.7 mL for men and 17.5 ± 4.2 mL for women [19]. Iodine deficiency goiter is not a significant problem in the United States because of iodine supplements in food.

- Thyroid volume is calculated by measuring each thyroid lobe and adding together the size of lobes calculated by using the formula: Volume = length × width × height × π/6 (0.52) (Fig. 9.12).
- Goiter is present when thyroid gland size exceeds 24.3 mL in men or 21.7 mL in women.
- A thyroid isthmus >10 mm thick is indicative of thyroid enlargement (Fig. 9.13).
- Iodine deficiency goiter shows diffuse parenchymal enlargement without abnormality of echogenicity.

Graves' Disease

Graves' disease (diffuse toxic goiter) is a chronic autoimmune disease that causes hyperthyroidism and goiter. Women are more commonly affected (7:1). Antibodies to thyroid stimulating hormone are present in the blood. Proptosis is commonly present.

- The thyroid gland is diffusely enlarged, frequently 2–3 times normal size.
- Thyroid echotexture may be homogeneous and normal, or diffusely hypoechoic.
- Color Doppler shows a characteristic pattern of pronounced increased blood flow ("thyroid inferno") manifest by multiple small dots of color signal throughout the gland during both systole and diastole [20].

Adenomatous Goiter

Multiple hyperplastic adenomatous nodules characterize adenomatous goiter (multinodular goiter).

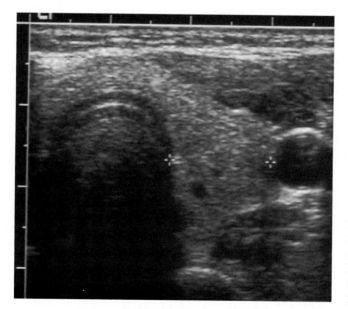

Figure 9.12 *Thyroid Measurement*. The calipers (+) indicate the transverse dimension of the left thyroid lobe of a normal thyroid gland. A colloid cyst is present.

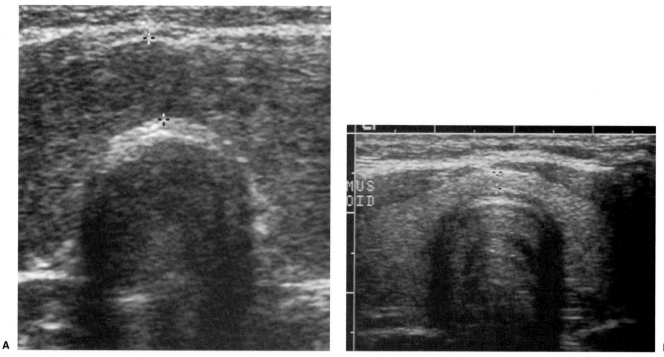

Figure 9.13 *Thickened Thyroid Isthmus. A.* The thyroid isthmus measured 13 mm (*between calipers,* +) confirming the sonologist's subjective impression of goiter. The thyroid parenchyma is mildly heterogeneous. *B.* A normal thyroid gland and thyroid isthmus (2 mm thick) is shown for comparison.

- The thyroid gland is enlarged, asymmetric, and heterogeneous in echotexture (Fig. 9.14).
- Multiple solid nodules of varying size and appearance are present. The nodules may be isoechoic, hypoechoic, hyperechoic, or mixed.
- The nodules commonly have cystic areas of colloid concentration, foci of necrosis and hemorrhage, and coarse calcifications present.

Hashimoto's Thyroiditis

This autoimmune process is the most common cause of hypothyroidism in the United States. Antithyroglobulin and antimicrosomal antibodies are present. The gland shows diffuse lymphocytic infiltration (chronic lymphocytic thyroiditis).

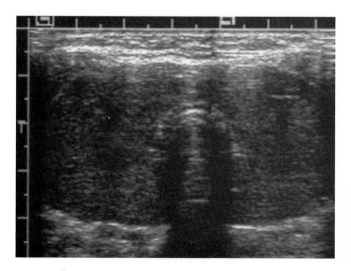

Figure 9.14 *Adenomatous Goiter.* Although this condition is commonly termed *multinodular goiter,* it frequently manifests as diffuse, heterogeneous thyroid enlargement without distinct nodules.

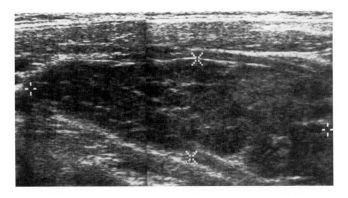

Figure 9.15 *Hashimoto's Thyroiditis.* Longitudinal image shows a diffusely abnormal gland (*between calipers, +, x*) with a pattern of innumerable ill-defined hypoechoic nodules.

- A diffuse micronodular pattern of the thyroid parenchyma is characteristic (Fig. 9.15). The micronodules are hypoechoic and most are 2–3 mm in size (range = 1–6 mm) [21].
- The gland is usually enlarged but may be normal in size.
- Hyperemia is marked on color Doppler.
- Radionuclide studies show little or no tracer uptake.
- Distinct nodules are occasionally present (Fig. 9.9).

Subacute (de Quervain's) Thyroiditis

Subacute (de Quervain's) thyroiditis is a self-limited granulomatous inflammation of the thyroid probably caused by a viral infection. Also more common in women (5:1), the gland becomes painful and tender 2–3 weeks after an upper respiratory infection. Severe destruction of the gland releases hormone, resulting in a period of hyperthyroidism, followed by a short period of hypothyroidism caused by hormone depletion. Most patients recover fully.

- The gland is initially enlarged but becomes atrophic as the disease progresses.
- Diffuse decreased parenchymal echogenicity is seen in half [22].
- The remainder show poorly defined hypoechoic nodules [22].

Atrophic Thyroiditis

Atrophic thyroiditis is an autoimmune disease that causes hypothyroidism in adults [23]. Circulating thyroid hormone levels are low, thyroid stimulating hormone levels are high, and autoantibodies to thyroid peroxidase and thyroglobulin are present in the patient's serum. The disease is distinguished from Hashimoto's thyroiditis by the small size of the gland.

- Echogenicity of the thyroid gland is diffusely low.
- The thyroid gland is atrophic. Combined volume of the thyroid lobes is <5.5 mL in males and <4.3 mL in females.

Acute Suppurative Thyroiditis

The thyroid is strikingly resistant to bacterial infection because of its copious blood supply, excellent lymphatic drainage, and high iodine content. Patients with suppurative thyroiditis present with fever and neck pain. US is used primarily to detect abscess. Congenital branchial pouch sinus tracts from the pyriform recess to the thyroid gland have been demonstrated in patients with recurrent suppurative thyroiditis [24].

- The gland is diffusely enlarged and hypoechoic due to inflammation.
- Focal fluid or air collections suggest abscess. Purulent fluid is commonly echogenic.
- A sinus tract to the pyriform fossa is suggested by an irregular tubular lucency extending into the neck [25].

PARATHYROID

HYPERPARATHYROIDISM

Primary hyperparathyroidism is caused in 80–90% of cases by a solitary parathyroid adenoma, in 10–20% of cases by multiple hyperplastic glands, and in 1% of cases by parathyroid carcinoma [26]. The role of US is to preoperatively localize parathyroid disease in the neck. Ectopic parathyroid glands are best localized by Tc-99m sestamibi or MR [4,5]. Ectopic locations include the mediastinum (commonly in the thymus), behind the trachea, and high in the carotid sheath. US does not demonstrate mediastinal parathyroid adenomas.

Secondary hyperparathyroidism occurs in patients with chronic renal failure and chronic hypocalcemia. Parathyroid surgery or alcohol ablation is required when dialysis and medical therapy is ineffective in controlling calcium levels and the resulting bone demineralization and soft tissue calcification. Multiple hyperplastic parathyroid glands are present.

PARATHYROID ADENOMA

Solitary adenomas arise in each of the four parathyroid glands with equal frequency. "Incidental" parathyroid adenomas are occasionally discovered during sonography of the thyroid [27].

■ Parathyroid adenomas are of low echogenicity, substantially less than thyroid parenchyma (Fig. 9.16). The adenomas are usually found between the dorsal aspect of the thyroid lobe and the longus colli muscle. Thyroid tissue may partially or completely

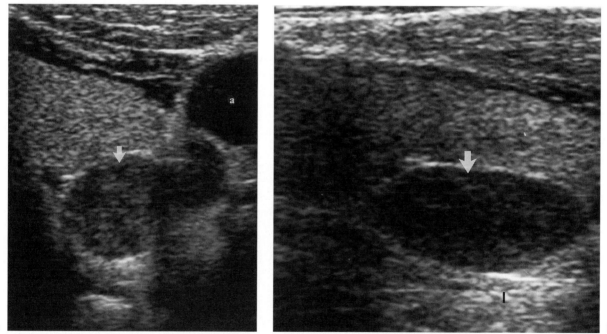

A   **B**

Figure 9.16 *Parathyroid Adenoma.* Transverse (A) and longitudinal (B) images show the characteristic, homogeneous, hypoechoic appearance of a well-defined parathyroid adenoma (*arrows*). Note the characteristic location deep to the thyroid gland and superficial to the longus colli muscle (l). a, common carotid artery.

envelop the parathyroid adenoma. Diffusely hyperechoic nodules or nodules with calcifications are much more likely to be thyroid, rather than parathyroid, nodules [28].

■ Most adenomas are 8–15 mm in size. Small lesions (<10 mm) are usually round, well defined, and nearly anechoic, but without accentuated through-transmission. Larger lesions tend to be oval, more heterogeneous, and lobulated in contour.

■ Giant parathyroid adenomas exceed 20 mm in size and are associated with greatly elevated levels of serum calcium and serum parathyroid hormone. These large tumors may develop cystic areas of necrosis and hemorrhage. Benign giant adenomas cannot be reliably differentiated from carcinomas.

■ Doppler demonstrates marked hypervascularity of the functioning adenomas. Prominent feeding vessels are evident [29].

■ Lymph nodes may mimic parathyroid adenomas. Lymph nodes are usually more intimately related to the carotid artery or are located inferior to the thyroid gland. Lymph nodes tend to have an echogenic center (see Fig. 9.18), whereas most parathyroid adenomas are uniformly hypoechoic.

■ Percutaneous fine needle aspiration with measurement of parathyroid hormone level is confirmatory of a parathyroid adenoma [30]. This procedure is particularly helpful when multiple thyroid nodules are present and identification of a parathyroid adenoma is uncertain.

MULTIPLE PARATHYROID GLAND HYPERPLASIA

Parathyroid adenomas are indistinguishable from parathyroid hyperplasia.

Multiple gland disease may be caused by multiple parathyroid adenomas or hyperplasia of multiple glands.

■ Hyperplastic glands and adenomas have an identical sonographic appearance (Fig. 9.17).

■ The individual glands are commonly asymmetrical in size. Careful examination should always include looking for multiple enlarged glands.

PARATHYROID CARCINOMA

Parathyroid carcinomas are rare and may be difficult to distinguish from adenomas even histologically. Invasion of adjacent structures and prominent fibrosis provides evidence of malignancy. The cancer is aggressive and metastasizes early resulting in unrelenting hypocalcemia.

■ Carcinomas are larger, more lobulated, and more heterogeneous than adenomas.

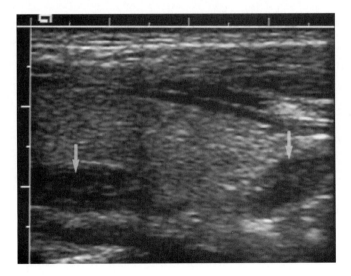

Figure 9.17 *Multiple Parathyroid Hyperplasia.* Longitudinal image through the left lobe of the thyroid demonstrates two enlarged hyperplastic parathyroid glands (*arrows*) in a patient with chronic renal failure and persistent elevation of serum calcium. Two more enlarged parathyroid glands were also seen on the right side.

- Most carcinomas are larger than 2 cm in size and may be indistinguishable from benign giant parathyroid adenomas.
- Cystic components and heterogeneous internal echogenicity are signs of malignancy.

NECK

LYMPH NODES

US is effective in demonstrating normal, enlarged benign, and malignant lymph nodes in the neck [31]. Differentiation of benign from malignant is often not possible but several US features are helpful in selecting nodes for biopsy.

- Normal nodes are flattened, oblong, and small (<10 mm in smallest diameter) [32]. Normal nodes are hypoechoic with an echogenic hilus [33].
- Benign, enlarged lymph nodes remain oblong in shape with a short-to-long axis ratio of 0.5 or less. Color or power Doppler reveals a normal vascular pattern of central vascularity radiating symmetrically from the hilum. The periphery of the node shows no vascularity [34]. Homogeneous echogenic fat extending from the hilum is a sign of benignancy (Fig. 9.18) [35]. Avascular nodes tend to be benign [34].
- Nodes involved with lymphoma tend to mimic the Doppler characteristics of benign nodes [34]. Lymphoma nodes tend to be enlarged and homogeneous in echogenicity.
- Malignant nodes are enlarged (>10 mm) with heterogeneous internal architecture and a round, rather than oblong, shape. Punctate calcifications and cystic changes are seen in metastatic nodes involved with papillary carcinoma of the thyroid. Color flow US shows deranged, irregular vascularity with decreased or absent hilar vessels and increased vascularity in the periphery [36].
- Lymph node metastases may be cystic appearing as fixed masses with nodular irregular wall [37].
- US can be used to guide fine needle aspiration biopsy of any questionable lymph nodes.

THYROGLOSSAL DUCT CYSTS

These are the most common congenital cystic lesions in the neck. They arise from segments of the thyroglossal duct that fail to regress. Thyroid tissue is commonly present in the wall. Most present in childhood and are readily diagnosed by their characteristic midline position.

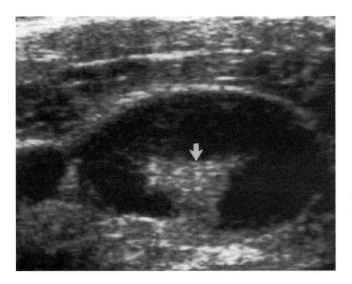

Figure 9.18 *Benign Lymph Node.* This enlarged cervical lymph node is markedly hypoechoic. Fat infiltrating the node from the hilum (*arrow*) is indicative of benignancy.

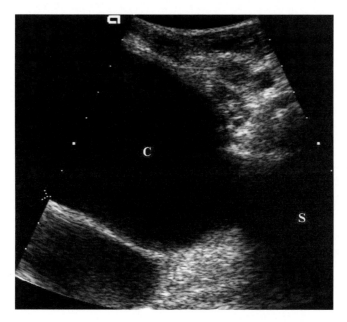

Figure 9.19 *Branchial Cleft Cyst.* Large mass (C) in the neck is filled with anechoic fluid and has a thin wall. Pathologic examination after surgical excision demonstrated respiratory epithelium lining the wall. S, shadowing from the spine.

- Cystic midline mass, usually at the level of the hyoid bone. They may be found in the midline from the tongue base to the suprasternal region.
- Classic appearance is an anechoic, well-defined, unilocular cyst with increased through-transmission. Size varies from a few mm to 2–3 cm [38].
- Many are hypoechoic with internal echoes, although nearly all show increased through-transmission [39].
- Infection causes thickening of the walls and internal septations.
- A soft tissue component within or around the cyst suggests the possibility of malignant degeneration (papillary carcinoma), a rare complication [40].

Branchial Cleft Cyst

These cysts are the congenital result of failure of obliteration of the embryonic branchial cleft in the eighth to ninth fetal week. Most (95%) arise from a remnant of the second branchial cleft [41]. They most often present in young adults.

- Cystic, thin-walled, round to oval mass, near the angle of the mandible (Fig. 9.19). Size ranges from 2–3 mm to 7 cm.
- The mass displaces the sternocleidomastoid muscle posteriorly, the CCA and IJV medially, and the submandibular salivary gland anteriorly.
- Infection is relatively common.

Cystic Hygroma

Most cystic hygromas (90%) enlarge rapidly after birth and are discovered before age 2. They result from congenital blockage of regional lymphatic drainage. Cystic hygroma is the common name for the cystic form of lymphangioma.

- Classic appearance is a thin-walled, multiseptated cyst in the posterior triangle of the neck. Septa are of variable thickness [42].
- Extension into the mediastinum is found in 3–10% of cases [37]. Lesions dissect through tissue planes as they expand.
- Lymph is anechoic. The presence of internal echoes suggests that hemorrhage has occurred.

TERATOMAS

Most teratomas in the neck originate within or near the thyroid gland [37]. Nearly all are benign, but they may cause respiratory obstruction.

- Dermoid cysts have internal echoes (from keratinous debris) with slight or no accentuated through-transmission [43]. The cysts are sharply defined with smooth borders. Absence of internal vascularity on Doppler US helps to confirm the cystic nature of the lesions.
- Solid teratomas are rare and are heterogeneous in appearance.

REFERENCES

1. Livraghi T, Paracchi A, Ferrari C, et al. Treatment of autonomous thyroid nodules with percutaneous ethanol injection: 4-year experience. Radiology 1994;190:529–533.
2. Lin J-D, Huang B-Y, Weng H-F, et al. Thyroid ultrasonography with fine-needle aspiration cytology for the diagnosis of thyroid cancer. J Clin Ultrasound 1997;25:111–118.
3. Takashima S, Fukuda H, Kobayashi T. Thyroid nodules: clinical effect of ultrasound-guided fine-needle aspiration biopsy. J Clin Ultrasound 1994;22:535–542.
4. Lee V, Spritzer C. MR imaging of abnormal parathyroid glands. AJR Am J Roentgenol 1998;170:1097–1103.
5. Perez-Monte J, Brown M, Shah A, et al. Parathyroid adenomas: accurate detection and localization with Tc-99m sestamibi SPECT. Radiology 1996;201:85–91.
6. Gordon BM, Gordon L, Hoang K, et al. Parathyroid imaging with 99mTc-sestamibi. AJR Am J Roentgenol 1996;167:1563–1568.
7. Brander A, Viikinkoski P, Nickels J, et al. Thyroid gland: US screening in a random adult population. Radiology 1991;181:683–687.
8. Tessler R, Tublin M. Thyroid sonography: current applications and future directions. AJR Am J Roentgenol 1999;173:437–443.
9. Brander A, Viikinkoski P, Nickels J, et al. Thyroid gland: US screening in middle-aged women with no previous thyroid disease. Radiology 1989;173:507–510.
10. Schlumberger M. Papillary and follicular thyroid carcinoma. N Engl J Med 1998;338:297–306.
11. Gagel RF, Goepfert H, Callender DL. Changing concepts in the pathogenesis and management of thyroid carcinoma. CA Cancer J Clin 1996;46:261–283.
12. Takashima S, Morimoto S, Ikezoe J, et al. Primary thyroid lymphoma: comparison of CT and US assessment. Radiology 1989;171:439–443.
13. Ellison E, Lapuerta P, Martin S. Psammoma bodies in fine-needle aspirates of the thyroid: predictive value for papillary carcinoma. Cancer 1998;84:169–175.
14. Takashima S, Fukuda H, Nomura N, et al. Thyroid nodules: re-evaluation with ultrasound. J Clin Ultrasound 1995;23:179–184.
15. Pacini F, Vorontsova T, Demidchik E, et al. Post-Chernobyl thyroid carcinoma in Belarus children and adolescents: comparison with naturally occurring thyroid carcinoma in Italy and France. J Clin Endocrinol Metab 1997;82:3563–3569.
16. Ahuja A, King W, Metreweli C. Clinical significance of the comet-tail artifact in thyroid ultrasound. J Clin Ultrasound 1996;24:129–133.
17. Clark KJ, Cronan JJ, Scola FH. Color Doppler sonography: anatomic and physiologic assessment of the thyroid. J Clin Ultrasound 1995;23:215–223.
18. Shimamoto K, Endo T, Ishigaki T, et al. Thyroid nodules: evaluation with color Doppler ultrasonography. J Ultrasound Med 1993;12:673–678.
19. Hegedüs L, Perrild H, Poulsen L, et al. The determination of thyroid volume by ultrasound and its relationship to body weight, age, and sex in normal subjects. J Clin Endocrinol Metab 1983;56:260–263.
20. Ralls PW, Mayekawa DS, Lee KP, et al. Color-flow Doppler sonography in Graves' disease: "thyroid inferno." AJR Am J Roentgenol 1988;150:781–784.
21. Yeh H-C, Futterweit W, Gilbert P. Micronodulaton: ultrasonographic sign of Hashimoto thyroiditis. J Ultrasound Med 1996;15:813–819.
22. Brander A. Ultrasound appearance in de Quervain's subacute thyroiditis with long-term follow-up. J Intern Med 1992;232:321–325.
23. Vitti P, Lampis M, Piga M, et al. Diagnostic usefulness of thyroid ultrasonography in atrophic thyroiditis. J Clin Ultrasound 1994;22:375–379.

24. Bar-Ziv J, Slasky B, Sichel J, et al. Branchial pouch sinus tract from the piriform fossa causing acute suppurative thyroiditis, neck abscess, or both: CT appearance and the use of air as a contrast agent. AJR Am J Roentgenol 1996;167:1569–1572.

25. Ahuja A, Griffiths J, Roebuck D, et al. The role of ultrasound and oesophagography in the management of acute suppurative thyroiditis in children associated with congenital pyriform fossa sinus. Clin Radiology 1998;53:209–211.

26. Van Heerden J, Beahrs O, Woolner L. The pathology and surgical management of primary hyperparathyroidism. Surg Clin North Am 1977;57:557–563.

27. Frasoldati A, Pesenti M, Toschik E, et al. Detection and diagnosis of parathyroid incidentalomas during thyroid sonography. J Clin Ultrasound 1999;27:492–498.

28. Gooding G. Parathyroid ultrasound: the why and the wherefore. Radiologist 2000;7:29–35.

29. Lane M, Desser T, Weigel R, et al. Use of color and power Doppler sonography to identify feeding arteries associated with parathyroid adenomas. AJR Am J Roentgenol 1998;171:819–823.

30. Sacks BA, Pallotta JA, Cole A, et al. Diagnosis of parathyroid adenomas: efficacy of measuring parathormone levels in needle aspirates of cervical masses. AJR Am J Roentgenol 1994;163:1223–1226.

31. Takashima S, Sone S, Nomura N, et al. Nonpalpable lymph nodes of the neck: assessment with US and US-guided fine-needle aspiration biopsy. J Clin Ultrasound 1997;25:283–292.

32. van den Brekel M, Stel H, Castelijns J, et al. Cervical lymph node metastasis: assessment of radiologic criteria. Radiology 1990;177:379–384.

33. Ying M, Ahuja A, Brook F, et al. Sonographic appearance and distribution of normal cervical lymph nodes in a Chinese population. J Ultrasound Med 1996;15:431–436.

34. Wu C-H, Chang Y-L, Hsu W-C, et al. Usefulness of Doppler spectral analysis and power Doppler sonography in the differentiation of cervical lymphadenopathies. AJR Am J Roentgenol 1998;171:503–509.

35. Ying M, Ahuja A, Metreweli C. Diagnostic accuracy of sonographic criteria for evaluation of cervical adenopathy. J Ultrasound Med 1998;17:437–445.

36. Na D, Lim H, Byun H. Differential diagnosis of cervical lymphadenopathy: usefulness of color Doppler sonography. AJR Am J Roentgenol 1997;168:1311–1316.

37. Som P, Sacher M, Lanzieri C, et al. Parenchymal cysts of the lower neck. Radiology 1985;157:399–406.

38. Noujaim S, Arpasi P, Fink-Bennett D, et al. Imaging thyroglossal duct anomalies. Radiologist 1997;4:235–241.

39. Wadsworth D, Siegel M. Thyroglossal duct cysts: variability of sonographic findings. AJR Am J Roentgenol 1994;163:1475–1477.

40. Bowell W. Thyroglossal duct carcinoma. Am Surgeon 1994;60:650–655.

41. Benson M, Dalen K, Mancuso A, et al. Congenital anomalies of the branchial apparatus: embryology and pathologic anatomy. RadioGraphics 1992;12:943–960.

42. Sheth S, Nussbaum A, Hutchins G, et al. Cystic hygromas in children: sonographic-pathologic correlation. Radiology 1987;162:821–824.

43. Yasumoto M, Shibuya H, Gomi N, et al. Ultrasonographic appearance of dermoid and epidermoid cysts in the head and neck. J Clin Ultrasound 1991;19:455–461.

NEONATAL NEUROSONOGRAPHY

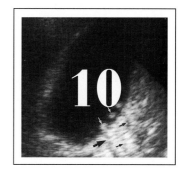

- Cranial Sonography
- Spine Sonography

Sonography provides a cost-effective, readily available method to image the infant brain. It is especially valuable because it can be performed at the bedside of premature or critically ill infants, keeping the infant within the protective environment of the neonatal intensive care unit. US is particularly accurate in the detection and follow-up of intracranial hemorrhage and is used to screen for a wide variety of congenital brain anomalies and for complications of central nervous system infection [1].

Spinal sonography is used to demonstrate the anatomy of the spinal canal and the position of the conus medullaris in infants at risk for a tethered spinal cord.

CRANIAL SONOGRAPHY

IMAGING TECHNIQUE

The anterior fontanelle provides an excellent sonographic window to image the infant brain. High-frequency 7.5-MHz sector or curved array transducers are utilized to examine the brain in angled sagittal and coronal planes. From the anterior fontanelle, the transducer is swept from the frontal to the occipital lobes in coronal orientation to obtain symmetrical images of the cerebral hemispheres and lateral ventricles. Care must be taken to orient the transducer properly to display the right side of the infant brain on the left side of the image. The transducer is turned 90 degrees for the sagittal plane. A midline sagittal view demonstrates the third ventricle, brain stem, and posterior fossa. The transducer is angled right and left from its midline sagittal position to examine each hemisphere and lateral ventricle in detail. The posterior fontanelle, the foramen magnum, and the thin squamous portion of the temporal bone may be utilized to provide supplementary images whenever indicated [2,3]. Lower-frequency transducers (3.5–5.0 MHz) may be needed to improve penetration in older and larger infants. Representative views of the cerebral hemispheres, lateral ventricles, third ventricle, choroid plexus, caudothalamic groove, corpus callosum, cavum septum pellucidum/vergae, fourth ventricle, and vermis of the cerebellum are documented [4]. US examination can routinely be performed up to approximately 12–14 months of age when the fontanelle becomes too small to serve as an effective window.

ANATOMY

Basic Infant Brain Anatomy

Several concepts of infant brain anatomy must be kept in mind when performing and interpreting sonography of the neonatal brain. The ventricles can be conceptualized as the easily identified "skeleton" of the brain. Their complex shape must be recognized in each plane of section. Surrounding structures are then identified with respect to their location relative to the ventricles. The **lateral ventricles** form the framework of each cerebral hemisphere. Each lateral ventricle has a frontal horn, body, atrium, occipital horn, and temporal horn. The lateral ventricles are commonly (in up to 70% of individuals) mildly asymmetric in size. Normal lateral ventricles may be tiny slits or form angulated or comma-shaped lucencies on coronal images [5]. The atrium or trigone is the junction of the temporal and occipital horns with the body of the lateral ventricle. The **choroid plexus** functions as the site of production of cerebrospinal fluid (CSF) and forms a prominent echogenic structure that lines the temporal horn, atrium, and body of each lateral ventricle. No choroid plexus is present in the frontal horns or occipital horns. This is most important to note because acute hemorrhage has the same echogenicity as the choroid plexus and is recognized primarily by location. Echogenic material in the anterior or occipital horns is hemorrhage, not choroid plexus. The choroid plexus is biggest in the atrium of each lateral ventricle. This prominent blob of choroid plexus in the atrium is called the **glomus**. The choroid plexus extends forward from the glomus to pass through the **foramen of Monro** and then reflects posteriorly along the roof of the third ventricle. The anterior-most portion of the choroid plexus in the roof of the third ventricle serves as a marker for the location of the foremen of Monro.

The **germinal matrix** is a group of loosely organized proliferating cells that give rise to the neurons of the cerebral cortex during embryologic development. The germinal matrix is exceptionally vascular with a network of thin fragile capillaries highly susceptible to injury by hypoxia. In early gestation, the germinal matrix lines the wall of the entire ventricular system, lying just beneath the **ependyma**, the thin membranous lining of the ventricular system. After 12 weeks gestation, the germinal matrix begins to regress. By 24 weeks, only the germinal matrix over the caudate nucleus persists. By full term at 40 weeks, the germinal matrix no longer exists. Thus hemorrhage of the germinal matrix is a disease of premature infants. It originates in the residual germinal matrix that overlies the caudate nucleus in the frontal horns of the lateral ventricles. The normal germinal matrix is not visualized by US.

A prominent fluid-filled structure is seen in the midline of the developing brain. This cystic structure is solitary and continuous, but for reasons unknown to me, it is given two unhandy names [6]. The anterior portion is called the **cavum septum pellucidum** whereas the posterior portion is called the **cavum vergae**. The foramen of Monro marks the divide between the two names. This structure involutes from back to front during fetal life and infancy. At full term, only the cavum septum pellucidum exists in most infants. This structure normally closes completely by 3–6 months of life. However, in approximately 5% of adults it persists as a residual fetal structure. The cavum septum pellucidum/vergae has been mistaken for hydrocephaly.

In premature infants, the surface of the cerebral hemispheres is smooth and flat [7]. With development between the equivalent of 24 and 40 weeks gestation, the sulci deepen, bend, and branch to form the prominent normal gyral pattern of full-term infants.

Although cisterns are by definition CSF-filled spaces around the brain, on US the cisterns are often echogenic rather than echolucent. The echogenicity is produced by reflection from folds of meninges that float in the fluid of the cisterns.

Coronal Plane Anatomy

In coronal plane, the most anterior section is obtained anterior to the frontal horns. This image documents the frontal lobes extending over the orbits (Fig. 10.1).

The next plane posterior documents the **frontal horns**, which appear as paired slit-like or comma-shaped anechoic structures (Fig. 10.2). The **caudate nuclei** form the angled

Differences in the anatomy of the brain of premature infants as compared to older children must always be kept in mind when interpreting neonatal brain sonograms.

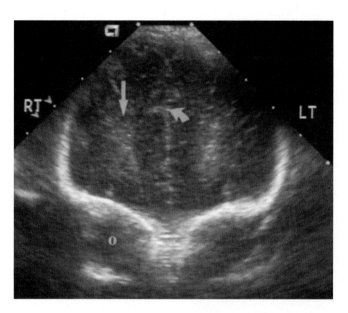

Figure 10.1 *Coronal Plane—Frontal Lobes.* This anatomic plane is just anterior to the frontal horns of the lateral ventricles. Normal periventricular echogenicity is evident centrally in each frontal lobe (*straight arrow*). The curved arrow indicates the midline sagittal fissure. o, orbit.

floors of the frontal horns and must be inspected in detail to detect small echogenic hemorrhages of the germinal matrix. The **cavum septum pellucidum** is the anechoic fluid-filled structure in the midline. The hypoechoic band extending between the cerebral hemispheres just above the cavum septum pellucidum is the **corpus callosum** [8]. The midline

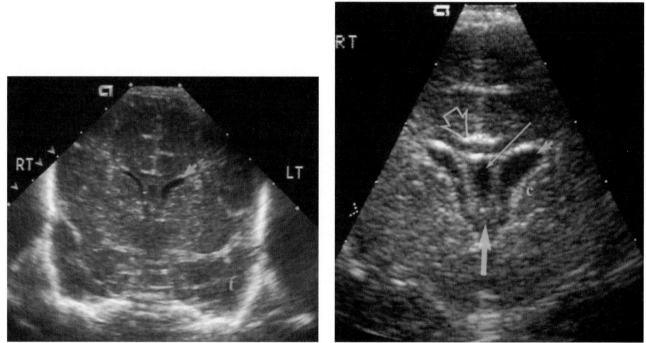

Figure 10.2 *Coronal Plane—Frontal Horns.* Images demonstrate the full field of view (*A*) and a coned down view (*B*) of the frontal horns (*shortest arrow*) in two different infants. The cavum septum pellucidum is the cystic space (*long thin arrow*) between the frontal horns. The lateral wall (the septum pellucidum) of the cavum septum pellucidum is the medial wall of the frontal horn. The corpus callosum (*open arrow*) is the hypoechoic white matter band that connects the two hemispheres and provides the floor of the sagittal fissure. The caudate nucleus (c) serves as the angled floor of the frontal horn. The echogenic blob of the choroid plexus in the roof of the third ventricle is absent (*large solid arrow*) indicating that this anatomic plane is anterior to the foramen of Monro. Echogenic foci in the caudate nuclei in this plane are indicative of germinal matrix hemorrhage. t, temporal lobe.

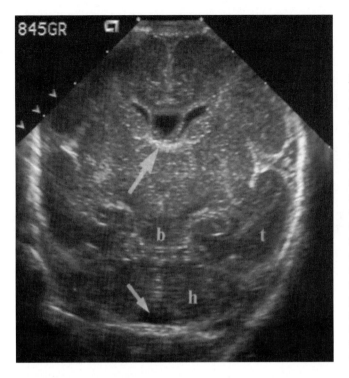

Figure 10.3 *Coronal Plane—Third Ventricle.* The echogenic choroid plexus (*large arrow*) is visible lying along the roof of the third ventricle just inferior to the cavum septum pellucidum. This landmark indicates the plane of section is posterior to the foramen of Monro. Echogenic choroid plexus may be seen normally overlying the caudate nucleus in the lateral ventricles in this plane of section. The third ventricle is usually slit-like and is not discretely visualized in coronal plane. Also seen on this image are a portion of the brainstem (b), the cerebellar hemisphere (h), the cisterna magna (*small arrow*), and the temporal lobes (t).

sagittal fissure extends to the level of the corpus callosum. Anterior cerebral arteries pulsate and are visible with color Doppler in the sagittal fissure. The tips of the temporal lobes are seen inferiorly and laterally.

Moving posteriorly to a direct coronal plane, the echogenic **choroid plexus** is visualized in the midline just below the cavum septum pellucidum (Fig. 10.3). The choroid plexus is normally present in both lateral ventricles in the same anatomic planes where the choroid is visualized in the roof of the third ventricle, but not in the frontal horns more anteriorly. The third ventricle is slit-like and may be seen as a linear lucency between the oval globes of the thalami. Commonly the normal third ventricle is not seen as a discrete structure. Portions of the hypoechoic brainstem are seen in the midline below the third ventricle and thalami.

A posteriorly angled coronal plane demonstrates the prominent echogenic **glomus of the choroid plexus** in atria of the lateral ventricles (Fig. 10.4). The glomus swings dependently toward the downside of the baby's head, commonly revealing a gap between the wall of the lateral ventricle and the choroid plexus. The tentorium may be seen as an echogenic wall between the cerebrum and cerebellum.

Further posterior angulation of the transducer produces an image of the occipital lobes above the level of the occipital horns (Fig. 10.5). Vague symmetric echogenicity should be evident bilaterally. The echogenicity is produced by sound reflection from **periventricular white matter tracts**. The acute hemorrhagic stage of periventricular leukomalacia (PVL) produces asymmetric or increased echogenicity in this area. Cystic change is easily seen in this plane during the later cystic stage of PVL.

Sagittal Plane Anatomy

A direct midline sagittal image demonstrates the **corpus callosum** as a well-defined, curving hypoechoic band above the cystic cavum septum pellucidum/vergae (Fig. 10.6) [8]. The anterior **genu** and posterior **splenium** are normally slightly thicker than the trunk of the corpus callosum. The entire corpus callosum should be visualized to avoid missing partial agenesis. Immediately inferior to the cavum septum pellucidum is the curving echogenic band of the **choroid plexus in the roof of the third ventricle**. The third ventricle is normally slit-like and is not distinctly visualized. The midline **cerebellar vermis** is seen as a rounded echogenic mass in the posterior fossa. The **fourth ventricle** is visualized as a

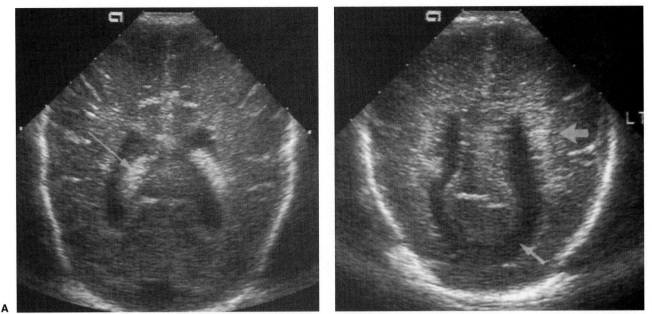

A   B

Figure 10.4 *Coronal Plane—Lateral Ventricles. A.* Posteriorly angled coronal view shows the prominent glomus (*arrow*) of the choroid plexus in the atrium of the lateral ventricles. When this scan was obtained, the infant was lying with the left side of his head down. The choroid plexus lies dependently against the left lateral wall of the ventricle. *B.* Image angled further posteriorly shows the occipital horns of the lateral ventricles (*small arrow*). The size of the occipital horns is commonly asymmetric. Note the prominent but symmetric echogenicity of the periventricular white matter tracts (*large arrow*).

triangular lucency at the mid-base of the echogenic vermis [9]. Anterior to the vermis is the hypoechoic and poorly defined **brainstem**. The pons is more echogenic than the remainder of the brainstem. Special note should always be made of the presence or absence of the **cisterna magna** inferior to the vermis. Obliteration of the cisterna magna is seen with Chiari malformation.

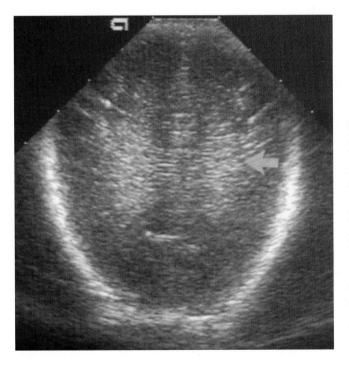

Figure 10.5 *Coronal Plane—Periventricular White Matter.* With the transducer held in coronal orientation at the anterior fontanelle, this image is obtained by angling the transducer far posteriorly approaching an axial plane. The prominent echogenic periventricular white matter (*arrow*) is demonstrated superior to the lateral ventricles. The normal echogenicity is symmetric. Asymmetry of the periventricular echogenicity suggests the early hemorrhagic stage of periventricular leukomalacia.

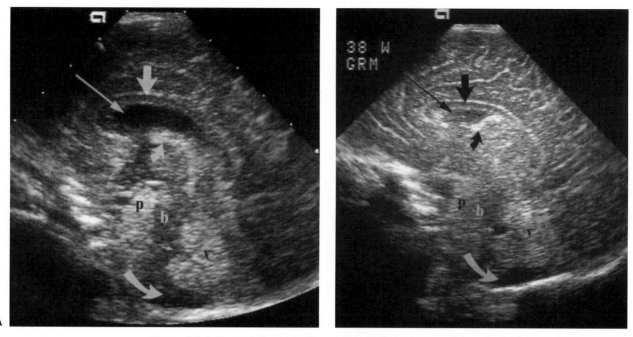

Figure 10.6 *Sagittal Plane—Midline.* Images of a premature (*A*) and a full-term (*B*) newborn infant demonstrate the important normal anatomic landmarks. The midline cystic cavum septum pellucidum (*long arrow*) and cavum vergae are prominent in the premature infant but are smaller and limited to only the cavum septum pellucidum in the full-term infant. Note the increased prominence of the gyri and sulci in the full-term infant compared to the relatively featureless brain of the premature. The corpus callosum (*fat arrow*) forms a curving hypoechoic band just above the cavum septum pellucidum. The choroid plexus (*short curved arrow*) in the roof of the third ventricle forms an echogenic band just below the cavum septum pellucidum. The vermis (v) of the cerebellum is a round echogenic mass in the posterior fossa. The fourth ventricle (*tiny arrow*) is seen as a triangular lucency indenting the vermis. Anterior to the vermis is the hypoechoic brainstem (b). The pons (p) is echogenic compared to the remainder of the brainstem. A normal fluid-filled cisterna magna (*long curved arrow*) should always be present. Absence of the cisterna magna is indicative of a Chiari defect.

Approximately 10 degrees of lateral angulation to each side will demonstrate the lateral ventricles (Fig. 10.7). Note that the frontal horns are slightly closer together than the atria of the lateral ventricles. To show the long axis of the ventricles, the posterior aspect of the transducer is angled slightly more laterally than the anterior portion. The important landmarks here are the round shape of the **thalamus** and the tongue shape of the **caudate nucleus**. These two structures are nearly isoechoic but are separated by a slight V-shaped defect and echogenic line called the **caudothalamic groove**. The caudothalamic groove marks the location of the foramen of Monro and the anterior-most location of the choroid plexus [10]. Echogenicity in the caudate nucleus anterior to the caudothalamic groove indicates hemorrhage in the germinal matrix. The lateral ventricle enlarges posteriorly and contains the **glomus** of the choroid plexus. The glomus is commonly lobulated in contour. The **occipital horns** may be seen further posteriorly. Their size is quite variable and they are commonly asymmetric. Remember no choroid plexus is present in the occipital horns, so echogenicity in the occipital horns usually represents intraventricular blood clot.

Further lateral angulation will demonstrate the ill-defined normal echogenicity of the **periventricular white matter tracts** (Fig. 10.8). Asymmetric or increased echogenicity suggests the hemorrhagic stage of PVL. This laterally angled image plane is best for demonstrating the cystic change of PVL as well.

Sonographic landmarks of the location of the foramen of Monro are the anterior-most aspect of the choroid plexus in the roof of the third ventricle and the caudothalamic groove.

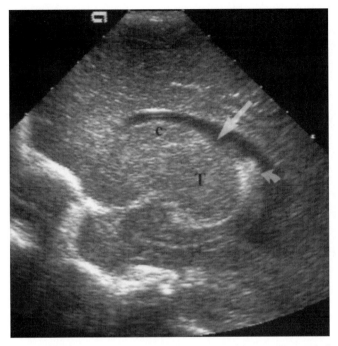

Figure 10.7 *Sagittal Plane—Lateral Ventricle.* Laterally angled, sagittally oriented image demonstrates the rounded mass of the thalamus (T) and the tongue-shaped structure of the caudate nucleus (c). The slight indentation between these two structures is the caudothalamic groove (*straight arrow*). The caudothalamic groove is the sagittal plane marker of the location of the foramen of Monro. Echogenic mass replacing the tip of the tongue of the caudate nucleus anterior to the caudothalamic groove is indicative of germinal matrix hemorrhage. The echogenic glomus of the choroid plexus (*curved arrow*) is seen in the atrium of the lateral ventricle. Echogenic choroid plexus extends anteriorly and inferiorly into the temporal horn.

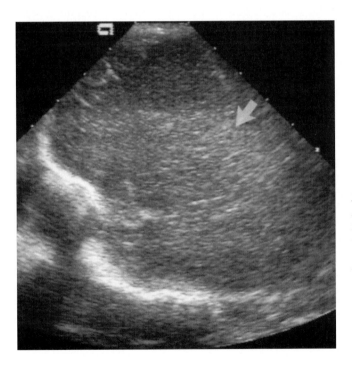

Figure 10.8 *Sagittal Plane—Periventricular White Matter.* Sagittally oriented view angled further laterally demonstrates the echogenic periventricular white matter (*arrow*). This view is utilized to detect periventricular leukomalacia. The echogenicity of the right side should be compared to the echogenicity of the left side.

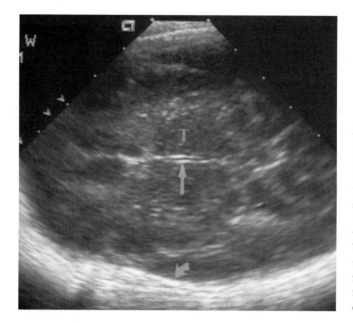

Figure 10.9 *Axial Plane—Third Ventricle.* An axial plane view obtained by imaging through the thin squamous portion of the temporal bone is optimal for demonstrating the third ventricle (*straight arrow*). The normal third ventricle is a slit-like structure between the two walnut-shaped thalami (T). The brain–cranium interface (*curved arrow*) should be noted to detect extra-axial fluid collections.

Axial Plane Anatomy

Axial plane images are a useful addition to routine examination. The squamous portion of the temporal bone is thin enough in infants to allow adequate US penetration. Two image planes are most useful.

A mid-thalamic plane, similar to the plane used to measure biparietal diameter in the fetus, demonstrates the **third ventricle** and **thalami** (Fig. 10.9). The third ventricle is normally a narrow slit. In axial plane the sound beam is perpendicular to the lateral walls of the third ventricle and shows the size of the ventricle better than the coronal or sagittal plane. Axial plane views also demonstrate the lateral interface between brain and cranium and are useful for detection of extra-axial fluid collections and abnormalities of the cerebral cortex.

Just inferior to the plane of the third ventricle is the plane of the **suprasellar cistern** (Fig. 10.10). The cistern has the appearance of a 5-pointed echogenic star. The **hypothalamus** is seen as an oval structure centered in the cistern. The arteries of the **circle of Willis** are clearly visualized as pulsating vessels encircling the cistern on real-time US. This is an excellent plane for Doppler evaluation of these vessels. Posterior to the cistern is the heart-shaped structure of the **cerebral peduncles**. In the midline posterior aspect of the peduncles courses the **cerebellar aqueduct**, seen as an echogenic dot with or without a central lucency.

HYPOXIC BRAIN INJURY

Premature infants are routinely screened for hypoxic brain injury 4–7 days after birth.

Hypoxia is a common event in the sick neonate, especially in the premature infant with underdeveloped lungs. Hypoxia may result in two basic types of infant brain injuries: germinal matrix hemorrhage (GMH) and PVL [11]. The prevalence of GMH in infants born before 32 weeks gestation or with birth weight less than 1500 g is 30–55%. The prevalence of PVL in these infants is 10–40%.

It is important to note that the arterial watershed areas are different in the infant brain than in the adult or older child. In the premature infant, the watershed areas most susceptible to hypoxic injury are in the regions of the periventricular white matter. Autoregulation of cerebral blood pressure is commonly lacking in the neonate, making the infant more susceptible to hypoxic injury and hemorrhage associated with hypotension or hypertension.

Germinal Matrix Hemorrhage

GMH is a disease confined to premature infants, because the germinal matrix resorbs and is no longer present at full term. GMH is also commonly called *subependymal hemorrhage*

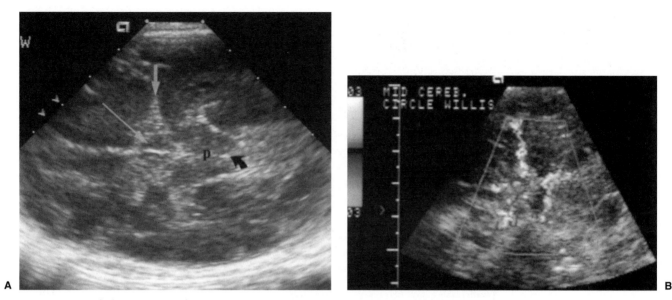

Figure 10.10 *Axial Plane—Suprasellar Cistern. A.* Axial plane view obtained more inferiorly demonstrates the suprasellar cistern as a 5-pointed-star-shaped echogenic structure (*short arrow*) surrounding the hypothalamus (*long arrow*). Posterior to the suprasellar cistern is the heart-shaped structure of the cerebral peduncles (p). The echogenic spot (*curved arrow*) at the apex of the "heart" is the cerebral aqueduct (of Sylvius). *B.* With color Doppler (*shown here in gray scale*), the circle of Willis is clearly visible in the suprasellar cistern.

because of the subependymal location of the germinal matrix, or is called *intraventricular hemorrhage* because extension of hemorrhage into the ventricles is common. The Papile classification of GMH is commonly utilized (Table 10.1) [12]. More severe grades of hemorrhage are predictive of worse neurological prognosis. GMH may result in cerebral palsy, developmental delays, and learning disabilities (see Fig. 10.14) [13]. Hemorrhages occur initially in the subependymal caudate nucleus in the frontal horn and then extend elsewhere in the brain [14].

- GMH may be unilateral or bilateral.
- Grade I GMH is seen as a small discrete focus of increased echogenicity in the region of the caudate nucleus (Fig. 10.11).
- Grade II GMH extends into the ventricular system and appears as an echogenic cast of a portion of, or the entire, lateral ventricle. The ventricle itself may be obscured by the

Table 10.1: Grading of Germinal Matrix Hemorrhage

Grade	Description	US Findings
I	Subependymal germinal matrix hemorrhage confined to region of caudate nucleus	Hemorrhage is hyperechoic compared to brain parenchyma and equal in echogenicity to choroid plexus.
II	Intraventricular extension of germinal matrix hemorrhage without ventriculomegaly	Echogenic clot makes a cast of the normal size ventricle. Clot is seen within the frontal or occipital horns of the lateral ventricle.
III	Intraventricular hemorrhage with hydrocephaly	Same as Grade II but with enlarged ventricles.
IV	Intraparenchymal hemorrhage	Echogenic clot within brain parenchyma.

Adapted from Papile L, Burstein J, Burstein R, et al. Incidence and evolution of subependymal and intraventricular hemorrhage: study of infants with birth weight less than 1500 grams. J Pediatr 1978;92:529–534, with permission.

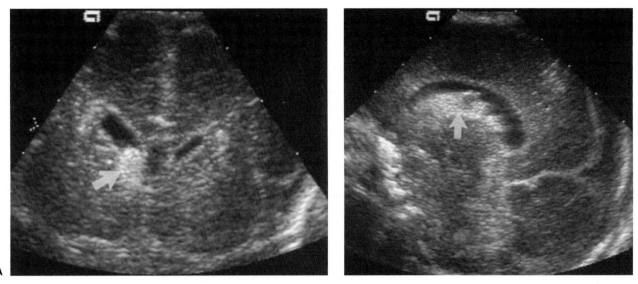

Figure 10.11 *Germinal Matrix Hemorrhage—Grade I. A. Coronal view. B. Sagittal view. Focal echogenicity* (*arrows*) *overlying the right caudate nucleus seen in two anatomic planes is indicative of germinal matrix hemorrhage, Grade I. The right ventricle is slightly larger than the left ventricle, but no evidence of blood is seen within the ventricular system.*

clot. Floating clot may be seen in the frontal or occipital horns. Blood may form a fluid level with CSF. The size of the ventricle remains normal (Fig. 10.12).

■ Grade III GMH is intraventricular hemorrhage with ventricular enlargement. The ventricles are measurably larger. The contour of the ventricles becomes rounded. Clot is seen within the ventricular system (Fig. 10.13).

■ Grade IV GMH is intraparenchymal hemorrhage caused by venous infarction complicating GMH (Fig. 10.14). Large GMH compresses and may thrombose subependymal veins that course through the area of hemorrhage. This results in hemorrhagic infarction of

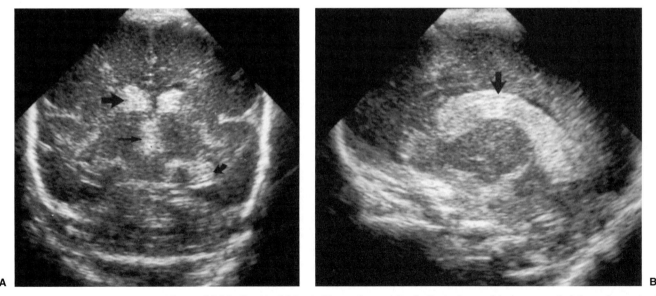

Figure 10.12 *Germinal Matrix Hemorrhage—Grade II. A. Coronal image reveals bilateral germinal matrix hemorrhages that extend into the normal sized ventricle system forming an echogenic cast of the lateral* (*fat arrow*) *and third* (*small arrow*) *ventricles. Clot is also evident in the temporal horn* (*curved arrow*) *of the left lateral ventricle. B. Sagittal view of the right lateral ventricle shows the ventricular cast* (*arrow*) *formed by clot.*

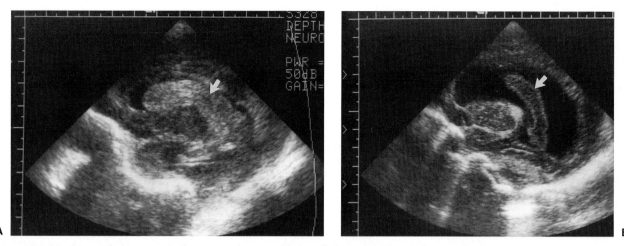

A   B

Figure 10.13 *Germinal Matrix Hemorrhage—Grade III—Evolution of Clot. A.* Initial sagittal image shows echogenic blood clot (*arrow*) filling and enlarging the lateral ventricle. Note the lucency surrounding the clot that confirms enlargement of the ventricle. *B.* Image of the same ventricle obtained 16 days later shows further enlargement of the ventricle and typical evolution of blood clot. The clot (*arrow*) is reduced in size and is decreased in echogenicity centrally while maintaining an echogenic rim.

periventricular brain parenchyma in the frontal to parieto-occipital lobes. Brain necrosis leads to porencephaly and results in spastic hemiparesis by disruption of the corticospinal motor tracts that course through the area of infarction. US shows echogenic clot in the involved parenchyma (Fig. 10.15).

- Blood clot shows characteristic evolution over time (Fig. 10.13) [15]. Following acute hemorrhage, clot is equal to or exceeds the echogenicity of choroid plexus. As the clot ages, it shrinks and becomes more echolucent centrally while remaining echogenic peripherally. As clot lyses, floating echogenic debris is seen within the ventricles. Clot fragments appear as larger floating masses. Clots may adhere to the walls of the ventricles and to the choroid plexus causing a "lumpy-bumpy" choroid (Fig. 10.15A).

- Chemical ventriculitis resulting from hemorrhage causes thickening and increased echogenicity of the ependymal lining, "ependymitis."

- Hydrocephaly commonly results from intraventricular hemorrhage (Fig. 10.16, Box 10.1). Clots may obstruct the foramen of Monro, the cerebral aqueduct, the outflow

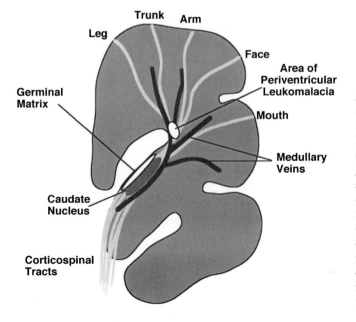

Figure 10.14 *Anatomy of the Corticospinal Tracts and Medullary Veins.* Line drawing of the left hemisphere in coronal plane orientation demonstrates how germinal matrix hemorrhage and periventricular leukomalacia can injure the corticospinal tracts and cause cerebral palsy. Germinal matrix hemorrhage can cause thrombosis of the nearby medullary veins that drain the motor cortex, resulting in hemorrhagic infarction in the parietal lobe.

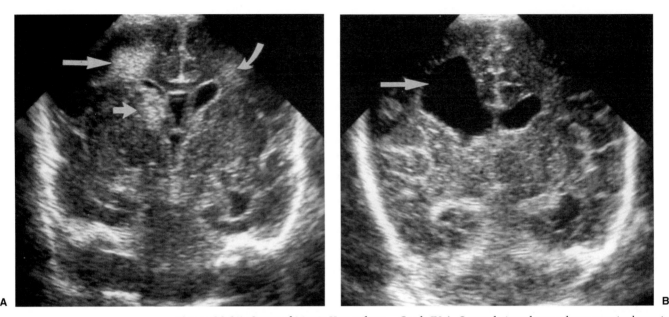

Figure 10.15 *Germinal Matrix Hemorrhage—Grade IV. A.* Coronal view shows a large germinal matrix hemorrhage (*short arrow*) that extends to involve the medullary veins, resulting in hemorrhagic parenchymal infarction (*large arrow*). Compare to the drawing in Figure 10.14. An area of increased echogenicity at the angle of the left frontal horn (*curved arrow*) represents coexistent hemorrhagic periventricular leukomalacia. *B.* Image of the same patient obtained approximately 3 weeks later shows a large defect of porencephaly (*arrow*) in the area of brain involved by the hemorrhagic infarction.

tracts of the fourth ventricle, or the arachnoid granulations. Shunting may be required if hydrocephaly is progressive, but most cases resolve spontaneously with lysis of the clots. Ventricular size can be followed by US measurement of the frontal horns.

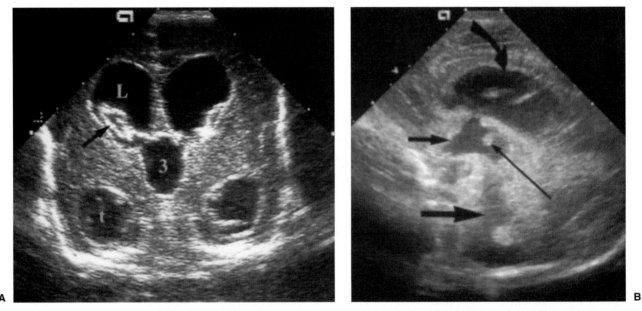

Figure 10.16 *Hydrocephaly Complicates Germinal Matrix Hemorrhage. A.* Coronal view demonstrates marked ventriculomegaly involving both lateral ventricles (L) and the third ventricle (3). The temporal horns (t) are markedly dilated. Resorbing clot (*arrow*) is seen in the lateral ventricles. *B.* Midline sagittal view shows the dilated third (*small arrow*) and fourth (*large arrow*) ventricles. The circular band (*long skinny arrow*) crossing the third ventricle is the massa intermedia. The dilated lateral ventricles are seen as a fluid-filled structures (*curved arrow*) above the third ventricle.

> ### *Box 10.1: Ultrasound Sequela of Germinal Matrix Hemorrhage*
>
> Subependymal cysts   Hydrocephalus
> Parenchymal cysts   Brain atrophy
> Porencephaly

- Subependymal and intraparenchymal cysts may occur in areas of necrosis caused by hemorrhage (Fig. 10.17). The cysts appear as the hemorrhage resolves usually 3–6 weeks after the acute event. These cystic areas do not communicate with the ventricles. The cysts may subsequently resolve completely or form a linear echogenic scar.

- Porencephaly describes the resorption of an area of infarcted brain parenchyma resulting in an area of absent brain tissue that communicates with the ventricular system (Figs. 10.15, 10.18). Porencephaly results from large intraparenchymal hemorrhages and is commonly associated with spastic paresis.

Periventricular Leukomalacia

PVL is infarction and necrosis of the periventricular white matter [16]. It results from severe hypoxia usually caused by episodes of hypotension. PVL occurs commonly in premature infants but also occurs in compromised full-term neonates. Long-term sequelae of PVL include spastic diplegia or quadriplegia, visual defects, developmental delays, and intellectual deficits [14].

- PVL is most commonly bilateral and symmetric. However, it may be unilateral (Fig. 10.19).

- Initial US examination is commonly normal because the injury is ischemic and without associated hemorrhage.

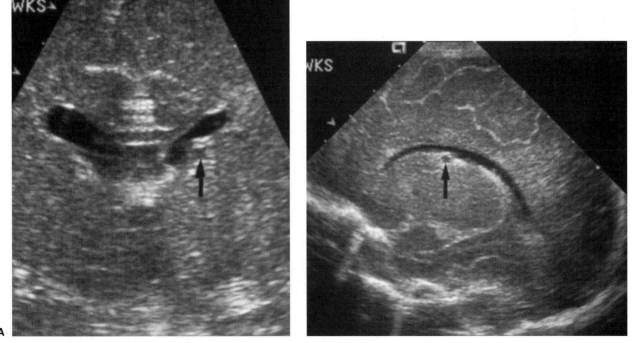

Figure 10.17 *Subependymal Cyst. A.* Coronal image. *B.* Sagittal image. Tiny subependymal cyst (*arrow*) is the only residual US finding of a Grade I germinal matrix hemorrhage.

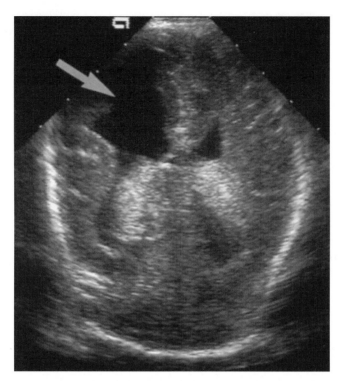

Figure 10.18 *Porencephaly.* Coronal image shows a large cystic area (*arrow*) of infarcted parietal lobe that communicates openly with the right lateral ventricle. Hemorrhage resulted in infarction, necrosis, and resorption of brain parenchyma.

■ Hemorrhage, which occurs with reperfusion of the injured area, causes increased echogenicity of periventricular white matter. This finding is commonly equivocal because the periventricular white matter is normally echogenic. Echogenicity that exceeds that of the choroid plexus is highly indicative of PVL (Fig. 10.19).

■ Cysts occur in periventricular white matter at 2–3 weeks following acute injury (Fig. 10.20). These cysts reflect necrosis and loss of white matter tracts. Cysts are usually multiple and cause a fenestrated appearance to the brain parenchyma. Cysts vary in size up to 1–2 cm.

■ Cysts resolve within several weeks to several months, resulting in a glial scar that is shown with high sensitivity by MR but not by US.

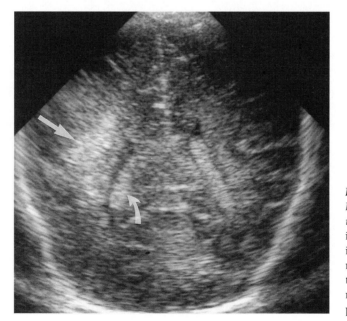

Figure 10.19 *Periventricular Leukomalacia—Early Hemorrhagic Stage.* Coronal plane image demonstrates asymmetric increased echogenicity in the right periventricular white matter (*straight arrow*). The echogenicity exceeds that of the choroid plexus (*curved arrow*).

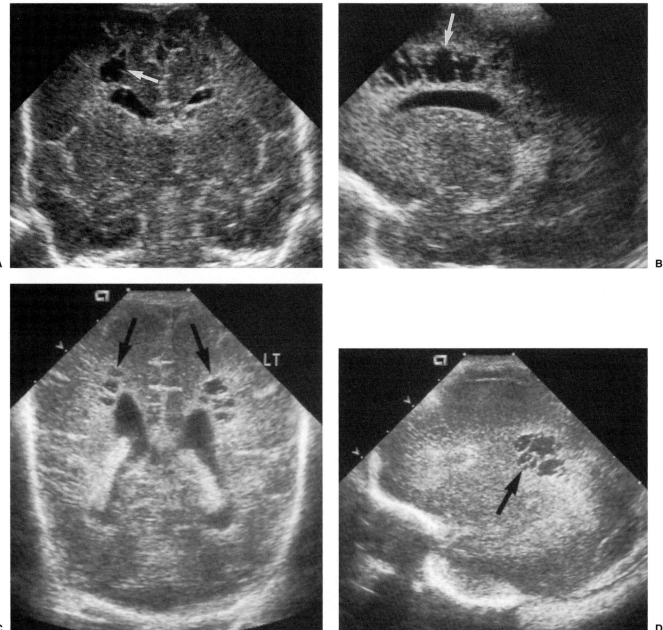

Figure 10.20 *Periventricular Leukomalacia.* Four examples of periventricular leukomalacia (*arrows*) in different patients are shown. Note the fenestrated cystic appearance and location of periventricular leukomalacia. Image *D* shows the value of the far lateral sagittal plane image. *A.* Coronal plane. *B.* Sagittal plane. *C.* Posterior coronal plane. *D.* Far lateral sagittal plane.

■ Because US examination may be normal in the acute phase of PVL, high-risk infants should be screened at approximately 3 weeks of age to detect the cystic change of PVL for which US is highly sensitive.

Diffuse Brain Edema

Severe hypoxia may cause diffuse brain swelling with or without acute hemorrhage in premature or full-term infants. This injury often occurs with asphyxia at birth.

■ The brain is mildly and diffusely increased in echogenicity with poor definition of anatomic structures.

- The ventricles are slit-like and the gyri appear compressed.
- If infarction occurs, brain atrophy becomes evident approximately 2 weeks after the acute event. Extra-axial fluid spaces become enlarged. Gyri and sulci appear prominent. Ventricles enlarge due to loss of brain parenchyma. Diffuse cystic encephalomalacia or porencephaly may be evident. Dystrophic calcifications may be seen in areas of destroyed brain parenchyma.
- This injury may be superimposed on findings of GMH and PVL.

CONGENITAL ANOMALIES

US is used to screen for and to classify major congenital brain malformations [17]. However, MR is commonly needed to confirm the classification and to detect subtle associated anomalies such as neuronal migration anomalies not evident on US examination.

Holoprosencephaly
Holoprosencephaly is a spectrum of malformations caused by failure of complete division of midline structures.

- Septo-optic dysplasia is the mildest form, with absence of the septum pellucidum and hypoplasia of the optic nerves. The frontal horns are flattened and the ventricles are characteristically downward pointing (Fig. 10.21).
- Lobar holoprosencephaly has fused frontal horns with absent septum pellucidum but has separated occipital horns. The frontal horns have a box-shaped appearance. The third ventricle is present.
- Semilobar holoprosencephaly consists of a single ventricle with some separation of the temporal and occipital horns. Incomplete falx and interhemispheric fissure are usually present. The thalami are partially separated and the third ventricle is rudimentary. The splenium of the corpus callosum is present but the remainder of the corpus callosum is absent.
- Alobar holoprosencephaly is the most severe and usually fatal form (see Fig. 7.45). Severe facial anomalies including cyclopia, cebocephaly, and midline clefts are usually present. A single, large, horseshoe-shaped ventricle is present with the surrounding cortex being thin and poorly developed. The cerebral hemispheres and thalami are fused. The corpus callosum, falx, interhemispheric fissure, and third ventricle are absent. The posterior fossa structures are often normal.

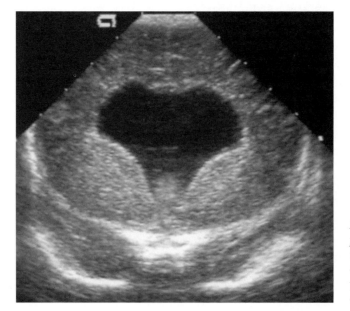

Figure 10.21 *Septo-Optic Dysplasia.* The frontal horns are fused and downward pointing on this coronal image. The corpus callosum and septum pellucidum are absent.

Hydranencephaly

Hydranencephaly is near complete destruction of the cerebral cortex caused by *in utero* occlusion of both internal carotid arteries or by other severely destructive processes.

- The calvarium is filled with CSF, but no peripheral brain tissue is evident (see Fig. 7.46).
- The falx is usually identifiable but often is incomplete. Visualization of even part of the falx helps differentiate this condition from alobar holoprosencephaly.
- The thalamus and posterior fossa structures are normal.
- Doppler shows no flow in the carotid arteries.

Congenital Hydrocephaly

Ventriculomegaly may be caused by obstruction to CSF flow, overproduction of CSF (choroid plexus tumor) or by loss of brain parenchyma (ex vacuo). Hemorrhage or infection may cause hydrocephaly by fibrosis of the foramen of Monro, the aqueduct, basal cisterns, or arachnoid granulations. Tumors or congenital malformations may obstruct the ventricles at any level.

- The ventricles are enlarged but maintain their normal shape.
- Peripheral cortex and midline structures are present.
- Dilatation of all ventricles suggests an extraventricular cause.
- Dilatation of the lateral and third ventricle with normal size of the fourth ventricle suggests aqueductal stenosis (Fig. 10.22). Aqueductal stenosis may be inherited as an X-linked recessive trait.

Dandy-Walker Malformation

Cystic anomalies of the posterior fossa are classified as Dandy-Walker malformations and variants [18].

- Classic Dandy-Walker malformation consists of dilatation of the fourth ventricle with direct communication with the cisterna magna (see Fig. 7.47). The posterior fossa is enlarged and the tentorium is elevated. The cerebellar vermis is absent or hypoplastic. The brainstem is compressed. Most cases have associated hydrocephalus (80%). The corpus callosum is usually absent (70%). Additional anomalies of brain development are commonly coexistent.

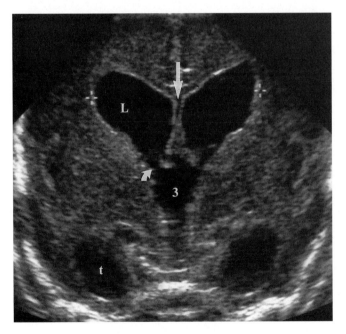

Figure 10.22 *Congenital Hydrocephalus—Aqueductal Stenosis.* Coronal image shows marked symmetric dilatation of the lateral (L) and third (3) ventricles and the foramina of Monro (*curved arrow*). The temporal horns (t) are prominently dilated. The fourth ventricle was normal in size, indicating congenital aqueductal stenosis as the most likely diagnosis. When the lateral ventricles are enlarged, the cavum septum pellucidum (*straight arrow*) is often compressed. Cursors (+) measure the biventricular diameter.

■ Dandy-Walker variant is a lesser degree of abnormality with hypoplasia of the vermis and lesser enlargement of the fourth ventricle. The posterior fossa is normal in size. No hydrocephalus is present.

■ Arachnoid cyst of the posterior fossa does not show communication of fourth ventricle and cisterna magna, although the fourth ventricle and brainstem may be displaced. A cyst wall may be visualized.

■ Mega cisterna magna is a normal variant with a normal fourth ventricle, brainstem, and cerebellum.

Chiari Malformations

Chiari malformations are a group of probably unrelated developmental anomalies that involve the posterior fossa.

■ Chiari I malformation is downward displacement of the cerebellar tonsils with or without displacement of the fourth ventricle or medulla. The cisterna magna is obliterated.

■ Chiari II malformations are the most common and are nearly always present in association with meningomyelocele (see Fig. 7.44). The posterior fossa is small and the tentorium is displaced downward. The cerebellar tonsils and vermis herniate into the spinal canal through an enlarged foramen magnum obliterating the cisterna magna. The fourth ventricle is elongated. Obstruction of the cerebellar aqueduct results in enlargement of the lateral and third ventricles. The septum pellucidum is usually partially or completely absent.

■ Chiari III is an encephalomeningocele in the high cervical region that contains the cerebellum, medulla, and fourth ventricle.

■ Chiari IV is severe hypoplasia of the cerebellum without displacement.

Agenesis of the Corpus Callosum

Agenesis of the corpus callosum may be partial or complete. It is commonly associated with other anomalies, but when isolated may have a normal prognosis [8].

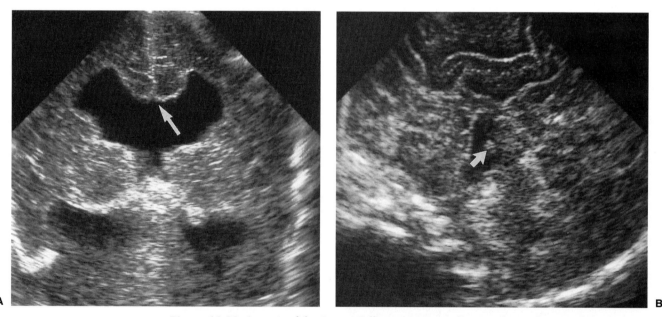

Figure 10.23 *Agenesis of the Corpus Callosum. A.* Coronal image shows absence of the hypoechoic band of the corpus callosum that crosses between the two hemispheres (*arrow*). The midline sagittal sinus extends all the way to the top of the fused frontal horns. The septum pellucidum is absent. *B.* Midline sagittal image confirms absence of the corpus callosum. The gyral pattern is somewhat disorganized in appearance. The massa intermedia (*arrow*) is seen in the third ventricle.

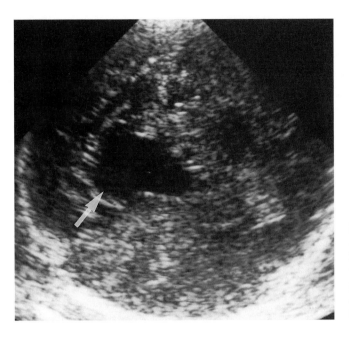

Figure 10.24 *Vein of Galen Aneurysm.* Posterior coronal image shows large cystic structure (*arrow*) that extends asymmetrically to the right. Doppler confirmed pulsatile turbulent blood flow.

- The well-defined hypoechoic band of the corpus callosum is partially or completely absent or is thinned (Fig. 10.23).
- The lateral ventricles are abnormally far apart.
- In coronal plane images, the frontal horns and bodies of the lateral ventricles have sharply angulated lateral peaks.
- The third ventricle is dilated and elevated. Its roof extends between the lateral ventricles and may extend to the interhemispheric fissure.
- Lipoma of the corpus callosum causes a highly echogenic mass that extends into both hemispheres. Dysgenesis of the corpus callosum is always present.

Vein of Galen Malformation
The vein of Galen malformation is the most common intracranial vascular anomaly presenting in the neonatal period. Multiple abnormal feeding vessels or an arteriovenous fistula with few feeding vessels drain into the vein of Galen, which becomes massively enlarged.

- The vein of Galen is greatly dilated, resulting in a large cystic mass posterior to the third ventricle (Fig. 10.24).
- Spectral or color flow Doppler reveals turbulent flow within the mass. Flow is pulsatile reflecting the arterial feeders.
- Blood flow in the more peripheral areas of the brain is decreased because of a vascular steal phenomenon shunting flow to the low resistance vascular malformation. Shunting of blood can result in brain atrophy and cortical calcifications.

INFECTION

Congenital Brain Infections
Congenital and perinatal brain infections are most commonly caused by *Toxoplasma gondii,* cytomegalovirus, rubella, and herpes simplex virus type II. All infections cause destructive lesions. Prenatal infections may cause developmental brain defects.

- Brain parenchymal calcifications are a major clue to the presence of congenital brain infection (Fig. 10.25). Calcifications may or may not cause acoustic shadowing. Effective treatment may result in resolution of the calcifications [19].

Parenchymal calcifications in the infant brain suggest congenital brain infection.

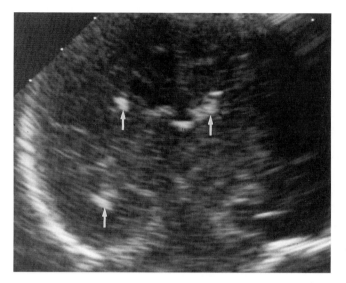

Figure 10.25 *Congenital Brain Infection.* Coronal image shows punctate periventricular calcifications (*arrows*), indicating high likelihood of congenital brain infection. Serum titers for cytomegalovirus were elevated.

- Toxoplasmosis results in periventricular and cortical calcifications, microcephaly, hydrocephaly, porencephaly, and diffuse brain atrophy.
- Cytomegalovirus causes periventricular calcifications, absent or small gyri, and hypoplasia of the cerebellum [20].
- Rubella causes calcifications in the periventricular white matter and basal ganglia, hydrocephaly, and microcephaly.
- Herpes simplex virus causes punctate or diffuse gyral calcifications, diffuse cerebral atrophy, and multicystic encephalomalacia.

Perinatal Meningitis

Meningitis is a serious illness in the neonate that can cause permanent neurological injury even if treated early in its course. Causative organisms include group B streptococcus, *Escherichia coli*, *Haemophilus influenzae*, *Streptococcus pneumoniae*, and *Neisseria meningitides*. Infections are usually hematogenously disseminated and cause ventriculitis and diffuse meningoencephalitis.

- US may be normal with early meningitis.

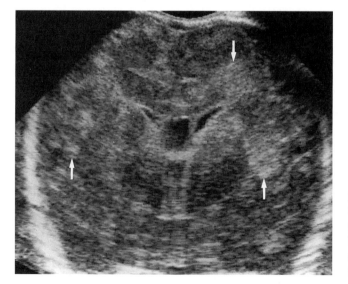

Figure 10.26 *Diffuse Cerebritis.* Candida septicemia in a premature infant caused diffuse cerebritis manifest as diffuse patchy areas of increased echogenicity (*arrows*).

■ Meningitis manifests as echogenic thickening of the meninges covering the gyri and sulci. Extraaxial fluid collections are usually present. Brain parenchyma echogenicity is focally or diffusely increased. Hydrocephalus may occur.

■ Ventricles are slit-like with early brain edema but onset of the ventriculitis causes ventricular enlargement with thickening and increased echogenicity of the lining ependyma. Echogenic fluid layers within the ventricles and avascular strands may cross the ventricular lumen.

■ Diffuse cerebritis appears as irregular patchy areas of increased and decreased parenchymal echogenicity (Fig. 10.26).

■ Brain abscess appears as a well-defined hypoechoic lesion containing echogenic, layering fluid. The wall is thick and echogenic. Mass effect displacing ventricles and brain structures is evident.

SPINE SONOGRAPHY

The primary indication for sonography of the infant spine is to detect a tethered spinal cord in infants who are clinically suspected of being at risk. US offers an easy, quick, readily available, and accurate method of examination [21]. The posterior elements of the infant spine are cartilage and can easily be penetrated by US up to age 12 weeks. Older infants should undergo MR imaging because posterior element ossification will obscure sonographic detail.

IMAGING TECHNIQUE

Available radiographs of the infant spine should be reviewed prior to examination. Note any evidence of segmentation anomalies or spinal dysraphism. A 7.0-MHz linear array transducer provides an optimal examination. The infant is placed in prone position with the upper body elevated slightly to distend the lower thecal sac with CSF. The spine is scanned in longitudinal and transverse planes. Vertebrae from T12 to S2 are identified and numbered. The location of any skin abnormality should be documented. The location of the tip of the conus medullaris is determined and documented. Any abnormalities of spine development or the surrounding soft tissues are shown on transverse and longitudinal images. A standoff pad is useful for examining subcutaneous abnormalities.

ANATOMY

The **spinal cord** is a hypoechoic rod that contains a central linear bright echo (Fig. 10.27). This **central bright echo** is not the central canal as originally believed but is caused by an acoustic interface between the myelinated ventral white commissure and the central portion of the anterior median fissure [22]. Nonetheless, this bright echo is adjacent to the central canal and serves as a useful marker of its location and as a landmark for the spinal cord itself. The spinal cord tapers to the **conus medullaris**, the tip of which is normally never lower than the L2–3 disc space [23]. The spinal cord ends as the **filum terminale**, a string-like structure that attaches to the first segment of the coccyx. The **cauda equina** is the group of nerve roots that surround and extend below the conus medullaris until they exit the spinal canal at their designated levels. The normal filum terminale is usually indistinguishable from the cauda equina. The spinal cord and cauda equina are surrounded by CSF and encased within the **thecal sac**. The thecal sac terminates at the S2 level. The anterior spinal artery may be seen pulsating in the anterior median fissure of the spinal cord. Smaller posterior spinal arteries pulsate on the dorsolateral aspect of the cord.

The key to US examination is determining the correct spinal levels by counting vertebrae. Landmarks used for counting vertebrae are listed in Box 10.2. Five sacral vertebrae make a curving arc that extends dorsally (Fig. 10.28). The vertebrae of the coccyx are not

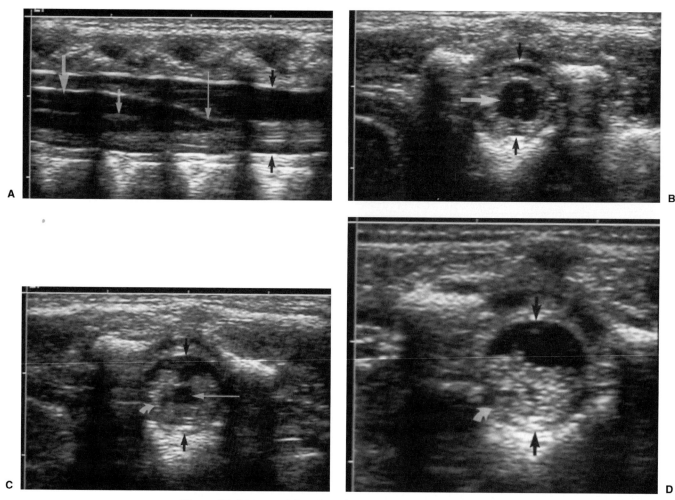

Figure 10.27 *Normal Spinal Cord. A.* Longitudinal image shows the normal distal spinal cord (*large arrow*) tapering to the conus medullaris (*long skinny arrow*). Note the echogenic central linear echo (*small arrow*) characteristic of the cord. The cauda equina is seen as linear echogenic strands around and below the conus medullaris. The cauda equina is formed by nerve roots that arise from the more superior cord and course within the thecal sac to their exit foramina. The thecal sac (*between black arrows*) is distended with cerebrospinal fluid. Posterior vertebral elements cast acoustic shadows across the thecal sac. This cord terminates normally at the top of L2. *B.* Transverse image shows the full diameter of the spinal cord (*white arrow*) centered within the thecal sac (*between black arrows*). *C.* Transverse image near the tip of the conus medullaris (*long skinny arrow*) shows the nerve roots of the cauda equina (*curved arrow*) and anechoic cerebrospinal fluid within the thecal sac (*between black arrows*). *D.* Transverse image below the conus medullaris shows the normal clumping of the nerve roots of the cauda equina (*curved arrow*). The thecal sac (*between black arrows*) is well distended because the baby's torso has been elevated to cause cerebrospinal fluid to flow to the lower sac to improve visualization.

Box 10.2: Landmarks Used to Count Vertebrae

5 sacral vertebrae are ossified, coccygeal
vertebrae are cartilaginous
—Count from S5
Lumbosacral junction at L5–S1

Top of the iliac crest at L4–5 interspace
Tip of the twelfth rib at L2
End of the thecal sac at S2

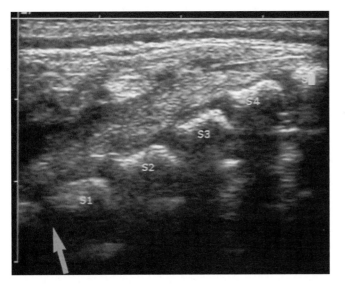

Figure 10.28 *Counting Vertebrae.* The sacral vertebrae are easily recognized in longitudinal plane by the dorsally directed, curving arc they make. Sacral vertebrae are ossified and echogenic while coccygeal vertebrae are cartilaginous and hypoechoic. The lumbosacral junction of L5–S1 is recognized by the angle (*arrow*) formed by the alignment of the lumbar and sacral vertebrae.

ossified but may be seen as hypoechoic structures [24]. Identify S5, then count vertebrae proceeding cranially. The lumbosacral junction (L5–S1) is at the angle between the relatively straight alignment of the lumbar vertebrae and the curving alignment of the sacral vertebrae. The top of the iliac crest marks the L4–5 disc space. The tip of the last rib is at L2.

TETHERED CORD

An abnormally low and fixed position of the spinal cord is associated with bowel, bladder, and lower limb dysfunction in childhood. The tethered cord suffers progressive injury caused by ischemia, stretching, and compression during normal activities. Muscle weakness, gait disturbances, back or perineal pain, and radiculopathy may not present clinically until age 5 to 15 years. Early diagnosis allows for surgical repair before progressive cord damage occurs. Clinical findings associated with tethered cord include low lumbar dimple or cleft; hairy patch, mass, or discolored skin in lumbosacral area; vertebral anomalies of the lower spine; abnormal neurological examination of the lower extremities; and abnormal rectum (imperforate anus, rectal stenosis, cloacal abnormality).

- Tip of the conus medullaris below the mid-portion of L2 is suspicious for tethered cord [23].
- Tip of the conus medullaris below the L2–3 interspace level is unequivocally a tethered cord.
- The tethered spinal cord is fixed dorsally in the spinal canal. The normal spinal cord is centered in the spinal canal and can move with changes in infant position.
- The conus medullaris is atypical in shape. It may be wedged or blunted.
- The filum terminale is thickened (>2 mm) and echogenic because of fat infiltration. The filum terminale is short providing abnormal fixation of the cord.
- Pulsations of the spinal cord are absent because of fixation.
- Intradural lipomas cause a focal echogenic mass enclosed within the dural sac. The bony spinal canal may be normal or focally enlarged when a lipoma is present.
- A cleft spinal cord (**diastematomyelia**) is split in the sagittal plane by a fibrous, cartilaginous, or bony septum. Transverse images show the two rounded, usually equal size, portions of the cord.

REFERENCES

1. Babcock DS. Sonography of the brain in infants: role in evaluating neurologic abnormalities. AJR Am J Roentgenol 1995;165:417–423.

2. Sudakoff G, Montazemi M, Rifkin M. The foramen magnum: the underutilized acoustic window to the posterior fossa. J Ultrasound Med 1993;4:205–210.

3. Anderson N, Allan R, Darlow B, et al. Diagnosis of intraventricular hemorrhage in the newborn: value of sonography via the posterior fontanelle. AJR Am J Roentgenol 1994;163:893–896.

4. American Institute of Ultrasound in Medicine. Guidelines for performance of the pediatric neurosonology examination. Rockville, Maryland: American Institute of Ultrasound in Medicine, 1991.

5. Patel MD, Cheng AG, Callen PW. Lateral ventricular effacement as an isolated sonographic finding in premature infants: prevalence and significance. AJR Am J Roentgenol 1995;165:155–159.

6. Shaw C, Alvord EJ. Cava septi pellucidi et vergae: their normal and pathological states. Brain 1969;92:213–224.

7. Worthen N, Gilbertson V, Lau C. Cortical sulcal development seen on sonography: relationship to gestational parameters. J Ultrasound Med 1986;5:153–156.

8. Babcock D. The normal, absent, and abnormal corpus callosum: sonographic findings. Radiology 1984;151:449–453.

9. Yousefzadeh D, Naidich T. US anatomy of the posterior fossa in children: correlation with brain sections. Radiology 1985;156:353–361.

10. Naidich T, Yousefzadeh D, Gusnard D, et al. Sonography of the internal capsule and basal ganglia in infants—Part II. Localization of pathologic processes in the sagittal section through the caudothalamic groove. Radiology 1986;161:615–621.

11. Carson SC, Hertzberg BS, Bowie JD, et al. Value of sonography in the diagnosis of intracranial hemorrhage and periventricular leukomalacia: a postmortem study of 35 cases. AJR Am J Roentgenol 1990;155:595–601.

12. Papile L, Burstein J, Burstein R, et al. Incidence and evolution of subependymal and intraventricular hemorrhage: study of infants with birth weight less than 1500 grams. J Pediatr 1978;92:529–534.

13. Roth SC, Baudin J, McCormick DC, et al. Relation between ultrasound appearance of the brain of very preterm infants and neurodevelopmental impairment at eight years. Developmental Medicine and Child Neurology 1993;35:755–768.

14. Volpe JJ. Current concepts of brain injury in the premature infant. AJR Am J Roentgenol 1989;153:243–251.

15. Bowerman RA, Donn SM, Silver T M, et al. Natural history of neonatal periventricular/intraventricular hemorrhage and its complications: sonographic observations. AJR Am J Roentgenol 1984;143:1041–1052.

16. Flodmark O, Roland E, Hill A, et al. Periventricular leukomalacia: radiologic diagnosis. Radiology 1987;162:119–124.

17. Carrasco CR, Stierman ED, Harnsberger HR, et al. An algorithm for prenatal ultrasound diagnosis of congenital CNS abnormalities. J Ultrasound Med 1985;4:163–168.

18. Kollias S, Ball WJ, Prenger E. Cystic malformations of the posterior fossa: differential diagnosis clarified through embryological analysis. RadioGraphics 1993;13:1211–1231.

19. Patel D, Holfels E, Vogel N, et al. Resolution of intracranial calcifications in infants with treated congenital toxoplasmosis. Radiology 1996;199:433–440.

20. Kapilivsky A, Garfinkle W, Rosenberg H, et al. US case of the day—congenital CMV infection. RadioGraphics 1995;15:239–242.

21. Rohrschneider W, Forsting M, Darge K, et al. Diagnostic value of spinal US: comparative study with MR imaging in pediatric patients. Radiology 1996;200:383–388.

22. Nelson MJ, Sedler J, Gilles F. Spinal cord central echo complex: histoanatomic correlation. Radiology 1989;170:479–481.

23. DiPietro M. The conus medullaris: normal US findings throughout childhood. Radiology 1993;188:149–153.

24. Beek F, Bax K, Mali W. Sonography of the coccyx in newborns and infants. J Ultrasound Med 1994;13:629–634.

VASCULAR ULTRASOUND

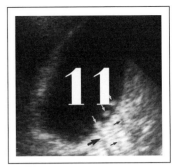

Vascular US is based upon the use of the Doppler effect first described in 1842 by the Austrian mathematician Johann Christian Doppler. As applied to diagnostic US, the Doppler effect describes the change in sound frequency that occurs when sound is reflected from a moving object. In medical diagnostics, the US beam is reflected by clumps of moving red blood cells (RBCs) within blood vessels. The resulting change in sound frequency (the Doppler shift) is carefully measured to determine the presence, direction, and velocity of blood flow. Doppler shifts may also be produced by microbubbles induced by ureteral peristalsis producing a ureteral jet that confirms patency of the ureter. Doppler shifts produced by movement of the patient (breathing, heartbeat, and bowel peristalsis) or by movement of the transducer produces Doppler artifacts.

UNDERSTANDING DOPPLER ULTRASOUND

The **Doppler shift** is the difference in sound frequency between the US beam transmitted into tissue and the echo produced by reflection from the moving RBCs. A Doppler interrogation beam is directed into tissue in a direction controlled by the operator. The Doppler beam intercepts moving blood within a blood vessel at an angle called the **Doppler angle**. Blood flow that is relatively toward the Doppler beam increases the frequency of the echo returning to the transducer (Fig. 11.1). The movement toward it compresses the Doppler sound wave. A "positive frequency shift" to a higher frequency indicates that blood flow is relatively toward the Doppler beam. A "negative frequency shift" to a lower frequency indicates that blood flow is relatively away from the Doppler beam. Doppler frequency shifts are fortuitously within the range of human hearing, so the sound of moving blood can be heard as well as measured by US.

The amount of frequency shift is proportional to the velocity of the moving RBCs. By using a mathematical formula (the **Doppler equation**) and the handy computer intrinsic to our US units, we can measure the Doppler shift and calculate blood flow velocity. It is most important to recognize that Doppler can accurately measure blood flow *velocity*, but is not

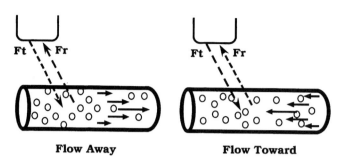

Flow Away   **Flow Toward**

Figure 11.1 *Doppler Frequency Shift.* Flow relatively away from the Doppler beam shifts the Doppler echo to a lower frequency. Flow relatively toward the Doppler beam shifts the Doppler echo to a higher frequency. **Ft** is the frequency of the transmitted Doppler beam. **Fr** is the frequency of the Doppler echo returned to the transducer.

accurate at measuring blood flow *volume.* Measurement of blood flow volume requires accurate measurement of the cross-sectional area of blood vessels. This measurement is difficult and constantly changing because of the pulsatile nature of blood flow.

The Doppler equation can be written in two ways:

$$\textbf{Doppler frequency shift} = Fr - Ft = \frac{2 \times Ft \times v \times \text{cosine } \theta}{C}$$

$$\textbf{Blood flow velocity} = V = \frac{(Fr - Ft) \times (C)}{2 \times (Ft) \times (\text{cosine } \theta)}$$

Ft is the frequency of the Doppler interrogation beam. **Fr** is the frequency of the echo shifted by the Doppler effect. **(Fr − Ft)** is the Doppler shift. **C** is the velocity of sound in human tissue, assumed to be constant at 1540 m/sec. **V** is the velocity of moving blood. The Doppler angle is indicated by the Greek letter theta (θ). The Doppler shift is proportional to the *cosine* function of the Doppler angle. The Doppler angle must be estimated by the operator and is communicated to the US unit by steering the "wing" of the Doppler angle indicator (Fig. 11.2).

For those mathematically inclined, the Doppler equation immediately demonstrates several important features of Doppler US. For those not mathematically inclined, just memorize the following facts:

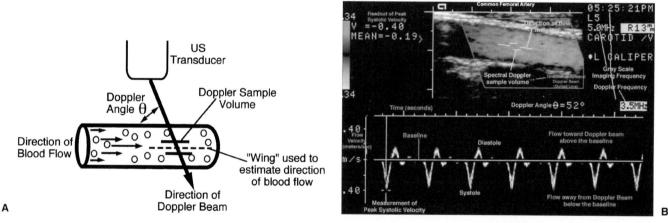

Figure 11.2 *Spectral Doppler Display. A.* Drawing illustrates the Doppler beam, Doppler angle, Doppler sample volume, and the operator-controlled "wing" used to communicate to the US computer the estimated direction of blood flow. *B.* In this illustration, color Doppler and gray-scale US are used to locate and display the vessel being interrogated in the box at the top of the image. The spectral Doppler sample volume, the direction of the spectral Doppler US beam, and the Doppler angle indicator are shown. The Doppler spectrum is shown at the bottom of the image. See text for explanation of the spectral Doppler display (see Color Figure 11.2B).

Table 11.1: Cosine Values

Doppler Angle (θ)	Cosine Value
0°	1
10°	0.98
20°	0.93
30°	0.87
40°	0.77
50°	0.64
60°	0.50
70°	0.34
80°	0.17
90°	0

- The Doppler frequency shift is the signal that we must optimize to obtain reliable blood flow velocity information. The Doppler signal is intrinsically weak, as little as 1/10,000 as strong as the gray-scale US signal. RBC reflectors in blood are very limited in number compared to innumerable sound reflectors within soft tissue. So, Doppler technique must always be optimized to produce useful and accurate information. The Doppler frequency shift is proportional to the Doppler transmission frequency. The higher the transmission frequency, the higher the Doppler shift. When blood flow velocity is slow, higher transducer frequency improves its detection. However, higher-frequency US is limited in penetration and lower frequencies must often be used to produce a Doppler signal from deep vessels.

- The Doppler frequency shift is proportional to the *cosine* of the Doppler angle. This has important implications as seen by inspection of the cosine values listed in Table 11.1. The maximum Doppler frequency shift will be obtained by directing the Doppler interrogation beam straight down the barrel of the vessel—the Doppler angle is 0 degrees. The cosine of 0 degrees is 1, the maximum cosine value. Unfortunately, most blood vessels course parallel to the skin and a zero Doppler angle is seldom obtainable. The cosine of 90 degrees is zero. No Doppler shift is obtained at precisely 90 degrees of interrogation to direction of blood flow. In practice, a weak Doppler signal is often obtained because the Doppler interrogation beam diverges slightly. However, this weak signal is misleading as to flow direction and is inaccurate in determining velocity.

- Acute Doppler angles (<60 degrees) must be created to obtain accurate Doppler information. Note from Table 11.1 that the cosine values change slowly at acute angles (10 degrees, 20 degrees) and change rapidly at larger angles (70 degrees, 80 degrees). The operator routinely assumes that blood flow is parallel to the walls of visualized blood vessels and aligns the Doppler angle "wing" to align with the wall of the vessel. However, blood vessels, especially diseased arteries, are commonly tortuous and the exact orientation of blood flow and the Doppler angle must be estimated. Erroneous estimates of the Doppler angle cause smaller errors in blood flow velocity calculations at acute angles than at angles close to 90 degrees. The Doppler shift diminishes to 50% of maximum at 60 degrees, and falls rapidly at larger angles, reducing the quality of Doppler information. A 60 degrees, or smaller, Doppler angle is obtainable, with effort, in nearly all imaging situations.

Continuous wave (CW) Doppler uses two US crystals, one as a transmitter and the other as a receiver, to continuously record all Doppler shift information along the entire path of the Doppler beam. CW Doppler is non-selective and combines all Doppler shift information from all blood vessels in its path. CW Doppler is used commonly in obstetrics to monitor fetal heart tones.

Pulsed wave Doppler is commonly used in conjunction with real-time gray-scale US imaging to perform **duplex Doppler US**. Duplex Doppler combines routine imaging with Doppler interrogation of visualized vessels. Excluding all signals obtained along the Doppler beam line-of-sight except those obtained from a small time window creates a **Doppler sample volume** (Fig. 11.2A). This sample volume can be precisely positioned within any vessel visualized to obtain selective blood flow information from one vessel or even just a portion of one vessel. The combination of gray-scale US, color Doppler, and spectral Doppler is sometimes called **triplex Doppler US** (Fig. 11.2).

Spectral Doppler displays Doppler shift information as a graph of velocity, or frequency shift, information displayed over time. Blood flow velocity can be displayed interchangeably with Doppler frequency shift information by solving the Doppler equation shown previously. The appearance of the Doppler spectrum remains the same; only the scale changes.

Color Doppler uses a larger sample volume to detect *mean* Doppler shifts within a larger visualized area. Moving blood is displayed in color superimposed upon the gray-scale image.

DOPPLER SPECTRAL DISPLAY

Echoes returning from the Doppler sample volume are analyzed for frequency shift information. A Fast Fourier Transform sorts the range and mixture of Doppler shift information into individual components and displays them as a function of time. Analysis is performed rapidly enough to display the information in real time corresponding to heartbeat (Fig. 11.2B).

- The horizontal scale (x-axis) is time in seconds.
- The vertical scale (y-axis) is flow velocity in m/sec or cm/sec, or is the Doppler frequency shift in kHz.
- Brightness of pixels in the spectrum corresponds to the relative number of RBCs moving at given velocity at a specific instant in time. The more RBCs moving at that specific velocity and time, the brighter the pixel.
- Flow relatively toward the Doppler beam is displayed above the zero baseline.
- Flow relatively away from the Doppler beam is displayed below the zero baseline.
- Spectral waveforms vary over time with cardiac contraction with highest flow velocities during systole and lowest flow velocities during diastole. Many vessels show reversed flow or no flow during diastole.

COLOR DOPPLER IMAGING DISPLAY

Color Doppler imaging (CDI) superimposes Doppler flow information on a standard gray-scale real-time US image. Color Doppler displays colors based on measurement of *mean* Doppler shifts (Fig. 11.3) [1].

- A color map is displayed adjacent to the image to indicate the colors used to display flow information [2]. A wide variety of color maps are available. The map in use must be analyzed to interpret the color information (Fig. 11.4).
- The color map is divided into two parts by a black bar that corresponds to the baseline or zero flow point on the Doppler spectral display. The color on the top of the map, above the baseline, is used to show flow relatively toward the Doppler beam. The color on the bottom of the map, below the baseline, shows flow relatively away from the Doppler beam. Red is commonly used to indicate flow toward the Doppler beam, whereas blue indicates flow away from the Doppler beam. Obviously, red and blue colors provide no direct indication of whether vessels are arteries or veins. Knowledge of anatomy, appearance of the vessel, and Doppler waveform analysis are used to differentiate various arteries and veins.
- Brighter colors are used to display higher mean velocities. Darker colors indicate lower mean velocities. Some color maps use different color shades for higher and lower velocities (Fig. 11.3). For instance, red may transition to yellow and blue may transition to green for higher flow velocities.
- Numbers at the top and bottom of the color map indicate the velocity scale setting the Nyquist limit. The velocity scale must be set appropriately to the blood flow velocity

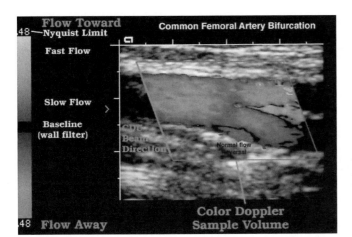

Figure 11.3 *Color Doppler Imaging Display.* The color map is shown on the left side of this image. See text for detailed explanation of the color Doppler display (see Color Figure 11.3).

encountered. A scale set too high will obscure slow flow. A scale set too low will alias. Aliasing and the Nyquist limit are discussed later in this chapter.

■ A color Doppler sample volume is specified and positioned on the gray-scale image by the US operator. The color Doppler sample volume box is usually etched in white. Only the tissue within the box will be analyzed for Doppler shift information. Keeping the sample volume small optimizes Doppler information gathering.

■ Note that in CDI the format of the transducer determines the direction of the Doppler beam. The Doppler angle may change with vessel orientation and produce color changes related only to changes in the Doppler angle and not to changes in blood flow.

■ As with spectral Doppler, color flow information will not be obtained when the Doppler angle is at or near 90 degrees.

■ The color displayed within blood vessels on CDI is a function of
 – Flow velocity
 – Doppler angle
 – Presence of aliasing
 – Color map utilized
 – Phase of the cardiac cycle

Color Doppler and spectral Doppler are complementary to each other. Color flow shows flow information based on measurement of mean Doppler shifts, whereas spectral Doppler displays the full range of detected Doppler shifts. Color flow imaging can be used to detect blood vessels and confirm presence and direction of blood flow, whereas spectral Doppler provides more detailed characterization of blood flow and precise velocity measurements to estimate stenosis.

COLOR DOPPLER ENERGY DISPLAY

Color Doppler energy (CDE) displays color flow information obtained from integration of the *power* of the Doppler signal, rather than the Doppler frequency shift itself [3]. Another name for this technique is **power Doppler**. CDE relates more directly to the *number* of mov-

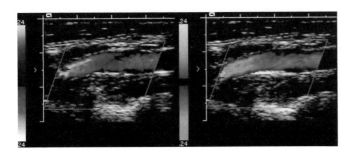

Figure 11.4 *Color Maps.* Inversion of the color map radically changes the appearance of the color image of a carotid artery. Choice and orientation of the color map are at the option of the US operator (see Color Figure 11.4).

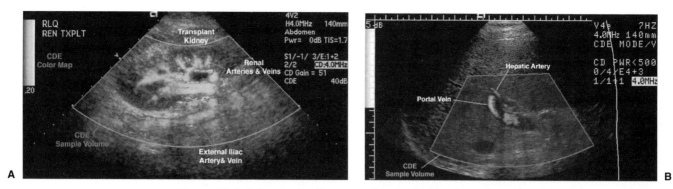

Figure 11.5 *Color Doppler Energy Display. A.* The blood vessels within and supplying a renal transplant are displayed on this color Doppler energy (CDE) (power Doppler) image. CDE shows the presence of blood flow with high sensitivity. However, direction of blood flow is not determined and adjacent arteries and veins with blood flow in opposite directions are shown in the same color. The CDE sample volume is adjusted by the operator to include the tissues of interest. *B.* CDE image of the liver shows flow in the portal vein and hepatic artery. In this example, the Doppler sample volume is shaded in color (see Color Figure 11.5).

ing RBCs than to their velocity. CDE is relatively angle-independent and is more sensitive to slow flow than is CDI. CDE is a useful adjunct to CDI, especially in technically challenging situations. CDE significantly improves evaluation of parenchymal flow and assessment of tumor vascularity (Fig. 11.5) [4,5].

- CDE provides no information on flow direction or velocity.
- Artifacts related to patient motion are significantly increased with CDE compared to CDI. Patients unwilling or unable to hold their breath or remain motionless may not be accurately imaged with CDE.
- Visualization of gray-scale anatomy is often limited within the CDE sample volume.
- CDE also displays a color map adjacent to the image. As with CDI, the colors chosen are arbitrary. However, no information on flow direction is obtained with CDE.
- The CDE sample volume may be shaded in a color different than that used to indicate blood flow.

BLOOD FLOW DYNAMICS

The major types of blood flow are laminar (parabolic), plug, disturbed, and turbulent [6].

LAMINAR BLOOD FLOW

Laminar blood flow is the normal blood flow found in arteries and in large veins (Fig. 11.6) [7]. The highest velocity RBCs are in the center of the blood vessels. Blood flow velocity progressively decreases closer to the vessel wall. Blood at the vessel wall is hardly moving. Laminar blood flow is sometimes called **parabolic** blood flow because a line connecting the levels of flow at differing velocities has the shape of a parabola. The characteristics of laminar flow are:

- Spectral Doppler shows a narrow range of velocities within the sample volume at any given instance in time. This is the normal "narrow spectrum" (Fig. 11.6B).
- A well-defined window is seen beneath the Doppler spectrum in systole reflecting the fact that detected RBCs accelerate uniformly during systole. This is called the "systolic window."
- Highest flow velocities are mid-stream with decreasing flow velocities closer to the vessel wall.

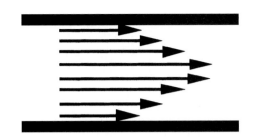

A Laminar Blood Flow

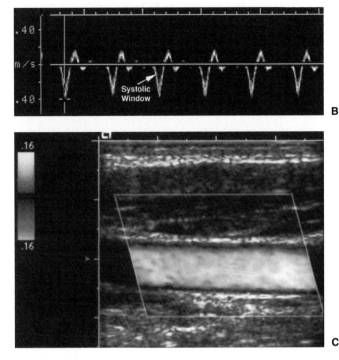

Figure 11.6 *Normal Laminar Blood Flow. A.* Arrows represent the orderly layers of red blood cells moving at different velocities that characterize laminar blood flow. The highest velocities are found in mid-stream. The lowest velocities are found adjacent to the vessel wall. *B.* Doppler spectral display shows the narrow spectrum characteristic of laminar flow in the common femoral artery. The systolic window (*arrow*), characteristic of laminar flow, is seen as the triangular space beneath the Doppler spectrum in systole. *C.* Color Doppler image of the common carotid artery at mid-systole shows bright color in mid-stream, indicating faster flow, and darker color near the vessel wall, indicating slower flow (see Color Figure 11.6C).

- Color Doppler shows the brightest color mid-stream with darker colors toward the vessel wall (Fig. 11.6C).
- Cardiac contraction causes flow velocity to increase rapidly to peak values during systole, then flow velocity decreases with diastole during which there may be no flow or flow may reverse in direction.
- The sound of laminar flow has a whistling quality.

PLUG FLOW

Plug flow is a type of normal flow seen in large diameter vessels such as the aorta. In mid-stream a wide band of RBCs is moving at the same speed, forming a plug-shaped velocity profile.

- The Doppler spectral is very narrow, reflecting RBCs all moving at the same speed throughout the cardiac cycle.

DISTURBED BLOOD FLOW

Disturbed blood flow occurs at vessel bifurcations and in areas of vessel stenosis. Disturbed flow no longer travels in a straight line but generally continues in a forward direction [8].

- Flow velocity is increased (Fig. 11.7).
- "Spectral broadening" indicates the disorganization characteristic of disturbed flow. The thickness (vertical height) of the Doppler spectrum is increased, indicating a broader range of the velocities within the sample volume at any given instant of time.

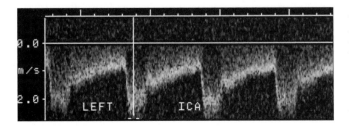

Figure 11.7 *Disturbed Blood Flow.* Spectral display of the waveform obtained in an area of high-grade stenosis of the internal carotid artery (ICA). Peak systolic velocity is increased to 270 cm/sec. The spectrum is broadened and ill-defined.

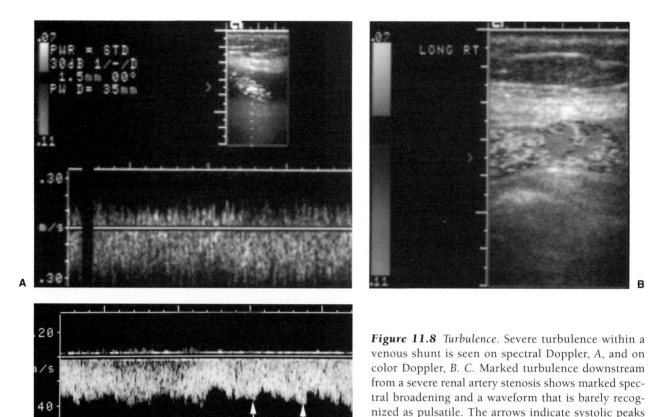

Figure 11.8 *Turbulence.* Severe turbulence within a venous shunt is seen on spectral Doppler, *A*, and on color Doppler, *B*. *C*. Marked turbulence downstream from a severe renal artery stenosis shows marked spectral broadening and a waveform that is barely recognized as pulsatile. The arrows indicate systolic peaks (see Color Figure 11.8B).

■ Increased spectral broadening indicates increased disturbance of flow. The systolic window characteristic of laminar flow is reduced in size and may be obliterated.

TURBULENT BLOOD FLOW

Turbulent blood flow is random and chaotic, with RBCs flowing in all directions. Turbulence is found downstream from high-grade stenosis and in areas where flow velocities are very high, such as within shunts and fistulas [8].

■ Spectral broadening is severe and the systolic window is obliterated (Fig. 11.8A).
■ With severe turbulence, flow is concentrated at lower velocities.
■ With severe stenosis, flow is less pulsatile.
■ Flow may be detected in both directions simultaneously, owing to the formation of eddy currents. Eddy currents occur downstream from high-grade obstructions where the blood vessel lumen widens after the stenosis.
■ Flow velocities fluctuate with time.
■ Color Doppler shows a mixture of colors with aliasing reflecting the high velocities (Fig. 11.8B).

Individual blood vessels may be characterized by their Doppler "signatures," a recognizable Doppler spectrum relatively unique to the vessel (Fig. 11.6B). A major determinant of the appearance of the Doppler spectrum is downstream resistance to blood flow. Blood vessels may be characterized as being "high resistance" or "low resistance" vessels.

HIGH RESISTANCE BLOOD VESSELS

When vessels show a high resistance pattern, small arteries and arterioles downstream are contracted, increasing resistance to blood flow and maintaining blood pressure at high

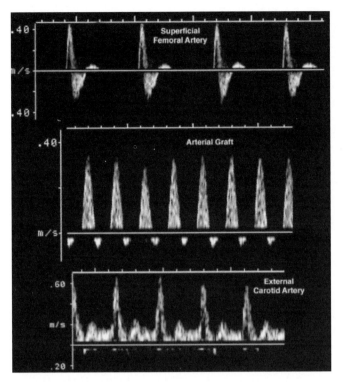

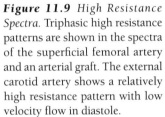

Figure 11.9 *High Resistance Spectra.* Triphasic high resistance patterns are shown in the spectra of the superficial femoral artery and an arterial graft. The external carotid artery shows a relatively high resistance pattern with low velocity flow in diastole.

levels. Pulse pressures traveling down the arterial tree are highly reflected resulting in little flow to the capillary bed during diastole. Arteries that supply systemic muscles are characteristically high resistance when the muscles are at rest. With exercise, arterioles open, blood flow increases, and the high resistance pattern converts to low resistance.

- A triphasic waveform characterizes arteries supplying skeletal muscles at rest (Fig. 11.9). Examples include the femoral artery, the external iliac artery, and the radial artery.
  - Velocity rises sharply with onset of systole and falls rapidly with cessation of ventricular contraction.
  - Flow reverses for a short time in early diastole.
  - The remainder of diastole shows little or no forward flow.
- Some arteries show relatively high resistance patterns. Examples include the external carotid artery (ECA) (Fig. 11.9) and the superior mesenteric artery (SMA) during fasting.
  - The rise to peak systolic velocity (PSV) is sharp with a rapid fall of velocity at the termination of systole.
  - Flow in diastole remains forward in direction but is at very low velocity.

LOW RESISTANCE BLOOD VESSELS

Low resistance blood vessels are characterized by forward flow throughout the cardiac cycle. These arteries supply vital organs like the brain and kidneys that demand a continuous supply of oxygenated blood. Arterioles within these organs are generally kept wide open.

- Low resistance arteries have characteristic biphasic waveforms. Examples include the internal carotid artery (ICA), the renal artery, the umbilical artery, and the SMA after eating (Fig. 11.10).
  - Velocity rises more slowly and falls more gradually during systole.
  - Flow is forward throughout the cardiac cycle.
  - Flow never reaches the zero velocity baseline.

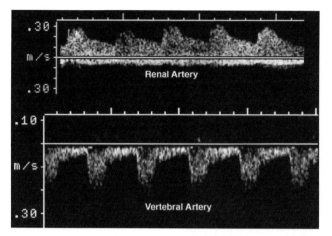

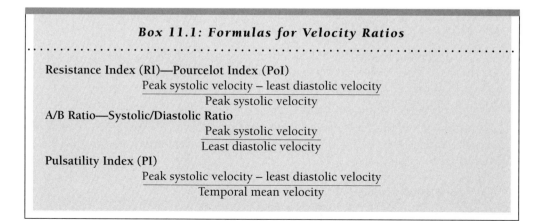

Figure 11.10 *Low Resistance Spectra.* The renal artery and vertebral artery show relatively high velocity flow in diastole characteristic of low resistance spectra seen in arteries that supply vital organs. Forward flow toward the organ is present throughout the cardiac cycle.

VELOCITY RATIOS

Many times a Doppler signal can be obtained from tiny blood vessels that cannot be discretely visualized. Intrarenal arteries are a common example. At other times the vessel is so tortuous that a Doppler angle cannot be accurately estimated, such as in the twisted umbilical artery in the umbilical cord. Without an accurate Doppler angle estimation, an accurate flow velocity cannot be determined. In these instances the Doppler equation can be solved using the measured Doppler frequency shift and a cosine θ value of 1. The velocity values will not be accurate, but the Doppler spectrum characterizes flow within the blood vessel. A variety of velocity ratios can be calculated from the displayed Doppler spectrum. The formulas for the commonly used velocity ratios are displayed in Box 11.1.

■ **Resistance index** is also called the *Pourcelot index.* It is calculated by subtracting end diastolic velocity from PSV and dividing the result by PSV. A high resistance index indicates high resistance to blood flow within the vessel. High resistance to blood flow may be produced by arteriole constriction or by limited arterial distensibility such as may be produced in an edematous obstructed kidney [9].
■ **Systolic/diastolic ratio** (A/B ratio) is calculated by dividing PSV by end-diastolic velocity.
■ **Pulsatility index** requires determination of temporal mean velocity and thus is more difficult to calculate. US computers allow the operator to trace the spectrum and the computer will calculate a mean velocity (Fig. 11.11). Pulsatility index is then calculated by subtracting end diastolic velocity from PSV and dividing the result by mean velocity.

Box 11.1: Formulas for Velocity Ratios

Resistance Index (RI)—Pourcelot Index (PoI)

$$\frac{\text{Peak systolic velocity} - \text{least diastolic velocity}}{\text{Peak systolic velocity}}$$

A/B Ratio—Systolic/Diastolic Ratio

$$\frac{\text{Peak systolic velocity}}{\text{Least diastolic velocity}}$$

Pulsatility Index (PI)

$$\frac{\text{Peak systolic velocity} - \text{least diastolic velocity}}{\text{Temporal mean velocity}}$$

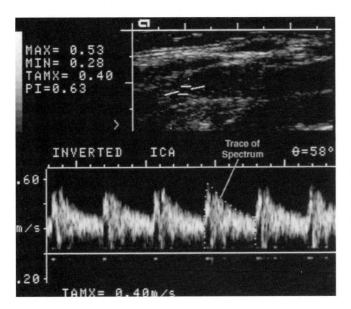

Figure 11.11 *Pulsatility Index.* The operator manually traces the outline of one cardiac cycle on the Doppler spectrum. From this tracing, the US computer determines the temporal mean velocity and calculates the pulsatility index (PI). The result is displayed in the upper left-hand corner of the image (PI = 0.63). ICA, internal carotid artery.

DOPPLER CHANGES CAUSED BY STENOSIS

A common use of Doppler US is to detect and characterize arterial stenosis. Gray-scale US will identify atherosclerotic plaques and vessel narrowing. The severity of stenosis is determined by correlation of Doppler findings with real-time imaging.

- Proximal to the stenosis, laminar flow is generally present unless the vessel is seriously diseased upstream (Fig. 11.12).
- Within the stenotic zone, flow velocity is increased but usually remains laminar. PSV correlates best with the severity of stenosis. The highest velocity may be found in a very small region of the stenosed vessel lumen. A careful search of the vessel with a small sample volume is needed.
- In the post-stenotic zone, spectral broadening occurs as flow spreads out to occupy the widened vessel lumen. Turbulence and eddy currents form downstream to severe stenosis. Maximum flow disturbance is usually found within 1 cm of the maximum stenosis.
- Downstream, the Doppler signal is dampened by severe stenosis. This results in the tardus parvus waveform.

TARDUS PARVUS WAVEFORM

The tardus parvus waveform is a sign of marked arterial stenosis that does not require direct evaluation of the stenosis [10]. The waveform is detected in arteries downstream from the

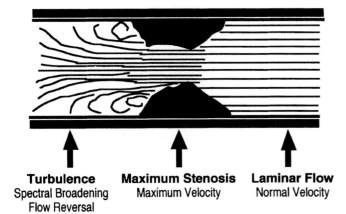

Turbulence
Spectral Broadening
Flow Reversal

Maximum Stenosis
Maximum Velocity

Laminar Flow
Normal Velocity

Figure 11.12 *Velocity Changes Across a Vessel Stenosis.* To maintain flow volume across an area of stenosis, velocity must increase through the stenotic segment. The maximal change in velocity occurs at the site of greatest narrowing. Doppler velocity measurements made at this site correlate best with the severity of stenosis. Beyond the stenosis, flow is disturbed and sampling shows spectral broadening, turbulence, and areas of flow reversal.

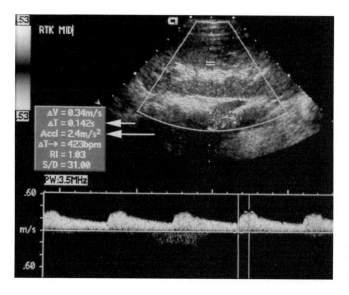

Figure 11.13 *Tardus Parvus Waveform.* Doppler of an intrarenal artery in a patient with surgically proven, renal artery stenosis shows a characteristic tardus parvus waveform. The acceleration time (ΔT) (*short arrow*) is 0.142 seconds. The acceleration index (Accl) (*long arrow*) is 2.4 m/sec^2. Note the blunted appearance of the waveform in systole.

stenosis. It is particularly useful in situations where visualization of the supplying artery is commonly difficult because of location of the artery or obscuration by bowel gas. Evaluation for stenosis of the renal artery or stenosis of an artery supplying a transplant are examples (Fig. 11.13) [11].

- **Tardus** refers to a slowed systolic upstroke. This can be measured by acceleration time, the time from end diastole to the first systolic peak. An acceleration time >0.07 sec correlates with >50% stenosis of the renal artery [12].
- **Parvus** refers to decreased systolic velocity. This can be measured by calculating the acceleration index, the change in velocity from end diastole to the first systolic peak. An acceleration index <3.0 m/sec^2 correlates with >50% stenosis of the renal artery [12].

VENOUS FLOW

Blood flow within veins is typically low velocity and non-pulsatile. However, venous spectra may be phasic when influenced by respiration, may vary in velocity when influenced by motion of the vein itself, or may be pulsatile when transmitting motion from the right side of the heart. These normal variations in venous flow must be recognized to avoid diagnostic errors (Fig. 11.14).

PORTAL VEIN

The portal vein is formed by the confluence of the splenic and superior mesenteric veins. It provides approximately 70% of the incoming blood to the liver.

- Normal blood flow velocity is 13–23 cm/sec with an average of 18 cm/sec.
- Flow velocity is commonly somewhat phasic because rocking motion of the liver caused by motion of the heart moves the portal vein under the Doppler sample volume (see Fig. 11.24).
- Slight phasicity may also be evident related to respiration.
- Normal blood flow direction is into the liver. Any reversal of blood flow direction is abnormal and usually indicative of portal hypertension.
- The portal vein is normally <13 mm in diameter. Increased diameter suggests portal hypertension.

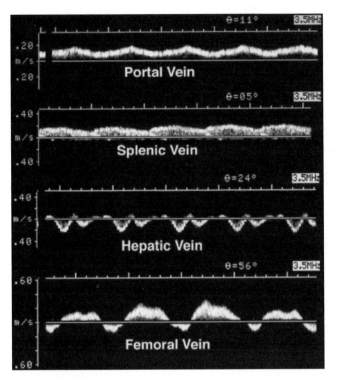

Figure 11.14 *Venous Waveforms.* Doppler spectra from the portal, splenic, hepatic, and femoral veins are shown. See text for discussion of the waveforms.

SPLENIC VEIN

The splenic vein drains the spleen and receives inflow from the inferior mesenteric vein. The splenic vein joins the superior mesenteric vein posterior to the neck of the pancreas to form the portal vein.

- The splenic vein shows low velocity forward flow toward the liver. Reversal of blood flow direction is seen with advanced portal hypertension.
- Slight respiratory variation is common.
- Normal diameter of the splenic vein is <10 mm. Increase in diameter is a sign of portal hypertension.

HEPATIC VEINS

Most individuals have three major hepatic veins that run a straight course to converge in the inferior vena cava just below the diaphragm and only approximately 1 cm from the right atrium. These three hepatic veins drain all of the liver except the caudate lobe. The appearance of the right, middle, and left hepatic veins and inferior vena cava has been likened to a Playboy bunny, a crow's foot, or a caribou with antlers.

- Pulsations of the right atrium are transmitted directly to the inferior vena cava and hepatic veins. None of these veins contains valves.
- The normal hepatic vein waveform is undulating and mirrors motion of the right heart. The A-wave (reversed flow) is produced by atrial contraction. Forward flow of atrial filling is interrupted by the C-wave caused by bulging of the tricuspid valve with onset of ventricular contraction. The dominant S-wave represents high velocity atrial filling during ventricular systole. The V-wave represents the end of atrial filling and the D-wave is produced by opening of the tricuspid valve and simultaneous filling of the right atrium and right ventricle.
- Color Doppler accurately demonstrates the normal flow direction changes characteristic of the hepatic vein (Fig. 11.15).

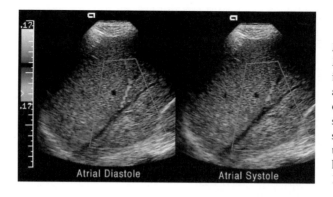

Figure 11.15 *Normal Hepatic Vein Flow.* Blood flow in the hepatic veins is normally toward the heart during atrial filling and away from the heart during atrial contraction. Note that a static color Doppler image represents only an instant in time during the cardiac cycle. Compare to the hepatic vein waveform in Figure 11.14 (see Color Figure 11.15).

PERIPHERAL VEINS

Venous flow from the extremities occurs in response to the effects of gravity and muscular contraction.

- Blood flow in peripheral veins is low velocity and may be appear to be absent if the Doppler velocity scale is set too high or if a large wall filter is used (see Fig. 11.21).
- Flow shows respiratory variation (Fig. 11.14) caused by changes in intra-abdominal pressure produced by motion of the diaphragm. With inspiration the diaphragm descends, increasing intra-abdominal pressure and decreasing venous flow from the legs. With expiration the diaphragm rises, intra-abdominal pressure decreases, and venous flow from the legs increases. If the patient holds his breath, venous flow usually stops. A Valsalva maneuver will reverse flow in the lower extremity veins. Squeezing the patient's calf will augment flow and improve detection of veins.

DOPPLER ARTIFACTS

Artifacts produce confusing alterations of the Doppler signal and affect both spectral Doppler and color flow imaging. Artifacts are produced by physical limitations of Doppler instrumentation and by incorrect instrument settings [13]. Recognition of artifacts and proper correction prevents misdiagnosis.

ALIASING

Aliasing is a performance limitation of *pulsed* Doppler US that is related to the pulse repetition frequency. Pulse repetition frequency is limited by depth. The greater the distance to the vessel of interest, the longer it takes to transmit and receive echoes from that vessel. The Doppler signal that must be measured is the echo of the transmitted Doppler pulse that has been changed in frequency by reflection from moving RBCs. To accurately measure the frequency of the Doppler echo, the pulse repetition frequency must be at least twice the frequency of the Doppler echo. For any given setting of the Doppler US instrument, the **Nyquist limit** is defined as the maximal Doppler shift frequency that can be accurately measured. Because Doppler shift frequency and blood flow velocity can be substituted for each other mathematically by use of the Doppler equation, the Nyquist limit can also be expressed as the maximal blood flow velocity that can be detected by Doppler for a given set of instrument settings.

- Aliasing produces a wrap-around effect on the Doppler display. On spectral Doppler, the peaks of the spectrum are cut off and displayed on the opposite side of the baseline (Figs. 11.16, 11.17).
- On color Doppler, aliasing projects the color of reversed flow within central areas of highest velocity (Fig. 11.18). The key to recognizing color aliasing is to observe that *no black stripe* surrounds the color change. Color change of aliasing involves the brightest

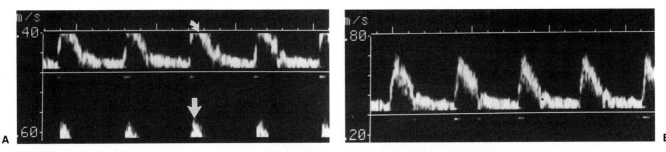

Figure 11.16 *Aliasing in Spectral Doppler.* A. Spectral Doppler shows the peaks (*curved arrow*) of the spectral display are cut off the top and are displayed on the bottom (*straight arrow*). B. With readjustment of the baseline to allow display of the 80 cm/sec peak systolic velocity, the aliasing is eliminated.

shades of the color display. Color change produced by true reversal of blood flow direction, or by changes in the Doppler angle, are etched in black and involve the darkest shades of the color display.

- On most Doppler instruments the pulse repetition frequency cannot be adjusted directly.
- Increasing the velocity scale, which increases the pulse repetition frequency, can eliminate aliasing. Changing the baseline setting or using a lower Doppler US frequency can also eliminate aliasing.
- Aliasing is not a feature of CDE (power Doppler) [14].

SPECTRAL BROADENING

Spectral broadening is an important spectral Doppler sign of abnormal blood flow. However, spectral broadening has a number of other causes that must be recognized and excluded before spectral broadening can be interpreted as a sign of abnormal blood flow.

- When the Doppler sample volume is large compared to the size of the blood vessel, the sample volume will include the full range of blood flow velocities from slow flow near the vessel wall to the fastest flow in midstream. Inclusion of all flow velocities will broaden the spectrum. Because the smallest sample volume available on most Doppler instruments is 1.0–1.5 mm, vessels of this size and smaller will inevitably show broadening of the displayed velocity spectrum.
- Placing the sample volume near the vessel wall instead of mid-stream will produce spectral broadening by inclusion of the slow-moving RBCs near the vessel wall. The highest flow velocities in mid-stream may be missed.
- Excessive Doppler gain falsely broadens the spectrum.

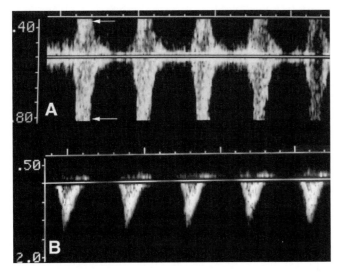

Figure 11.17 *Aliasing in Spectral Doppler.* A. In an example of more severe aliasing, both the top and bottom (*arrows*) of the spectrum are cut off. Direction of blood flow cannot be determined from this spectrum. B. Adjustment of baseline and scale results in appropriate display of the spectrum.

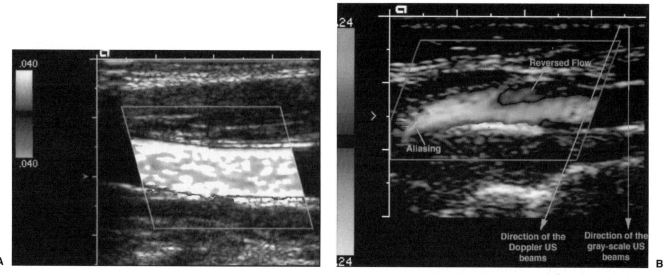

Figure 11.18 Aliasing in Color Doppler. A. The dominant color displayed within this vessel is yellow from the top side of the color map. Yellow indicates flow toward the Doppler beams, or in this case, from right to left. The splotches of green color are areas of aliasing. Note the absence of a black border. The color velocity scale is set low with a Nyquist limit of 0.040 m/sec. When the detected mean blood flow velocity exceeds this limit, aliasing occurs and color from the bottom portion of the color map is displayed. Aliasing must be recognized, but in this case may be useful by providing identification of highest velocity flow. *B.* This color Doppler image of the internal carotid artery demonstrates the appearance of true reversal of blood flow direction as indicated by the black border around the region of color shift. A small area of flow reversal is a normal finding opposite the flow divider at the bifurcation of the common carotid artery. Note that the direction of the Doppler beams is different than the direction of the gray-scale image beams (see Color Figure 11.18).

INCORRECT DOPPLER GAIN

When the color or spectral Doppler gain is set too low, Doppler information may be lost and blood flow may not be detected. The color image with gain set too high demonstrates color in non-flow areas and random color noise. Correct gain settings are attained by turning up the gain setting until noise appears on the color image or spectral display, then gain is reduced slowly until the noise disappears.

- Gain set too low shows no spectral display or color flow on the image.
- Color gain set too high shows color bleed beyond the limits of the vessel, color signal in non-flow areas, and random color noise.
- Spectral gain set too high shows random noise on the spectral display, false spectral broadening, and commonly displays a mirror image of the spectrum on the opposite side of the baseline (Fig. 11.19).

VELOCITY SCALE ERRORS

Errors in the setting of the Doppler velocity scale may obscure slow flow or cause aliasing. Velocity scale and baseline settings must be adjusted to be appropriate to the velocity of blood flow in the interrogated vessel.

- Too high settings of velocity scale obscure low velocity flow on both color flow and spectral Doppler (Fig. 11.20). The small signal may be obliterated by the wall filter (Fig. 11.21). Vessels with slow flow may be judged to be thrombosed.
- When velocity scale settings are too low, aliasing occurs (Figs. 11.16–11.18).

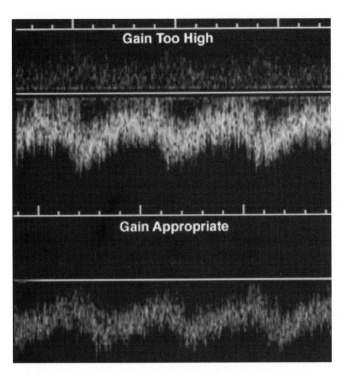

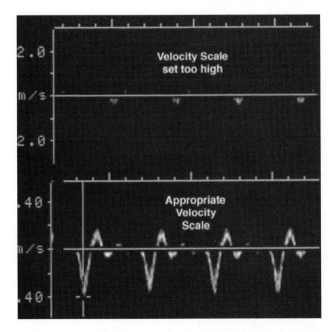

Figure 11.19 *Gain Error.* Doppler gain set too high causes artifactual spectral broadening of the true Doppler spectrum and displays a mirror image of the Doppler spectrum on opposite sides of the baseline. Turning down the Doppler gain to an appropriate setting corrects the artifacts.

INCORRECT WALL FILTER

Motion of the vessel wall produced by pulsatile blood flow causes a low-velocity but very high-intensity Doppler shift. To prevent wall motion from being displayed as blood flow, *wall filters* are included in Doppler instrumentation for both spectral and color Doppler. The spectral Doppler wall filter produces a thin black line on either side of the baseline. The black bar in the color map represents the color Doppler wall filter.

- A wall filter set too high will obscure low-velocity blood flow (Fig. 11.21).
- The wall filter on color Doppler is included in the black bar in the center of the color map (Fig. 11.3) and may not be obvious as a cause of absent color signal in a vessel.

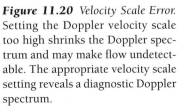

Figure 11.20 *Velocity Scale Error.* Setting the Doppler velocity scale too high shrinks the Doppler spectrum and may make flow undetectable. The appropriate velocity scale setting reveals a diagnostic Doppler spectrum.

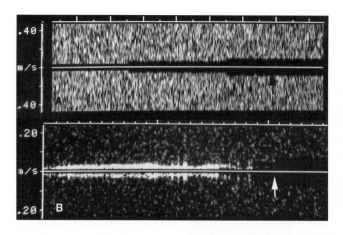

Figure 11.21 Wall Filters. A. Wall filters (*arrow*) set at three different levels obliterate all low-velocity spectral signals near the baseline. B. Spectral waveform of low-velocity flow within a vein is obliterated by a wall filter set too high (*arrow*).

DOPPLER MIRROR IMAGE ARTIFACT

Mirror image duplication of the color flow US display may be produced by strong reflectors such as the surface of the air-filled lung or even the wall of a blood vessel.

- Carotid ghost artifact duplicates the color image of the carotid artery in deeper cervical tissue [15].
- Mirror images of the CDI of the subclavian artery and vein may be produced by reflection from the aerated apex of the lung (Fig. 11.22) [16].
- Color display of hepatic vessels may be included in the gray mirror image of the liver displayed above the diaphragm.
- Mirror images of the Doppler spectrum are displayed on the opposite side of the baseline by Doppler gain set too high or by large Doppler angles near 90 degrees (Fig. 11.19).

TISSUE VIBRATION ARTIFACT

Vibration may produce color display in perivascular solid tissue, indicating blood flow where none is present. Tissue vibration artifact is produced in non-flow areas by turbulence caused by severe stenosis, arteriovenous fistulas, and shunts [17]. A color bruit at the site of arterial stenosis is indicative of a severe stenosis.

- The artifact appears as a mixture of red and blue colors in perivascular soft tissues (Fig. 11.23). The artifact is more prominent during systole and less prominent during diastole.

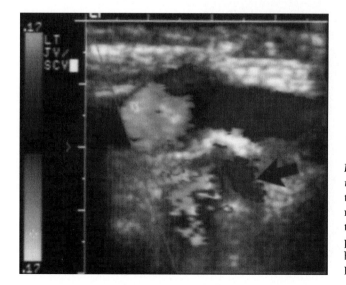

Figure 11.22 Color Doppler Mirror Image. Intense reflection from the surface of the lung causes a mirror image reflection (*arrow*) of the subclavian artery to be displayed over the lung where no blood vessel is present (see Color Figure 11.22).

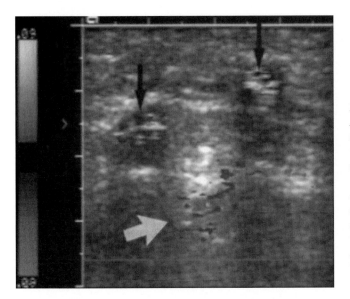

Figure 11.23 *Tissue Vibration Artifact.* Turbulent blood flow in a hemodialysis shunt produces a "visible bruit" of tissue vibration artifact seen as a random pattern (*white arrow*) of red and blue color displayed over the soft tissues adjacent to the shunt. The random color pattern within the two limbs of the shunt (*black arrows*) is indicative of turbulent blood flow (see Color Figure 11.23).

VESSEL MOTION ARTIFACT

Artifactual pulsatility may be introduced into a spectral Doppler tracing when the vessel under interrogation is moving. The portal vein and its branches move with cardiac contraction that rocks the liver. The rocking motion of the vessel displaces the Doppler sample volume from regions of higher velocity to regions of lower velocity, simulating pulsatility or periodic motion in the venous flow spectrum (Fig. 11.24). This artifact is decreased by increasing the size of the Doppler sample volume or by changing the Doppler angle.

DIRECTIONAL AMBIGUITY

When a Doppler interrogation beam intercepts a vessel at a Doppler angle near 90 degrees, the direction of blood flow is difficult to determine (Fig. 11.25). The Doppler spectrum is commonly displayed both above and below the baseline. The ambiguity is corrected by adjusting the approach to the vessel to create a more acute Doppler angle.

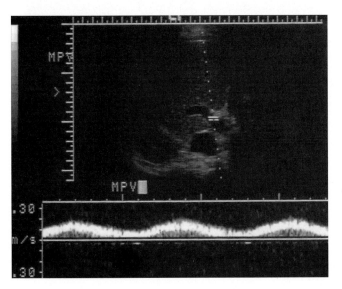

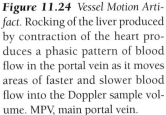

Figure 11.24 *Vessel Motion Artifact.* Rocking of the liver produced by contraction of the heart produces a phasic pattern of blood flow in the portal vein as it moves areas of faster and slower blood flow into the Doppler sample volume. MPV, main portal vein.

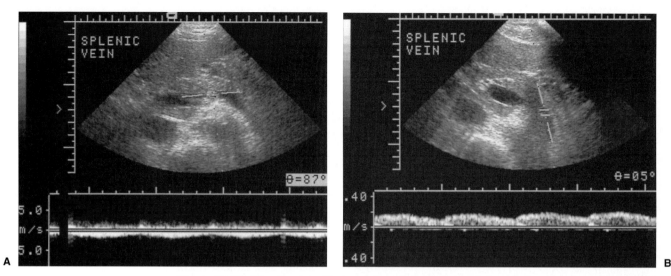

Figure 11.25 *Directional Ambiguity. A.* Doppler spectrum of the splenic vein obtained with a Doppler angle of 87 degrees shows signal on both sides of the baseline. Direction of blood flow cannot be determined. *B.* By readjusting position and angulation of the transducer, an acute Doppler angle of 5 degrees is created, and an unambiguous spectrum is produced. Blood flow in the normal direction toward the liver is confirmed.

COLOR FLASH—COLOR IN NON-VASCULAR STRUCTURES

Any motion of non-vascular tissue will produce a Doppler shift and may result in false color display. Cardiac contraction and highly pulsatile vessels, such as the aorta, cause motion of adjacent tissues which produces a splash of color that obscures blood flow information (Fig. 11.26). Most color Doppler instruments incorporate motion discriminators to suppress this artifact. However, in hypoechoic regions, such as within cysts or ducts, the artifact suppression is limited. Thus color flash may be particularly prominent, or be seen solely, within these lucent structures, falsely simulating blood flow. Color flash is particularly prominent with CDE (power Doppler) imaging. Color flash is reduced by lowering color sensitivity, increasing the velocity scale, and by lowering the gain setting.

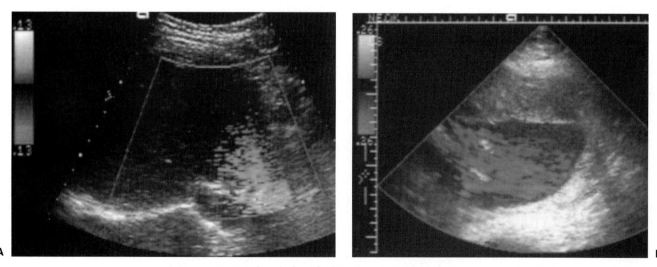

Figure 11.26 *Color Flash—Fluid Motion. A.* Cardiac motion causes color flash artifact and obscures the junction of hepatic veins and inferior vena cava. *B.* A kicking motion by a baby *in utero* moves the amniotic fluid to produce a prominent color flash artifact (see Color Figure 11.26).

FLUID MOTION

Color signal can be produced during CDI by motion of fluids other than flowing blood. Motion by fluid within cysts, by moving bowel contents, and by ureteral peristalsis may be misinterpreted as blood flow.

- Bowel peristalsis with moving gas bubbles can result in rectangular or comet tail areas of false color display.
- Movement of a fetus stirs the amniotic fluid and produces color artifact (Fig. 11.26).
- Visualization of ureteral jets from squirts of urine into the bladder caused by ureteral peristalsis is good evidence of ureteral patency (see Fig. 3.4) [18].

COLOR DOPPLER INTERPRETATION

INTERPRETATION OF COLOR DOPPLER IMAGES

To interpret the meaning of the colors displayed on a color Doppler image, the following parameters must be analyzed:

- **Color Map.** The colors chosen for forward flow (top of the map) and for reversed flow (bottom of the map) must be noted (Figs. 11.3, 11.4). The velocity scale is indicated by the Nyquist limit velocities displayed at the top and bottom of the map. When these mean velocities are exceeded, the color display will be aliased. The velocity scale must be set appropriately for the blood flow velocity in the vessel imaged.
- **Transducer Format and Color Doppler Sample Volume.** The format of the transducer in use determines the direction of color Doppler interrogation beams. Sector and curved array transducers have diverging beams that may intersect a vessel at continuously changing Doppler angles (Fig. 11.27). With linear array transducers, the color Doppler

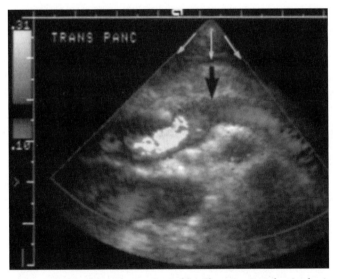

Figure 11.27 *Color Change Caused by Changing Doppler Angle.* A sector transducer is used to produce a color image of the splenic vein as it curves through the pancreas (PANC). The sector transducer sends diverging Doppler beams (*tiny white arrows*) through the pancreas. On the right side of the image, the red color in the splenic vein indicates flow toward the Doppler beams. In the mid-portion of the image (*black arrow*), the Doppler beams intersect the moving blood at a 90-degree angle; therefore no color is displayed in this portion of the vein. On the left side of the image, the blue color indicates blood flow away from the Doppler beams. The yellow color without a black border indicates aliasing caused by an unbalanced velocity scale as shown on the color map. In summary, the color changes indicate normal flow in the splenic vein toward the portal confluence and the liver (see Color Figure 11.27).

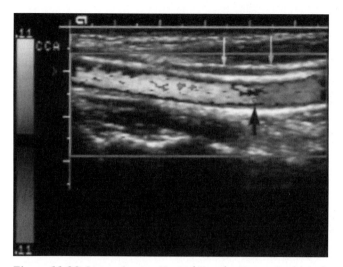

Figure 11.28 *Linear Array—Vertical Doppler Beams.* In this color image, the Doppler beams are vertical (*tiny white arrows*) and parallel to the gray-scale US beams. The common carotid artery (CCA) has a gently curving course through the color field of view. On the right side of the image, the blue color indicates flow relatively away from the Doppler beams. On the left side of the image, the red/yellow color indicates flow relatively toward the Doppler beams. In summary, blood flow is from left to right, indicating normal flow direction toward the brain. Note the black border of transition between the red and blue colors (*black arrow*) where the color changes because of change in Doppler angle. Aliasing is indicated by patches of green without a black border in the yellow colored flow (see Color Figure 11.28).

beams may be aligned parallel to the vertical beams of the gray-scale image or be steered to create more acute Doppler angles (Figs. 11.18B, 11.28). In this circumstance the gray-scale beams are vertical whereas the color Doppler beams are angled parallel to the sides of the color sample volume.

- **Doppler Angle.** The Doppler angle must be analyzed for each portion of the color image (Figs. 11.27, 11.28). The Doppler angle commonly changes because of divergence of the Doppler US beams or because the vessel curves within the field of view.
- **Blood Flow Physiology.** The physiology of blood flow (laminar, disturbed, turbulent) must be interpreted in concert with the technical analysis of the color image. Color images will change constantly throughout the cardiac cycle (Figs. 11.15, 11.29).
- **True color changes** from red to blue shades are etched in black and result from either changes in the Doppler angle or from reversal of blood flow direction (Figs. 11.18B, 11.27, 11.28).
- **Color changes caused by aliasing** are not etched in black and involve the brightest colors on the color scale (Figs. 11.18, 11.27, 11.28).

The final interpretation of the color image is based upon piece-by-piece analysis of each of the items listed.

TO OPTIMIZE COLOR DOPPLER IMAGES

Because the Doppler signal is intrinsically weak, color Doppler images are frequently difficult to obtain. Gray-scale and color Doppler information is obtained sequentially, each taking a finite length of time that depends upon the depth of the image and the width of the field of view. To produce a duplex color and gray-scale image requires 10–20 sweeps through the color field of view for every sweep through the gray-scale field of view. To optimize the color image, adjust the following instrument settings:

- **Doppler Gain Setting.** Turn the Doppler gain up until noise, seen as a random pattern of red and blue dots, covers the image. Then slowly decrease the gain setting until the noise is eliminated.

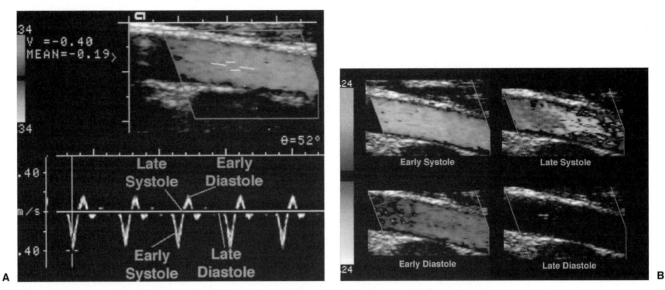

Figure 11.29 *Color Changes in the Cardiac Cycle. A.* Spectral Doppler shows the characteristic changes of the Doppler spectrum of the common femoral artery during the cardiac cycle. *B.* Color Doppler images show the corresponding changes in color images that correspond to phases of the cardiac cycle (see Color Figure 11.29).

- **Power.** Color Doppler commonly requires that the Doppler power setting be set to the maximum setting (Fig. 11.30).
- **Transducer Frequency.** Higher transmit frequencies (5.0–10.0 MHz) provide the greatest Doppler shift. However, high frequency is very limited in tissue penetration. Particularly when encountering difficulties in obtaining Doppler signals from deep in the abdomen, a lower transmit frequency must be utilized to obtain adequate penetration (Fig. 11.30).
- **Doppler Angle.** Doppler signals are very weak at large angles (>60 degrees) and are absent at 90 degrees. Therefore, even in color Doppler, the color signal will be increased and the color image will be improved by adjusting the angle of scanning to produce more acute Doppler angles relative to the vessel imaged.
- **Color Doppler Field of View.** To limit color information gathering time and to improve the quality of the color image, narrow the color field of view and reduce its depth to the minimum needed to visualize the vessel of interest.

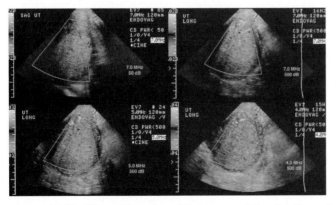

Figure 11.30 *Effect of Transducer Frequency and Doppler Power Settings.* This series of transvaginal images of a uterus containing a first trimester molar pregnancy provides graphic example of the effect of transducer frequency and power settings on the color Doppler image. The best color image is obtained using the lowest transducer frequency (4 MHz) with the highest power setting (500 dB) (see Color Figure 11.30).

- **Gray-Scale US Field of View.** Narrowing the gray-scale field of view and reducing its depth provides a minor improvement in the color image by decreasing the gray-scale information gathering time.
- **Color-Write Priority.** Many color Doppler US instruments allow the operator to manually adjust the color-write priority. The quality of the gray-scale image may be sacrificed to produce a better quality color image. Increasing the color-write priority setting devotes more time to color Doppler information gathering and less time to gray-scale information gathering.

CAROTID ULTRASOUND

A major use of vascular US is in the detection of significant stenosis of the ICA that can lead to stroke. Approximately 76% of all strokes are caused by atherosclerotic disease at the carotid bifurcation. Because it is non-invasive and relatively inexpensive, carotid US is the initial study of choice for detection and characterization of extracranial carotid disease.

ULTRASOUND TECHNIQUE

Carotid sonography requires a thorough and methodical examination utilizing gray-scale US, color flow US, and spectral Doppler. Examination should always include both carotid systems and both vertebral arteries.

- The patient is positioned supine with head turned slightly away from the side being examined. The neck may be hyperextended slightly by placing a pillow under the patient's shoulders. Both patient and examiner must be comfortable because the examination routinely takes 20–40 minutes.
- The examiner sits at the head of the table and is able to rest the examining arm on the table for stability and comfort. High-frequency (7.5–10 MHz) linear array transducers are used for the examination.
- The carotid bifurcation is identified usually 1–2 cm below the angle of the jaw. The bifurcation is easiest to locate by scanning in the transverse plane.
- Gray-scale US is used to detect and evaluate the appearance of carotid plaque. Plaques are always evaluated in both longitudinal and transverse planes.
- Color Doppler or power Doppler is used to identify vessels, assess the presence of blood flow, and to identify the presence and location of plaque and carotid wall thickening.
- Spectral Doppler is used to evaluate the severity of stenosis. The Doppler angle must be kept at <60 degrees to minimize measurement error. All Doppler spectra must be angle corrected to obtain accurate velocity measurements. The Doppler angle indicator is aligned parallel to the wall of the vessel at the location of Doppler sampling. The Doppler sample volume must be kept at less than half of the vessel diameter. Usually the sample volume is kept at 1.5 mm and is positioned in the middle of the flow channel. Doppler spectra are obtained from the common carotid artery (CCA), ECA, and ICA. A careful search is made to ensure that the highest velocity in the area of stenosis is detected and recorded. Doppler spectra are compared to spectra obtained upstream and downstream to the narrowed area of the artery.
- Both vertebral arteries are routinely examined to assess patency and direction of blood flow (Fig. 11.31) [19].

NORMAL CAROTID ULTRASOUND

Findings that differentiate the ICA from the ECA are listed in Table 11.2. Characteristic Doppler spectra are shown in Figure 11.32.

- The CCA is the source of blood for both the ICA and ECA. The Doppler spectrum of the CCA combines characteristics of both ICA and ECA proportional to their relative blood

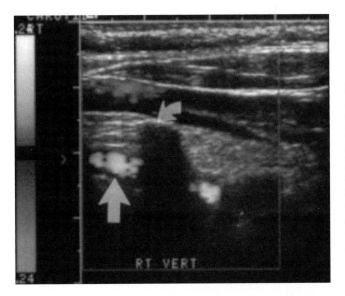

Figure 11.31 *Normal Vertebral Artery.* A normal vertebral artery (*straight arrow*) is seen on color Doppler US between the acoustic shadows cast by the transverse processes (*curved arrow*) of the cervical spine. The vertebral artery is imaged by aligning the transducer with the common carotid artery and then looking deeper for the shadows of the transverse processes. The vertebral arteries are evaluated for patency and flow direction.

flow (70% to the ICA and 30% to the ECA). Normal PSV is 50–100 cm/sec. Symmetric bilateral low CCA velocity is caused by low cardiac output (congestive heart failure) or wide diameter arteries. Symmetric bilateral high CCA velocity is caused by hypertension, bradycardia, hyperthyroidism, or small diameter arteries.

- The ECA supplies the head and face. Its Doppler spectrum is relatively high resistance. Flow velocity returns to baseline during diastole. PSV is greater than the ICA and less than the CCA. The ECA is the smallest of the carotid arteries and has visible branches. Tapping the temporal artery with a finger distorts the ECA spectrum and confirms its identification (Fig. 11.33).
- The ICA supplies the brain and has a low resistance Doppler spectrum. PSV is lower than both the CCA and ECA. Flow is antegrade toward the brain throughout the cardiac cycle. The artery is larger than the ECA and is usually lateral to the ECA.
- Normal reversed flow is seen in the proximal ICA opposite the flow divider at the bifurcation.

Table 11.2: Characteristics of the Internal versus the External Carotid Artery

Internal Carotid Artery	External Carotid Artery
Gray-scale US	**Gray-scale US**
Larger vessel lumen (~6 mm)	Smaller vessel lumen (~3–4 mm)
Postero-lateral location	Antero-medial location
Courses posteriorly toward mastoid	Courses anteriorly toward face
No branch vessels	Has branch vessels
Carotid bulb is at origin	**Color flow US**
Color flow US	Color flow is intermittent during the cardiac cycle
Continuous color flow is seen throughout the cardiac cycle	**Spectral Doppler US**
Spectral Doppler US	High systolic velocity
Low systolic velocity	Sharp, narrow systolic peak
Broad systolic peak	Low-velocity diastolic flow
High-velocity diastolic flow	Diastolic velocity approaches zero baseline
Diastolic velocity does not return to baseline	Tapping on the temporal artery disturbs the Doppler spectrum
Tapping on the temporal artery has no effect on the Doppler spectrum	

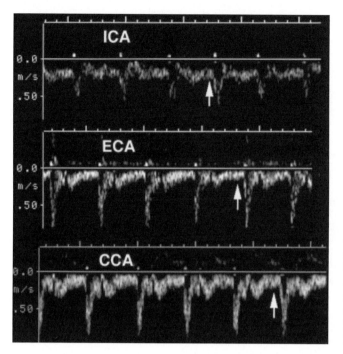

Figure 11.32 *Normal Doppler Spectra of the Carotid Arteries.* See text for description. Arrows indicate end-diastole for each carotid waveform. CCA, common carotid artery; ECA, external carotid artery; ICA, internal carotid artery.

THICKNESS OF THE CAROTID WALL

Thickness of the wall of the carotid artery is a physiologic marker for atherosclerotic disease and may be used to follow the progression of atherosclerosis and to assess the effectiveness of medical therapies (Fig. 11.34) [20,21].

■ Diffuse thickening of the carotid wall, measurable by the intima-media thickness, may be atherosclerotic or non-atherosclerotic in origin. By definition, intima-media thickness is measured on the far arterial wall as the distance between the echogenic lumen-intima interface and the hypoechoic media-adventitia interface [22]. This US appearance of the intima and media has been called the *double line pattern*. Because of gain-dependent reverberation artifact, measurements of the near arterial wall are not accurate.

■ Diffuse increase in intima-media thickness, as measured in the CCA or ICA, has been correlated with symptomatic coronary artery disease, obstructive peripheral artery disease, and increased risk of stroke [23–27]. This measurement is useful in assessing the effects of lifestyle intervention (cessation of cigarette smoking, low-fat diet, etc.) and in the use of medications (antihypertensives and lipid-lowering drugs) [28,29]. Significant thickening is defined differently in various studies. Thickening >1.0–1.3 mm is generally considered abnormal. An increase of 0.1–0.2 mm in thickness over time is considered evidence of significant disease progression.

■ Hypertension is the primary cause of non-atherosclerotic diffuse thickening of the vessel wall. Thickening results primarily from hypertrophy of the media [30].

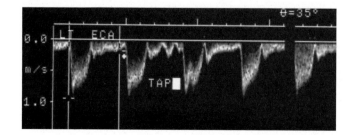

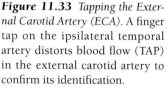

Figure 11.33 *Tapping the External Carotid Artery (ECA).* A finger tap on the ipsilateral temporal artery distorts blood flow (TAP) in the external carotid artery to confirm its identification.

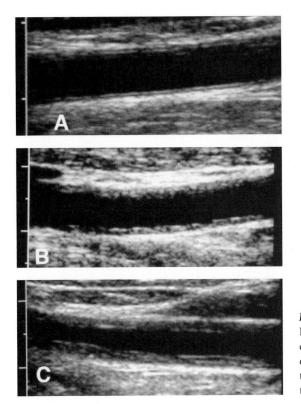

Figure 11.34 *Carotid Wall Thickness.* Images of the common carotid artery demonstrate normal thickness and appearance of the arterial wall in *A*, mild intima-media thickening in *B*, and severe intima-media thickening in *C*.

PLAQUE CHARACTERIZATION

Atherosclerotic plaque may be homogeneous, heterogeneous, or calcified (Fig. 11.35). Heterogeneous plaque is associated with intraplaque hemorrhage and an increased risk of subsequent stroke [27].

■ Focal thickening of the arterial wall, found primarily near vessel bifurcations, corresponds to atherosclerotic plaque.

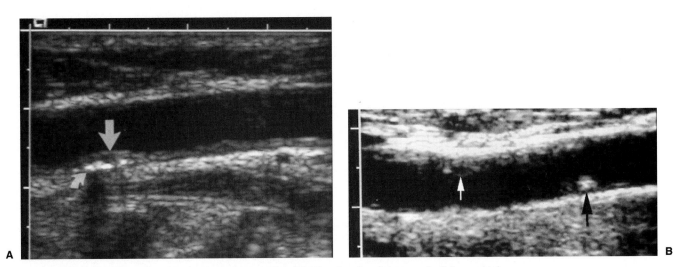

Figure 11.35 *Carotid Plaques. A.* A plaque is seen as a focal thickening (*straight arrow*) of the arterial wall. This plaque would be classified as homogeneous because of its uniform echogenicity. The presence of calcifications (*curved arrow*) within the plaque does not affect its classification. *B.* Image of another common carotid artery shows a heterogeneous plaque with central lucency (*white arrow*) and a focal densely calcified plaque (*black arrow*).

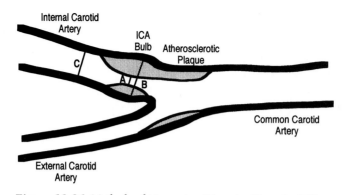

Figure 11.36 *Methods of Measuring Diameter Stenosis.* Different methods of measuring diameter stenosis on arteriograms lead to different calculations of percent diameter stenosis. The traditional method, used by the European Carotid Surgery Trial (ECST), uses the diameter of the carotid bulb, B, as the diameter of reference. Percent diameter stenosis is calculated as (B − A)/B. The North American Carotid Endarterectomy Trial (NASCET) used C, the diameter of the internal carotid artery (ICA) distal to the bulb as the diameter of reference. Percent diameter stenosis is calculated as (C − A)/C. If A is 4 mm, B is 10 mm, and C is 8 mm, ECST would calculate diameter stenosis as 60% [(10 − 4)/10], while NASCET would calculate diameter stenosis as 50% [(8 − 4)/8]. A, diameter of the internal carotid artery (ICA) lumen at the point of maximal narrowing. B, diameter of the disease-free ICA distal to the bulb. C, estimated normal diameter of the bulb of the ICA.

- Homogeneous plaque consists of uniform, low-level echoes comparable in echogenicity to muscles in the neck. The surface of the plaque is smooth. Homogeneous plaque corresponds pathologically to dense, fibrous, laminated, connective tissue.
- Heterogeneous plaque is complex in appearance and contains at least one distinct focal sonolucent area that represents intraplaque hemorrhage or amorphous lipid deposits. An irregular plaque surface classifies plaque as heterogeneous. However, heterogeneous plaque may have a smooth or irregular surface. Although an irregular surface suggests the possibility of plaque ulceration, it is not a reliable criterion for ulceration. No US sign is reliable in detecting ulceration.
- Calcification may be seen in either homogeneous or heterogeneous plaque and is not considered as a criterion for classifying plaque.

Table 11.3: University of Washington Criteria for Internal Carotid Artery Stenosis

Diameter Stenosis (Percent)[a]	Peak Systolic Velocity (cm/sec)	End Diastolic Velocity (cm/sec)	Spectral Broadening	Plaque Visualized
0	<125	<140	No	No
1–15	<125	<140	During systolic deceleration	Yes
16–49	<125	<140	Throughout systole	Yes
50–79	>125	<140	Extensive	Yes
80–99	>125	>140	Extensive	Yes
Occlusion	No flow detected			

Note that each category of stenosis is characterized by presence of an additional criterion.
[a]Percent diameter stenosis is calculated in the traditional manner using the diameter of the bulb of the internal carotid artery as the diameter of reference. These criteria are *not* applicable to the 60% and 70% stenosis cutoffs of the North American Carotid Endarterectomy Trial and the Asymptomatic Carotid Atherosclerosis Study. Source: Fell G, Phillips DJ, Chikos PM, et al. Ultrasonic duplex scanning for disease of the carotid artery. Circulation 1981;64:1191–1195 and Carotid Research Laboratory, University of Washington, Seattle, WA.

Table 11.4: Criteria for Internal Carotid Artery Stenosis Used at the University of Utah

Diameter Stenosis (Percent)[a]	Peak Systolic Velocity (cm/sec)	End Diastolic Velocity (cm/sec)	ICA/CCA Ratio PSV-ICA/PSV-CCA[b]
≥60%	>260	>70	>3.5
≥70%	>325	>110	>4.0

[a]Percent diameter stenosis is calculated by the North American Carotid Endarterectomy Trial standard using the diameter of the distal internal carotid artery as the diameter of reference. These criteria are applicable to the 60% and 70% stenosis cutoffs of the North American Carotid Endarterectomy Trial and the Asymptomatic Carotid Atherosclerosis Study.
[b]Internal carotid artery/common carotid artery ratio equals peak systolic velocity in the area of maximal stenosis in the internal carotid artery divided by peak systolic velocity in a normal segment of the common carotid artery.
Source: Zwiebel WJ. New Doppler parameters for carotid stenosis. Semin Ultrasound CT MRI 1997;18:66–71; and University of Utah School of Medicine and Department of Radiology, Veterans Affairs Medical Center, Salt Lake City, UT [37].

CAROTID STENOSIS

As a result of the North American Carotid Endarterectomy Trial (NASCET) and the European Carotid Surgery Trial, endarterectomy is currently routinely recommended for 70–99% diameter stenosis of the ICA in symptomatic patients [31,32]. It is important to note that percent diameter stenosis was calculated differently in these two studies (Fig. 11.36) [33]. A 70% European Carotid Surgery Trial stenosis is equivalent to a 50% NASCET stenosis. Care must be taken to note the method used to calculate stenosis when evaluating any published study and when using published US parameters to determine stenosis (Tables 11.3–11.5) [34]. The NASCET method yields a consistently lower percentage stenosis.

Because perioperative risk of stroke is high, prophylactic endarterectomy is routinely recommended for asymptomatic patients with >75% stenosis who are undergoing major surgery such as coronary artery bypass grafting. Management is controversial for asymptomatic patients with significant carotid stenosis (≥60%). The Asymptomatic Carotid Atherosclerosis Study (ACAS) demonstrated a decreased stroke risk for asymptomatic patients with ≥60% stenosis treated with endarterectomy [35]. Although the improvement in stroke incidence was not as dramatic as in the NASCET study, many vascular surgeons quote this

Table 11.5: Criteria for Internal Artery Stenosis Recommended by Grant et al.[a]

Percent Diameter Stenosis[b]	Peak Systolic Velocity (cm/sec)	ICA/CCA Ratio PSV-ICA/PSV-CCA[c]
≥70% Symptomatic patients	175	2.5
≥60% Asymptomatic patients	200	3.0

[a]These criteria separate patients into those with (symptomatic) and those without (asymptomatic) neurological symptoms. All patients were considered at risk for generalized atherosclerotic disease.
[b]Percent diameter stenosis is calculated by the North American Carotid Endarterectomy Trial standard using the diameter of the distal internal carotid artery as the diameter of reference. These criteria are applicable to the 60% and 70% stenosis cutoffs of the North American Carotid Endarterectomy Trial and the Asymptomatic Carotid Atherosclerosis Study.
[c]Internal carotid artery/common carotid artery ratio equals peak systolic velocity (PSV) in the area of maximal stenosis in the ICA divided by PSV in a normal segment of the CCA.
Source: Grant EG, Duerinckx AJ, Saden SE, et al. Doppler sonographic parameters for detection of carotid stenosis: Is there an optimum method for their selection? AJR Am J Roentgenol 1999;172:1123–1129.

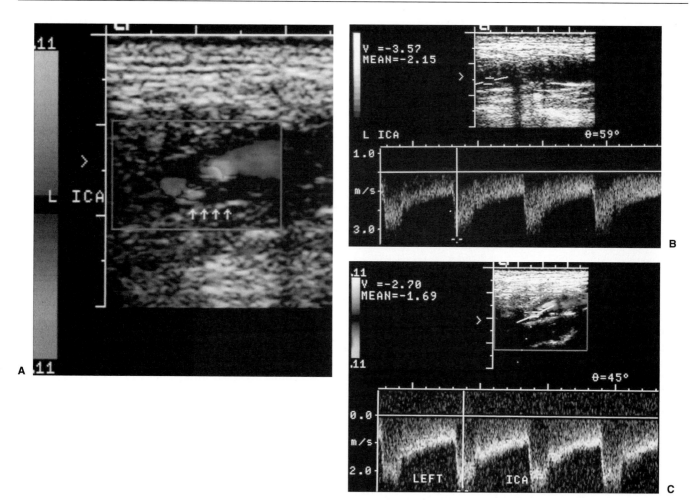

Figure 11.37 *Carotid Stenosis >70%. A.* Color Doppler identifies a large plaque (*arrows*) in the left internal carotid artery (L ICA). Flow as shown by color display is narrowed to a trickle in the area of maximum stenosis (see Color Figure 11.37A). *B.* Doppler spectrum in the area of maximal stenosis shows spectral broadening and elevated peak systolic velocity measured at 3.57 m/sec. End diastolic velocity is approximately 1.30 m/sec. Using the criteria from the University of Utah (Table 11.4) Doppler assessment indicates significant stenosis of >70%. *C.* Downstream from the plaque, flow velocities have decreased but turbulence is prominent.

study as justification for performing endarterectomy in asymptomatic patients. The ACAS used the NASCET method for measuring stenosis.

US parameters used to determine categories of carotid stenosis remain under debate. Historically, the University of Washington criteria (Strandness) (Table 11.3) have been widely accepted and utilized. However, these criteria do not match the 70% and 60% threshold levels of the NASCET and ACAS used to justify carotid endarterectomy in symptomatic and asymptomatic patients. In addition, the percent stenosis of the University of Washington criteria was determined by traditional angiographic methods using the diameter of the "normal" carotid bulb as the standard of reference. A wide range of new criteria matched to NASCET and ACAS criteria and using the NASCET method of determining percentage stenosis have been published and are being used (Tables 11.4, 11.5) [36–38]. Each US laboratory must correlate the criteria used with patient outcomes (Fig. 11.37).

The method of angiographic measurement used to determine percent diameter stenosis must be known to interpret severity of carotid disease as determined by US.

■ PSV in the area of maximum narrowing has the best statistical correlation with percent diameter stenosis as determined by carotid arteriography. Note that PSV continues to increase until critical stenosis is reached at approximately 60–70% diameter stenosis (Fig. 11.38). With increasing stenosis beyond this level, both blood flow volume and blood flow velocity fall rapidly.

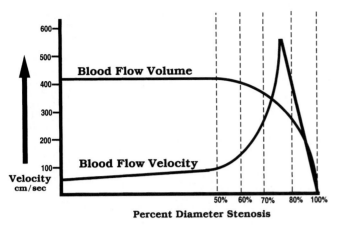

Figure 11.38 *Velocity vs. Flow and Percent Stenosis.* As the diameter of the vessel decreases (from left to right), the velocity in the area of maximum stenosis increases. Peak velocities occur at approximately 60–70% diameter stenosis. Thereafter, the velocity falls off rapidly to zero. Blood flow, however, remains stable until diameter stenosis of 50–60% is reached. Thereafter, blood flow falls off rapidly to zero.

- Carotid disease is classified in categories of stenosis (i.e., 50–79% or ≥60%), not as a specific percent diameter stenosis (i.e., 72%).
- CCA stenosis has no established parameters. ICA criteria are usually used to estimate severity of CCA stenosis.
- ECA stenosis has no established parameters and has limited clinical significance except for explanation of the presence of a carotid bruit. ECA stenosis can be estimated by using PSV. Mild stenosis is indicated by PSV >130 cm/sec, moderate stenosis by PSV >200 cm/sec, and severe stenosis by PSV >300 cm/sec.

OCCLUSION OF THE INTERNAL CAROTID ARTERY

Occlusion of the ICA may be asymptomatic if blood supply to the brain is adequate through collaterals of the circle of Willis (Fig. 11.39).

- Color and spectral Doppler signals are absent in the ICA.
- The CCA spectrum is identical in appearance to the ECA spectrum with low flow velocity in diastole.
- The ECA may show a Doppler waveform more characteristic of the ICA if it supplies collateral vessel connections to reconstitute the intracranial ICA.
- The ICA lumen is filled with echogenic thrombus.
- The ICA lumen is sub-normal in size.
- The wall of the ICA does not expand with pulsations.
- "Stump flow" may be seen at the proximal end of the occlusion. The spectrum shows brief systolic spikes caused by the "thumping" of blood against the occlusion.
- Doppler US does not reliably differentiate high-grade stenosis with a trickle of flow from complete occlusion. This differentiation is critical because near-occlusion is potentially correctable by endarterectomy whereas total occlusion is not reversible. Angiography is needed to confirm total occlusion.

SUBCLAVIAN STEAL

Occlusion of the innominate or subclavian artery proximal to the origin of the vertebral artery will "steal" blood from the intracranial circulation to supply the affected arm. Flow in the ipsilateral vertebral artery is retrograde and the patient may experience symptoms of cerebral ischemia, especially with muscle activity of the arm.

- Flow is reversed in the ipsilateral vertebral artery away from instead of toward the intracranial circulation (Fig. 11.40).
- Partial subclavian steal, caused by high-grade stenosis of the innominate or subclavian artery, results in reversed flow in the vertebral artery (away from the brain) during systole and forward flow (toward the brain) during diastole.

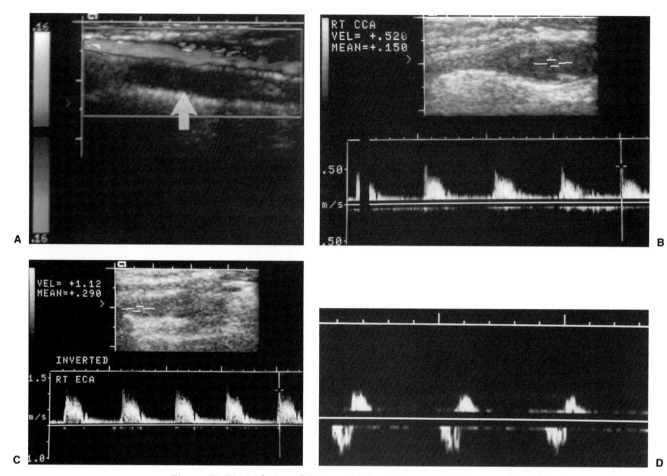

Figure 11.39 *Occlusion of the Internal Carotid Artery.* *A.* Color Doppler image shows no flow in the internal carotid artery (*arrow*). The lumen is filled with hypoechoic thrombus (see Color Figure 11.39A). *B.* Doppler spectrum of the common carotid artery (CCA) shows a high resistance spectrum identical to that of the external carotid artery (ECA) shown in *C. D.* Doppler spectrum obtained at the origin of the internal carotid artery shows "stump flow."

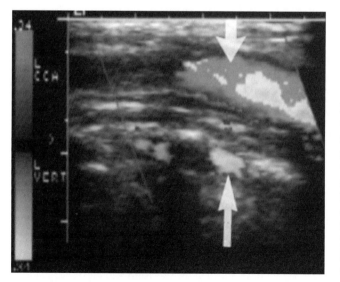

Figure 11.40 *Subclavian Steal.* Color Doppler image of the common carotid artery (CCA) (*short arrow*) and the vertebral artery (*long arrow*) shows colors on opposite sides of the color map indicating blood flow in different directions. The vertebral artery is flowing away from the brain while the CCA shows normal blood flow direction toward the brain (see Color Figure 11.40).

- Early subclavian steal with continued antegrade flow in the vertebral artery is suggested when a sharp decline in flow velocity is noted in early systole [39].

PERIPHERAL ARTERIES

PERIPHERAL ARTERY STENOSIS

No criteria for characterizing stenosis of peripheral arteries are firmly established by clinical studies [25]. The following criteria are generally used [40,41].

- PSV are determined in area of maximal stenosis and compared as a ratio to PSV obtained upstream to the stenosis. As illustrated in Figure 11.12, the artery should be examined with gray-scale and Doppler US upstream from any visualized plaque, at the area of maximal narrowing, and downstream from the visualized plaque. Normal PSV in peripheral arteries is <150 cm/sec.
- PSV (stenosis)/PSV (upstream) <2.0 indicates <50% stenosis. PSV is <200 cm/sec.
- PSV (stenosis)/PSV (upstream) >2.0 indicates >50% stenosis. PSV is 200–400 cm/sec.
- PSV (stenosis)/PSV (upstream) >3.5 indicates >70% stenosis. PSV is >400 cm/sec. Diastolic velocity in the area of stenosis is increased compared to upstream spectra. Flow reversal in diastole is lost because of the pressure drop across the severe stenosis. This feature is highly indicative of a severe stenosis. Severe downstream turbulence is usually present. Dampened waveforms may be characteristic of tardus parvus.
- Occlusion is manifest by absence of blood flow and visualization of enlarged collateral vessels. Tardus parvus waveforms are common in reconstituted distal vessels.

ABDOMINAL AORTA

NORMAL AORTA

The normal abdominal aorta is visualized from the diaphragm through the bifurcation into the common iliac arteries. The aorta lies on the left side of the lumbar spine.

- The normal aorta gradually tapers as it proceeds distally giving off its branches. The origins of the celiac axis and SMA from the anterior aorta can usually be visualized (see Fig. 2.10).
- Spectral Doppler of the infrarenal aorta shows a triphasic, high-resistance pattern with reversal of flow in early diastole.

ATHEROSCLEROTIC CHANGE OF THE AORTA

Atherosclerosis is the most common disease of the aorta.

- Atheromatous plaques cause the wall of the aorta to appear irregular and focally asymmetric. Calcification in the plaques produces bright, discontinuous, linear echoes that may case acoustic shadows and obscure the aortic lumen (Fig. 11.41).
- The aorta commonly becomes tortuous. Care must be taken to measure the aortic diameter in true transverse section and not be fooled by tortuosity simulating dilatation.

ANEURYSM OF ABDOMINAL AORTA

US is the screening method of choice to document the presence of, and to follow, abdominal aortic aneurysms (AAA) because of low cost, high accuracy, and noninvasive nature [42]. Complications of AAA include rupture, which is often catastrophic, distal embolism, fistula to adjacent structures, thrombosis, and dissection.

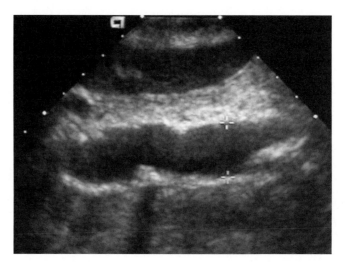

Figure 11.41 *Atherosclerotic Disease of the Abdominal Aorta.* Longitudinal US image of the aorta (*between cursors,* +) shows an irregular wall and calcified atherosclerotic plaques, some of which cast acoustic shadows.

- Focal or diffuse enlargement of the diameter of the abdominal aorta greater than 3 cm is an aneurysm (Fig. 11.42). The luminal diameter of the aorta is measured from inner wall to inner wall.
- Enlargement of the distal aorta to 1.5 times the diameter of the adjacent, more proximal aorta is considered to be an aneurysm even if the aortic diameter is less than 3 cm.
- Common iliac arteries are aneurysmal when the diameter exceeds 1.5 cm (Fig. 11.43) [43].
- Mural thrombus is commonly present within AAA. Thrombus is hypoechoic and is best identified by using color Doppler to show the patent lumen.
- Approximately 90–95% of AAA are confined to the infrarenal aorta.
- Aneurysms that involve the aorta at the level of origin of the renal arteries change surgical management and must be diagnosed preoperatively. The renal arteries may be difficult to visualize; however, both arise within 2 cm of the origin of the SMA. Therefore, if a normal caliber aorta is documented at least 2 cm below the origin of the SMA, the AAA is confirmed to be infrarenal. Aneurysms that involve the renal artery origins are frequently extensions of aneurysms of the thoracic aorta.
- AAA are usually not repaired until they exceed 4–5 cm in maximum diameter. The risk of rupture within 5 years is 25% at 5-cm diameter and rises to 75% at 7-cm diameter. AAA smaller than 5 cm have a 3% risk of rupture over 10 years [44].
- US is used to monitor the rate of enlargement of AAA. The average increase in diameter is 2 mm per year.

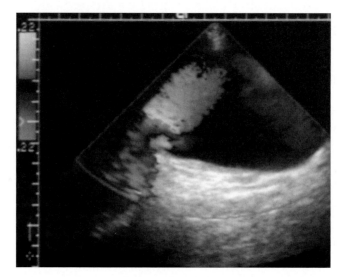

Figure 11.42 *Aneurysm of the Abdominal Aorta.* Longitudinal color Doppler image shows swirling blood flow within a 5-cm-diameter aneurysm (see Color Figure 11.42).

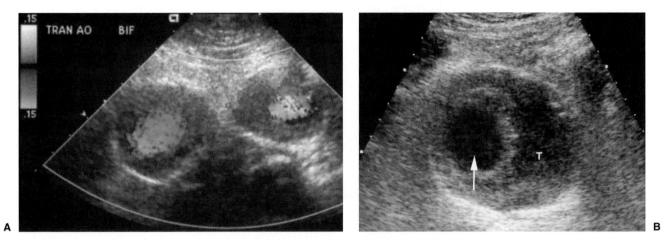

Figure 11.43 *Aneurysms of the Common Iliac Arteries. A.* Transverse plane color Doppler image (*shown here in gray scale*) below the aortic bifurcation (AO BIF) shows bilateral aneurysms of the common iliac arteries. *B.* Enlarged view of the right common iliac artery shows the large amount of intraluminal thrombus (T) commonly found in aneurysms of the aorta and iliac arteries. The patent lumen is indicated by the arrow.

- Leakage or rupture of an AAA is suggested by demonstration of fluid or hematoma around the aorta. However, spiral CT is the method of choice for diagnosis because US has unacceptably low sensitivity and specificity.
- AAA may obstruct the ureters by direct compression or by perianeurysmal fibrosis. Routine survey of the kidneys for hydronephrosis is indicated when US is used to follow AAA.

ENDOVASCULAR AORTIC STENTS

Endovascular repair of AAA is a new and rapidly expanding procedure that may replace standard surgical repair [45]. Aortic stent grafts are expandable intraluminal grafts that consist of a metal framework cage covered by synthetic graft material. These grafts are compressed within a catheter and guided under fluoroscopy to be placed within the AAA and expanded to the optimal size of the aorta. Ideally, all blood flow is excluded from the AAA allowing thrombosis of the AAA outside of the stent graft. Spiral CT or Doppler US are used to follow the integrity of stent grafts.

- US examination must determine
  - Patency of the stent graft
  - Size of the AAA
  - Presence of endoleaks, seen as blood flow within the aneurysm outside of the stent
  - Change in diameter of the vessels at the sites of endograft attachment
  - Presence of new aneurysms [45]

ULTRASOUND OF DEEP VENOUS THROMBOSIS

Compression US is the imaging procedure of choice for diagnosis of deep venous thrombosis (DVT) in the lower extremities [46]. US is highly accurate in the diagnosis of DVT involving the proximal leg veins with sensitivity exceeding 95% and specificity exceeding 98% [47]. DVT is the major risk factor for life-threatening pulmonary emboli.

ULTRASOUND TECHNIQUE

US examination consists of visualizing deep veins with gray-scale US, supplemented by color flow and spectral Doppler, and then using the transducer to compress the vein until opposing walls touch.

- The patient is examined in supine position with the head of the bed raised 20 degrees to 30 degrees to promote venous pooling in the legs. The leg is rotated externally and flexed slightly at the knee.
- A 7–10-MHz linear array transducer is utilized. Doppler capability greatly aids the examination but is not a requirement.
- The common femoral vein is identified medial to the common femoral artery in the groin at the crease of the thigh.
- Transducer pressure is used to compress and flatten the vein until the anterior and posterior walls are touching and the lumen is obliterated. Compression should always be performed transverse to the vein because the transducer may slide off the vein with compression in the longitudinal plane.
- Thrombus makes compression of vein impossible with force less than that required to compress the adjacent artery.
- The vein is followed distally and compressed every centimeter of its course to the bifurcation of the popliteal vein into posterior tibial and peroneal branches.
- In the adductor canal, the superficial femoral vein is deep and may be difficult to compress. Placing one hand under the medial aspect of the thigh allows the vein to be pushed to a more superficial location where it can be compressed between the fingers and the transducer.
- Having the patient perform a Valsalva maneuver will decrease venous return to the chest and distend the leg veins to make identification easier. Blood flow can also be augmented by gently squeezing the calf.
- Evaluation of the calf veins is considerably more difficult and time consuming, and has a much higher rate of inadequate examination. Because calf vein thrombosis is not a direct risk factor in the development of pulmonary embolus, most clinicians do not treat calf vein thrombosis and consider examination of the calf veins to be unnecessary [48].

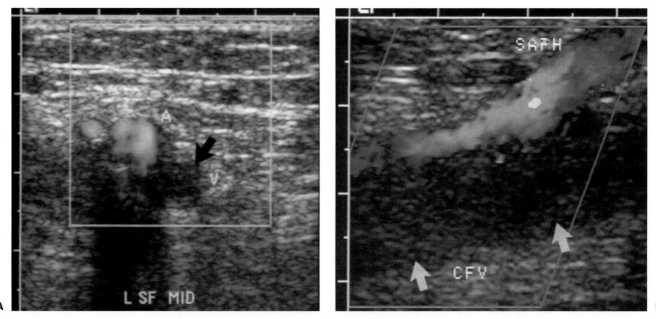

Figure 11.44 *Deep Venous Thrombosis—Lower Extremity.* A. Transverse power Doppler image with transducer compression applied shows flow in the femoral artery (A) and no flow in the femoral vein (V, *arrow*). The vein does not compress with transducer pressure, indicating intraluminal thrombus. B. Longitudinal color Doppler image of the junction of the greater saphenous vein (SAPH) with the common femoral vein (CFV, *arrows*) shows enlargement of the common femoral vein with intraluminal thrombus. Note the flow of blood around the thrombus above the venous junction (see Color Figure 11.44).

■ If the initial US study is negative, but the patient remains symptomatic or highly suspect for DVT clinically, the US examination should be repeated in 1 week. This follow-up study is intended to detect patients with calf vein thrombosis that has propagated to involve the deep venous system [46].

ACUTE DEEP VENOUS THROMBOSIS

Lack of venous compressibility is the hallmark of US diagnosis of DVT (Fig. 11.44).

■ Acute thrombus is hypoechoic and is commonly indistinguishable from flowing blood. Inability to compress the vein and obliterate the lumen is prime evidence of the presence of thrombus.
■ The vein is distended when DVT is acute.
■ Color Doppler reveals absence of blood flow or a trickle of blood flow around the thrombus.
■ Duplication of the normally solitary deep veins of the thigh is a potential pitfall [49]. One of the paired veins may be patent while the other has thrombus. A clue to this diagnosis is unusually small size of the visualized patent vein.
■ The radiographic report must specify the diagnosis of DVT when present. Some clinicians are unaware that the superficial femoral vein is actually a deep vein.

CHRONIC DEEP VENOUS THROMBOSIS

DVT is slow to resolve and is prone to recur. Involved deep veins return to normal appearance and compressibility in only 50% of patients by 12–24 months. In some patients, US evidence of DVT persists indefinitely. Diagnosis of new acute thrombus in a patient with known previous DVT is a challenge.

■ Thrombus becomes increasingly echogenic with time and may even calcify (Fig. 11.45).
■ The chronic clot is often discontinuous and only partially occlusive with intervening areas of normal appearing vein.
■ The chronic clot is usually adherent to the vein wall.
■ With chronic DVT, the wall of the vein thickens and stiffens, becoming more resistant to compression.
■ Re-examining high-risk patients after completion of their anticoagulant therapy is useful in establishing a new baseline on which to base diagnosis of recurrent DVT.

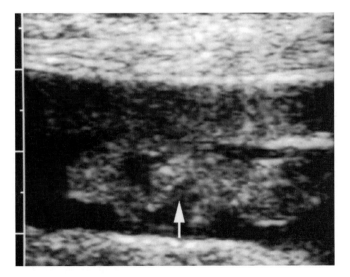

Figure 11.45 Chronic Deep Venous Thrombosis. Longitudinal image shows a very echogenic lobulated clot (*arrow*) in the common femoral vein. Increased echogenicity of the clot is evidence of chronicity.

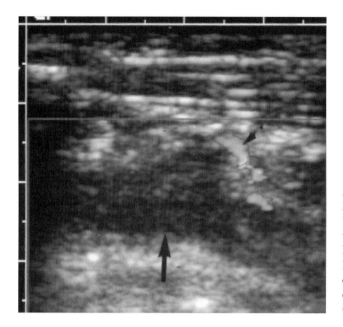

Figure 11.46 *Deep Venous Thrombosis—Upper Extremity.* Color Doppler image of the subclavian vein (*long arrow*) shows that the lumen is distended with thrombus. No blood flow in the vein is evident. Flow is present in an adjacent artery (*short arrow*) (see Color Figure 11.46).

UPPER EXTREMITY DEEP VENOUS THROMBOSIS

Upper extremity DVT may also result in pulmonary embolus. Patients at risk include chronically ill or cancer patients with indwelling catheters in the upper extremity veins and young patients with idiopathic thrombus [50].

- Compression US of the subclavian, axillary, basilic, and cephalic veins is performed in a manner similar to examination of the lower extremity. Doppler is exceptionally valuable in evaluating portions of the veins that are not easily accessible, such as the subclavian vein where covered by the clavicle [51].
- Diagnostic findings are identical to those used in the lower extremity (Fig. 11.46).

VASCULAR LESIONS OF THE EXTREMITIES

PSEUDOANEURYSM

Pseudoaneurysms occur as a complication of penetrating injuries to arteries. Many occur as complications of percutaneous interventional vascular procedures such as coronary or peripheral angioplasty [52]. A pseudoaneurysm is a perivascular hematoma that maintains a channel of flowing blood in communication with the parent artery. They are initially bounded by clotted blood but eventually form a fibrous capsule. Unlike true aneurysms, the wall does not contain any normal arterial wall layers (Fig. 11.47) [53].

- Gray-scale US shows a complex perivascular mass with a variable amount of echogenic thrombus. Multiple compartments may be evident.
- Color flow US shows swirling internal flow and a fistulous communication to the adjacent artery. The entire mass must be carefully examined because only a portion of the mass may show blood flow while the rest of the mass is thrombus.
- Spectral Doppler confirms arterial pulsations within the mass and a distinctive "to and fro" spectral pattern at the communication. Blood flows into the pseudoaneurysm during systole and out of the pseudoaneurysm during diastole [54].
- US-guided manual compression of the pseudoaneurysm is commonly curative, resulting in stable thrombosis [55]. The transducer is oriented to optimally visualize the neck of the pseudoaneurysm [56]. Firm compression is applied with the transducer with pressure sufficient to obliterate flow to the pseudoaneurysm. Compression is continued for

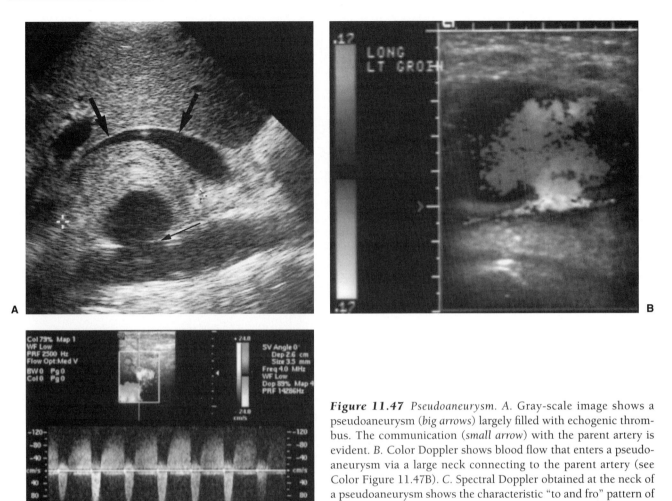

Figure 11.47 *Pseudoaneurysm. A.* Gray-scale image shows a pseudoaneurysm (*big arrows*) largely filled with echogenic thrombus. The communication (*small arrow*) with the parent artery is evident. *B.* Color Doppler shows blood flow that enters a pseudoaneurysm via a large neck connecting to the parent artery (see Color Figure 11.47B). *C.* Spectral Doppler obtained at the neck of a pseudoaneurysm shows the characteristic "to and fro" pattern of blood flow.

one or more 10-minute periods. Pressure is released after 10 minutes to assess for complete thrombosis. Patients on anticoagulant therapy commonly fail to respond to US-guided compression therapy. Surgery is usually required when guided compression fails.

PERIVASCULAR HEMATOMA

Hematomas may form adjacent to areas of vascular injury (Fig. 11.48) [52].

- Hematomas are masses of variable echogenicity that change in appearance and shrink in size over time. Differentiation from pseudoaneurysm requires careful Doppler evaluation.
- Internal blood flow is not present on spectral or color flow Doppler.
- Tissue vibration artifact from adjacent blood vessels may be mistaken for flow in a pseudoaneurysm especially when the hematoma is echolucent.

ARTERIOVENOUS FISTULA

Simultaneous arterial and venous puncture may result in a fistulous tract between the two vessels [53]. Arterial blood is preferentially shunted to the venous circulation and may result in distal limb ischemia [57].

- High-velocity diastolic flow is seen in the artery proximal to the fistula.
- Increased flow velocity with arterial pulsations are seen in the vein near the fistula. Turbulence is often prominent near the fistula.

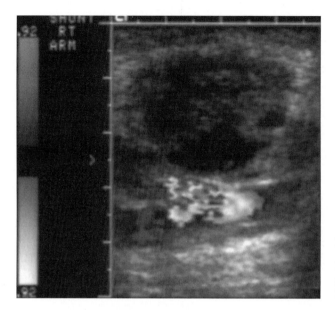

Figure 11.48 *Hematoma.* Color Doppler reveals no flow in a hematoma adjacent to a dialysis shunt graft in the arm (see Color Figure 11.48).

- The fistula may be visualized with color flow US as a tiny track extending between the artery and vein (Fig. 11.49).
- Perivascular tissue vibration artifact (a visible bruit) may be prominent on color Doppler US.

ARTERIOVENOUS MALFORMATION

Arteriovenous malformation is a congenital vascular anomaly made up of a network of direct communications between arteries and veins (Fig. 11.50) [58].

- Supplying arteries and draining veins are dilated.
- Color Doppler shows the subcutaneous network of abnormal intercommunicating arteries and veins [59].
- Tissue vibration artifact may be prominent in surrounding soft tissues.
- The supplying artery shows a low-resistance spectrum.

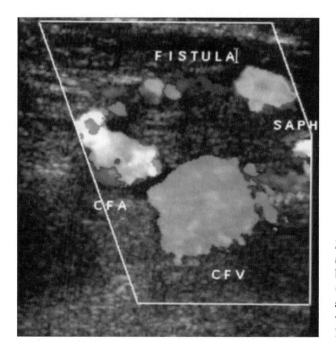

Figure 11.49 *Arteriovenous Fistula.* Color Doppler shows a fistula between the greater saphenous vein (SAPH) and the common femoral artery (CFA). The common femoral vein (CFV) is also seen (see Color Figure 11.49).

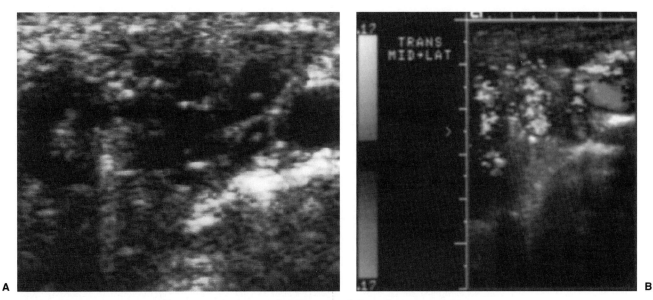

Figure 11.50 *Arteriovenous Malformation. A.* Gray-scale US image of the soft tissues of the upper chest shows a network of tubular structures in the subcutaneous tissues. *B.* Color Doppler confirms blood flow in the tubular structures, representing a complex of vessels of an arteriovenous malformation (see Color Figure 11.50B).

PERIPHERAL VASCULAR GRAFTS

US is an ideal modality to survey peripheral vascular grafts for complications [60]. US examination includes real-time gray-scale survey of the entire graft and spectral and color Doppler examination of blood flow [61].

- Focal fluid collections at the site of graft anastomoses are common, not pathologically significant, and generally resolve within a few months of surgery.
- US-guided aspiration can easily be performed if infection of a perigraft fluid collection is suspected.
- Grafts may show diffuse wall thickening caused by intimal hyperplasia or focal stenosis deemed significant if PSV in the area of stenosis is two times PSV in the more proximal graft.
- Arteriovenous fistulas may develop as a result of surgery or graft puncture for arteriography.
- Pseudoaneurysms are common at sites of graft anastomosis and are distinguished from hematomas and lymph nodes by use of color flow US.

HEMODIALYSIS ACCESS GRAFTS

Prosthetic and native vein arteriovenous grafts are in common use for vascular access for hemodialysis [62]. Progressive stenosis and thrombosis are common events with graft occlusion rates of 17–45% during the first year [63]. Routine US surveillance for developing graft stenosis with subsequent angioplasty of high-grade stenosis can prolong graft patency. The entire graft is inspected with gray-scale and color flow US. Any areas of stenosis are evaluated with spectral Doppler [62–64].

- Spectral Doppler of normal grafts show low-resistance waveforms with PSV of 100–400 cm/sec with end-diastolic velocities of 60–200 cm/sec [62].
- Focal elevation of PSV 2.0–2.9× PSV in the more proximal graft correlates with 50–79% stenosis. Focal 3× elevation of PSV indicates ≥75% stenosis [64]. Arteriography of the graft is routinely performed when US detects stenosis of ≥50% [63].

■ Infection of the graft is common (10–15% of synthetic grafts) and necessitates removal of the graft [62]. US demonstrates perigraft fluid collections in patients with fever and positive blood cultures. US-guided aspiration is used to confirm graft infection.

■ Aneurysms and pseudoaneurysms are common complications of repeated graft puncture [62]. Small pseudoaneurysms (<5 mm) tend to be stable and not clinically significant. Pseudoaneurysms >5 mm usually enlarge progressively and should be embolized or repaired surgically. Pseudoaneurysms at the site of graft anastomosis tend to be complications of graft infection. Aneurysmal dilatation of the graft is common and is usually not treated.

REFERENCES

1. Powis RL. Color flow imaging. Radiographics 1994;14:415–428.
2. Green IR, Dudley NJ, Gravill N. Presentation of colour flow maps of the peripheral circulation. British J Radiology 1994;67:689–694.
3. Murphy KJ, Rubin JM. Power Doppler: It's a good thing. Semin Ultrasound CT MRI 1997;18:13–20.
4. Hamper UM, DeJong MR, Caskey CI, et al. Power Doppler imaging: clinical experience and correlation with color Doppler US and other imaging modalities. Radiographics 1997;17:499–513.
5. Fleischer AC. Sonographic depiction of tumor vascularity and flow: from in vivo models to clinical applications. J Ultrasound Med 2000;19:55–61.
6. Kremkau FW. Doppler principles. Semin Roentgen 1992;27:6–16.
7. Zwiebel WJ, Fruechte D. Basics of abdominal and pelvic duplex: instrumentation, anatomy, and vascular Doppler signatures. Semin Ultrasound CT MRI 1992;13:3–21.
8. Burns PN. The physical principles of Doppler and spectral analysis. J Clin Ultrasound 1987;15:567–590.
9. Murphy ME, Tublin ME. Understanding the Doppler RI: impact of renal arterial distensibility on the RI in a hydronephrotic ex vivo rabbit kidney model. J Ultrasound Med 2000;19:303–314.
10. Bude RO, Rubin JM, Platt JF, et al. Pulsus tardus: its cause and potential limitations in detection of arterial stenosis. Radiology 1994;190:779–784.
11. Dodd GDI, Mernel DS, Zajko AB, et al. Hepatic artery stenosis and thrombosis in transplant recipients: Doppler diagnosis with resistive index and systolic acceleration time. Radiology 1994;192:657–661.
12. Stavros AT, Parker SH, Yakes WF, et al. Segmental stenosis of the renal artery: pattern recognition of tardus and parvus abnormalities with duplex sonography. Radiology 1992;184:487–492.
13. Mitchell DG. Color Doppler imaging: principles, limitations, artifacts. Radiology 1990;177:1–10.
14. Rubin JM, Bude RO, Carson PL, et al. Power Doppler US: a potentially useful alternative to mean frequency-based color Doppler US. Radiology 1994;190:853–856.
15. Middleton WD, Melson GL. The carotid ghost—a color Doppler ultrasound duplication artifact. J Ultrasound Med 1990;9:487–493.
16. Reading CC, Charboneau JW, Allison JW, et al. Color and spectral Doppler mirror-image artifact of the subclavian artery. Radiology 1990;174:41–42.
17. Middleton WD, Erickson S, Melson GL. Perivascular color artifact: pathologic significance and appearance on color Doppler US images. Radiology 1989;171:647–652.
18. Cox IH, Erickson SJ, Foley WD, et al. Ureteral jets: evaluation of normal flow dynamics with color Doppler sonography. AJR Am J Roentgenol 1992;158:1051–1055.
19. Gooding GAW. Vascular ultrasound: the vertebral and subclavian arteries. Radiologist 1998;5:219–225.
20. Bluth EI. Evaluation and characterization of carotid plaque. Semin Ultrasound CT MRI 1997;18:57–65.
21. Linhart A, Gariepy J, Massonneau M, et al. Carotid intima-media thickness: the ultimate surrogate end-point of cardiovascular involvement in atherosclerosis. Applied Radiology 2000;March 2000:25–39.
22. Pignoli P, Tremoli E, Poli A, et al. Intimal plus medial thickness of the arterial wall: a direct measurement with ultrasound imaging. Circulation 1986;74:1399–1406.
23. Chambless LE, Heiss G, Folsom AR, et al. Association of coronary heart disease incidence with carotid arterial wall thickness and major risk factors: the Atherosclerosis Risk in Communities (ARIC) Study, 1987–1993. Am J Epidemiol 1997;146:483–494.

24. O'Leary DH, Polak JF, Kronmal RA, et al. Carotid-artery intima and media thickness as a risk factor for myocardial infarction and stroke in older adults. Cardiovascular Health Study Collaborative Research Group. N Engl J Med 1999;340:14–22.

25. Polak JF. Arterial sonography: efficacy for the diagnosis of arterial disease of the lower extremity. AJR Am J Roentgenol 1993;161:235–243.

26. Polak JF, O'Leary DH, Kronmal RA, et al. Sonographic evaluation of carotid artery atherosclerosis in the elderly: relationship of disease severity to stroke and transient ischemic attack. Radiology 1993;188:363–370.

27. Polak JF, Shemanski L, O'Leary DH, et al. Hypoechoic plaque at US of the carotid artery: an independent risk factor for incident stroke in adults aged 65 years or older. Cardiovascular Health Study. Radiology 1998;208:649–654.

28. Blankenhorn DH, Selzer RH, Crawford DW, et al. Beneficial effects of colestipol-niacin therapy on the common carotid artery. Two- and four-year reduction of intima-media thickness measured by ultrasound. Circulation 1993;88:20–28.

29. Zanchetti A, Rosei EA, Dal Palu C, et al. The Verapamil in Hypertension and Atherosclerosis Study (VHAS): results of long-term randomized treatment with either verapamil or chlorthalidone on carotid intima-media thickness. J Hypertens 1998;16:1667–1676.

30. Armentano RL, Graf S, Barra JG, et al. Carotid wall viscosity increase is related to intima-media thickening in hypertensive patients. Hypertension 1998;31:534–539.

31. North American Symptomatic Carotid Trial Collaborators. Beneficial effect of carotid endarterectomy in symptomatic patients with high-grade carotid stenosis. N Engl J Med 1991;325:445–453.

32. European Carotid Surgery Trialist's Collaborative Group. MRC European carotid surgery trial: interim results for symptomatic patients with severe (70–99%) or with mild (0–29%) carotid stenosis. Lancet 1991;337:1235–1243.

33. Fox AJ. How to measure carotid stenosis. Radiology 1993;186:316–318.

34. Rothwell PM, Gibson SJ, Slattery J, et al. Equivalence of measurements of carotid stenosis. A comparison of three methods on 1001 angiograms. Stroke 1994;25:2435–2439.

35. Executive Committee for the Asymptomatic Carotid Atherosclerosis Study. Endarterectomy for asymptomatic carotid artery stenosis. JAMA 1995;273:1421–1428.

36. Fell G, Phillips DJ, Chikos PM, et al. Ultrasonic duplex scanning for disease of the carotid artery. Circulation 1981;64:1191–1195.

37. Zwiebel WJ. New Doppler parameters for carotid stenosis. Semin Ultrasound CT MRI 1997;18:66–71.

38. Grant EG, Duerinckx AJ, Saden SE, et al. Doppler sonographic parameters for detection of carotid stenosis: Is there an optimum method for their selection? AJR Am J Roentgenol 1999;172:1123–1129.

39. Kliewer MA, Hertzberg BS, Kim DH, et al. Vertebral artery Doppler waveform changes indication of subclavian steal physiology. AJR Am J Roentgenol 2000;174:815–819.

40. Cossman DV, Ellison JE, Wagner WH, et al. Comparison of contrast arteriography to arterial mapping with color-flow duplex imaging in the lower extremities. J Vasc Surgery 1989;10:522–529.

41. Sacks D, Robinson ML, Marinelli D, et al. Peripheral arterial Doppler ultrasonography: diagnostic criteria. J Ultrasound Med 1992;11:95–103.

42. Gooding GAW. Vascular ultrasound: abdominal aorta and mesenteric arteries. Radiologist 2000;7:71–80.

43. Pedersen OM, Aslaken A, Vik-Mo H. Ultrasound measurement of the luminal diameter of the abdominal aorta and iliac arteries in patients without vascular disease. J Vasc Surg 1993;17:596–601.

44. Reed WW, Hallett JW Jr, Damiano MA, et al. Learning from the last ultrasound. A population-based study of patients with abdominal aortic aneurysm. Arch Intern Med 1997;157:2064–2068.

45. Kaufman JA, Geller SC, Brewster DC, et al. Endovascular repair of abdominal aortic aneurysms: current status and future directions. AJR Am J Roentgenol 2000;175:289–302.

46. Fraser JD, Anderson DR. Deep venous thrombosis: recent advances and optimal investigation with US. Radiology 1999;211:9–24.

47. Kearon C, Julian JA, Newman TE, et al. Noninvasive diagnosis of deep venous thrombosis: McMaster diagnostic imaging practice guidelines initiative. Ann Intern Med 1998;128:663–667.

48. Gottlieb RH, Widjaja J, Mehra S, et al. Clinically important pulmonary emboli: does calf vein US alter outcomes? Radiology 1999;211:25–29.

49. Screaton NJ, Gillard JH, Berman LH, et al. Duplicated superficial femoral veins: a source of error in the sonographic investigation of deep venous thrombosis. Radiology 1998;206:397–401.

50. Wechsler RJ, Spirn PW, Conant EF, et al. Thrombosis and infection caused by thoracic venous catheters: pathogenesis and imaging findings. AJR Am J Roentgenol 1993;160:467–471.

51. Longley DG, Finlay DE, Letourneu JG. Sonography of the upper extremity and jugular veins. AJR Am J Roentgenol 1993;160:957–962.

52. Foshager MC, Finlay DE, Longley DG, et al. Duplex and color Doppler sonography of complications after percutaneous interventional vascular procedures. Radiographics 1994;14:239–253.

53. Liu J-B, Merton DA, Mitchell DG, et al. Color Doppler imaging of the iliofemoral region. Radiographics 1990;10:403–412.

54. Abu-Yousef MM, Wiese JA, Shamma AR. The "to and fro" sign: duplex Doppler evidence of femoral artery pseudoaneurysm. AJR Am J Roentgenol 1988;150:632–634.

55. Paulson EK, Kliewer MA, Hertzberg BS, et al. Ultrasonographically guided manual compression of femoral artery injuries. J Ultrasound Med 1995;14:653–659.

56. Fellmeth BD, Roberts AC, Bookstein JJ, et al. Postangiographic femoral artery injuries: nonsurgical repair with US-guided compression. Radiology 1991;178:671–674.

57. Roubidoux MA, Hertzberg BS, Carroll BA, et al. Color flow and image-directed Doppler ultrasound evaluation of iatrogenic arteriovenous fistulas in the groin. J Clin Ultrasound 1990;18:463–469.

58. Donnelly LF, Adams DM, Bisset GSI. Vascular malformations and hemangiomas: a practical approach in a multidisciplinary clinic. AJR Am J Roentgenol 2000;174:597–608.

59. Paltiel HJ, Burrows PE, Koazkewich HPW, et al. Soft-tissue vascular anomalies: utility of US for diagnosis. Radiology 2000;214:747–754.

60. Gooding GAW. A primer of vascular ultrasound: in situ saphenous vein graft surveillance. Radiologist 1995;2:323–329.

61. Buth J, Idu MM. Postoperative graft surveillance using color-flow duplex. Semin Vasc Surg 1993;6:103–110.

62. Finlay DE, Longley DG, Foshager MC, et al. Duplex and color Doppler sonography of hemodialysis arteriovenous fistulas and grafts. Radiographics 1998;13:983–999.

63. Older RA, Gizienski TA, Wilkowski MJ, et al. Hemodialysis access stenosis: early detection with color Doppler US. Radiology 1998;207:161–164.

64. Robbin ML, Oser RF, Allon M, et al. Hemodialysis access graft stenosis: US detection. Radiology 1998;208:655–661.

CHEST ULTRASOUND

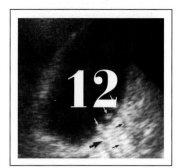

- Imaging Technique
- Anatomy
- Pleural Space
- Lung Parenchyma
- Mediastinum

Sonography is complementary to chest radiography and CT in the evaluation of pathologic processes in the thorax. US commonly reveals abnormalities not shown by other imaging methods (Fig. 12.1) [1–3]. Although limited by air and bone, US visualization is made possible by the pathologic processes creating a sonographic window. Pleural effusion, pulmonary consolidation, atelectasis, and mediastinal tumors are sonographic portals to the thorax. US can be performed at the bedside of critically ill patients, avoiding the necessity of moving them and all their life support equipment to the radiology department [4]. US is excellent for guidance of diagnostic and therapeutic invasive procedures in the chest [5].

IMAGING TECHNIQUE

The first step in US examination of the thorax is to review the chest radiograph. The chest radiograph or chest CT provides a guide for sonography. The examination is then directed to answer the specific questions raised. Two basic approaches are used to examine the chest with US. The direct approach utilizes the intercostal spaces. Linear or curved array transducers with frequencies of 5.0–7.5 MHz are used to examine the pleura and structures in the near field-of-view. For large pleural effusions and for structures deeper in the chest a 3.5-MHz sector transducer may be used. However, the near field is obscured by reverberation artifact with sector transducers, and important findings related to the pleura and chest wall may be missed if only sector transducers are used (Fig. 12.2). The second approach to examination of the thorax is the transabdominal technique. A 3.5-MHz sector transducer is angled superiorly through the liver or spleen to examine the diaphragm and lower thorax (Figs. 12.3, 12.4).

Always review any available chest radiographs or CT scans prior to US examination of the chest.

The sector transducer can also be used to examine the mediastinum by angling downward from the sternal notch or by angling centrally from parasternal positions. Placing the patient in right or left lateral decubitus positions helps to enlarge the parasternal window [6]. Doppler is essential when examining the mediastinum to evaluate major vessels and to diagnose vascular lesions [7].

ANATOMY

The pleural space is bounded by a continuous serosal membrane that forms the **visceral pleura**, covering the lungs and forming the interlobar fissures, and the **parietal pleura** that

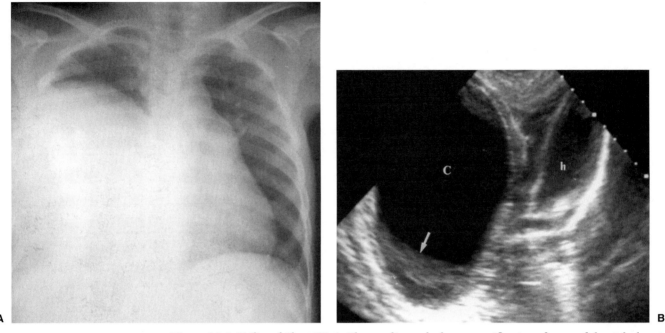

A   B

Figure 12.1 *Utility of Chest US. A.* Chest radiograph shows opacification of most of the right hemi-thorax but yields little information as to its nature. *B.* Transverse US image of the lower right thorax shows a large cystic mass (C) that displaces and compresses the heart (h). The cystic mass is thick-walled and contains layering echogenic debris (*arrow*). This proved to be a large pulmonary hydatid cyst. The layering echogenic debris is hydatid sand.

covers the mediastinum, diaphragm, and inner surface of the chest wall. The total thick-ness of both pleural membranes is only 0.2–0.4 mm. US does not directly demonstrate the normal pleura but rather shows the **interface** of the pleura with pleural fluid and the inter-face of the surface of the air-filled lung (Fig. 12.5). These interfaces serve as the sono-

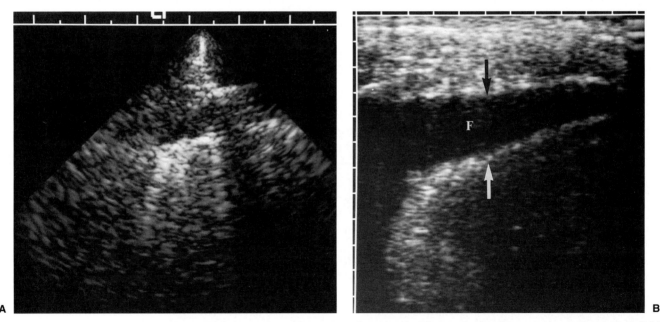

A   B

Figure 12.2 *Limitation of Sector Transducers in the Thorax. A.* 3.5-MHz sector transducer. Near-field artifact characteristic of sector transducers obscures the pleural space. *B.* 5.0-MHz linear array trans-ducer. Use of a linear array transducer in the same intercostal space clearly reveals a pleural effusion (F). The interface of the parietal pleura (*black arrow*) and the visceral pleura/lung interface (*white arrow*) are well demonstrated.

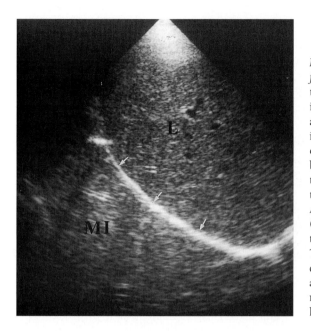

Figure 12.3 *Normal Mirror Image Artifact*. Longitudinal image obtained through the liver (L) shows the bright interface of the diaphragm (*arrows*) with air-filled lung above it. The soft tissue-air interface at the level of the diaphragm causes near-complete sound reflection back into the liver. Further reflection of the sound beam within the liver delays the return of the echoes to the transducer. As a result, an artifactual mirror image (MI) of the liver is displayed further from the transducer and above the diaphragm. The mirror image of the liver above the diaphragm should be recognized as an artifact, but also provides evidence that normal air-filled lung is present at the lung base. Compare to Figure 12.4.

graphic landmarks for evaluation of the pleura. The chest wall is identified by the characteristic appearance of the ribs. Ribs cause a bright surface echo and a dense acoustic shadow. Intercostal muscles extend between the ribs, providing an effective intercostal window. Subcutaneous fat is of variable thickness, so the ribs provide the best landmark for identification of the parietal pleura, which is approximately 1 cm deep to the surface echo of the rib. Between the parietal pleura and the chest wall is fatty connective tissue of variable thickness but rarely exceeding a few millimeters. The normal pleural space contains 1–5 mL of pleural fluid seen as a thin echolucent line between the two pleural interfaces (Fig. 12.6) [8]. Normal pleural fluid lubricates the pleural space easing motion of the lung with breathing. It also aids in providing an adhesive force that holds the lung open and against the chest wall. Pleural fluid, mass, or air breaks this adhesive seal and allows the lung to retract, resulting in atelectasis. The pleural space is easy to identify by observing the respiratory motion of the visceral pleura/lung interface, the "gliding sign" [9]. The bright, linear surface echo slides back and forth with inspiration and expiration. With breathing, streaks of bright reverberation artifacts emanate from the boundary of the visceral pleura and air-filled lung [10].

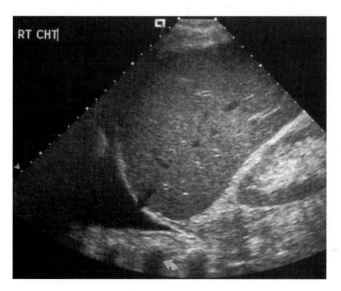

Figure 12.4 *Pleural Effusion Seen from the Abdomen*. Longitudinal image through the liver and right kidney shows a wedge of anechoic pleural fluid (*black arrow*) above the diaphragm. The sound wave penetrates the fluid and reveals the chest wall, recognized by rib shadows (*white arrow*). These findings are pathognomonic of pleural effusion.

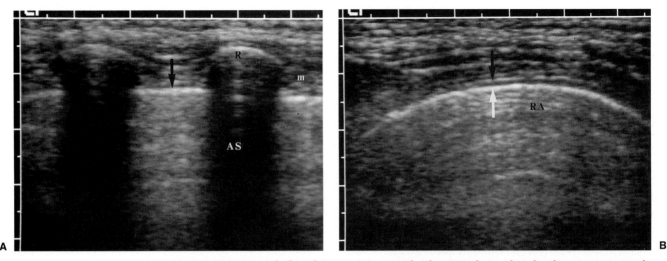

Figure 12.5 *Normal Pleural Space. A.* Longitudinal image obtained with a linear array transducer applied directly to the thorax demonstrates the bright surface echo produced by the ribs (R) and the dense acoustic shadow (AS) resulting from marked sound absorption by bone. The bright linear echo (*arrow*) produced by the interface of visceral pleura and air-filled lung indicates the location of the pleural space in this normal patient. This interface is observed on real-time scanning to move with respiration, the "gliding sign." Note that the pleural space is within 1 cm of the rib surface echo. Intercostal muscles (m) are seen between the ribs. *B.* Turning the transducer to align with the intercostal space produces this transverse image. The gliding sign identifies the location of the parietal pleura (*black arrow*) and the visceral pleura (*white arrow*). Air-filled lung is obscured by reverberation artifact (RA).

The normal lung is air-filled and is seen only as the bright linear surface echo and an intense reverberation artifact (Figs. 12.5, 12.6). Disease in the lung replaces air with fluid, inflammatory cells, or tumor, or collapses the air spaces of the lung to produce a solid structure that can be penetrated with US. Disease that is completely surrounded by air-filled lung will not be visible to US.

When scanning the thorax from an abdominal approach, the air-filled lung causes complete sound reflection and the curving surface of the diaphragm causes multipath reflection

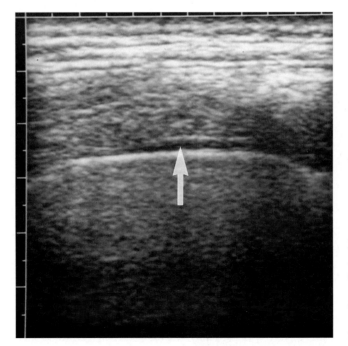

Figure 12.6 *Normal Pleural Fluid.* Intercostal image shows a sliver of normal pleural fluid (*arrow*) separating the parietal and visceral pleural surfaces. A tiny volume of pleural fluid is normally present.

of the US beam. This results in the striking **mirror-image artifact** described in Chapter 1. The image of the liver or spleen is duplicated above the diaphragm (Fig. 12.3). The presence of a mirror image artifact indicates that normal air-filled lung is above the diaphragm. Absence of the mirror image artifact is evidence of pathology in the lung base or pleural space.

PLEURAL SPACE

The pleura is involved by pathologic processes that occur as isolated disease or as a complication of diseases of the lung, chest wall, or abdomen. Chest radiographs accurately detect pleural disease but are limited in providing characterization of the disease. Disease in the pleura provides an excellent window for US evaluation [10]. US is exceptionally valuable in guiding aspiration, biopsy, and catheter drainage procedures in the pleural space [11].

PLEURAL EFFUSION

Pleural effusion is an abnormal increase in the volume of pleural fluid. Fluid escapes from the blood vessels and lymphatics of the pleural surface as a result of a pathologic process. US is excellent in diagnosing the presence and volume of pleural fluid, and in assessing whether the fluid is amenable to aspiration [12]. Pleural effusions may be characterized as to whether they are transudates or exudates [13].

> Pleural effusion and lower lobe pneumonia may be unexpected findings that can be routinely diagnosed during US examination of the abdomen.

- A layer of anechoic or hypoechoic pleural fluid separates the visceral and parietal pleura (Fig. 12.7).
- On transabdominal scanning the mirror image artifact is absent. Fluid is seen above the diaphragm and the inside of the chest wall is visualized through the fluid layer. The chest wall is recognized by the acoustic shadows that emanate from ribs (Figs. 12.4, 12.8).
- Atelectasis is always present with pleural effusion (Fig. 12.8). An abnormal volume of pleural fluid releases the adhesive tension that holds the surface of the lung against the chest wall and the lung reflexly collapses. The atelectatic lung is seen as a wedge-shaped echogenic mass moving with respiration within the pleural fluid.

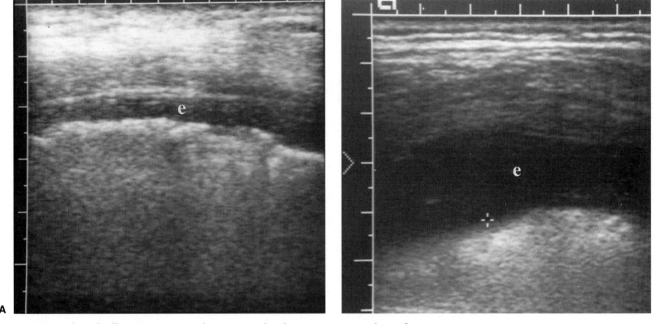

A   B

Figure 12.7 *Pleural Effusions.* Intercostal images with a linear array transducer from two patients (*A, B*) show small pleural effusions (e). Cursor (+) measures the distance to the lung surface.

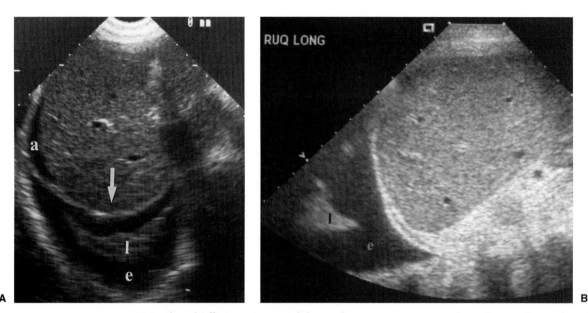

Figure 12.8 *Pleural Effusions. A.* Transabdominal image in transverse plane shows a large pleural effusion (e) with a wedge of echogenic collapsed lung (l). Atelectasis always accompanies pleural effusion. A small volume of ascites (a) is also evident. Note the bare area of the liver (*arrow*). *B.* Transabdominal image in longitudinal plane in a different patient shows a large pleural effusion (e) and right lower lobe atelectasis (l).

- Signs that indicate that a pleural lesion is fluid that can be aspirated are: (a) change in shape of the lesion with respiration, (b) floating echodensities, and (c) moving fibrous strands [12].
- The volume of pleural fluid can be estimated by US measurement of the distance between parietal and visceral pleura. The measurement is made with the patient supine and holding breath in maximal inspiration. Transverse scans are obtained in the intercostal space at the posterior axillary line just above the diaphragm. The maximum width of the fluid space is measured and related to the data shown in Table 12.1 [14].

Table 12.1: Quantification of Pleural Effusion Volume

Thickness of Effusion Measured by US (mm)	Mean Effusion Volume (mL)	Range of Effusion Volume (mL)
0	5	0–90
5	80	20–170
10	170	50–300
15	260	90–420
20	380	150–660
30	550	210–1060
40	1000	490–1670
50	1420	650–1840

Adapted from Eibenberger KL, Dock WI, Amman ME, et al. Quantification of pleural effusions: sonography versus radiography. Radiology 1994;191:681–684.
Reprinted from Brant WE. Chest. In McGahan JP, Goldberg BB. Diagnostic Ultrasound—A Logical Approach. Lippincott-Raven. Philadelphia, 1998.

■ Anechoic fluid may be either transudate or exudate. Aspiration and chemical analysis of the fluid is needed to differentiate the type of effusion [13].

■ Fluid that contains floating debris or has septations or fibrous strands is always an exudate [13].

■ US is exceptionally valuable in localizing pleural fluid and in guiding diagnostic or therapeutic thoracentesis.

Thoracentesis is needed to determine the exact nature of a pleural effusion.

TRANSUDATIVE PLEURAL EFFUSION

A transudative pleural effusion is a simple serous pleural effusion. Transudates are ultrafiltrates of plasma from normal pleural membranes [13]. Transudates result from an underlying disease, such as congestive heart failure, that increases capillary hydrostatic pressure or causes a decrease in colloid osmotic pressure [8,15]. Additional causes of transudative pleural effusion include cirrhosis, nephrotic syndrome, hypoalbuminemia, constrictive pericarditis, and superior vena cava obstruction.

■ Transudative pleural effusions are anechoic without floating debris (Figs. 12.4, 12.7B) [13].

■ The fluid changes shape with respiration and positioning.

EXUDATIVE PLEURAL EFFUSION

Exudative pleural effusions are complicated effusions with high protein content (>3.0 gm/100 mL) and may contain blood, pus, chyle, or malignant cells. The pleura is abnormal and is directly involved with an inflammatory or neoplastic process. Causes include empyema and parapneumonic effusion, neoplasms involving the pleura, hemothorax, tuberculous pleurisy, and intraabdominal inflammatory processes such as abscess or pancreatitis.

■ Floating echogenic debris is seen within the pleural fluid (Fig. 12.9).

■ Homogeneous floating echodensities are indicative of hemorrhagic effusion parapneumonic effusion, or empyema [13].

■ Moving debris within the fluid scatters the US beam and produces color signals within the fluid—the fluid color sign [16]. This finding aids in the differentiation of echogenic pleural fluid from pleural thickening.

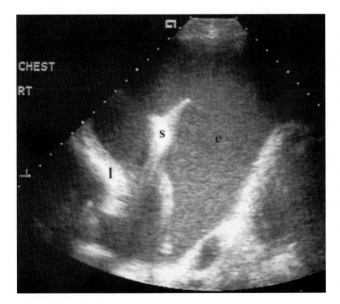

Figure 12.9 *Exudative Parapneumonic Pleural Effusion.* Transverse image shows a large echogenic pleural effusion (e). Real-time imaging revealed swirling motion of the particulate matter within the effusion. Echogenic particulate matter in a pleural effusion is indicative of an exudative effusion. This patient's chest radiograph revealed a right lower lobe pneumonia in association with the large effusion. Thoracentesis confirmed the absence of bacteria within the exudative effusion. l, partially collapsed right lower lobe; rt, right; s, coarse septation within the effusion.

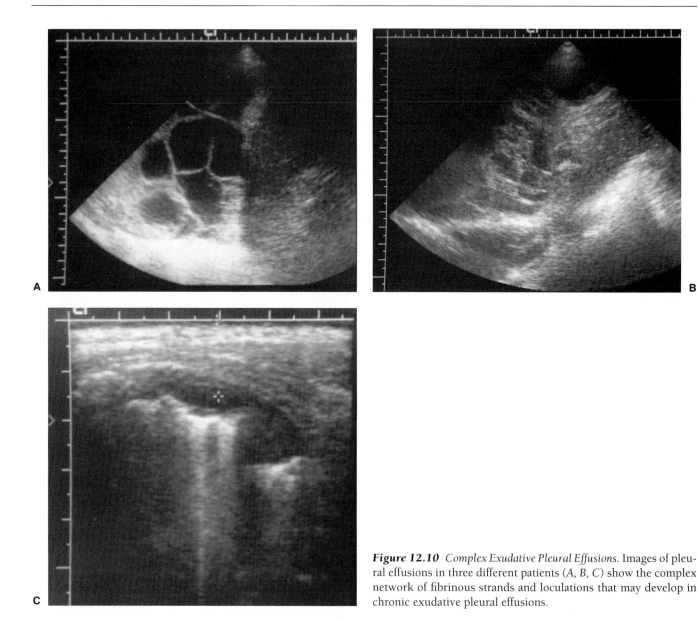

Figure 12.10 *Complex Exudative Pleural Effusions.* Images of pleural effusions in three different patients (*A, B, C*) show the complex network of fibrinous strands and loculations that may develop in chronic exudative pleural effusions.

- Linear fibrous bands form with organization of the exudative fluid (Fig. 12.10). These thin echogenic septa move to-and-fro with respiration and may cause loculation of the fluid. A honeycomb appearance is indicative of high likelihood of inability to drain the effusion with a small-bore catheter. These septa, seen easily with US, are not seen on chest radiographs and are often not apparent on CT.
- The presence of thickened pleura or associated lung consolidation or masses are associated with exudative effusion (Fig. 12.11) [13].

EMPYEMA AND PARAPNEUMONIC EFFUSION

Empyema is the presence of pus in the pleural cavity. Parapneumonic effusions are exudative effusions that complicate pneumonia and lung abscess. No US findings are specific for these conditions. Diagnosis is based upon analysis of the pleural fluid aspirated. Empyema is diagnosed when (a) the fluid is grossly purulent, (b) bacteria are identified on Gram's stain or culture, or (c) the white blood cell count in the fluid exceeds 15,000/mL [17].

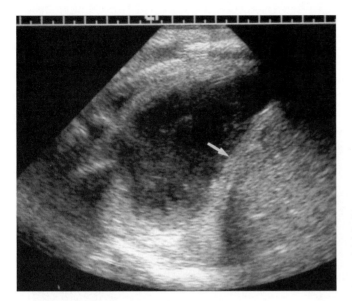

Figure 12.11 *Chronic Empyema.* Intercostal image shows a loculated, echogenic pleural fluid bounded by thickened pleura (*arrow*). US-guided aspiration confirmed chronic empyema.

PNEUMOTHORAX

Contrary to popular belief, pneumothorax can be reliably detected by US.

- Absence of visualization of the gliding visceral pleura (Fig. 12.12) and absence of the streak-like reverberation artifacts that emanate from the lung surface during breathing are evidence of pneumothorax [18].
- During US-guided invasive procedures sudden loss of visualization of the target lesion is evidence of pneumothorax [19].
- Because air in the pleural space will move to the non-dependent thorax, US is not reliable in excluding pneumothorax [20].
- Hydropneumothorax may be recognized by the presence of an air-fluid level with air shadow above a layer of fluid (Fig. 12.13). Microbubbles may be seen within the pleural fluid [21].

PLEURAL PLAQUES

Pleural plaques are localized thickenings of the pleura caused by inflammation or infarction. Asbestos exposure is a common cause of pleural plaques that frequently calcify.

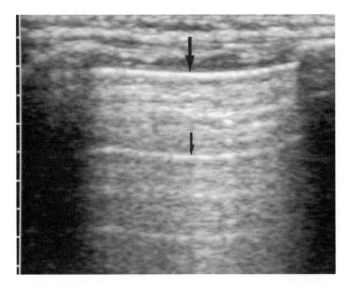

Figure 12.12 *Pneumothorax.* Intercostal image shows the bright reflection (*large arrow*) and the reverberation artifact caused by air in the pleural space. Real-time US is required to see the absence of the "gliding pleura sign" that confirms pneumothorax. On static images, pneumothorax cannot be differentiated from normal lung reflection (compare to Figure 12.4). Repeated sound reflection between the air interface and the surface of the transducer reproduces the image of the air interface deeper in the image (*small arrow*).

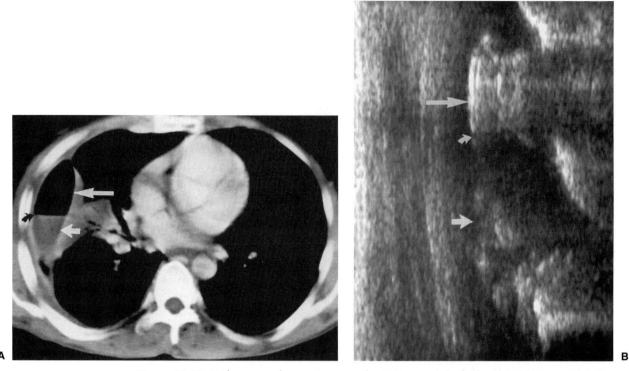

Figure 12.13 *Hydropneumothorax.* Compare the CT image (*A*) of a loculated hydropneumothorax to the US image (*B*) oriented to match the CT scan. With the patient supine, fluid (*smaller arrow*) gravitates to the dependent portion of the cavity while air (*larger arrow*) occupies the non-dependent portion of the cavity. Air in the pleural space produces a brightly reflective echo, while sound penetrates and shows the detail within the dependent fluid. The air-fluid level (*curved arrow*) is seen on US as the sharp area of transition between the bright air echo and the fluid echo.

- Plaques appear as focal hypoechoic thickening of the pleura. Thickness is usually in the 5–12-mm range [22].
- Calcified plaques are highly echogenic and cause acoustic shadowing [22].

FIBROTHORAX

Fibrothorax is a rind of thickened pleura that restricts lung motion.

- Fibrothorax appears as echogenic solid pleural thickening (Fig. 12.14). The surface of the pleura may undulate because of variation in the amount of thickening.
- No fluid color sign is present in the thickened pleura.
- Loculation of pleural fluid is commonly also present.

LOCALIZED FIBROUS TUMOR OF THE PLEURA

Benign mesothelioma is now called *localized fibrous tumor of the pleura*. The tumors are fibrous and of mesenchymal origin with areas of dense collagen tissue [23].

- US shows a well-defined hyperechoic mass with lobulated contours (Fig. 12.15) [10, 23]. The mass forms obtuse angles where it meets the chest wall. Most are found in the lower thorax.

MALIGNANT PLEURAL MESOTHELIOMA

Malignant pleural mesothelioma is a rare tumor related to occupational asbestos exposure. The tumor has a dismal prognosis [24].

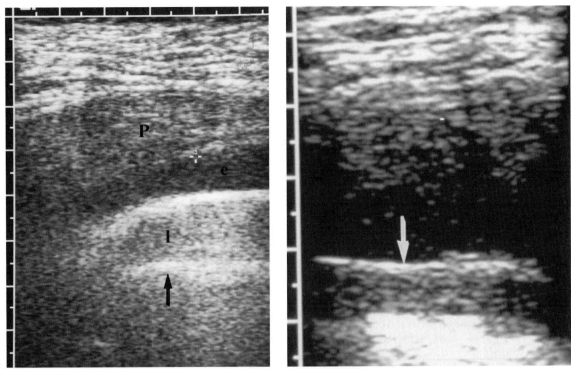

Figure 12.14 *Fibrothorax—Thickened Pleura. A.* Intercostal image shows marked thickening of the parietal pleura (P) and a small echogenic pleural effusion (e). Reverberation artifact obscures the lung (l). The visceral pleura-lung interface is duplicated as a reverberation artifact (*arrow*). The cursor (+) marks the interface between parietal pleura and pleural effusion. *B.* Intercostal image through a pleural effusion in another patient shows thickening of the visceral pleura (*arrow*) overlying air-filled lung.

- Multiple tumor masses on the visceral and parietal pleura are the most common pattern [24].
- The masses may grow to become confluent, encasing the lung with lobulated thickened pleura.
- Large pleural effusions are present in 60% of patients.

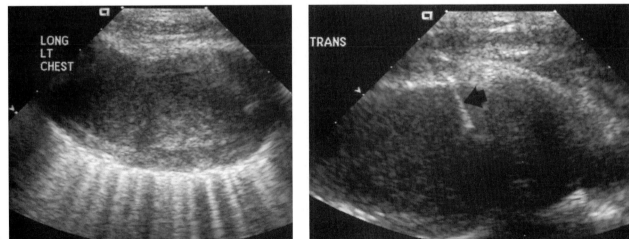

Figure 12.15 *Localized Fibrous Tumor of the Pleura. A.* A large solid tumor of the pleural space is evident. *B.* US was used to guide core needle (*arrow*) biopsy of the lesion to confirm a benign localized fibrous tumor of the pleura.

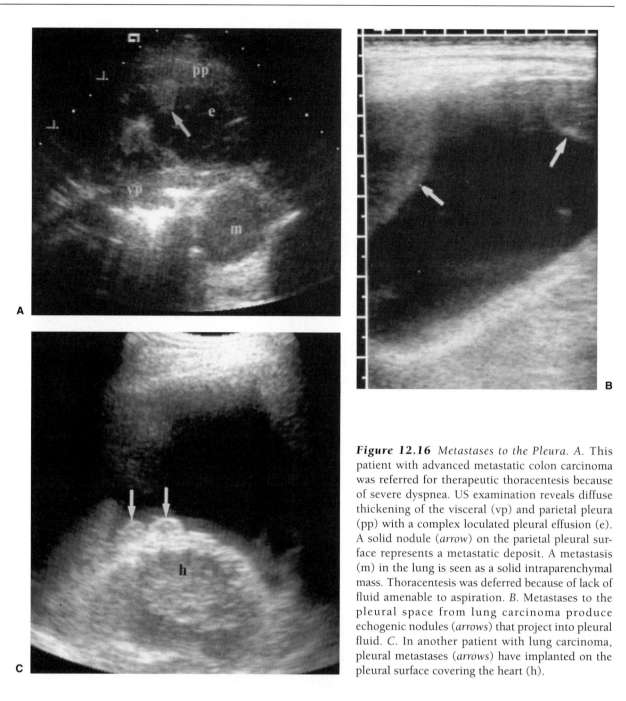

Figure 12.16 *Metastases to the Pleura. A.* This patient with advanced metastatic colon carcinoma was referred for therapeutic thoracentesis because of severe dyspnea. US examination reveals diffuse thickening of the visceral (vp) and parietal pleura (pp) with a complex loculated pleural effusion (e). A solid nodule (*arrow*) on the parietal pleural surface represents a metastatic deposit. A metastasis (m) in the lung is seen as a solid intraparenchymal mass. Thoracentesis was deferred because of lack of fluid amenable to aspiration. *B.* Metastases to the pleural space from lung carcinoma produce echogenic nodules (*arrows*) that project into pleural fluid. *C.* In another patient with lung carcinoma, pleural metastases (*arrows*) have implanted on the pleural surface covering the heart (h).

- Calcified pleural plaques are found in 20% of patients.
- US-guided core biopsy is a highly effective method of confirming the diagnosis (Fig. 12.15) [25].

METASTASES TO THE PLEURA

Metastatic disease to the pleura arises most commonly from lung carcinoma (40%), breast carcinoma (20%), and lymphoma (10%) [26].

- Diffuse pleural thickening >1 cm is highly indicative of pleural metastases (Fig. 12.16).
- Multiple hypoechoic tumor nodules typically involve the parietal pleura (Fig. 12.16). Appearance is indistinguishable from malignant mesothelioma.

- Exudative pleural effusion is commonly present and provides a sonographic window for visualization of the tumor nodules and diffuse nodular pleural thickening [27]. Malignant pleural effusion is second only to congestive heart failure as the most common cause of pleural effusion in patients older than age 50 [28].
- US is commonly used to guide diagnostic and therapeutic thoracentesis. Cytology of pleural fluid obtained by thoracentesis yields a specific diagnosis in approximately two-thirds of cases [28].

LUNG PARENCHYMA

CONSOLIDATION

Consolidation is the replacement of alveolar air by fluid, inflammatory or neoplastic cells, or blood. This solidification of the lung allows US evaluation. Consolidation may be caused by pneumonia, pulmonary edema, hemorrhage, or neoplasm such as lymphoma or bronchoalveolar cell carcinoma.

- The consolidated lung is homogeneous and hypoechoic but retains its wedge shape (Fig. 12.17).
- The border of the consolidated lung is sharply defined by the visceral pleura (Figs. 12.17, 12.18).
- Consolidation tends to be ill defined centrally where the consolidation is discontinuous and patchy.
- Sonographic air alveolograms are produced by isolated foci of air-filled alveoli surrounded by consolidated lung. The air-filled groups of alveoli are brightly echogenic but irregular in shape and size (Fig. 12.19) [9].
- Sonographic air bronchograms are produced by retained air in small bronchi surrounded by areas of consolidation (Fig. 12.17). Air-filled bronchi appear as intensely echogenic, linear, often branching structures that converge toward the lung hilum and are surrounded by hypoechoic lung [29].

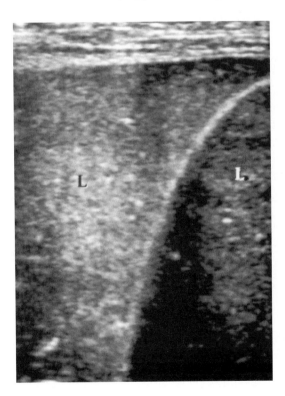

Figure 12.17 *Consolidation.* Complete filling of the alveoli with fluid, inflammatory cells, and debris has "solidified" the lung (*black L*) making it more echogenic than the liver (*white L*).

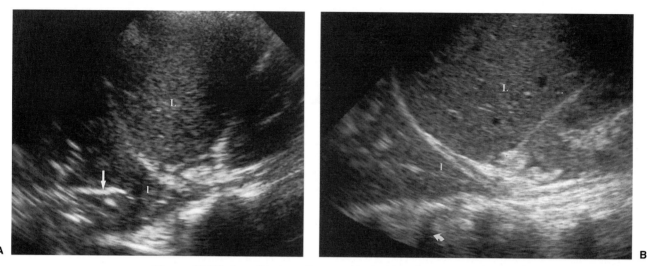

Figure 12.18 *Consolidation—Sonographic Air Bronchograms.* Transabdominal longitudinal images (*A, B*) show complete consolidation of the right lower lobe (l). The lung is "solidified" and now equal in echogenicity to the liver (L). Note the wedge shape of the lower lobe is maintained. Shadows from ribs (*curved arrow*) are evident. Prominent sonographic air bronchograms (*straight arrow*) are seen as highly echogenic branching linear echoes in the consolidated lung parenchyma. The lack of bronchial crowding indicates that the process is primarily consolidation, not atelectasis. No pleural effusion is present.

- Ring-down artifact and acoustic shadowing may be seen in association with sonographic air alveolograms and bronchograms.
- Sonographic fluid bronchograms are fluid-filled bronchi surrounded by consolidated lung. They appear as hypoechoic, linear, branching, tubular structures that converge toward the hilum [30].
- Doppler shows pulmonary vessels with normal spacing extending through the consolidated lung.
- The lung shows appropriate motion with respiration.

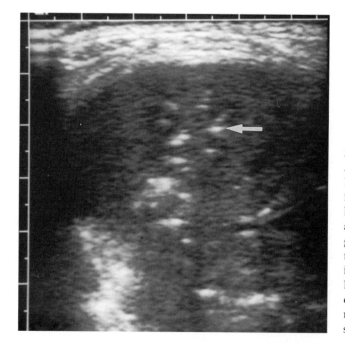

Figure 12.19 *Consolidation— Sonographic Air Alveolograms.* Intercostal image shows bright foci (*arrow*) within consolidated hypoechoic lung. The bright foci are caused by air trapped within groups of alveoli, which are surrounded by airless fluid- or inflammatory cell–filled alveoli. Note the irregular deep border of consolidation as compared to the rounded borders of lung tumor as shown in Figure 12.23.

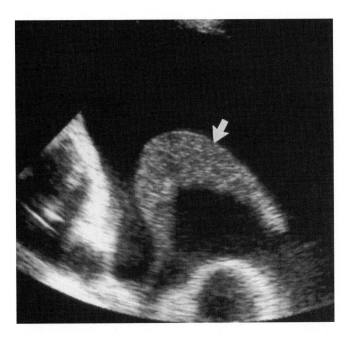

Figure 12.20 *Atelectasis.* Intercostal sonogram shows a wedge of collapsed lung (*arrow*) suspended in a large pleural effusion. The visceral pleura provides a sharp boundary for the atelectatic lung.

ATELECTASIS

Atelectasis describes the loss of lung volume with collapse of the lung. The complete or partial absence of air in the lung creates a solid tissue mass that can be penetrated with US. Causes of atelectasis are obstruction (endobronchial tumor), passive relaxation (pleural effusion or pneumothorax), compression (by lung mass or bulla), scarring (radiation fibrosis), or adhesive atelectasis (respiratory distress of the newborn).

All pleural effusions are associated with some degree of lung atelectasis.

- Atelectatic lung is flattened and wedge-shaped, reflecting volume loss. Boundaries are sharply defined by the visceral pleura (Figs. 12.8, 12.20).
- Atelectasis is seen by US most commonly in association with pleural effusion. The atelectatic lung is echogenic compared to pleural fluid.
- Sonographic fluid bronchograms may be evident.
- Pulmonary blood vessels and fluid-filled bronchi are crowded together reflecting volume loss.
- The lung shows appropriate motion with respiration.

LUNG ABSCESS

Lung abscess is a pulmonary parenchymal cavity that results from necrosis of lung tissue. Causes include necrotizing lung infection, pulmonary infarction, septic emboli, and necrotic neoplasms. Because most lung abscesses abut the pleural surface most can be evaluated with US (Fig. 12.21) [31].

- An echogenic, irregularly thickened wall surrounds a lung cavity that may be filled with fluid, inflammatory or necrotic debris, or air.
- Air in the abscess cavity may be in bubbles, discrete pockets, or in large collections that form air-fluid levels. Air may obscure visualization of portions of the abscess cavity and produce reverberation or comet tail artifacts and acoustic shadowing.
- With inspiration the entire circumference of the abscess cavity expands. Whereas with empyema only the lung-bordered portion of the loculated fluid collection moves with respiration.
- US guidance is used for aspiration and catheter drainage when indicated [31].

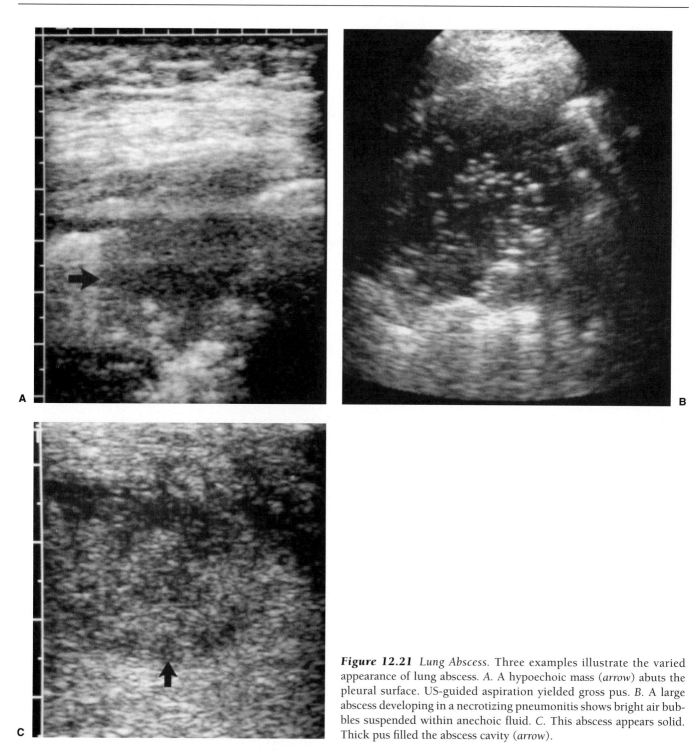

Figure 12.21 *Lung Abscess.* Three examples illustrate the varied appearance of lung abscess. *A.* A hypoechoic mass (*arrow*) abuts the pleural surface. US-guided aspiration yielded gross pus. *B.* A large abscess developing in a necrotizing pneumonitis shows bright air bubbles suspended within anechoic fluid. *C.* This abscess appears solid. Thick pus filled the abscess cavity (*arrow*).

LUNG TUMORS

Primary and metastatic lung neoplasms that abut the pleural surface may be evaluated and biopsied by US. Intraparenchymal tumors may also be seen if they are surrounded by consolidation or atelectasis.

- Lesions stand out as hypoechoic masses surrounded by brightly echogenic and reflective air-filled lung (Fig. 12.22).

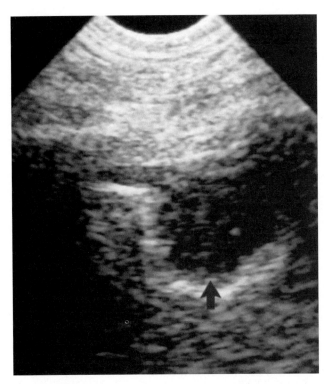

Figure 12.22 *Lung Tumor.* A round lung neoplasm (*arrow*) stands out as a hypoechoic mass surrounded by echogenic air-filled lung. US-guided biopsy confirmed large cell carcinoma.

- The bright surface reflection echo of air-filled lung is focally absent over the hypoechoic mass [32].
- The deep boundary of the mass is usually rounded and well defined as compared to the ill-defined deep border of consolidation (Fig. 12.23) [32].
- Absence of tapered edges helps to differentiate lung mass from pleural mass.
- Tumors are usually hyperechoic relative to hypoechoic surrounding lung consolidation [33].
- Calcifications with lung tumors are seen as echogenic foci with shadowing.

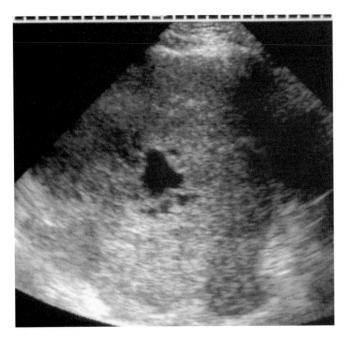

Figure 12.23 *Large Lung Cancer.* This large lung mass was found in a patient who was severely short of breath in the supine position and could not tolerate CT. US was used to define the tumor and to guide percutaneous biopsy, which yielded poorly differentiated squamous cell carcinoma. Note the rounded and relatively well-defined deep borders characteristic of tumor as compared to the ill-defined deep borders of lung consolidation seen in Figure 12.19.

- Tumor invasion of the chest wall is manifest by disruption of the pleura and fixation of the tumor during breathing. Invasion of tumor through the pleura and into the intercostal muscles may be seen.
- US is a valuable alternative method for guiding biopsy of lung lesions abutting the pleura [34].

PULMONARY SEQUESTRATION

Pulmonary sequestration is a mass of nonfunctioning lung parenchyma that lacks connection to the bronchial tree [35]. Intralobar sequestrations (75%) share a covering of visceral pleura with normal lung. Extralobar sequestrations (25%) are enclosed in their own separate pleura. All sequestrations receive systemic blood from an anomalous artery that usually arises from the aorta. Approximately 5% of sequestrations are retroperitoneal in location [36].

- US demonstrates a complex echogenic mass that may be homogeneously solid or solid with a few or many cysts [37]. The appearance is very similar to that of cystic adenomatoid malformation (CAM) [38]. Pulmonary sequestrations may have areas of CAM within them.
- Demonstration by color flow imaging of an anomalous supplying artery arising from the aorta is diagnostic of sequestration and provides unequivocal differentiation from CAM [39].

CYSTIC ADENOMATOID MALFORMATION

CAM is believed to be the result of premature arrest of alveolar development at approximately 6 weeks gestational age. The malformed lung consists of multiple cysts of varying size that maintain communication to the bronchial tree [40]. CAM accounts for approximately 25% of all congenital lung malformations. CAM closely resembles pulmonary sequestration pathologically and sonographically.

- Type I CAM (50%) involves only part of one lobe and consists of one or more large cysts 2–10 cm in size surrounded by numerous smaller cysts. Demonstration of one or more large cysts within an echogenic mass is diagnostic.
- Type II CAM (40%) also involves only part of one lobe and consists of numerous small cysts less than 2 cm in size. US shows an echogenic mass with uniform small cysts smaller than 2 cm.
- Type III CAM (10%) is a large lesion that involves an entire lobe or the whole lung. Cysts are tiny, 3–5 mm in diameter. US shows a very echogenic mass with the cysts being too small to demonstrate.

MEDIASTINUM

US evaluation of the mediastinum is particularly valuable in the supra-aortic, pericardial, peritracheal, and prevascular regions that are most accessible to examination [41]. Masses can be characterized by the organ of origin, cystic and solid characteristics, and vascularity (Fig. 12.24). Tortuous brachiocephalic vessels and retrosternal goiter are easily evaluated.

NORMAL THYMUS

The normal thymus is a prominent structure in the superior mediastinum of children up to 8 years of age [42,43].

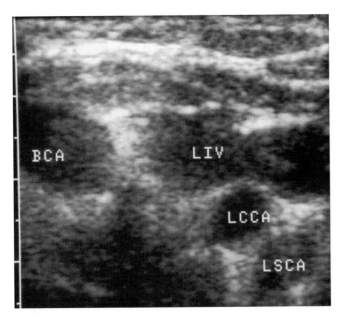

Figure 12.24 *Normal Mediastinum—Suprasternal Approach.* A transverse image of the mediastinum obtained by angling a sector transducer behind the manubrium from a suprasternal approach shows major mediastinal blood vessels. Arteries and veins are differentiated by position and Doppler characteristics. BCA, brachiocephalic artery; LCCA, left common carotid artery; LIV, left innominate vein; LSCA, left subclavian artery.

- The normal thymus has two well-defined lobes that are teardrop or triangular in shape. Echogenicity is homogeneous and slightly less than the echogenicity of the thyroid gland (Fig. 12.25).
- Average dimensions are 1.4 cm anteroposterior and 2.5–2.9 cm in longitudinal plane [43].
- The normal thymus is in close contact with upper mediastinal blood vessels and may partially or completely encircle them (Fig. 12.25).
- Fatty replacement of the thymus, which is usually complete by age 8 years, makes the thymus non-detectable by US in adults and older children. A visible thymus in an adult suggests replacement of the thymus by tumor [44].

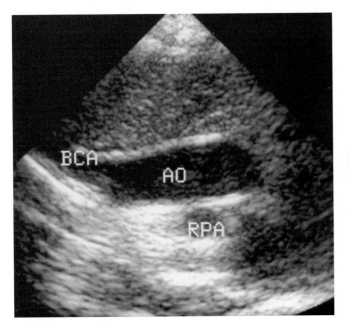

Figure 12.25 *Normal Thymus.* Longitudinal right parasternal image in an infant shows normal thymus partially enveloping the ascending aorta (AO) and brachiocephalic artery (BCA). Note the homogeneous mid-level echogenicity of the normal thymus. The right pulmonary artery (RPA) is seen in cross section just posterior to the ascending aorta.

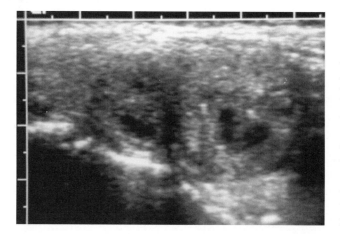

Figure 12.26 *Mediastinal Goiter.* A chest radiograph showed rightward displacement of the trachea by a mediastinal mass at the thoracic inlet. US demonstrated an enlarged thyroid with multiple nodules characteristic of multinodular goiter that extended into the upper mediastinum and caused mass effect on the trachea and aortic arch vessels. This is a longitudinal paramanubrial image.

MEDIASTINAL THYROID

Extension of thyroid tissue into the anterior mediastinum is one of the most common causes of a mediastinal mass. Multinodular goiter is most common, but any thyroid lesion may extend into the mediastinum.

- US confirms contiguity of the mediastinal mass with the thyroid gland (Fig. 12.26).
- Appearance varies with the nature of the thyroid pathology. The thyroid parenchyma may be normal, multinodular, or neoplastic.

THYMOMA

Thymomas generally occur in adults (>age 40) and are the most common primary tumor of the thymus [45]. Most thymomas (50%) present as an asymptomatic mediastinal mass discovered on chest radiography. Approximately 25–30% present with symptoms of compression of mediastinal structures. The remaining 20–25% present with myasthenia gravis or other parathymic syndromes such as red cell aplasia, hypogammaglobulinemia, or other endocrine or connective tissue disorders.

- Thymomas are sharply defined, oval, round, or lobulated hypoechoic masses that occupy the anterior mediastinum [46].
- Tumors are slow growing and vary in size from 5–10 cm up to 34 cm [45].
- Hemorrhage and necrosis may occur within the tumor, resulting in cystic areas that may be the dominant feature of the tumor [45].
- Most tumors are well encapsulated but up to one-third show local invasion of mediastinal fat, lung, pericardium, heart, or mediastinal blood vessels [45].
- Thin peripheral calcifications may occur within the tumor capsule.
- Rare hematogenous metastases may go to liver, bone, kidneys, or brain.

LYMPHADENOPATHY/LYMPHOMA

Normal lymph nodes in the mediastinum are not visualized by US [46]. Visualized lymph nodes should be considered enlarged by an inflammatory or neoplastic process.

- Lymphomas are homogeneous and hypoechoic (Fig. 12.27) [46]. Large nodes commonly coalesce into bulky masses that infiltrate the mediastinum and displace and encase blood vessels.
- Sonography can be used to determine response of lymphoma to therapy. Responding nodes demonstrate a measurable decrease in size. Persistence of small nodes suggests incomplete remission. Complete response is evidenced by disappearance of all nodes. Reappearance of lymph nodes after complete remission is indicative of recurrence [47].

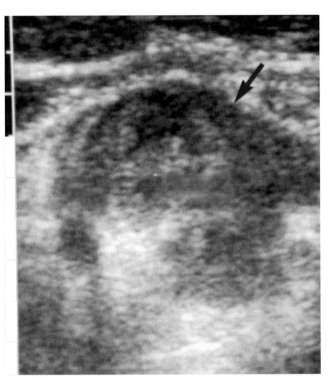

Figure 12.27 *Mediastinal Lymphoma*. A chest radiograph of a pregnant woman showed mediastinal widening suspicious for adenopathy. US demonstrates enlarged and confluent mediastinal lymph nodes (*arrow*) and guided percutaneous biopsy, which confirmed lymphoma.

- Calcified lymph nodes have echogenic foci with acoustic shadowing. Lymphomatous nodes may calcify after therapy.

THYMIC LYMPHOMA

Involvement of the thymus accompanies mediastinal lymphoma in 50% of cases of Hodgkin's disease and is the sole site of mediastinal disease in 20% [48].

- Lymphoma in the thymus may appear hypoechoic, hyperechoic, or cystic [46].
- Internal structure is usually nodular.
- Many patients have adenopathy elsewhere in the mediastinum.

THYMIC CYSTS

Thymic cysts are rare lesions. Most are congenital and asymptomatic [48].

- Thymic cysts may be solitary, multiple, or multiloculated. Borders are smooth, round or oval, and well-defined. Cyst walls are thin and contain thymic tissue.
- Anechoic serous fluid is contained within the cysts.

PERICARDIAL CYSTS

Pericardial cysts may arise from any portion of the pericardium.

- Cysts are round, well defined, and thin walled.
- Internal fluid is usually anechoic but may become echoic with hemorrhage.

BRONCHOGENIC CYSTS

Bronchogenic cysts are the most common intrathoracic foregut anomaly. Cysts are lined with respiratory epithelium.

- Bronchogenic cysts are characteristically located along the right wall of the trachea or near the carina.
- The cysts are thin walled and usually contain echogenic fluid caused by mucinous secretions [46].

VASCULAR MASSES

Tortuous vessels, aneurysms, anomalies of the aortic arch, and thrombosis of the superior vena cava are common causes of mediastinal abnormalities. Doppler is essential in confirming the diagnosis.

- A tortuous ectatic brachiocephalic artery is a common cause of a right upper mediastinal mass with tracheal deviation on a chest radiograph. US examination with Doppler performed from a suprasternal approach confirms this diagnosis.
- Dilatation of the aorta may represent aneurysm, post-stenotic dilatation of aortic stenosis, or dissection.
- Anomalies of the aortic arch can be evaluated with use of Doppler to confirm the identity of arteries and veins.
- Real-time and Doppler US can confirm thrombosis of the superior vena cava or brachiocephalic veins. Hypoechoic thrombus is visualized within the lumen. Blood flow is absent or diverted around the clot.

REFERENCES

1. Brant WE. Interventional procedures in the thorax. In: McGahan JP, ed. Interventional Ultrasound. Baltimore: Williams & Wilkins, 1990:85–100.
2. Brant WE. The Thorax. In: Rumack CM, Wilson SR, Charboneau JW, eds. Diagnostic Ultrasound. 2nd ed. St. Louis: Mosby, 1998:575–597.
3. Brant WE. Chest. In: McGahan JP, Goldberg BB, eds. Diagnostic Ultrasound—A Logical Approach. Philadelphia: Lippincott-Raven, 1998:1063–1086.
4. Yu C, Yang P, Chang D, et al. Diagnostic and therapeutic use of chest sonography: value in critically ill patients. AJR Am J Roentgenol 1992;159:695–701.
5. Klein JS, Schultz S, Heffner JE. Interventional radiology of the chest: image-guided percutaneous drainage of pleural effusions, lung abscesses, and pneumothorax. AJR Am J Roentgenol 1995;164:581–588.
6. Wernecke K, Pötter R, Peters P, et al. Parasternal mediastinal sonography: sensitivity in the detection of anterior mediastinal and subcarinal tumors. AJR Am J Roentgenol 1988;150:1021–1026.
7. O'Laughlin M, Huhta J, Murphy DJ. Ultrasound examination of extracardiac chest masses in children—Doppler diagnosis of a vascular etiology. J Ultrasound Med 1987;6:151–157.
8. Müller N. Imaging of the pleura. Radiology 1993;186:297–309.
9. Targhetta R, Chavagneux R, Bourgeois J, et al. Sonographic approach to diagnosing pulmonary consolidation. J Ultrasound Med 1992;11:667–672.
10. Wernecke K. Sonographic features of pleural disease. AJR Am J Roentgenol 1997;168:1061–1066.
11. O'Moore P, Mueller P, Simeone J, et al. Sonographic guidance in diagnostic and therapeutic interventions in the pleural space. AJR Am J Roentgenol 1987;149:1–5.
12. Marks W, Filly R, Callen P. Real-time evaluation of pleural lesions: new observations regarding the probability of obtaining free fluid. Radiology 1982;142:163–164.
13. Yang PC, Luh KT, Chang DB, et al. Value of sonography in determining the nature of pleural effusion: analysis of 320 cases. AJR Am J Roentgenol 1992;159:29–33.
14. Eibenberger K, Dock W, Ammann M, et al. Quantification of pleural effusions: sonography versus radiography. Radiology 1994;191:681–684.
15. Chetty K. Transudative pleural effusions. Clin Chest Med 1985;6:49–54.
16. Wu R, Yang P, Kuo S, et al. Fluid color sign: a useful indicator for discrimination between pleural thickening and pleural effusion. J Ultrasound Med 1995;14:767–769.
17. Hanna J, Reed J, Choplin R. Pleural infections: a clinical-radiologic review. J Thor Imaging 1991;6:68–79.

18. Wernecke K, Galanski M, Peters P, et al. Pneumothorax: evaluation by ultrasound—preliminary results. J Thorac Imag 1987;2:76–78.

19. Targhetta R, Bourgeois J, Chavagneux R, et al. Diagnosis of pneumothorax by ultrasound immediately after ultrasonically guided aspiration biopsy. Chest 1992;101:855–856.

20. Sistrom C, Reiheld C, Gay S, et al. Detection and estimation of the volume of pneumothorax using real-time sonography: efficacy determined by receiver operating characteristic analysis. AJR Am J Roentgenol 1996;166:317–321.

21. Targhetta R, Bourgeois J, Chavagneux R, et al. Ultrasonographic approach to diagnosing hydropneumothorax. Chest 1992;101:931–934.

22. Morgan R, Pickworth F, Dubbins P, et al. The ultrasound appearance of asbestos-related pleural plaques. Clinical Radiology 1991;44:413–416.

23. Ferretti G, Chiles C, Choplin R, et al. Localized benign fibrous tumors of the pleura. AJR Am J Roentgenol 1997;169:683–686.

24. Miller B, Rosado-de-Christenson M, Mason A, et al. Malignant pleural mesothelioma: radiologic-pathologic correlation. Radiographics 1996;16:613–644.

25. Heilo A, Stenwig A, Solheim O. Malignant pleural mesothelioma: US-guided histologic core-needle biopsy. Radiology 1999;211:657–659.

26. Dynes M, White E, Fry W, et al. Imaging manifestations of pleural tumors. Radiographics 1992;12:1191–1201.

27. Goerg C, Schwerk WB, Goerg K, et al. Pleural effusion: an "acoustic window" for sonography of pleural metastases. J Clin Ultrasound 1991;19:93–97.

28. Matthay R, Coppage L, Shaw C, et al. Malignancies metastatic to the pleura. Invest Radiol 1990;25:601–619.

29. Weinberg B, Diakoumakis E, Kass E, et al. The air bronchogram: sonographic demonstration. AJR Am J Roentgenol 1986;147:593–595.

30. Dorne H. Differentiation of pulmonary parenchymal consolidation from pleural disease using the sonographic fluid bronchogram. Radiology 1986;158:41–42.

31. Yang P, Luh K, Lee Y, et al. Lung abscesses: US examination and US-guided transthoracic aspiration. Radiology 1991;180:171–175.

32. Targhetta R, Bourgeois JM, Marty-Double C, et al. Peripheral pulmonary lesions: ultrasonic features and ultrasonically guided fine needle aspiration biopsy. J Ultrasound Med 1993;12:369–374.

33. Yang P, Luh K, Wu H, et al. Lung tumors associated with obstructive pneumonitis: US studies. Radiology 1990;174:717–720.

34. Sheth S, Hamper U, Stanley D, et al. US guidance for thoracic biopsy: a valuable alternative to CT. Radiology 1999;210:721–736.

35. Hang J, Guo Q, Chen C, et al. Imaging approach to the diagnosis of pulmonary sequestration. Acta Radiologica 1996;37:883–888.

36. Hernanz-Schulman M, Johnson J, Holcomb GI, et al. Retroperitoneal pulmonary sequestration: imaging findings, histopathologic correlation, and relationship to cystic adenomatoid malformation. AJR Am J Roentgenol 1997;168:1277–1281.

37. West M, Donaldson J, Shkolnik A. Pulmonary sequestration—diagnosis by ultrasound. J Ultrasound Med 1989;8:125–129.

38. Kim O, Kim W, Kim M, et al. US in the diagnosis of pediatric chest disease. Radiographics 2000;20:653–671.

39. Hernanz-Schulman M, Stein S, Neblett W, et al. Pulmonary sequestration: diagnosis with color Doppler sonography and a new theory of associated hydrothorax. Radiology 1991;180:817–821.

40. Stocker J, Madewell J, Drake R. Congenital cystic malformation of the lung: classification and morphologic spectrum. Hum Pathol 1977;8:155–171.

41. Wernecke K, Vassallo P, Pötter R, et al. Mediastinal tumors: sensitivity of detection with sonography compared with CT and radiography. Radiology 1990;175:137–143.

42. Han B, Babcock D, Oestreich A. Normal thymus in infancy: sonographic characteristics. Radiology 1989;170:471–474.

43. Adam E, Ignotus P. Sonography of the thymus in healthy children: frequency of visualization, size, and appearance. AJR Am J Roentgenol 1993;161:153–155.

44. Ikezoe J, Morimoto S, Arisawa J, et al. Percutaneous biopsy of thoracic lesions: value of sonography for needle guidance. AJR Am J Roentgenol 1990;154:1181–1185.

45. Rosado-de-Christenson M, Galobardes J, Moran C. Thymoma: radiologic-pathologic correlation. Radiographics 1992;12:151–168.

46. Wernecke K, Diederich S. Sonographic features of mediastinal tumors. AJR Am J Roentgenol 1994;163:1357–1364.

47. Wernecke K, Vassallo P, Hoffman G, et al. Value of sonography in monitoring the therapeutic response of mediastinal lymphoma: comparison with chest radiography and CT. AJR Am J Roentgenol 1991;156:265–272.

48. Tashjian J, Teel G, Engeler C, et al. The radiographic spectrum of thymic lesions. The Radiologist 1996;3:167–177.

MUSCULOSKELETAL ULTRASOUND

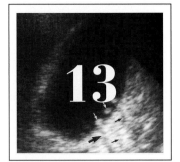

- Imaging Technique
- Anatomy
- Musculoskeletal Masses
- Cystic Lesions
- Infection, Inflammation, and Trauma
- Hernias

US evaluation of the musculoskeletal system is a rapidly expanding area of sonographic diagnosis. Indications include assessment of soft tissue infections, detection and characterization of soft tissue masses, and the evaluation of muscle, tendon, and joint abnormalities [1–3]. This chapter highlights some of these areas of musculoskeletal sonography [4].

IMAGING TECHNIQUE

Most structures imaged are superficial; therefore, high-frequency (7–10 MHz) linear array transducers are most useful [4]. Interaction between the patient and the examining physician is essential to accurate examination. Consider the history and precise location of symptoms. Correlate the examination with point tenderness and location of pain with motion. Real-time observation during compression with the transducer yields vital additional information about the nature of visualized structures. Comparison with normal structures on the opposite side of the body may be extremely helpful. Color flow and spectral Doppler provide vital information about the vascularity of masses and inflammatory processes. Anisotropic artifact (see Chapter 1) is a prominent feature of US examination of tendons and ligaments. Because of their longitudinal fibrillar structure, tendons and ligaments appear echogenic when imaged perpendicular to the US beam and appear hypoechoic when imaged at an angle to the US beam [5].

The examining physician must be familiar with the US appearance of normal structures to recognize abnormalities [1].

ANATOMY

SUBCUTANEOUS FAT

Subcutaneous fat is found just below the covering layer of skin.

- Subcutaneous fat is hypoechoic and interspersed with thin linear septations of connective tissue. Thickness is related to the patient's state of obesity (Fig. 13.1).

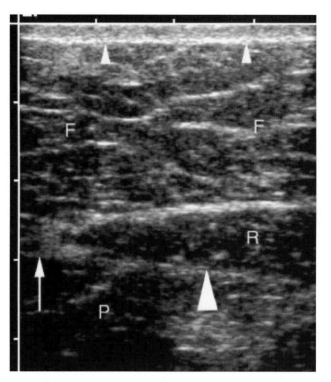

Figure 13.1 *Normal Subcutaneous Fat.* Transverse image of the abdominal wall near the midline shows the rectus abdominis muscle (R), the linea alba (*arrow*), the parietal peritoneum (*large white arrowhead*) and the peritoneal cavity (P). Superficial to the rectus muscle is the subcutaneous fat (F), which appears hypoechoic and septated. The skin (dermal layer) is seen as a thin echogenic layer (*small white arrowheads*) in contact with the transducer.

SKELETAL MUSCLE

Skeletal muscle fibers are grouped into bundles defined by fibroadipose septa [4]. Dense connective tissue covers the entire muscle and additional thick fascia separates individual muscles.

- On longitudinal scans, muscles are hypoechoic with a pattern of fine echogenic strands in an oblique orientation. These strands correspond to fibroadipose septations (Fig. 13.2).
- On transverse scans, the septa appear punctate or linear and are diffusely scattered over the hypoechoic background of muscle tissue (Fig. 13.2).
- Doppler shows moderate blood flow within muscle tissue.
- Dynamic imaging during contraction and relaxation illustrates function and aids in the detection of abnormalities.
- Diffuse fat infiltration of muscle occurs with obesity and diffusely increases the echogenicity of muscle [6].

TENDONS

Tendons in all areas of the body have a fairly uniform, clearly recognizable appearance.

- In longitudinal plane, tendons have a fine, linear, fibrillar internal pattern of parallel hyperechoic lines (Fig. 13.3). Higher frequency US shows more detail with finer and more numerous fibrillar echoes [7].
- On transverse section, tendons are hyperechoic and round or oval in shape.
- Synovial sheaths cover many tendons and appear as a thin (1–2 mm) hypoechoic rim surrounding the echogenic tendon (Fig. 13.3B). The long biceps tendon of the shoulder and the tendons of the wrist and ankle have synovial sheaths. The rotator cuff, Achilles, patellar, gastrocnemius, and semimembranous tendons do not have sheaths [4].
- Tendons will routinely demonstrate the anisotropic effect (Fig. 13.3A) [5].

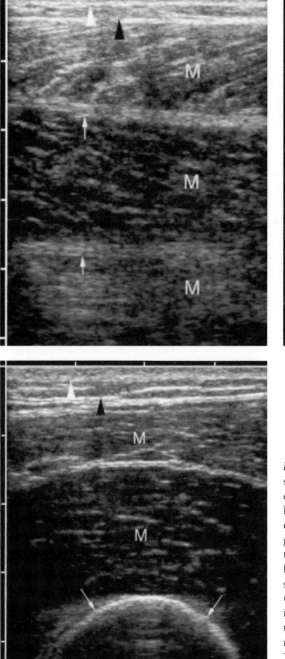

Figure 13.2 *Normal Muscle. A.* Longitudinal image of the calf shows three muscles (M) with oblique muscle fibers oriented in different directions. The dermal layer (*white arrowhead*) and a thin layer of subcutaneous fat (*black arrowhead*) are also evident. Layers of thick fascia (*arrows*) separate the individual muscles. *B.* Longitudinal image of the thigh shows longitudinal muscle fibers in two muscles (M) of differing echogenicity. The surface of the femur (*arrow*) is brightly echogenic and casts a dense acoustic shadow. The dermal layer (*white arrowhead*) and subcutaneous fat (*black arrowhead*) are identified. *C.* Transverse image of the thigh in the same location as *B* shows the more speckled appearance of the fibroadipose septations in the two visualized muscles (M). The round surface (*arrows*) of the mid-shaft of the femur is evident. The arrowheads identify the dermal (*white arrowhead*) and subcutaneous fat (*black arrowhead*) layers.

LIGAMENTS

Ligaments attach bone to bone to provide stabilization.

- Ligaments appear similar to tendons but have a more compact hyperechoic fibrillar pattern. Collagen fibers are most interweaved and more irregular in appearance than tendons.

PERIPHERAL NERVES

Larger peripheral nerves can be accurately seen by US [8,9].

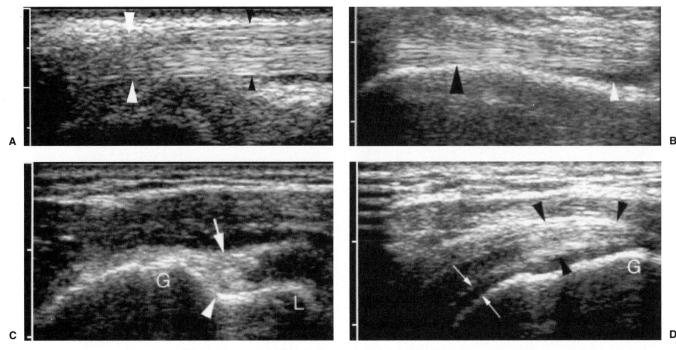

Figure 13.3 *Normal Tendons. A.* Longitudinal image of a flexor tendon of the hand shows the characteristic pattern of linear echogenic strands (*black arrowheads*) where the tendon is imaged perpendicular to the US beam. Where the tendon curves away and the US beam strikes the tendon at an angle, the tendon (*white arrowheads*) appears hypoechoic, and the linear pattern of echogenic strands is lost. *B.* Longitudinal view of the long head of the biceps tendon (*black arrowhead*) in the bicipital groove of the humerus shows the characteristic fibrillar pattern. A small volume of fluid (*white arrowhead*) is seen within the biceps tendon sheath. *C.* Transverse view of the biceps tendon (*arrow*) near the humeral head shows the characteristic "dot" pattern of tendons when imaged transverse to their long axis. The bicipital groove (*arrowhead*) separates the greater (G) and lesser (L) tuberosities of the humerus. *D.* Transverse view of the left shoulder shows the supraspinatus tendon (*black arrowheads*) coursing to its attachment on the greater tuberosity (G). The hyaline cartilage of the humerus is seen as a thin hypoechoic line (*white arrows*) covering the bone surface.

■ Nerves appear as tubular, echogenic structures slightly less echogenic than tendons and ligaments. Multiple, parallel, linear internal echoes are characteristic.

Synovial Bursa

Bursa are potential spaces than normally contain only a tiny volume of fluid.

■ Normal bursa appear as flattened hypoechoic structures 1–4 mm in thickness in characteristic locations.

Bone Cortex

Because bone avidly absorbs sound energy, only the superficial surface of bone is evaluated by US.

■ Bone cortex appears as a bright echogenic surface with prominent posterior shadowing (Figs. 13.2B, C; 13.3C, D).

Hyaline Articular Cartilage

Hyaline cartilage covers the articular cortical surface of bone.

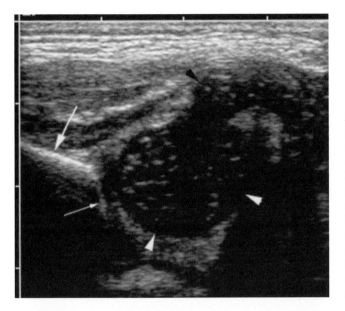

Figure 13.4 *Normal Cartilage.* Coronal plane image of the hip in a newborn infant shows the characteristic appearance of the cartilaginous head (*white arrowheads*) and greater trochanter (*black arrowhead*) of the femur. The iliac bone (*larger arrow*) and roof of the normal acetabulum (*smaller arrow*) are also seen. US is an excellent imaging method to diagnose developmental dysplasia of the hip in infants.

■ Cartilage is seen as a thin hypoechoic rim that covers the echogenic bone cortex (Fig. 13.3D).

HYALINE EPIPHYSEAL CARTILAGE

Sound transmits well through hyaline cartilage, allowing US evaluation of developing bone such as the infant hip [10,11].

■ In the newborn infant the femoral head and trochanters consist entirely of cartilage. The hyaline cartilage appears diffusely hypoechoic with a pattern of echogenic dots scattered throughout its substance (Fig. 13.4). A pattern of echogenic vertical or spiral columns may also be seen. The nucleus of ossification appears as a highly echogenic focus in the center of the hypoechoic head. This focus progressively enlarges as ossification advances [12].

MUSCULOSKELETAL MASSES

US can characterize the cystic or solid nature and vascularity of a mass but, with few exceptions, US cannot determine whether a solid mass is benign or malignant. US is effectively used to guide biopsy of soft tissue masses [13,14]. Soft tissue masses are described as to location, size, shape, margins, vascularity, deformability, and number of lesions.

US is used to confirm or refute the presence of a suspected soft tissue mass.

LIPOMA

Lipomas are a common mass of the superficial soft tissues. The tumor is benign and consists entirely of fat bounded by a thin capsule. The tumor may be lobulated in contour and divided by fibrous septa.

■ Knowing that fat in the abdomen is usually quite echogenic, it is somewhat surprising to recognize that subcutaneous lipomas appear moderately hypoechoic. Echogenicity is homogeneous. Lipomas may be isoechoic or mildly hyper- or hypoechoic compared to subcutaneous fat (Fig. 13.5) [15].
■ Lipomas appear well defined when surrounded by fibrous tissue or muscle but their margins are often indistinct when surrounded by fatty tissue.
■ Lipomas are oval in shape with the long axis of the tumor parallel to the skin [15].

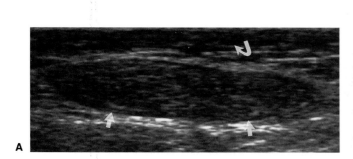

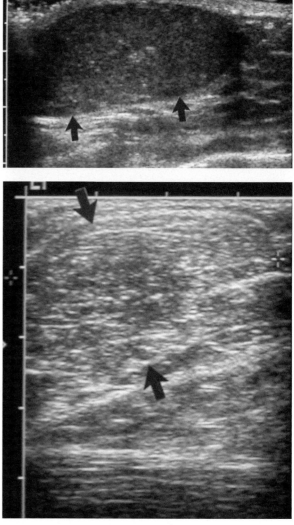

Figure 13.5 Lipomas. *A.* This lipoma (*straight arrows*) is well defined by surrounding echogenic fibrous tissue. It is oval in shape with long axis parallel to the skin. Its echogenicity is homogeneous and equal to subcutaneous fat (*curved arrow*). Palpation revealed a fluctuant mass that was easily compressible by gentle transducer pressure. *B.* This lipoma (*arrows*) is slightly echogenic compared to adjacent fat and is well marginated by a thin, but distinct, fibrous capsule. *C.* Because it is surrounded by isoechoic fat, this lipoma (*arrows*) is difficult to differentiate from surrounding tissues. Correlation with simultaneous physical examination confirms its size and nature.

- Correlation with physical examination is useful to define the borders of the mass and to confirm the soft fluctuant nature of fat.
- Tumor heterogeneity, large size, and prominent lobulations are signs that suggest malignancy (liposarcoma).

HEMANGIOMA

Hemangioma is the second most common benign tumor of muscle and subcutaneous tissues. Hemangiomas consist of endothelial-lined vascular spaces of varying size with a variable amount of intervening fibrofatty tissue [16].

- Hemangiomas are heterogeneous masses with tortuous blood vessels often visible coursing through the mass (Fig. 13.6).
- Color flow Doppler shows prominent blood flow. A high vessel density (more than 5 vessels/cm^2) and high flow velocity is characteristic [17].
- Shadowing punctate echogenic foci represent phleboliths, which are characteristically present.

NERVE TUMORS

Tumors arising from peripheral nerves are usually classified as *schwannomas* (also called *neurinoma* or *neurilemoma*) or neurofibromas. Malignant tumors are sarcomas that arise

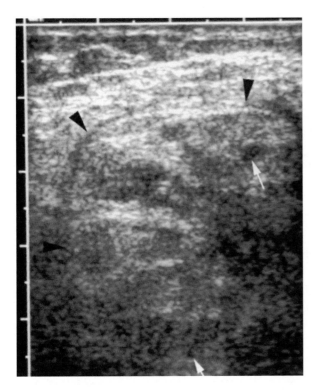

Figure 13.6 *Hemangioma.* A soft tissue mass in the thigh proved to be a hemangioma. The mass (*black arrowheads*) is well defined but heterogeneous in echogenicity. Several small blood vessels (*white arrows*) are visible within the mass.

from neurofibromas. Von Recklinghausen neurofibromatosis is characterized by widespread neurofibromas that present as skin nodules [9,18].

- Nerve tumors appear as well-defined, fusiform, hypoechoic masses. Lesions may be solitary, multiple, or elongated plexiform masses. A neurogenic origin is confirmed if careful scanning confirms that the soft tissue mass is connected to a nerve bundle at its proximal and distal poles [9].
- Schwannomas tend to be more eccentric to the nerve and appear homogeneous with posterior acoustic enhancement. Doppler shows prominent vascularity. Cystic changes may occur.
- Neurofibromas are more echogenic and coarse in appearance. Doppler shows low vascularity. A sonographic target appearance with peripheral low echogenicity surrounding central higher echogenicity has been described [19]. This sonographic finding corresponds to the MR target sign of high intensity peripherally and low intensity centrally seen on T2-weighted images.
- US cannot reliably differentiate benign from malignant nerve sheath tumors. Findings that suggest malignancy include rapid growth, indistinct tumor margins, and invasion of adjacent tissue. Fine needle aspiration biopsy can be performed with US guidance. Needle insertion into the nerve causes intense pain.
- Morton's neuroma is not a true neuroma but is a benign mass of perineural fibrosis arising along the plantar interdigital nerve. The characteristic location is between the second and third, or third and fourth metatarsals. They appear as well-defined, ovoid, hypoechoic nodules. Doppler shows prominent vascularity [20].

US cannot reliably differentiate benign from malignant solid soft tissue masses.

SUPERFICIAL METASTASES

- Superficial melanoma metastases are usually well-defined hypoechoic nodules with smooth or lobulated borders. The lesions have mild to moderate heterogeneity and demonstrate accentuated through-transmission. Doppler shows internal flow in most lesions [21].
- Kaposi's sarcoma produces superficial nodules, which are hypoechoic with ill-defined margins (Fig. 13.7) [22].

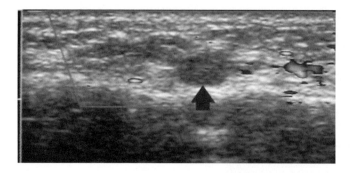

Figure 13.7 *Kaposi's Sarcoma.* Multiple small subcutaneous nodules were palpated in this patient with AIDS. US revealed small, ill-defined hypoechoic masses (*arrow*) corresponding to the palpable nodules. Biopsy confirmed Kaposi's sarcoma. (This color Doppler image is shown here in gray scale.)

SOFT TISSUE SARCOMAS

Soft tissue sarcomas develop most commonly in the extremities. The two most frequent sarcomas are liposarcoma and malignant fibrous histiocytoma.

- Liposarcomas are predominantly echogenic and heterogeneous.
- All other soft tissue sarcomas are hypoechoic (Fig. 13.8). They may be relatively well circumscribed or ill defined and infiltrative. Normal muscle and subcutaneous structure is disrupted. Areas of necrosis, cystic change, and calcification may be evident.
- Sarcoma recurrences appear as small, round or oval, hypoechoic nodules in the area of surgical resection [23].

LYMPHOMA

- Cutaneous lymphoma appears as diffuse echogenic thickening of both dermal and subcutaneous layers with ill-defined margins [22].
- Lymph nodes involved by lymphoma show diffuse low echogenicity. Nodes may appear almost cystic because of uniform cellularity and commonly demonstrate accentuated through-transmission (Fig. 13.9).

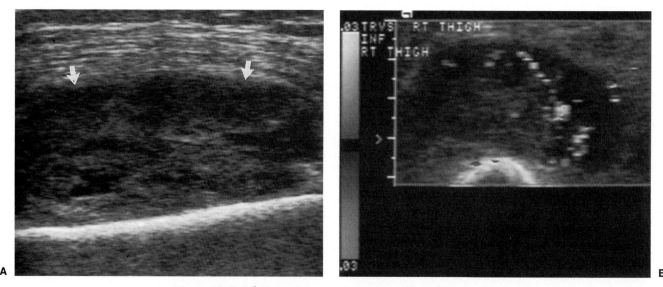

Figure 13.8 *Soft Tissue Sarcoma.* An 85-year-old woman presented with a tender enlarging mass in the right thigh. She noticed the mass after bumping her leg on a table. *A.* Gray scale US reveals a relatively well-defined, but heterogeneous mass (*arrows*). *B.* Color Doppler US shows prominent internal vascularity indicating this mass is a tumor, not a hematoma (see Color Figure 13.8).

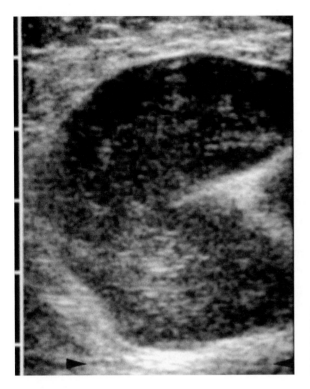

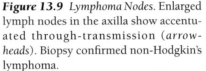

Figure 13.9 *Lymphoma Nodes.* Enlarged lymph nodes in the axilla show accentuated through-transmission (*arrowheads*). Biopsy confirmed non-Hodgkin's lymphoma.

FOREIGN BODIES

US is excellent for determining the presence and location of foreign bodies, especially those that are non-radiopaque. Fragments of glass, wood, or metal may be identified with US [24].

- All foreign bodies are echogenic compared to surrounding tissue (Fig. 13.10). Shape will obviously depend on nature of the object. Examination concentrates on the area of the wound. Acoustic shadowing, comet tail artifacts, and reverberation echoes may be seen depending on the nature and shape of the foreign body [24].
- Bleeding or inflammatory changes may be present adjacent to the foreign body. Air in the soft tissues may obscure detection of the foreign body.

CYSTIC LESIONS

POPLITEAL CYST

Popliteal (Baker's) cysts are common findings associated with internal derangement of the knee. A weakening in the posteromedial wall of the joint capsule allows a synovial commu-

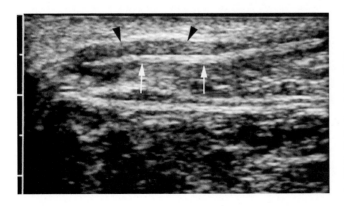

Figure 13.10 *Foreign Body.* A wood splinter embedded in the soft tissues of the calf appears as a well-defined, linear, brightly echogenic object (*white arrows*). A hypoechoic granulomatous reaction (*black arrowheads*) has developed around the foreign body that had been in place several weeks.

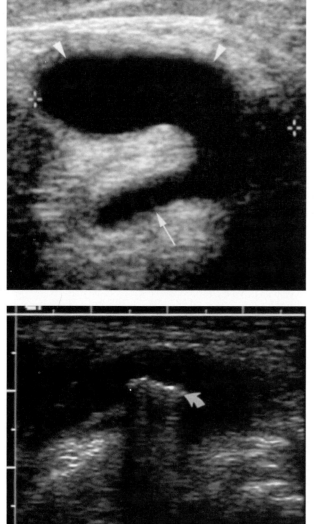

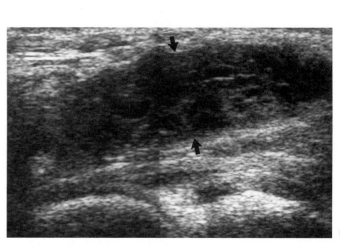

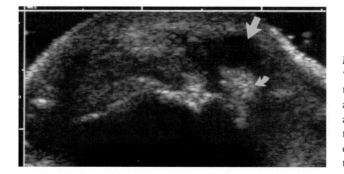

Figure 13.11 *Baker's Cysts. A.* An uncomplicated Baker's cyst (*arrowheads, between cursors, +*) appears as a cystic mass containing anechoic fluid in popliteal fossa. A component of the cyst (*arrow*) extends toward the knee joint space. *B.* A large Baker's cyst (*arrows*) in a patient with rheumatoid arthritis contains echogenic debris and pannus. *C.* An osteochondral fragment (*arrow*) from traumatic knee injury has migrated into a Baker's cyst appearing as an echogenic shadowing mass within the cyst.

nication with the gastrocnemius-semimembranosus bursa, forming a cystic mass filled with joint fluid. Any disease process that increases fluid volume in the joint space may cause a Baker's cyst. The cyst causes symptoms by internal hemorrhage, rupture, or pressure effects on adjacent structures.

■ The cyst occurs in a characteristic anatomic location in the popliteal fossa between the medial head of the gastrocnemius and the distal semimembranosus muscles (Fig. 13.11).
■ Uncomplicated Baker's cysts contain anechoic joint fluid.

Figure 13.12 *Ganglion.* A "bump" on the ventral surface of the great toe is shown by US to be a ganglion (*straight arrow*) attached to the tendon sheath of the extensor hallucis longus tendon (*curved arrow*) shown on a transverse image.

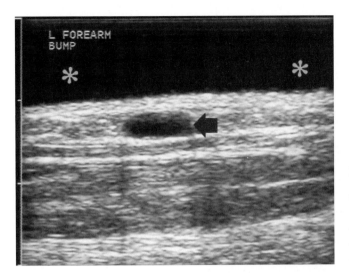

Figure 13.13 *Sebaceous cyst.* A "bump" on the forearm is shown by US to be a sebaceous cyst (*arrow*) extending from the dermal layer. An anechoic standoff pad (**) improves visualization of superficial structures. L, left.

- Complications of Baker's cysts include hemorrhage, pannus formation, dissection, rupture, and loose bodies [25]. Complicated Baker's cysts may be septated and contain echogenic fluid and debris. The cyst may dissect into the muscles of the calf. Osteochondral fragments form as loose bodies in the knee joint that may migrate into the Baker's cyst. Synovial proliferation (pannus) is seen with rheumatoid arthritis and pigmented villonodular synovitis.
- US provides clear distinction from other masses in the popliteal fossa, such as aneurysm of the popliteal artery or soft tissue mass.

GANGLION CYST

Ganglion cysts are the most common soft tissue mass in the wrist and hand [26]. Ganglions are mucin-filled cysts lined by fibrous tissue. Their etiology is uncertain; however, some may be caused by trauma. The cysts are attached to tendon sheaths, muscles, or cartilage. Unlike synovial cysts, they are not lined by synovium and rarely communicate with the joint space [27].

- Ganglion appear as well-defined anechoic masses with acoustic enhancement (Fig. 13.12). They are firm masses that do not compress.
- Some contain layering echogenic debris. They may be multiloculated.

SKIN CYSTS

Skin cysts are best visualized by US with a standoff pad (Fig. 13.13).

- Sebaceous cysts are very superficial within the dermal layer. They are round, well-defined and contain diffusely echogenic fluid [22].
- Mucinous cysts are oval, well-defined, and located superficially between subcutaneous fat and the dermal layer. Fluid is anechoic or hypoechoic [22].

INFECTION, INFLAMMATION, AND TRAUMA

CELLULITIS

Bacterial infections of the soft tissues show a spectrum of abnormalities that range from cellulitis to tissue necrosis to liquefaction to a well-formed abscess [28,29]. The most common causative organisms are *Staphylococcus aureus* and *Streptococcus pyogenes* [30]. US-guidance is utilized to aspirate any fluid collections for analysis and culture.

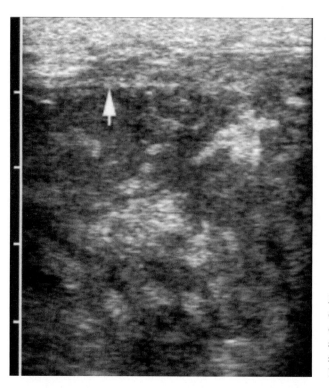

Figure 13.14 Cellulitis. Cellulitis causes diffuse and irregular thickening of the skin (*arrow*) and edematous disruption of the pattern of subcutaneous tissue. Compare to Figure 13.1.

■ Cellulitis appears as diffuse thickening and increased echogenicity of the involved soft tissues with numerous hypoechoic edematous strands that create a network pattern through the tissues (Fig. 13.14). The edematous strands represent distended lymphatic channels [30,31].
■ Diffuse skin edema may have a similar appearance [30].

ABSCESS

Soft tissue abscesses have a variable appearance [30]. Any discrete fluid collection is suspicious in a patient with cellulitis.

■ Abscesses range in appearance from anechoic fluid to complex, heterogeneous, echogenic masses. Internal debris, septations, and loculations are commonly evident (Fig. 13.15).
■ Demonstration of an aspiratable or drainable fluid collection is the key to US examination. Echogenic fluid is best recognized by observation of swirling motion of suspended material during ballottement with the US transducer [32].
■ Doppler will usually show a peripheral rim pattern of prominent blood flow [33].

US is excellent for use in guiding aspiration of soft tissue fluid collections.

NECROTIZING FASCIITIS

Necrotizing fasciitis is a rapidly progressive bacterial infection of skin and subcutaneous tissue associated with extensive tissue loss, severe systemic toxicity, and sometimes, death [34]. It presents clinically as a localized cellulitis but with prominent systemic symptoms including fever, tachycardia, tachypnea, and profound malaise. The infection dissects along fascial layers causing extensive tissue necrosis that undermines surrounding structures. Early surgical excision of necrotic tissue is required to preserve tissue and prevent mortality.

■ Characteristic US findings are [34]:
 – Irregular fascial thickening with fluid accumulation.
 – Loculated abscess within a fascial plane.

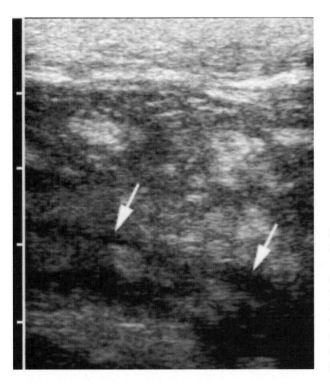

Figure 13.15 *Abscess.* Image from the same patient as shown in Figure 13.14 but in a different area shows a subcutaneous fluid collection (*arrows*). Ballottement with the transducer causes swirling of the echoes within fluid, confirming the liquid nature of the collection. US-guided aspiration yielded a small volume of gross pus.

- Subcutaneous tissue swelling.
- Air bubbles are commonly present in soft tissue.

HEMORRHAGE

Soft tissue trauma may cause discrete hematomas, intramuscular hemorrhage, subcutaneous fat necrosis, soft tissue inflammation, and myositis ossificans. Hemorrhage provides a fertile site for development of infection. US is used to detect fluid components and to guide aspiration to diagnose infection or to relieve pressure symptoms.

- Hematoma are usually well marginated and confined to one compartment (Fig. 13.16). Acute clotted blood is homogeneously echogenic. With time and clot dissolution, the collection becomes more heterogeneous and eventually predominantly cystic. Subacute hemorrhage shows mixed areas of increased and decreased echogenicity. Liquefied hematomas or seromas are predominantly cystic with echogenic fibrinous strands and internal debris.

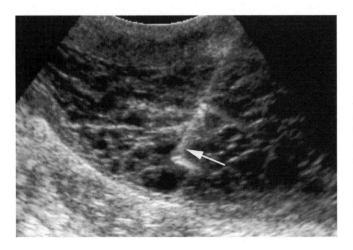

Figure 13.16 *Hematoma.* A subcutaneous hematoma approximately 9 days old has a partially cystic, partially solid appearance. US-guided needle aspiration was performed to exclude infection. The needle tip (*arrow*) is well visualized within the hematoma. Only old blood was aspirated.

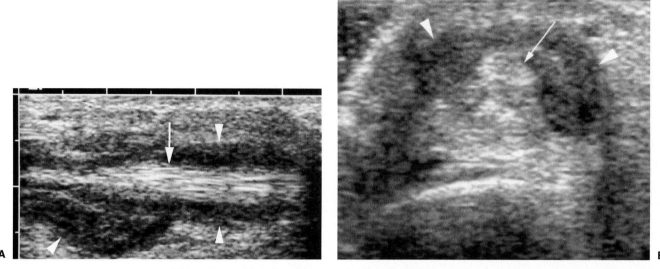

Figure 13.17 *Tenosynovitis. A.* Longitudinal view of the extensor hallucis longus tendon shows marked swelling of the tendon sheath (*arrowheads*) with diffuse thickening of the tendon (*arrow*). *B.* Transverse view confirms the irregular swollen echogenic tendon (*arrow*) and the large amount of fluid in the tendon sheath (*arrowheads*).

- Intramuscular hemorrhage appears infiltrative and mass-like, disrupting the normal uniform fascicular pattern of skeletal muscle. Comparison with adjacent muscles or with the same muscle on the opposite side is helpful in recognizing the hemorrhagic changes. Color Doppler is used to detect abnormal vascularity. Look carefully for a tumor nodule that might have hemorrhaged. If the history of trauma is equivocal or an intramuscular mass is suspected, follow-up US or MR examination is recommended.

TENOSYNOVITIS

Tenosynovitis refers to inflammation of the tendon or synovial tendon sheath. Causes include overuse, connective tissue disorders, and infection [35]. Infection usually results from puncture or penetrating injury. Septic tenosynovitis requires prompt drainage to avoid tendon necrosis or joint contamination [30].

- US shows excessive fluid in the tendon sheath with or without swelling of the tendon (Fig. 13.17) [30,35].
- Acute tendonitis appears as a swollen and hypoechoic tendon with ill-defined margins.
- Doppler demonstrates increased blood flow surrounding the tendon sheath. More prominent blood flow is seen in patients with more pronounced symptoms [36].
- Focal tendon sheath masses may be caused by rheumatoid nodules or pigmented villonodular synovitis.
- Calcifications are seen within tendons in chronic tendonitis. They appear as echogenic foci with acoustic shadowing. Small calcifications may show comet tail artifacts.

BURSITIS

Bursitis most often involves the subdeltoid, patellar, olecranon, or calcaneal bursa. Bursitis is caused by trauma, infection, or crystal-induced arthropathies.

- The inflamed bursa is distended and fluid-filled (Fig. 13.18). Fluid may be anechoic but more commonly contains echogenic debris. Margins may be indistinct. Septations are often present. The nearby joint is often unaffected. Aspiration of the bursa is required if infection is suspected [30,31].
- Chronic bursitis may show calcifications in the wall of the bursa.

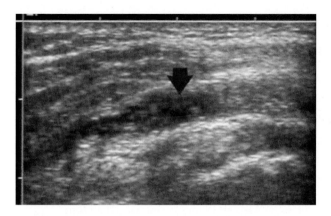

Figure 13.18 *Bursitis.* The subdeltoid bursa (*arrow*) is distended with echogenic fluid in this patient with a rotator cuff tear.

MUSCLE INJURIES

Muscle injuries are caused by excessive pulling force (distraction) or by direct blunt trauma [35].

■ Distraction injury disrupts a variable number of muscle fibers. Small injuries produce small, linear, flame-shaped fluid collections between the muscle fibers. Partial or complete muscle rupture results in disrupted muscle fibers surrounded by larger fluid collections. Muscle fibers are seen to be discontinuous. These injuries are associated with acute functional impairment of the involved muscle [35].

■ Blunt force injuries result in intramuscular bleeding without extensive disruption of muscle fibers. Small hemorrhages are usually called *contusions* whereas larger hemorrhages are called *intramuscular hematomas.*

■ Rhabdomyolysis is necrosis of muscle fibers caused by ischemia that may be induced by crush injury, drug toxicity, or extreme overuse. Myoglobin and muscle enzymes are released into the blood stream. US shows areas of decreased echogenicity and nonhomogeneous muscle texture.

■ Fibrous muscle scars produce focal echogenic areas in the damaged muscle. Acoustic shadowing may be evident.

TENDON RUPTURE

Tendon injuries are usually classified as partial or complete tendon ruptures.

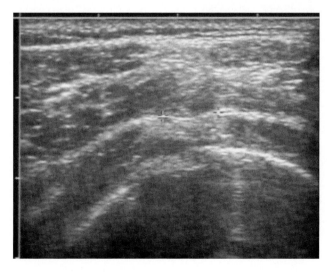

Figure 13.19 *Partial Tendon Tear.* The infraspinatus tendon shows a focal area of thinning (*between cursors, +*) with increased echogenicity of the tendon, indicating a chronic tendon injury.

■ Complete tendon rupture is usually evident clinically. US shows a discontinuous tendon with the two fragments separated by hypoechoic blood or granulation tissue. Absence of visualization of a normally visualized tendon may be the only sign.

■ Partial tendon ruptures are seen as focal hypoechoic defects within the echogenic tendon or as focal thinning of the tendon (Fig. 13.19). Care must be taken to avoid calling tendon anisotropy a partial tendon tear. The tendons must always be imaged as near to perpendicular to the US beam as possible. Tendons routinely examined by US include the rotator cuff tendons, Achilles tendon, and the quadriceps and patellar tendons.

■ When a tendon sheath is present, partial ruptures appear as an anechoic cleft in the tendon with fluid distention of the tendon sheath [4].

■ Subluxation or dislocation of a tendon is documented by demonstrating absence of the tendon in its normal location [4]. This finding is often best demonstrated during dynamic imaging as the tendon and joint are moved through the normal range of motion.

HERNIAS

Hernias of the abdominal wall are common and are frequently a diagnostic challenge especially in obese patients. Hernias may present as a superficial soft tissue mass and must be differentiated from other musculoskeletal masses. US is very effective in the diagnosis of hernias. Abdominal wall hernias are classified as incisional, linea alba, umbilical, or Spigelian hernias. Groin hernias are classified as inguinal (indirect or direct) or femoral. Complications of hernia include pain, which may be positional, incarceration, and strangulation. Incarceration means that the hernia is not reducible but the blood supply is not compromised. Strangulation means that the blood supply to the hernia contents is reduced and that the tissue involved in the hernia is ischemic. Strangulation is an indication for immediate surgical repair [37].

■ The US diagnosis of a hernia is based upon visualization of abdominal contents protruding through tissue planes (Figs. 13.20–13.22). For abdominal wall hernias the parietal peritoneum is identified by visualization of moving bowel beneath it. The presence of ascites makes identification of the parietal peritoneum easy. Hernia contents are then observed to *move* through the parietal peritoneum and into the abdominal wall. The Valsalva maneuver promotes motion of hernia contents and increases the size of the hernia. Some herniations occur only in the standing position. If a hernia is not present

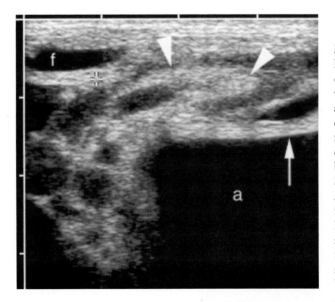

Figure 13.20 *Incisional Hernia.* A hernia through a surgical wound created during cholecystectomy is well visualized in a patient with ascites (a). The ascites clearly defines the layer of parietal peritoneum (*arrow*) lining the peritoneal cavity. Omentum containing fluid between its layers herniates (*arrowheads*) into the abdominal wall. Ascites fluid (f) has also dissected into the hernia sac. The size of the hernia defect is measured by a cursor (+). Omentum is differentiated from bowel by absence of peristalsis and lack of continuity with bowel in the peritoneal cavity.

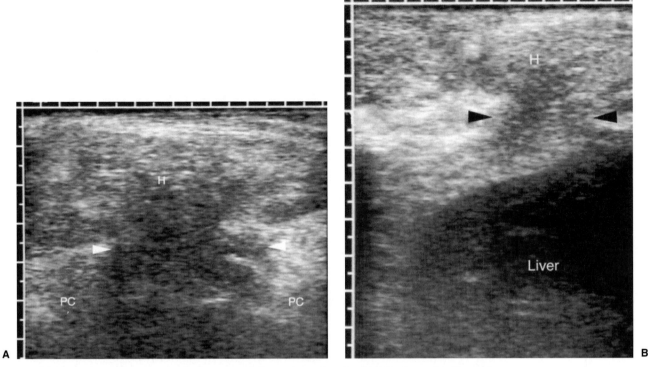

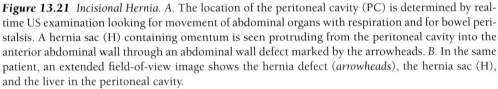

Figure 13.21 *Incisional Hernia. A.* The location of the peritoneal cavity (PC) is determined by real-time US examination looking for movement of abdominal organs with respiration and for bowel peristalsis. A hernia sac (H) containing omentum is seen protruding from the peritoneal cavity into the anterior abdominal wall through an abdominal wall defect marked by the arrowheads. *B.* In the same patient, an extended field-of-view image shows the hernia defect (*arrowheads*), the hernia sac (H), and the liver in the peritoneal cavity.

in the area of concern with the patient supine, the US examination should be repeated with the patient standing [37,38].

■ The contents of hernias vary (Figs. 13.20, 13.21). Most hernias diagnosed by US contain fat and membranes (omentum or properitoneal fat) rather than bowel. Peritoneal fluid may also be present in the hernia sac.

■ The size of the hernia neck should be estimated. Small hernia necks increase the risk of incarceration and strangulation.

■ US signs of strangulation include edema, thickening of the wall of the hernia sac, thickening of bowel wall and absence of peristalsis in bowel contained within the hernia, and absent blood flow in hernia sac contents on Doppler examination.

■ **Incisional hernias** occur through surgical incisions in the anterior abdominal wall (Figs. 13.20, 13.21). Any abdominal wound may be a site of hernia development.

■ **Linea alba hernias** protrude through the fascia of the linea alba in the midline of the abdomen.

■ **Umbilical hernias** are common and usually congenital caused by failure of complete closure of the abdominal wall around the umbilical cord. The hernia bulges at the umbilicus.

■ **Spigelian hernias** occur in characteristic location along the linea semilunaris (Fig. 13.22) [39]. Spigelian hernias are rare but difficult to diagnose and have a high risk of incarceration. The aponeuroses of the internal oblique, external oblique, and transversus abdominis muscles in the flank fuse along the medial edge of the three muscles forming the linea semilunaris. This fused aponeurosis divides medially to pass both anterior and posterior to the rectus muscle in the upper abdomen. In the lower abdomen, midway between the umbilicus and the symphysis pubis, the aponeurosis of the three flank muscles passes only anterior to the rectus muscle, leaving a weakened fascial

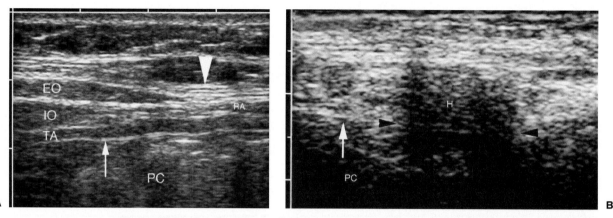

Figure 13.22 *Spigelian Hernia. A.* Transverse image of the anterior abdominal wall shows the fascia layers used as anatomic landmarks for identification of the weak fascial area where Spigelian hernias occur. The fascia of the external oblique (EO), internal oblique (IO), and transversus abdominis (TA) muscles fuse medially to join the fascia of the rectus abdominis (RA) muscle. The fascia is weakest lateral to the rectus and medial to the flank muscles (*arrowhead*) in the lower abdomen below the level of the umbilicus. The arrow indicates the location of the parietal peritoneum. *B.* A Spigelian hernia (H) protrudes through a defect (*arrowheads*) in the abdominal wall. The arrow indicates the location of the parietal peritoneum. PC, peritoneal cavity.

layer involving the lower one-fourth of the edge of the rectus muscle. Spigelian hernias form along this weak fascia plane.

- **Indirect inguinal hernias** extend into the deep inguinal ring and a variable distance down the inguinal canal as far as the scrotum or labia. Indirect hernias lie medial to the inferior epigastric artery and anterior to the spermatic cord. Color Doppler aids in the identification of the inferior epigastric artery and in the differentiation of indirect and direct inguinal hernias [40].

- **Direct inguinal hernias** develop as a result of weakening of the transversalis fascia. The fascia may tear or just stretch and bulge. Direct hernias lie lateral to the inferior epigastric artery and posterior and medial to the spermatic cord.

- **Femoral hernias** are uncommon and difficult to diagnose because they lie deep within the femoral canal. Femoral hernias also occur because of weakening of the transversalis fascia often related to pregnancy. Thus, they are more common in women. The hernia sac protrudes through the femoral canal posterior to the inguinal ligament and medial to the common femoral vein.

REFERENCES

1. Lin J, Fessell DP, Jacobsen JA, et al. An illustrated tutorial of musculoskeletal sonography: Part I, introduction and general principles. AJR Am J Roentgenol 2000;175:637–645.
2. McGahan JP, Brant WE, Gerscovich EO. Ultrasound of the extremities and soft tissue masses. Semin Orthopedics 1991;6:145–155.
3. Kaplan PA, Matamoros A, Jr., Anderson JC. Sonography of the musculoskeletal system. AJR Am J Roentgenol 1990;155:237–245.
4. Hashimoto BE, Kramer DJ, Wiitala L. Applications of musculoskeletal sonography. J Clin Ultrasound 1999;27:293–318.
5. Crass JR, van de Vegte GL, Harkavy LA. Tendon echogenicity: ex vivo study. Radiology 1988;167:499–501.
6. Reimers K, Reimers CD, Wagner S, et al. Skeletal muscle sonography: a correlative study of echogenicity and morphology. J Ultrasound Med 1993;2:73–77.
7. Martinoli C, Derchi LE, Pastorino C, et al. Analysis of echotexture of tendons with US. Radiology 186;186:839–843.
8. Fornage BD. Peripheral nerves of the extremities: imaging with US. Radiology 1988;167:179–182.

9. Martinoli C, Bianchi S, Derchi LE. Ultrasonography of peripheral nerves. Semin Ultrasound CT MRI 2000;21:205–213.

10. Hubbard AM, Dormans JP. Evaluation of developmental dysplasia, Perthes disease, and neuro-muscular dysplasia of the hip in children before and after surgery: an imaging update. AJR Am J Roentgenol 1995;164:1067–1073.

11. Gerscovich EO. Practical approach to ultrasound of the hip in developmental dysplasia. Radiologist 1998;5:23–33.

12. Yousefzadeh DK, Ramilo Jl. Normal hip in children: correlation of US with anatomic and cryomicrotome sections. Radiology 1987;165:647–655.

13. Konermann W, Wuisman P, Ellermann A, et al. Ultrasonographically guided needle biopsy of benign and malignant soft tissue and bone tumors. J Ultrasound Med 2000;19:465–471.

14. Logan PM, Connell DG, O'Connell JX, et al. Image-guided percutaneous biopsy of musculoskeletal tumors: an algorithm for selection of specific biopsy techniques. AJR Am J Roentgenol 1996;166:137–141.

15. Fornage BD, Tassin GB. Sonographic appearances of superficial soft tissue lipomas. J Clin Ultrasound 1991;19:215–220.

16. DuBois J, Garel L, Grignon A, et al. Imaging of hemangiomas and vascular malformations in children. Acad Radiol 1998;5:390–400.

17. DuBois J, Patriquin HB, Garel L, et al. Soft-tissue hemangiomas in infants and children: diagnosis using Doppler sonography. AJR Am J Roentgenol 1998;171:247–252.

18. Murphey MD, Smith WS, Smith SE, et al. Imaging of musculoskeletal neurogenic tumors: radiologic-pathologic correlation. Radiographics 1999;19:1253–1280.

19. Lin J, Jacobsen JA, Hayes CW. Sonographic target sign in neurofibromas. J Ultrasound Med 1999;18:513–517.

20. Quinn TJ, Jacobson JA, Craig JG, et al. Sonography of Morton's neuromas. AJR Am J Roentgenol 2000;174:1723–1728.

21. Nazarian LN, Alexander AA, Kurtz AB, et al. Superficial melanoma metastases: appearances on gray-scale and color Doppler sonography. AJR Am J Roentgenol 1998;170:459–463.

22. Nessi R, Betti R, Bencini PL, et al. Ultrasonography of nodular and infiltrative lesions of the skin and subcutaneous tissues. J Clin Ultrasound 1990;18:103–109.

23. Pino G, Conzi GF, Murolo C, et al. Sonographic evaluation of local recurrences of soft tissue sarcomas. J Ultrasound Med 1993;12:23–26.

24. Shiels WE, II, Babcock DS, Wilson JL, et al. Localization and guided removal of soft-tissue foreign bodies with sonography. AJR Am J Roentgenol 1990;155:1277–1281.

25. Lin J, Fessell DP, Jacobsen JA, et al. An illustrated tutorial of musculoskeletal sonography: Part 3, lower extremity. AJR Am J Roentgenol 2000;175:1313–1321.

26. Lin J, Jacobsen JA, Fessell DP, et al. An illustrated tutorial of musculoskeletal sonography: Part 2, upper extremity. AJR Am J Roentgenol 2000;175:1071–1079.

27. Teefey SA, Middleton WD, Boyer MI. Sonography of the wrist and hand. Semin Ultrasound CT MRI 2000;21:192–204.

28. Loyer EM, DuBrow RA, David CL, et al. Imaging of soft-tissue infections: sonographic findings in cases of cellulitis and abscess. AJR Am J Roentgenol 1996;166:149–152.

29. Chao H-C, Lin S-J, Huang Y-C, et al. Sonographic evaluation of cellulitis in children. J Ultrasound Med 2000;19:743–749.

30. Bureau NJ, Chhem RK, Cardinal E. Musculoskeletal infections: US manifestations. Radiographics 1999;19:1585–1592.

31. Lin J, Jacobsen JA, Fessell DP, et al. An illustrated tutorial of musculoskeletal sonography: Part 4, musculoskeletal masses, sonographically guided interventions, and miscellaneous topics. AJR Am J Roentgenol 2000;175:1711–1719.

32. Loyer EM, Kaur H, David CL, et al. Importance of dynamic assessment of the soft tissues in the sonographic diagnosis of echogenic superficial abscesses. J Ultrasound Med 1995;14:669–671.

33. Latifi HR, Siegel MJ. Color Doppler flow imaging of pediatric soft tissue masses. J Ultrasound Med 1994;13:165–169.

34. Chao H, Kong M, Lin T. Diagnosis of necrotizing fasciitis in children. J Ultrasound Med 1999;18:277–281.

35. Lund PJ, Nisbet JK, Valencia FG, et al. Current sonographic applications in orthopedics. AJR Am J Roentgenol 1996;166:889–895.

36. Breidahl WH, Stafford Johnson DB, Newman JS, et al. Power Doppler sonography in tenosynovitis: significance of the peritendinous hypoechoic rim. J Ultrasound Med 1998;17:103–107.

37. Rapp C, Stavros AT, Kaske TI. Ultrasound of abdominal wall hernias. J Diag Med Sonography 1999;15:231–235.
38. Wechsler RJ, Kurtz AB, Needleman L, et al. Cross-sectional imaging of abdominal wall hernias. AJR Am J Roentgenol 1989;153:517–521.
39. Mufid MM, Abu-Yosef MM, Kakish ME, et al. Spigelian hernia: diagnosis by high-resolution real-time sonography. J Ultrasound Med 1997;16:183–187.
40. Korenkov M, Paul A, Troidl H. Color duplex sonography: diagnostic tool in the differentiation of inguinal hernias. J Ultrasound Med 1999;18:565–568.

Ultrasound of Organ Transplants and Transjugular Intrahepatic Portosystemic Shunt

RENAL TRANSPLANTS

Sonography plays a central role in the initial evaluation and long-term follow-up of renal transplants. US is used to detect early and late complications and to guide aspiration of fluid collections and biopsies of the transplanted kidney. Doppler US is used to screen for vascular complications, which are then usually confirmed and often treated by angiographic techniques [1,2].

SURGICAL TECHNIQUE

Transplant kidneys are most often placed in the iliac fossa in a retroperitoneal position. When combined with pancreas transplantation, the renal transplant is intraperitoneal in position. The renal pelvis and ureter are routinely positioned anteriorly to allow for easier access if subsequent intervention is necessary. For this reason a right donor kidney is usually turned over and placed in the recipient's left iliac fossa. A left donor kidney is usually placed in the right iliac fossa. The transplant renal artery may be connected to either the internal or external iliac artery. End-to-side anastomosis to the external iliac artery is often preferred because of a lower incidence of postoperative stenosis. Cadaver kidneys are commonly removed with the renal artery intact and still attached to a portion of the aorta. The aorta is trimmed to an oval or round shape (a Carrel patch) and is sutured end-to-side to the external iliac artery of the recipient. Arteries of living donor kidneys are harvested without an aortic patch and are anastomosed directly to the recipient artery. Connection to the internal iliac artery is made end-to-end. Multiple renal transplant arteries require additional anastomoses. The transplant renal vein is connected end-to-side to the external iliac vein with special care taken to ensure that the vein is mobile and is not kinked. The transplant ureter is usually connected to the bladder directly by ureteroneocystostomy. Occasionally the transplant ureter is connected to a native ureter or to an ileal conduit. US examination is commonly performed within the first 24 hours to provide a baseline scan for comparison with future studies.

Knowledge of surgical anatomy and the precise nature and location of the vascular anastomosis is most helpful in performing an accurate US evaluation of the transplant.

RENAL TRANSPLANT SCAN PROTOCOL

Because the renal transplant is usually superficial, a high-frequency 5.0–7.0-MHz curved array transducer is preferred. For larger patients with deeper transplant kidneys, a 3.5–4.0-MHz sector transducer may be used. The kidney is scanned in its long and transverse axes. Measurements are made of its greatest length, width, and anteroposterior (AP) dimensions. Renal volume is calculated by the standard formula (volume = length × width × AP dimension × 0.523). Renal size is an important parameter to follow to assess for pathologic changes. The echogenicity of the cortex, medulla, and renal sinus is carefully evaluated and compared to images from previous US examinations. The perirenal areas are scanned for fluid collections, hematomas, solid masses, and adenopathy. A full bladder is preferred to displace overlying bowel out of the pelvis and away from the transplant. If hydronephrosis is present, the bladder should be emptied to see if the dilatation is caused by bladder distention. A dilated ureter should be searched for.

Doppler evaluation is an essential part of every US evaluation of transplanted organs.

Patency of the transplant arteries and vein should be confirmed with color and spectral Doppler. Spectral waveforms of intrarenal arteries at the upper pole, mid-kidney, and lower pole are obtained and resistance index (RI) calculated from the waveforms. Intrarenal arteries are identified by flashes of color on color flow imaging. A small spectral Doppler sample volume is placed over the flashing color signal and is moved until an adequate spectral tracing is obtained. Because the intrarenal arteries are usually not discretely visualized, no attempt is made to determine Doppler angle. Power Doppler provides evaluation of vascular perfusion of the transplant kidney and is used to detect focal flow defects.

US imaging is highly cost-effective as a screening tool to detect complications. Examinations should be interpreted with a low threshold for abnormalities, which are then confirmed by additional testing [1].

NORMAL RENAL TRANSPLANT

The following features characterize a normal renal transplant:

- The echogenicity of the renal cortex is equal to or slightly greater than the echogenicity of the medulla. Absence of corticomedullary differentiation is a normal finding seen in many transplants.
- The echogenicity of the cortex and medulla is uniform throughout the kidney. Focal areas of increased or decreased echogenicity suggest edema, hemorrhage, infection, ischemia, or infarction.
- Renal size measurements are compared to previous scans. In transverse plane the kidney is elliptical in shape with the width being greater than the AP dimension. Rounding of the kidney with AP dimension equal to transverse dimension is a sign of diffuse renal swelling. However, the volume of normal renal transplants may increase up to 20% in the first 2–3 weeks after transplantation [3].
- The renal sinus should be obvious and is distinctly more echogenic than the renal parenchyma.

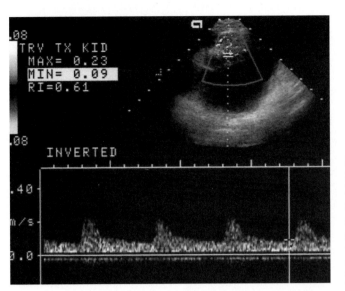

Figure 14.1 *Normal Transplant Resistance Index.* The normal Doppler spectrum of an intrarenal artery of a renal transplant shows relatively high velocity flow throughout diastole. Resistance index (RI) in this case is 0.61. A peritransplant fluid collection is present.

- Mild pelviectasis is a common and usually normal finding. Calyectasis is a relatively reliable sign of obstruction.
- Doppler of the normal renal artery shows a low resistance pattern with forward flow into the kidney throughout the cardiac cycle. The range of normal peak systolic velocity is broad (60–203 cm/sec, mean 132 cm/sec) [4].
- Renal vein flow is flat with low velocity and flow away from the kidney.
- RI of intrarenal arteries is normally <0.80 (Fig. 14.1).
- Normal perfusion as shown by power Doppler is characterized as a high vessel density in cortical tissue, in the intrarenal septa, and peripheral parenchyma (Fig. 14.2). Vessels may be absent in the medullary pyramids [5].

Complications of Renal Transplantation

Peritransplant Fluid Collections. Fluid collections adjacent to the transplant are very common (approximately 40% of transplants) and may be lymphoceles, urinomas, seromas, hematomas, or abscesses [6]. US determines the size, location, and appearance of the fluid collection. Although each entity shows some characteristic findings, differentiation is confirmed by US-guided aspiration of the fluid. Small fluid collections are often observed and usually resolve over time without compromising the transplant.

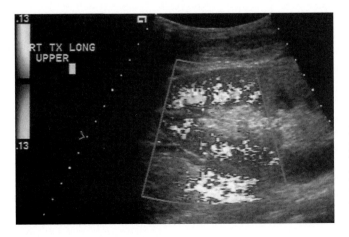

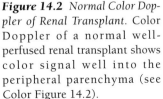

Figure 14.2 *Normal Color Doppler of Renal Transplant.* Color Doppler of a normal well-perfused renal transplant shows color signal well into the peripheral parenchyma (see Color Figure 14.2).

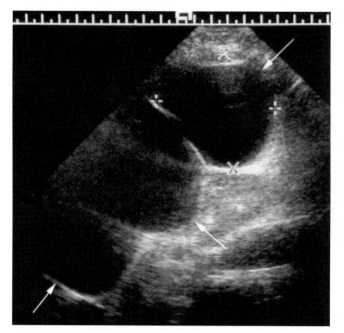

Figure 14.3 *Lymphocele.* Peritransplant fluid collection (*between arrows*) shows several thin septations. US-guided fluid aspiration confirmed a lymphocele. Calipers (*+, x*) measure the size of a loculation.

- **Lymphoceles** are most common, affecting up to 15% of transplants. They are accumulations of lymph in the extraperitoneal space and usually result from interruption of the recipient's lymphatic channels.
    - Fluid collections are anechoic, often large in size, and most (80%) have thin septations (Fig. 14.3).
    - Lymphoceles are most common 4–8 weeks after transplantation.
    - Small lymphoceles are usually asymptomatic and require no therapy.
- **Hematomas and seromas** are common but usually small and insignificant in the immediate postoperative period. Large hematomas may result from injury to the vascular pedicle of the kidney or rupture of the transplant.
    - Acute hematomas are hypoechoic, solid, and often lobulated perirenal collections (Fig. 14.4).
    - An increase in size of the hematoma indicates continued bleeding and a need for intervention.
    - Old hematomas are most variable and show solid-appearing areas of clotted blood and cystic areas of seroma. Septations are common.
- **Abscess** is usually an early complication (first 3 weeks), presenting with postoperative fever and pain.
    - US shows a fluid collection of mixed echogenicity with internal echoes representing pus and debris.
    - Gas within the fluid collection is highly indicative of infection.
- **Urinoma** is also usually an early complication but is relatively rare. Urine leaks may develop due to faulty anastomosis or be caused by ischemic necrosis of the collecting system. Ischemic necrosis most commonly involves the distal ureter, but may involve the entire ureter and collecting system.
    - The collection is purely cystic, anechoic, and usually without septations (Fig. 14.5).
    - Large urinomas may cause urinary obstruction.
    - Large urinomas require aspiration or drainage.
    - Small urinomas regress spontaneously.
    - Radionuclide imaging shows progressive accumulation of radiotracer in the collection when a urine leak is present.
- In women, **ovarian cysts** must be considered as an additional cause of a peritransplant fluid collection.

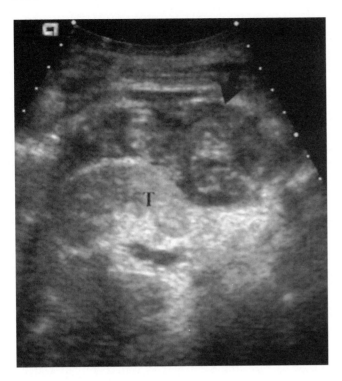

Figure 14.4 *Peritransplant Hematoma.* A postoperative hematoma (*arrow*) appears as a lobulated hypoechoic solid mass adjacent to the transplant kidney (T) seen in transverse section.

Diminished Renal Function. Elevation of serum creatinine is a common clinical problem indicative of impaired transplant function. Causes are listed in Box 14.1. US is used to detect urinary obstruction, pathologic fluid collections, and vascular complications. However, the most common causes are acute rejection, acute tubular necrosis, and cyclosporine toxicity.

■ US findings are non-specific. The following findings may be evident with each of the conditions listed. US-guided core biopsy is usually performed to confirm the diagnosis.
  − The kidney is often enlarged and has increased thickness of the cortex. The AP diameter is equal to or exceeds the transverse diameter.
  − Pyramids may be prominent or corticomedullary differentiation may be lost.

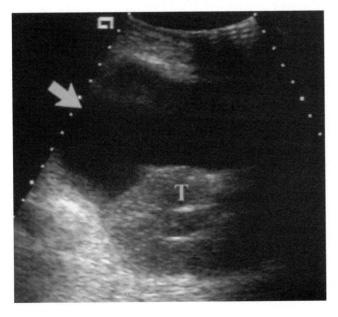

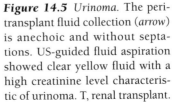

Figure 14.5 *Urinoma.* The peritransplant fluid collection (*arrow*) is anechoic and without septations. US-guided fluid aspiration showed clear yellow fluid with a high creatinine level characteristic of urinoma. T, renal transplant.

> **Box 14.1: Causes of Impaired Function of Renal Transplant**
>
> Acute tubular necrosis   Drug nephrotoxicity
> Rejection   Cyclosporine
>   Acute   Ureteral obstruction
>   Chronic   Infection
>   Arterial stenosis

Elevated resistance index is a nonspecific finding of transplant dysfunction.

  – The renal cortex may show increased or decreased echogenicity (Fig. 14.6).
  – The walls of the collecting system may be thickened.
  – The central renal sinus may be effaced and its normal high echogenicity is absent.
  – RI of the intrarenal arteries >0.8 is a nonspecific finding of renal dysfunction. Occasionally reversal of blood flow direction is seen in diastole.

- **Acute tubular necrosis** results in the postoperative period from prolonged ischemia and reperfusion injury. Cold storage of the donor kidney for longer than 24–30 hours increases the probability of acute tubular necrosis. The condition is uncommon when the kidney is obtained from a living related donor.
- **Acute rejection** occurs in the first year in up to 50% of transplant recipients. Presentation includes malaise, fever, and a painful kidney. However, cyclosporine therapy may mask all symptoms. Acute rejection is rare immediately post-transplant but usually becomes apparent on serial follow-up. Acute rejection is rare after the first year.
- **Chronic rejection** is the most common cause of late transplant loss. Loss of renal function is progressive to complete transplant failure.
  – US shows diminished renal size, thinning of the cortex, and often mild hydronephrosis.
- **Drug nephrotoxicity** may be caused by many of the drugs used to suppress rejection, but cyclosporine toxicity is most common. Toxicity is dose dependent and function often improves with reduction of dose.

Vascular Complications. Vascular complications are an uncommon (<10%) but important cause of impaired graft function [7]. They have a high incidence of morbidity and mortality but are usually easily repaired when detected. US with spectral Doppler and color flow imaging is used to screen the transplant for vascular complications. Positive screening studies are routinely followed by angiography for confirmation and therapy.

- **Renal artery stenosis** is the most common vascular complication (1.5–4.0% of transplants). Patients present with an audible bruit or severe hypertension unresponsive to

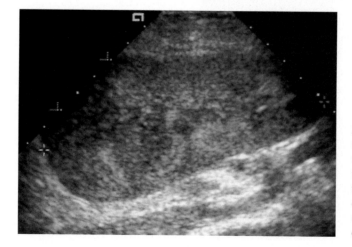

Figure 14.6 *Chronic Rejection—Renal Transplant.* A failing transplant shows diffusely increased parenchymal echogenicity. US-guided core biopsy confirmed chronic rejection. Calipers (+) measure the length of the transplant kidney.

treatment usually within the first 3 years after transplantation. Moderate hypertension due to non-renovascular causes is common (65% of transplant patients), and usually not a sign of renal artery stenosis. Stenosis at the anastomosis is usually related to surgical technique, but stenosis anywhere along the renal artery may be caused by rejection [8].

– The renal artery is examined throughout its length with color and spectral Doppler looking for zones of high velocity flow and for zones of aliasing on color Doppler.
– Peak systolic velocity >200 cm/sec suggests significant stenosis.
– Velocity gradient >2:1 between stenotic and prestenotic segments indicates significant stenosis.
– Marked turbulence is seen downstream from the area of narrowing.
– Tardus parvus waveform is highly indicative of significant stenosis but is often not present. Identification of this waveform is important because the entire course of the artery is not always seen.

■ **Renal vein thrombosis** is rare and usually occurs in the first week after transplantation. Renal vein thrombosis commonly results in infarction that necessitates removal of the transplant.
– The kidney is hypoechoic and swollen because of edema.
– The arterial waveform shows reversed flow throughout diastole.
– No venous flow is present.

■ **Renal artery occlusion** occurs in the early postoperative period. Infarction leads to graft loss. The surgical anastomosis is usually faulty.
– No arterial or venous flow is detected by Doppler US.
– Severe acute rejection may mimic this finding. If in doubt, an arteriogram should be performed.

■ **Intrarenal arteriovenous fistula** is a complication of biopsy of the transplant when an adjacent artery and vein are lacerated. Small fistulas are incidental and resolve spontaneously. Large fistulas may shunt so much blood that the transplant becomes ischemic.
– Most arteriovenous fistulas are not evident on gray-scale US.
– Color flow shows turbulence, aliasing, and tissue vibration artifact in the area of the fistula (Fig. 14.7).
– High-velocity, low-resistance waveforms are seen on the arterial side.
– Draining veins show arterial pulsations.
– Tissue vibration artifact, caused by the turbulent blood flow, is shown with high sensitivity by power Doppler [9].
– Rupture of the fistula results in a large perirenal hematoma.

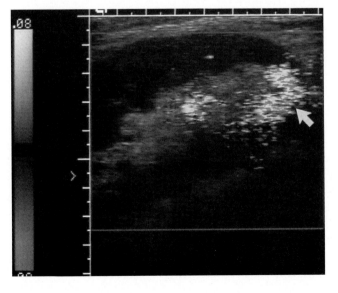

Figure 14.7 *Arteriovenous Fistula—Renal Transplant.* Biopsy of the renal transplant too close to the hilum has caused an arteriovenous fistula (*arrow*) seen as a focus of abnormal turbulent color flow. This color Doppler image is reproduced in gray scale only.

■ Pseudoaneurysms result from isolated arterial laceration during biopsy.
 – Pseudoaneurysms appear as a bubble-like mass within the parenchyma.
 – Doppler confirms turbulent blood flow within the mass.
 – The neck of the pseudoaneurysm connecting to the injured artery may be seen when the pseudoaneurysm is large.

Urinary Obstruction. Urinary obstruction can be found during sonography for a failing renal transplant. In the immediate postoperative period, temporary obstruction may result from edema at the ureterovesical anastomosis or temporarily impaired peristalsis of the transplanted ureter [6,10].

■ Mild hydronephrosis (splaying of the pelvis without calyectasis) is common and is most likely due to non-obstructive causes such as overhydration or bladder distention [1].
■ Moderate (dilated pelvis and calyces) to severe (marked distention of the pelvis and calyces) hydronephrosis is a reliable sign of significant urinary obstruction [1]. Obstruction should be confirmed by excretory urography or radionuclide renography [11].
■ A dilated ureter should be searched for to determine the location of obstruction.
■ Peritransplant fluid collections, adenopathy or mass associated with posttransplantation lymphoproliferative disorder (PTLD), intraluminal calculus or blood clot, and ureteral fibrosis are causes of obstruction [6].

Urine Leaks. Most urine leaks are evident in the immediate postoperative period and are caused by faulty anastomosis or ureteral necrosis resulting from impaired blood supply. Late leaks are associated with ureteral graft rejection.

■ Urine leak is suspected if a peritransplant fluid collection shows an increase in volume or if a new fluid collection occurs. Radionuclide renography is then indicated to confirm the leak.

PANCREAS TRANSPLANTS

The primary indication for pancreas transplantation is to provide an intrinsic source of insulin for patients with severe insulin-dependent diabetes mellitus. Because many of these patients also have diabetic nephropathy, pancreas transplant is commonly (~90% of pancreas transplants) combined with simultaneous renal transplant. Ideal candidates are patients with type I diabetes who are younger than age 45 and have little or no atherosclerotic disease. Most pancreatic transplants are whole organ transplants harvested intact from cadavers, which may also be the source of the renal transplant. Live donor grafts are always segmental, have a smaller mass of beta cells and have a higher risk of thrombosis.

SURGICAL TECHNIQUE

Traditional whole organ pancreatic transplantation involves arterial anastomosis of the celiac axis/splenic artery with the external iliac artery, systemic venous drainage with anastomosis of the splenic/portal vein to the external iliac vein, and drainage of pancreatic exocrine secretions into the bladder through an attached segment of duodenum [12]. Vascular anastomoses are usually made end-to-side. The donor splenic and superior mesenteric arteries may be joined in a Y-graft and then anastomosed to the iliac artery. The transplanted pancreas is usually intraperitoneal in location. This procedure has been associated with a variety of urologic complications, reflux graft pancreatitis, and hematuria. Systemic venous drainage is associated with hyperinsulinemia and peripheral insulin resistance. Usually the pancreas is placed in one iliac fossa and the kidney is placed in the other iliac fossa.

To combat complications of the traditional procedure, another technique with venous drainage to the portal system and exocrine drainage to the intestinal tract is used at some institutions [13]. The pancreas is placed in the lower abdomen surrounded by bowel and mesentery.

PANCREAS TRANSPLANT SCAN PROTOCOL

The goals of imaging are to detect and characterize complications, to guide aspiration of fluid collections, and to guide biopsy of the transplanted pancreas. Sonography is indicated for routine follow-up and whenever transplant dysfunction or complication is suspected. All US examinations should include Doppler evaluation of the parenchyma and its vascular connections. Knowledge of the vascular anastomoses of the specific transplant examined is most helpful in its evaluation.

- The pancreas is evaluated for parenchymal echogenicity, location, and orientation.
- Measurement of the size of the graft should be made to establish a baseline for detection of enlargement that is associated with acute rejection and acute pancreatitis.
- A careful search for peripancreatic fluid collections is undertaken.
- Arterial and venous flow is carefully evaluated with color flow and spectral Doppler.

NORMAL PANCREAS TRANSPLANT

- In the immediate postoperative period, the transplanted pancreas commonly shows focal abnormalities related to handling and surgical trauma. The graft may appear focally or diffusely hypoechoic, even though the pancreas is functioning normally. The graft appearance should be normal within 2–4 weeks provided no complications intervene.
- Normal pancreatic parenchyma shows homogeneous mid-level echogenicity slightly greater than muscle (Fig. 14.8).
- Doppler confirms venous and low resistance arterial flow.

Complications of Pancreas Transplantation

Complications are common and are associated with significant morbidity and mortality [12].

Fluid Collections. Peripancreatic fluid collections are the most common complication [14]. Fluid collections are associated with an increased risk of graft dysfunction and may coexist with other complications.

- Small fluid collections are common in the postoperative period. Most are clinically insignificant and resolve spontaneously in 7–10 days [14].

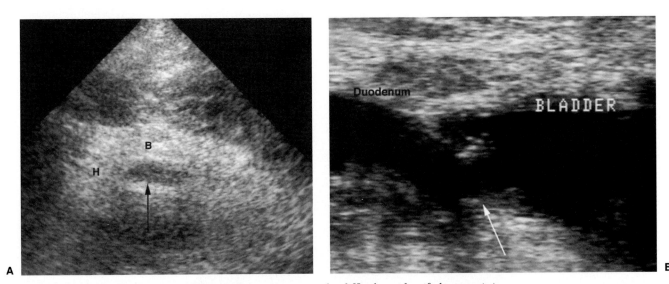

Figure 14.8 *Normal Pancreas Transplant. A.* The pancreas may be difficult to identify because it is surrounded by bowel and mesentery. This image shows the head (H) and body (B) of the transplant, as well as the splenic vein (*arrow*). *B.* The anastomosis (*arrow*) of the duodenum to the bladder is well shown.

- Free ascites is commonly present in varying volume. Ascites associated with pancreatitis is usually large in volume. The diagnosis is confirmed by paracentesis with fluid showing elevated amylase.
- Pancreatic or peripancreatic abscess is life-threatening and affects 8–22% of patients.
  – The presence of gas bubbles in a fluid collection is highly indicative of infection.
- **Hematoma**, **seroma**, **urinoma**, and **lymphocele** have the same appearances as described for renal transplants. Imaging diagnosis is confirmed by US-guided fluid aspiration.
- **Pancreatic pseudocysts** may form as a complication of pancreatitis.
- **Anastomotic leaks** are common. The presence of digestive enzymes promotes development of anastomotic leaks and impairs their healing. The presence of a leak is suggested by US identification of a fluid collection in the region of the anastomosis. The diagnosis of leak at the bladder anastomosis is confirmed by retrograde cystography with fluoroscopic or CT imaging [15]. Enteric anastomotic leaks are difficult to confirm by imaging methods because of inability to directly fill the recipient bowel loops.

Transplant Rejection. Rejection is the most common cause of transplant failure, affecting up to 35% of pancreas transplants. Elevation of serum creatinine suggests possible rejection of both the renal and pancreas transplants. Pancreatic graft failure is suspected when the urine amylase level drops. Beta cells are affected late so serum glucose may remain normal until rejection is severe.

- The pancreas enlarges and the parenchyma appears inhomogeneous with diffuse or focal hypoechoic or anechoic areas (Fig. 14.9).
- RI of intraparenchymal arteries >0.70 is found with acute rejection. However, many patients with rejection have normal arterial indices [16].
- Percutaneous US-guided biopsy of the pancreas transplant is indicated to confirm rejection [17].
- Chronic rejection is associated with diffuse decrease in size of the pancreas and a diffuse increase in parenchymal echogenicity.

Acute Pancreatitis. Mild transient pancreatitis is almost universal in the first few days after transplantation. Urinary reflux is the most common cause of pancreatitis after immediate postoperative period. Pain and tenderness in the transplant region and increasing serum amylase are the usual presenting features.

- The pancreas is enlarged and edematous with decreased parenchymal echogenicity focally or globally.

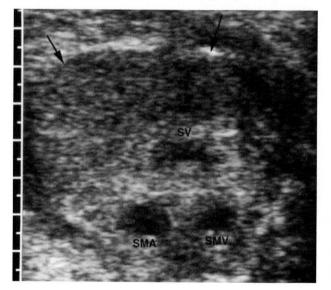

Figure 14.9 *Acute Rejection of Pancreas Transplant.* The pancreas (*arrows*) is enlarged and heterogeneously hypoechoic. This oblique view shows the splenic vein (SV), superior mesenteric artery (SMA), and superior mesenteric vein (SMV).

- Dilatation of the pancreatic duct is strong evidence of pancreatitis. A duct >2 mm diameter is considered dilated.
- Pancreatitis-related fluid collections may be anechoic or complex.

Vascular Complications. Vascular complications affect 13–20% of pancreas grafts [18].

- Arterial thrombosis usually occurs within days of surgery.
    - Doppler signals are absent in the pancreatic parenchyma and in the graft vessels. The transplant must be removed.
- Venous thrombosis is also most common in the first week after transplantation [19].
    - Venous signals are absent in veins that drain the graft.
    - Arterial signals are usually preserved but show a high resistance pattern often with flow reversal in diastole [20,21].
- Pseudoaneurysms and arteriovenous fistulas are uncommon [22]. Pseudoaneurysm may occur as a complication of pancreatitis as well as of pancreas biopsy.

Urologic Complications. Drainage of digestive enzymes into the bladder causes a variety of complications. Cystoscopy is the diagnostic method of choice.

- Transient hematuria is almost universal after bladder anastomosis. Postoperative hematuria resolves spontaneously within a week.
- Continuing hematuria suggests enzyme-induced cystitis, which is further complicated by the neurogenic bladder dysfunction so common in the diabetic patient.
- Ulceration of duodenum is another cause of persisting hematuria.
- Urethritis and stricture complicate approximately 3% of pancreas transplants.

LIVER TRANSPLANTS

Liver transplantation is performed in adult and pediatric patients with severe acute or chronic liver failure for which no other therapy is available. US is performed preoperatively to detect contraindications to transplantation and conditions that will alter surgical technique. US is performed serially after surgery to detect complications. US guidance is preferred to aspirate fluid collections and to guide parenchymal biopsies performed to diagnose rejection.

SURGICAL TECHNIQUE

Orthotopic liver transplantation involves removal of the native liver and replacement with a donor liver. This procedure requires four vascular anastomoses: hepatic artery, inferior vena cava (IVC) above and below the liver, and portal vein. A variety of hepatic artery anastomoses may be performed. The donor hepatic artery may include a variable length of the celiac axis or even a portion of the aorta (Carrel patch). The actual anastomosis is usually end-to-end with a dilated or fish-mouth configuration [23]. Anastomoses to the IVC are usually made end-to-end just above and below the intrahepatic cava. Portal vein anastomosis is made end-to-end between recipient and donor portal veins. If the recipient portal vein is thrombosed a venous jump graft is made between the donor portal vein and the recipient superior mesenteric vein (SMV). The biliary anastomosis is made end-to-end between donor and recipient common bile ducts near the porta hepatis [23]. The gallbladder is routinely resected prior to transplantation.

Because of the shortage of cadaveric livers for transplantation, a newer procedure allows healthy adults to donate the right lobe of their liver. The procedure requires that the liver be healthy and without evidence of fatty infiltration. At least 35% of the donor liver volume must be left in place for the donor to continue to have normal liver function [24].

PREOPERATIVE SONOGRAPHY OF THE RECIPIENT

Preoperative US is performed to identify conditions that preclude transplantation or require modification of the surgical technique [25,26].

- Doppler is used to confirm patency of the portal vein, hepatic veins, and IVC. Measure and report the size of the portal vein and SMV.
  - Because the patient has end-stage liver disease, signs of portal hypertension are evident.
  - Reflecting portal hypertension, the size of the portal vein is usually >12 mm. Collateral veins in the porta hepatis seen with portal vein thrombosis and cavernous transformation are seldom larger than 4–5 mm.
  - Thrombosis of the portal vein associated with thrombosis of the SMV precludes liver transplantation.
  - Thrombosis of the portal vein, with or without cavernous transformation but with a patent SMV, allows transplantation but requires a venous jump graft from donor portal vein to recipient SMV.
- Doppler is used to identify anomalies of the hepatic artery such as origin of the right hepatic artery from the superior mesenteric artery.
- The liver parenchyma is carefully inspected for evidence of hepatoma or cholangiocarcinoma. CT or MR may be needed to improve tumor detection. Any mass without imaging features of cyst or hemangioma should be biopsied. Most surgeons consider the presence of cholangiocarcinoma to be a contraindication to liver transplant, while liver transplant is feasible but controversial in patients with hepatoma. Resected livers commonly contain small hepatomas that are not detected preoperatively.
- The presence and function of any therapeutic shunts must be evaluated because these shunts must be ligated or removed prior to transplantation.

POSTOPERATIVE SONOGRAPHY OF THE RECIPIENT

Postoperative sonography is performed to detect a wide variety of complications. Most institutions perform a baseline examination within 24 hours of transplant surgery.

- Examine the perihepatic regions and abdominal cavity for fluid collections and ascites.
- Examine the liver and porta hepatis for biliary dilatation. Show the full length of the common bile duct to its anastomosis. Measure its diameter.
- Use color flow and spectral Doppler to examine the following vessels for patency and direction, velocity, and character of blood flow:
  - Main, right, and left hepatic artery. Show the anastomosis.
  - Main, right, and left portal vein. Show the anastomosis.
  - Right, middle, and left hepatic vein. Confirm phasic flow.
  - IVC within, above, and below the liver. Show suprahepatic and infrahepatic anastomoses.
- The liver parenchyma should be homogeneous. Hypoechoic zones suggest infarction related to vascular complications. Solitary or multiple focal masses suggest development of hepatocellular carcinoma or post-transplant lymphoproliferative disorder.

NORMAL LIVER TRANSPLANT

- The normal hepatic artery shows a relatively low resistance Doppler spectrum with RI of 0.5–0.7 [27]. Normal systolic acceleration time is <0.1 sec.
- Flow in the portal vein is flat and toward the liver [27].
- Flow in the hepatic veins is multiphasic reflecting cardiac contractions. Flow is into the IVC.
- A margin of the liver may be irregular or ill-defined if partial resection was performed to allow the liver to "fit" in the recipient. This is especially common in children [28].

- The biliary tree has a normal non-dilated appearance. A T-tube is usually left in place crossing the biliary anastomosis postoperatively. Air may be seen in the biliary tree if the anastomosis is a choledochojejunostomy.
- Periportal edema is normally present (~21%) in the postoperative period [28].
- Right adrenal hemorrhage occurs in ~4% of patients because of clamping of the adrenal vein during creation of the IVC anastomosis. These resolve spontaneously without treatment [28].

Complications of Liver Transplantation

Vascular Complications. Vascular complications are routinely detected on US examination and are confirmed by angiography [23,27].

Vascular complications are a common and serious cause of patient morbidity and mortality in liver transplantation.

- **Hepatic artery thrombosis** is the most common vascular complication affecting 4–22% of adults and up to 42% of pediatric patients [23]. Most cases occur in the first 3 months after surgery. The condition is a life-threatening emergency that usually requires retransplantation.
  - Blood flow in the proper hepatic and intrahepatic arteries is absent.
  - Because the donor bile duct depends entirely on the hepatic artery for its blood supply, arterial thrombosis is associated with bile duct ischemia, infarction, bile leaks, and bilomas.
  - Hepatic infarction and intrahepatic abscess may be present.
  - False positive diagnosis may occur with severe rejection or high-grade stenosis with very slow intrahepatic flow. Angiographic confirmation of the diagnosis of hepatic artery thrombosis is recommended.
  - False negative diagnosis occurs when collateral arteries have developed and flow remains present in intrahepatic arteries. Tardus parvus waveform in the intrahepatic arteries suggests this possibility.
- **Hepatic artery stenosis** (~11% of transplants) usually occurs at the anastomotic site. Balloon angioplasty has been reported to be successful in treatment.
  - Focal velocities >2–3 m/sec with associated turbulence are found at or just distal to the arterial anastomosis.
  - Tardus parvus waveform in intrahepatic arteries is highly indicative of hepatic artery stenosis [29]. This finding is particularly valuable when the hepatic artery anastomosis is not adequately visualized and when angle-corrected velocities in the hepatic artery cannot be obtained. Acceleration time is >0.1 sec and RI is <0.5 [30].
  - Biliary complications are significantly more common in patients with hepatic artery stenosis [31].
- **Portal vein thrombosis** is less common (3%) and may be complete or partial.
  - With complete thrombosis, clot fills and distends the portal vein. Doppler shows no blood flow.
  - With partial thrombosis, Doppler shows a channel of flowing blood around the intraluminal thrombus.
- **Portal vein stenosis** results from faulty surgical technique or a mismatch in size of the donor and recipient veins.
  - US shows focal narrowing of the portal vein (<2.5 mm) [32].
  - Doppler shows aliasing flow jet formation at the site of narrowing with a 3–4-fold increase in venous flow velocity.
  - Flow direction may be reversed in the SMV and splenic vein.
  - Enlarged porto-systemic collateral veins may be visualized.
- **IVC thrombosis** shows intraluminal clot and absent blood flow.
- **IVC stenosis** occurs at either anastomotic site.
  - Aliasing and increased flow velocity is evident at or just beyond the stenosis.
  - Hepatic veins and the intrahepatic IVC show a loss of their normal phasic pattern when the stenosis is suprahepatic. Hepatic veins may be dilated [33].

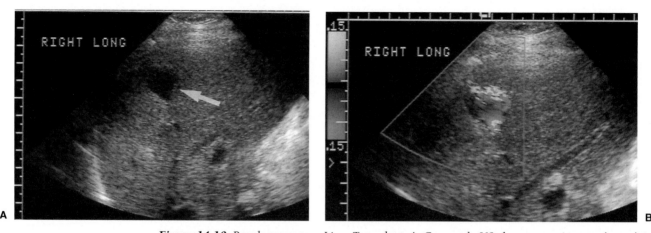

Figure 14.10 *Pseudoaneurysm—Liver Transplant. A.* Gray-scale US shows a cystic mass (*arrow*) in the liver. *B.* Color Doppler confirms swirling blood flow in the cystic mass. The pseudoaneurysm was a complication of biopsy of the liver transplant (see Color Figure 14.10).

     – The liver is commonly enlarged and edematous with stenosis at the upper anastomosis.
     – Stenosis at the lower anastomosis is less common and may present with lower extremity edema.
■ **Pseudoaneurysms** occur at the hepatic artery anastomosis or are intrahepatic resulting as a complication of needle biopsy of the transplant [27].
     – US shows a cystic structure containing arterial blood flow (Fig. 14.10).

Biliary Complications. Biliary complications occur in 13–25% of liver transplants with a significantly higher incidence in children [23,34].

> The hepatic artery is the only source of blood flow to the common bile duct in liver transplants.

■ **Bile leaks** usually occur at the site of biliary anastomosis. Fluid collections form at the site of the leak. Bile leaks are confirmed by cholangiography or scintigraphy. A T-tube is routinely placed during transplantation to allow healing of the anastomosis and easy access to the biliary tree. A stent may be placed endoscopically across the leak site to allow healing [35]. Hepatic artery stenosis decreases blood supply to the bile duct and may result in ischemic necrosis and bile leak.
■ **Bile duct strictures and obstruction** are twice as common as bile leaks [36]. Most are caused by ischemia or scarring and are also most common at the anastomotic site. Stones may form proximal to the stricture. Bile duct ischemia may result in strictures that start in the hilum and extend to the intrahepatic bile duct. Bile ducts are usually dilated above the stricture.
■ **Biliary sludge and stones** develop because of altered bile composition after transplantation or because of biliary stasis. Stones and debris may obstruct the biliary tree [37]. Endoscopic techniques including sphincterotomy are usually used for treatment [35].

Transplant Rejection. Rejection cannot be definitively diagnosed by imaging or laboratory methods. US is used to guide biopsy for histologic diagnosis.

Fluid Collections. The presence of a fluid collection is an indication for US-guided aspiration to determine its nature.

■ **Ascites** is commonly present in the postoperative period and has little significance.
■ **Bilomas** appear as anechoic fluid collections in the porta hepatis or near the biliary anastomosis.
■ **Hematomas and seromas** have the appearance previously described.
■ **Abscesses** contain echogenic fluid and commonly gas.

POSTTRANSPLANTATION LYMPHOPROLIFERATIVE DISORDERS

Immunosuppression increases the risk of cancer and is associated with a unique disease called posttransplantation lymphoproliferative disorder (PTLD) [38]. The prevalence of naturally occurring cancer is increased as much as one-hundred-fold in recipients of organ transplants. The most common tumors are squamous cell carcinoma of the skin, cervical and rectal carcinomas, and Kaposi's sarcoma.

PTLD affects approximately 2% of all organ transplants [39,40]. PTLD describes a disease of unregulated lymphoid proliferation that encompasses a spectrum from polyclonal lymphoid hyperplasia to aggressive monoclonal malignant lymphoma. The condition is associated with the presence and proliferation of the Epstein-Barr virus and the use of immunosuppressive drugs, especially cyclosporine [39,41]. PTLD may occur with any solid organ transplant but the highest rates of disease are found with lung, heart, and heart-lung transplants probably related to the requirement for greater immunosuppression. PTLD occurs more commonly with transplants in children than with transplants in adults [39]. The disease usually presents in the first year after transplantation with non-specific symptoms of fever, malaise, or dysfunction of the involved organs. The patient may be asymptomatic and the disease is discovered during routine surveillance imaging. Lymphocyte proliferation has a marked predilection for extranodal sites. The disease may affect the transplanted organ or any organ system with abdominal sites of disease being most frequent. Treatment consists of reduction or cessation of immunosuppressive therapy, acyclovir or ganciclovir to suppress the Epstein-Barr virus, and conventional antineoplastic therapy including surgical resection and anti-lymphoma chemotherapy. Untreated, PTLD is usually fatal. Even with treatment, monoclonal non-Hodgkin's lymphoma is fatal in up to 90% of adults.

> Solitary or multiple solid masses occurring within a transplanted organ suggest the possibility of PTLD.

- Extranodal disease in the abdomen is 3–4 times more common than nodal disease [39].
- Hypoechoic nodules 1–4 cm in size in the liver, kidney, spleen, or pancreas is the most common pattern of disease.
- Diffuse infiltrative disease results in hepatomegaly or liver failure.
- Infiltration of the biliary tree resulting in biliary obstruction is found only in liver transplant patients.
- Renal involvement is usually unilateral with a solitary solid hypoechoic mass.

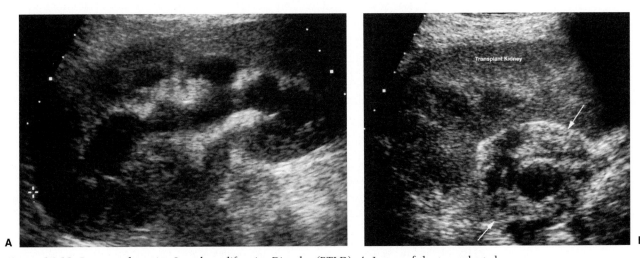

Figure 14.11 *Posttransplantation Lymphoproliferative Disorder (PTLD). A.* Image of the transplanted kidney shows hydronephrosis. Cursor (+) marks the upper pole of the transplant kidney. *B.* Image adjacent to the transplant shows a heterogeneous solid mass (*arrows*). Surgical excision confirmed a mass of confluent enlarged lymph nodes representing PTLD.

- The gastrointestinal tract is involved in 30% of cases and presents with circumferential wall thickening, aneurysmal dilatation of the bowel lumen, ulceration, and even perforation [42,43].
- Abdominal, retroperitoneal, or pelvic lymph nodes are involved in 20% of cases (Fig. 14.11). The omentum and mesentery are involved in 10% of cases [39]. Nodes are enlarged to 2–3 cm and commonly coalesce to form larger masses. Areas of internal necrosis are common. The omentum and mesentery are involved.
- Definitive diagnosis requires tissue biopsy.

TRANSJUGULAR INTRAHEPATIC PORTOSYSTEMIC SHUNT

Transjugular intrahepatic portosystemic shunt (TIPS) has proven to be effective therapy directed at treating complications of portal venous hypertension [44]. Accepted indications for placement of a TIPS are variceal bleeding not controlled by medical therapy and refractory ascites not responsive to maximal medical therapy [45]. Because TIPS are relatively short-lived, TIPS is most appropriate for patients who are candidates for liver transplantation. Contraindications for TIPS placement are intractable right heart failure with markedly elevated central venous pressure, advanced polycystic liver disease, and severe hepatic failure with encephalopathy [44].

TECHNIQUE

TIPS involves creation of a shunt between the portal vein and hepatic vein by use of a metallic vascular stent [44]. TIPS placement is generally performed via the right jugular vein, although the left jugular vein can usually be used if the right jugular vein is occluded. A 9-French, 40-cm-long angiographic sheath with 30-degree distal angulation is placed into the IVC. Fluoroscopy is used to guide the catheter into the appropriate hepatic vein. The hepatic vein of adequate diameter and angle to the portal vein is chosen for the shunt. The right hepatic vein is usually the vessel of choice, although the middle and left hepatic veins may be used. The catheter is then replaced with a transjugular hepatic puncture needle. US is commonly used to target the portal vein for puncture. The needle is advanced anteromedially and caudally 4–5 cm through the hepatic parenchyma and into the portal vein. When the portal vein is entered, the track is dilated and the flexible TIPS stent is positioned between the hepatic and portal veins. Angiography is performed to assess the filling and size of varices after shunt flow is established. Large varices may be embolized. Occasionally a second TIPS may be placed from a different hepatic vein to reduce portal pressures below 12 mm Hg. Technical success rates are reported at 95–97%. Successful control of acute or recurrent variceal hemorrhage is reported at rates of 81–94%. Ascites resolves or significantly improves in 50–83% [44].

PRE-TIPS SONOGRAPHY

Preprocedure sonography is performed to confirm patency and flow direction of the portal vein, splenic vein, SMV, hepatic veins, and jugular vein. Pre-TIPS evaluation provides a vascular roadmap for the procedure, documents the baseline vascular status for postprocedure comparison, and identifies vascular anomalies and pathology that may affect the technique [46].

- A complete abdominal sonogram is performed to assess liver size, parenchymal masses, status of the biliary system and gallbladder, spleen size, presence and severity of ascites, and presence of large portosystemic collateral vessels.
- Doppler US examination is used to document vessel size, patency, flow direction, and flow velocity of the following vessels:

- Main, right, and left portal veins.
- Right, middle, and left hepatic veins.
- Main, right, and left hepatic arteries.
- Right jugular vein. If the right jugular vein is thrombosed, the left jugular vein and left innominate vein should be evaluated for use as an alternative route of vascular access.
- While liver disease is the most common cause of ascites (80%), sonologists should carefully evaluate the patient for alternative causes, such as peritoneal carcinomatosis (caused by ovarian, colon, or pancreatic cancer), metastatic disease to the liver, and heart failure [47].

POST-TIPS SONOGRAPHY

Post-procedure US scans are usually performed at 24 hours to document shunt patency and to establish baseline flow velocities within the shunt [48]. Regular follow-up scans are performed at the request of the interventional radiologist to detect shunt stenosis and other complications.

- The liver is examined for fluid collections (hematomas, bilomas) that may occur as immediate complications of the procedure.
- The volume of ascites is compared subjectively to the pre-procedure ascites volume.
- Size of the spleen is compared to pre-procedure spleen size.
- Doppler US is used to evaluate the configuration, patency, and flow velocities in the stent.
  - Stents appear as highly echogenic fenestrated tubes 8–10 mm in diameter and 4–7 cm in length.
  - Flow velocities are obtained at the portal venous end, mid-portion, and hepatic venous end of the shunt. Angle correction is mandatory to obtain accurate flow velocity measurements.
- Doppler US is used to evaluate patency and flow direction in the portal veins and IVC. The main, right (anterior branch), and left portal veins are evaluated.

NORMAL TIPS

- The ends of the shunt protrude slightly into the portal vein and hepatic vein (Fig. 14.12).
- Color Doppler shows flow filling of the shunt from wall to wall (Fig. 14.12).
- Flow direction is continuously toward the heart. Moderate turbulence and spectral broadening are expected and are normal (Fig. 14.13).
- Normal peak velocity in well-functioning shunts is 135–200 cm/sec [49].
- Flow velocity in the portal vein is normally increased (to ~40 cm/sec) compared to pre-procedure measurements (~20 cm/sec) [49].

COMPLICATIONS OF TIPS

Procedure-Related Complications
Mortality may be as high as 3–15% within 30 days of TIPS placement, reflecting the critically ill status of many patients prior to shunt placement [50].

- Intraperitoneal hemorrhage may result from puncture of the liver capsule or injury to the hepatic artery.
- Encephalopathy occurs or worsens in 25% of TIPS patients but is usually controllable by dietary protein restriction.
- Injury to the bile ducts may cause intrahepatic bilomas or bile leaks. Fistulas between the biliary tract and the shunt may develop [51].

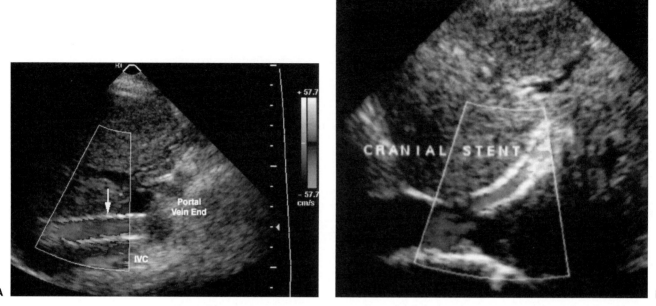

Figure 14.12 *Normal Transjugular Intrahepatic Portosystemic Shunt.* Color Doppler images show the portal (*A*) and hepatic (*B*) ends of the shunt. Note the bright wall of the shunt (*arrow*) caused by the metallic mesh (see Color Figure 14.12). IVC, inferior vena cava.

Vascular Complications

Granulation tissue covered by endothelial cells grows in to line the shunt surface within 3 weeks. Hyperplasia of this pseudointima is a primary cause of shunt stenosis. Shunt stenosis leading to shunt occlusion is the major cause of shunt failure [51].

- **Shunt stenosis** is common within 6 months of shunt placement. Shunt stenosis can often be effectively treated by balloon angioplasty, preserving shunt function. Shunt stenosis may occur anywhere but is most common at the hepatic venous end.
  - Localized increase in flow velocity with associated severe turbulence is a primary sign of shunt stenosis. Peak venous velocity ≥250 cm/sec is reliable evidence of shunt stenosis [52].
  - Reduced flow velocities throughout the shunt as compared to baseline values is additional reliable evidence of shunt stenosis. Velocities ≤50 cm/sec or maximum velocity ≤two-thirds of baseline values are indicative of stenosis [52].

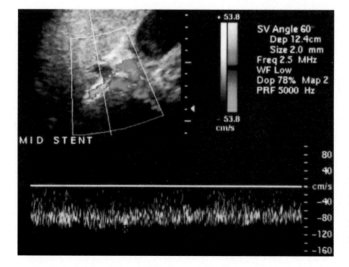

Figure 14.13 *Normal Transjugular Intrahepatic Portosystemic Shunt Spectral Doppler.* Spectral Doppler tracing obtained in the mid-portion of the shunt shows normal turbulent venous flow (see Color Figure 14.13).

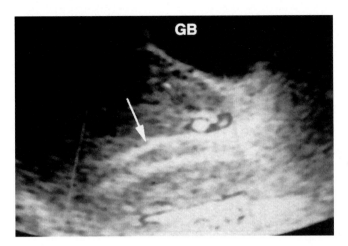

Figure 14.14 *Occluded Transjugular Intrahepatic Portosystemic Shunt.* Color Doppler image shows echogenic thrombus and no blood flow in the shunt (*arrow*) (see Color Figure 14.14). GB, gallbladder.

- A reversal of flow direction in the portal vein to hepatofugal flow (away from the liver) is a sign of severe shunt stenosis.

■ **Shunt occlusion** is irreversible and terminates function of the shunt. Occlusion commonly occurs within 2 years of the procedure.

- Thrombus fills the shunt and Doppler US detects no flow within the shunt (Fig. 14.14). Low-velocity "trickle" flow should be carefully searched for with power Doppler and spectral Doppler. Flow velocities may be very low with severe stenosis. Shunt occlusion is generally confirmed angiographically.

- Portal vein flow returns to pre-procedure direction and velocity.

REFERENCES

1. Gottlieb RH, Voci SL, Cholewinski SP, et al. Sonography: a useful tool to detect the mechanical causes of renal transplant dysfunction. J Clin Ultrasound 1999;27:325–333.
2. Brown ED, Chen MYM, Wolfman NT, et al. Complications of renal transplantation: evaluation with US and radionuclide imaging. Radiographics 2000;20:607–622.
3. Lachance SL, Adamson D, Barry JM. Ultrasonically determined kidney transplant hypertrophy. J Urol 1988;139:497–501.
4. Loubeyre P, Abidi H, Cahen R, et al. Transplanted renal artery: detection of stenosis with color Doppler US. Radiology 1997;203:661–665.
5. Martinoli C, Crespi G, Bertolotto M, et al. Interlobular vasculature in renal transplants: a power Doppler US study with MR correlation. Radiology 1996;200:111–117.
6. Kumar R, Wilson DD, Santa-Cruz FR. Postoperative urological complications of renal transplantation. Radiographics 1984;4:531–547.
7. Finlay DE, Letourneau JG, Longley DG. Assessment of vascular complications of renal, hepatic, and pancreatic transplantation. Radiographics 1992;12:981–996.
8. Dodd GD, III, Tublin ME, Shah A, et al. Imaging of vascular complications associated with renal transplants. AJR Am J Roentgenol 1991;157:449–459.
9. Claudon M, Lefevre F, Hestin D, et al. Power Doppler imaging: evaluation of vascular complications after renal transplantation. AJR Am J Roentgenol 1999;173:41–46.
10. Benedetti E, Hakim NS, Perez EM, et al. Renal transplantation. Acad Radiol 1995;2:159–166.
11. Shah AN. Radionuclide imaging in organ transplantation. Radiol Clin North Am 1995;33:473–492.
12. Low RA, Kuni CC, Letourneau JG. Pancreas transplant imaging: an overview. AJR Am J Roentgenol 1990;155:13–21.
13. Dachman AH, Newmark GM, Thistlewaite JRJ, et al. Imaging of pancreatic transplantation using portal venous and enteric exocrine drainage. AJR Am J Roentgenol 1998;171:157–163.
14. Patel BK, Garvin PJ, Aridge DL, et al. Fluid collections developing after pancreatic transplantation: radiologic evaluation and intervention. Radiology 1991;181:215–220.
15. Longley DG, Dunn DL, Gruessner R, et al. Detection of pancreatic fluid and urine leakage after pancreas transplantation: value of CT and cystography. AJR Am J Roentgenol 1990;155:997–1000.

16. Nelson NL, Largen PS, Stratta RJ, et al. Pancreas allograft rejection: correlation of transduodenal core biopsy with Doppler resistive index. Radiology 1996;200:91–94.
17. Wong JJ, Krebs TL, Klassen DK, et al. Sonographic evaluation of acute pancreatic transplant rejection: morphology—Doppler analysis versus guided percutaneous biopsy. AJR Am J Roentgenol 1996;166:803–807.
18. Snider JF, Hunter DW, Kuni CC, et al. Pancreatic transplantation: radiologic evaluation of vascular complications. Radiology 1991;178:749–753.
19. Hanto DW, Sutherland DER. Pancreas transplantation: clinical considerations. Radiol Clin North Am 1987;25:333–343.
20. Boiskin I, Sandler MP, Fleisher AC, et al. Acute venous thrombosis after pancreas transplantation: diagnosis with duplex Doppler sonography and scintigraphy. AJR Am J Roentgenol 1990;154:529–531.
21. Foshager MC, Hedlund LJ, Troppman C, et al. Venous thrombosis of pancreatic transplants: diagnosis by duplex sonography. AJR Am J Roentgenol 1997;169:1269–1273.
22. Keener TS, Cyr DR, Mack LA, et al. Sonographic diagnosis of arteriovenous fistula in pancreas transplant. J Ultrasound Med 1995;14:149–152.
23. Nghiem HV, Tran KT, Winter TC, III, et al. Imaging of complications in liver transplantation. Radiographics 1996;16:825–840.
24. Kawasaki S, Machuuchi M, Maatsunami H, et al. Living-related liver transplantation in adults. Ann Surg 1998;227:269–274.
25. Redvanly RD, Nelson RC, Stieber AC, et al. Imaging in the preoperative evaluation of adult liver-transplant candidates: goals, merits of various procedures, and recommendations. AJR Am J Roentgenol 1995;164:611–617.
26. Longley DG, Skolnick ML, Zajko AB, et al. Duplex Doppler sonography in the evaluation of adult patients before and after liver transplantation. AJR Am J Roentgenol 1988;151:687–696.
27. Glockner JF, Forauer AR. Vascular or ischemic complications after liver transplantation. AJR Am J Roentgenol 1999;173:1055–1059.
28. Westra SJ, Zaninovic AC, Hall TR, et al. Imaging in pediatric liver transplantation. Radiographics 1993;13:1081–1099.
29. De Gaetano AM, Cotroneo AR, Maresca G, et al. Color Doppler sonography in the diagnosis and monitoring of arterial complications after liver transplantation. J Clin Ultrasound 2000;28:373–380.
30. Platt JF, Yutzy GG, Bude RO, et al. Use of Doppler sonography for revealing hepatic artery stenosis in liver transplants. AJR Am J Roentgenol 1997;168:473–476.
31. Orons PD, Sheng R, Zajko AB. Hepatic artery stenosis in liver transplant recipients: prevalence and cholangiographic appearance of associated biliary complications. AJR Am J Roentgenol 1995;165:1145–1149.
32. Lee J, Ben-Ami T, Yousefzadeh D, et al. Extrahepatic portal vein stenosis in recipients of living-donor allografts: Doppler sonography. AJR Am J Roentgenol 1996;167:85–90.
33. Rossi AR, Pozniak MA, Zarvan NP. Upper inferior vena caval anastomotic stenosis in liver transplant recipients: Doppler US diagnosis. Radiology 1993;187:387–389.
34. Kok T, Van der Sluis A, Klein JP, et al. Ultrasound and cholangiography for the diagnosis of biliary complications after orthotopic liver transplantation: a comparative study. J Clin Ultrasound 1996;24:103–115.
35. Keogan MT, McDermott VG, Price SK, et al. The role of imaging in the diagnosis and management of biliary complications after liver transplantation. AJR Am J Roentgenol 1999;173:215–219.
36. Letourneau JG, Hunter DW, Payne WD, et al. Imaging of and intervention for biliary complications after hepatic transplantation. AJR Am J Roentgenol 1990;154:729–733.
37. Sheng R, Ramirez CB, Zajko AB, et al. Biliary stones and sludge in liver transplant patients: a 13-year experience. Radiology 1996;198:243–247.
38. Hoover R, Fraumeni JF. Risk of cancer in renal-transplant recipients. Lancet 1973;2:55–57.
39. Pickhardt PJ, Siegel MJ, Hayashi RJ, et al. Posttransplantation lymphoproliferative disorder in children: clinical, histopathologic, and imaging features. Radiology 2000;217:16–25.
40. Craig FE, Gulley ML, Banks PM. Posttransplantation lymphoproliferative disorders. Am J Clin Pathol 1993;99:265–276.
41. Dusenberry D, Nalesnik MA, Locker J, et al. Cytologic features of post-transplantation lymphoproliferative disorder. Diagn Cytopathol 1997;16:489–496.
42. Pickhardt PJ, Siegel MJ. Abdominal manifestations of posttransplantation lymphoproliferative disorder. AJR Am J Roentgenol 1998;171:1007–1013.

43. Strouse PJ, Platt JF, Francis IR, et al. Tumorous intrahepatic lymphoproliferative disorder in transplanted livers. AJR Am J Roentgenol 1996;167:1159–1162.

44. Kerlan RK, Jr., LaBerge JM, Gordon RL, et al. Transjugular intrahepatic portosystemic shunts: current status. AJR Am J Roentgenol 1995;164:1059–1066.

45. Crenshaw WB, Gordon FD, McEniff NJ, et al. Severe ascites: efficacy of the transjugular intrahepatic portosystemic shunt in treatment. Radiology 1996;200:185–192.

46. Foshager MC, Ferral H, Finlay DE, et al. Color Doppler sonography of transjugular intrahepatic portosystemic shunts (TIPS). AJR Am J Roentgenol 1994;163:105–111.

47. Thoeni RF. The role of imaging in patients with ascites. AJR Am J Roentgenol 1995;165:16–18.

48. Surratt RS, Middleton WD, Darcy MD, et al. Morphologic and hemodynamic findings at sonography before and after creation of a transjugular intrahepatic portosystemic shunt. AJR Am J Roentgenol 1993;160:627–630.

49. Foshager MC, Ferral H, Nazarian GK, et al. Duplex sonography after transjugular intrahepatic portosystemic shunts (TIPS): normal hemodynamic findings and efficacy in predicting shunt patency and stenosis. AJR Am J Roentgenol 1995;165:1–7.

50. Freedman AM, Sanyal AJ, Tisnado J, et al. Complications of transjugular intrahepatic portosystemic shunts: a comprehensive review. Radiographics 1993;13:1185–1210.

51. Saxon RR, Ross PL, Mendel-Hartvig J, et al. Transjugular intrahepatic portosystemic shunt patency and the importance of stenosis location in the development of recurrent symptoms. Radiology 1998;207:683–693.

52. Zizka J, Elias P, Krajina A, et al. Value of Doppler sonography in revealing transjugular intrahepatic portosystemic shunt malfunction: a 5-year experience in 216 patients. AJR Am J Roentgenol 2000;175:141–148.

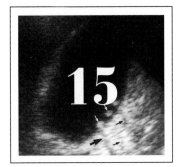

PROSTATE AND SEMINAL VESICLE ULTRASOUND

- Imaging Technique
- Anatomy
- Prostate Cancer
- Benign Prostatic Hypertrophy
- Inflammation
- Cystic Lesions

The initial enthusiasm for transrectal US (TRUS) imaging of the prostate to screen for and stage prostate cancer has dimmed considerably. Currently, in most practices, TRUS is primarily used to guide prostate biopsy and for a few specific indications, such as evaluation of male infertility and diagnosis and drainage of prostatic abscesses [1,2]. TRUS is an excellent technique for examining the seminal vesicles for diseases associated with infertility, perineal and ejaculatory pain, and hematospermia [3]. Transabdominal US imaging of the prostate through a urine-filled bladder has limited utility, but can be used to estimate prostate size.

The major indication for transrectal US of the prostate is to accurately guide prostate biopsy.

IMAGING TECHNIQUE

Using a transabdominal approach, the prostate is imaged through the fluid-distended bladder (Fig. 15.1). A 3.5–4.0-MHz sector transducer is positioned on the lower abdomen just above the symphysis pubis with the sound beam directed caudally. The prostate is examined in transverse and longitudinal planes. Prostate size is estimated and abnormalities, such as calcifications, can be demonstrated.

The transrectal approach allows the use of high-frequency 5–10-MHz transducers that provide the most detailed US examination. If transrectal biopsy is planned, the patient is routinely premedicated with antibiotics. No other patient preparation, such as an enema, is usually needed. The patient is placed in left lateral decubitus position with both knees flexed toward his chest and his head comfortably positioned on a pillow. Digital rectal examination is performed to judge the size of the prostate and to detect any palpable abnormalities. The endorectal transducer is coated heavily with US gel and is sheathed in a condom, which is also generously coated with US gel. The probe is gently placed into the rectum with the tip initially directed toward the sacrum to follow the curve of the rectum. Most endorectal transducers are end-fire sector format. Side-fire linear array transducers

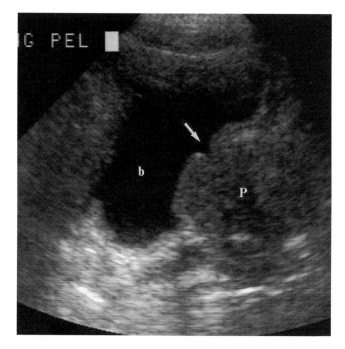

Figure 15.1 *Transabdominal US of Prostate*. Midline sagittal view through the urine-distended bladder (b) shows the enlarged prostate (P) at the bladder base. The urethral orifice (*arrow*) appears as a V-shaped notch in the prostate.

provide excellent images, but cannot be used to direct transrectal biopsy. The prostate, seminal vesicles, and periprostatic tissues are examined in transverse and sagittal planes. Color Doppler may be used to detect the vascular changes associated with prostate cancer and inflammatory conditions [4]. Images are routinely viewed inverted with the transducer

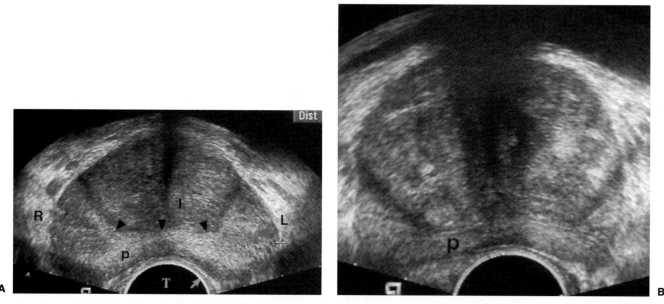

Figure 15.2 *Transrectal US of Prostate*. *A*. Transverse image of the prostate is viewed inverted with the intrarectal transducer (T) positioned at the bottom of the image. This orientation corresponds to images of the prostate as seen on CT or MR with the patient in supine position. The patient's right side (R) is displayed on the left side of the image. This scan through the mid-prostate shows the normal peripheral zone (p) to be well demarcated from and more echogenic than the hypertrophied inner gland (I). Arrowheads mark the surgical capsule. The wall of the rectum (*arrow*) is seen adjacent to the transducer. Cursors (+) measure the transverse dimension of the gland. L, patient's left side. *B*. Transverse image obtained closer to the base of the prostate in another patient shows excellent demarcation of the peripheral zone (p) from the inner gland. Compare (*A*) and (*B*) to observe that the peripheral zone is thinner near the base and thicker near the apex. The prostates of both men show the inner gland changes of BPH.

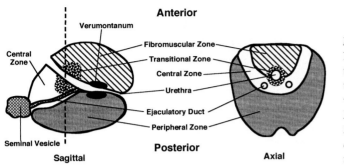

Figure 15.3 *Prostate Anatomy.* Drawing demonstrates prostatic anatomy in sagittal and transverse planes. (*Adapted with permission from Brant WE, Helms CA. Fundamentals of Diagnostic Radiology. Lippincott-Williams & Wilkins, Baltimore, 1999.*)

position at the bottom of the image (Fig. 15.2). The patient's right side is depicted on the left side of the image.

ANATOMY

The prostate is shaped like a rounded, inverted pyramid and sits on the urogenital diaphragm, just behind the symphysis pubis (Fig. 15.3). The broader **base** of the prostate supports the base of the bladder (base to base). The tapered **apex** rests on the muscular urogenital diaphragm. The **seminal vesicles** lie in the posterior groove between the bladder and the prostate. The seminal vesicles are convoluted tubes coiled to form a lobulated sac (Fig. 15.4). The terminal **ampullary portion of the vas deferens** passes medial to and joins the seminal vesicle to form the **ejaculatory duct** (see Fig. 15.6). The ejaculatory ducts course from superolateral to inferomedial in the upper half of the prostate and empty into the urethra at the verumontanum. The **urethra** runs through anterior prostate in an arching course from the bladder neck to the prostate apex. In cross-section, the urethra is horseshoe-shaped with a posterior ridge that forms the **verumontanum**. In the mid-portion of the verumontanum is a 6-mm, blind-ending sac—the **utricle**. The utricle is the müllerian remnant that forms the uterus and vagina in the female. Prostatic ducts empty into the length of the intraprostatic urethra. The prostate is enveloped by a thin but tough fibrous capsule and is surrounded by fat and a prominent plexus of **periprostatic veins**.

The prostate gland is divided into three anatomic zones and an anterior non-glandular area (Fig. 15.3). The zones of the prostate can be likened to a catcher's mitt holding a softball. The "mitt" is posterior and represents the **peripheral zone** (PZ). The PZ at the base of the prostate is thin, like the finger portion of the catcher's mitt. The PZ thickens toward the apex like the bottom portion of the catcher's mitt. The PZ encompasses only the posterolateral rectal surface of the gland, and does not extend circumferentially around the gland. The PZ contains 70% of the glandular tissue. The softball represents the "inner gland," which consists of the periurethral **transitional zone** (TZ) and the pyramidal-shaped **central zone** (CZ). The TZ constitutes only 5% of the total glandular tissue in young men, but is the site of **benign prostatic hypertrophy** (BPH) and enlarges substantially in most older men. The CZ is largest at the prostate base and tapers toward the apex, constituting 25% of

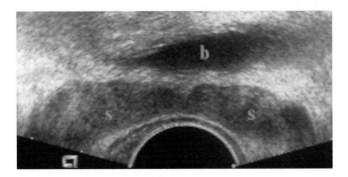

Figure 15.4 *Normal Seminal Vesicles.* Transverse image shows both seminal vesicles (s) with the normal "bow-tie" appearance. Slight asymmetry in size is a normal variant. b, bladder.

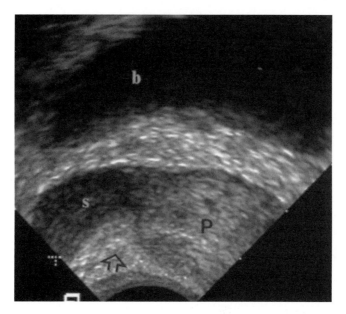

Figure 15.5 *Normal Seminal Vesicle Angle.* Lateral sagittal image shows the normal fat-filled acute angle (*arrow*) between the hypoechoic seminal vesicle (s) and the more echogenic base of the prostate (P). The bladder (b) is partially filled with urine.

the total glandular tissue. With BPH, the enlarging TZ compresses the CZ and thins the PZ. The anterior surface of the prostate consists only of fibrous and muscular tissue without acini. It is termed the **anterior fibromuscular stroma** and is not a site of disease.

Most cancer (70%) occurs in the PZ. Approximately 10% arise in the CZ and 20% in the TZ. Transurethral resection of the prostate consists of resection of the periurethral TZ tissue above the verumontanum, leaving a cavity that is continuous with the bladder lumen. Cancer in the TZ is often discovered incidentally in the tissue resected by transurethral resection of the prostate.

TRUS demonstrates the **seminal vesicles** as oval hypoechoic structures 3–5 cm long and 1–2 cm diameter. In axial plane, the two seminal vesicles have a bow-tie appearance (Fig. 15.4). Mild asymmetry in size is common. Marked asymmetry suggests tumor involvement in patients with prostate cancer. An acute angle between the posterior seminal vesicles and the base of the prostate is invested with echogenic fat. Loss of this acute angle suggests tumor invasion into the seminal vesicles (Fig. 15.5). The thickened ampullary portion of the vas deferens can often be seen separately from the seminal vesicles (Fig. 15.6).

In young men, the PZ is isoechoic with the TZ and CZ. With aging and hypertrophy of the TZ, the inner gland becomes enlarged and heterogeneous. The PZ then appears relatively hyperechoic and distinct. The tissue boundary between the PZ and the inner gland is termed the **surgical capsule** (Fig. 15.2). The urethra is identified in the midline of the prostate by looking for its V-shaped orifice at the bladder base (Fig. 15.7).

Estimates of prostate weight can be made by digital rectal examination. Measurement of prostate volume by US is easily related to weight because 1 cm³ equals 1 gm. Prostate

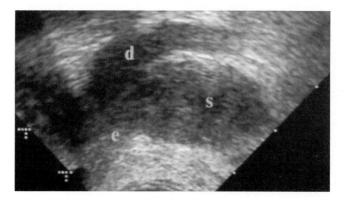

Figure 15.6 *Normal Ampullary Portion of the Vas Deferens.* Angled coronal image of the left seminal vesicle (s) shows the ampullary portion of the vas deferens (d). The junction of the vas deferens and seminal vesicle is the commencement of the ejaculatory duct (e).

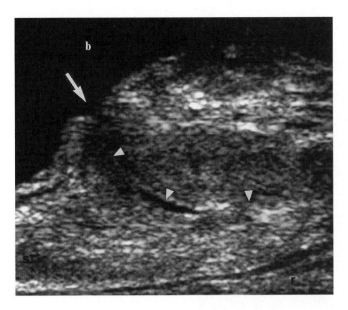

Figure 15.7 *Normal Prostatic Urethra.* Sagittal midline image of the prostate using an endorectal linear array transducer shows the prostatic urethra (*arrowheads*) and the urethral orifice (*arrow*) at the base of the bladder (b). r, wall of the rectum; s, seminal vesicle.

volume is calculated by the formula (length × width × height × 0.52 = volume). In young men the normal gland is 20 gm. In older men, the prostate is considered enlarged when it exceeds 40 gm.

PROSTATE CANCER

Prostate cancer is the most commonly diagnosed cancer in men. American men have approximately a 10% lifetime risk of having the disease and a 3% lifetime risk of dying from the disease. The incidence of prostate cancer is higher in African-American men and in men with a positive family history. TRUS was initially promoted as an effective imaging method to screen men for prostate cancer. However, its proven sensitivity in the range of 50–70% and specificity in the range of 40–60% makes it inadequate as a screening method [5]. Current American Cancer Society Guidelines for screening recommend yearly prostate-specific antigen (**PSA**) testing and digital rectal examination for all men older than age 50, and for men older than age 45 who are African-American or have family history of prostate cancer [6]. TRUS-guided biopsy is often recommended for PSA values >4 ng/mL and for palpable abnormalities [6,7].

Normal, hyperplastic, and neoplastic prostatic epithelium produce PSA. Cancers raise serum PSA 10 times as high as an equal volume of BPH tissue. PSA is organ-specific but not disease-specific. In addition to cancer, BPH, prostatitis, prostate infarction, biopsy, and surgery increase serum PSA. Serum PSA values of 0–4 ng/mL are considered normal, although up to 25% of men with prostate cancer will have PSA values in this range [6]. Values of 4–10 ng/mL are considered borderline and carry approximately a 20% risk of cancer. Values exceeding 10 ng/mL have a 67% risk of cancer. In attempts to increase the specificity of PSA, PSA density and PSA velocity calculations are used [8]. **PSA density** is determined by the ratio of serum PSA to prostate volume with values >0.12 interpreted as at risk for cancer. **PSA velocity** refers to the rate of increase of serum PSA over time. A 20% increase in serum PSA over baseline in 1 year or an absolute increase of 0.75 ng/mL in 1 year have been used as indications for biopsy.

TRUS-guided biopsy is performed using 18-gauge, spring-loaded, automated biopsy needles [9]. Because the biopsy is performed transrectally, patients are premedicated with antibiotics. Any lesions considered suspicious by digital rectal or US examination are biopsied, and 6–10 random biopsies are taken in an organized pattern to sample all areas of the gland (Fig. 15.8). Potential complications of the biopsy include hematuria, hematospermia, and infection.

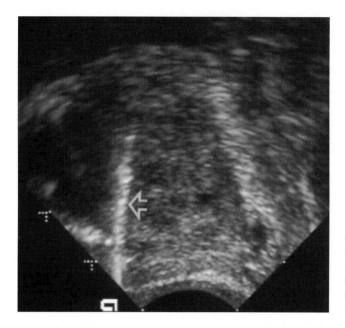

Figure 15.8 *TRUS-Guided Prostate Biopsy.* Sagittal image of the left lateral prostate shows the needle (*arrow*) in the left base region during a random pattern biopsy of the prostate.

Prostate cancer spreads by direct invasion through its capsule into the periprostatic tissues and seminal vesicles, by lymphatics to regional lymph nodes, and by venous invasion to the spine. Further hematogenous spread may extend to any organ. Findings of prostate cancer include

- Discrete nodule in the PZ.
  - Hypoechoic nodules (70%) (Fig. 15.9) are not specific for cancer. See Box 15.1 for differential diagnosis.
  - Hyperechoic/heterogeneous nodule (30%).
- Infiltrative zone in prostate glandular tissue.
  - Hypoechoic ill-defined mass is common (Fig. 15.10).
  - Cancers are isoechoic and difficult to detect by US in up to 25% of all cancers. Some lesions show mass effect, contour abnormality, asymmetry of gland size or shape, or loss of PZ differentiation from the central gland. However, most isoechoic tumors are detected only by random US-guided biopsy.

The US appearance of prostate cancer is nonspecific, and many cancers are not detected by US examination.

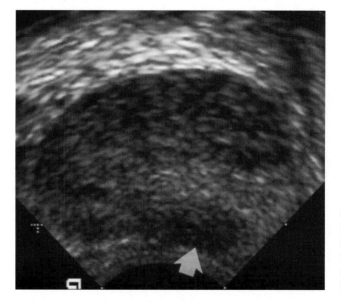

Figure 15.9 *Hypoechoic Nodule in Peripheral Zone.* Sagittal image shows an ill-defined hypoechoic nodule (*arrow*) in the peripheral zone of the prostate. Biopsy confirmed adenocarcinoma.

> ### *Box 15.1: Hypoechoic Prostate Lesion*
>
> Adenocarcinoma (20–35%)
> Benign hyperplasia, rare in peripheral zone
> Acute or chronic prostatitis
> Prostate infarction/atrophy
> Hematoma
>
> Cluster of retention cysts
> Normal prostate tissue
> Smooth muscle
> Ejaculatory duct
> Fibrosis

- Cystic lesions are very rare. Nodular soft tissue tumor is seen within a cystic mass [10].
- Focal abnormal vascularity on color Doppler US may identify cancers in the absence of gray scale US abnormalities. Focal increased vascularity or abnormal tangled vessels are signs of malignancy [11].

BENIGN PROSTATIC HYPERTROPHY

Benign hyperplasia of prostatic adenomatous tissue begins as early as age 40 and continues throughout life. By age 80, 90% of men have BPH. Starting at age 50, prostate weight doubles approximately every 10 years. Symptoms relate more to the pattern of hypertrophy than to the absolute volume of enlargement. So-called "median lobe hypertrophy" of periurethral prostatic tissues at the bladder base is primarily responsible for symptoms of hesitancy, decreased force and caliber of urine stream, dribbling, frequency, nocturia, and incomplete bladder emptying. Tissue hypertrophy occurs in the periurethral TZ and usually compresses the CZ and thins the PZ, so that the majority of the gland appears involved. The term **inner gland** is often used to describe the hypertrophied TZ and indistinguishable CZ. US diagnosis is based on the following findings [12]:

- Enlarged prostate >40 gm. The inner gland is hypoechoic compared to the PZ (Fig. 15.2). The CZ is compressed and is often not discernible.
- Inhomogeneous inner gland. The echogenicity of the inner gland is heterogeneous and the echotexture is coarse (Fig. 15.11).
- Multiple nodules. Most nodules are hyperechoic; some are hypoechoic or isoechoic.
- Calcifications. Prostatic calculi form primarily along the surgical capsule, the boundary between the hypertrophied tissue and the PZ (Fig. 15.12).
- Cystic changes. Cystic degeneration of hyperplastic nodules and retention cysts are common (Fig. 15.11).

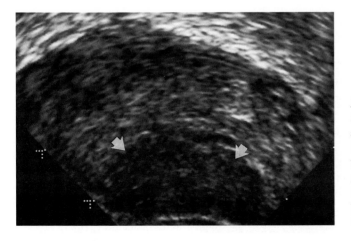

Figure 15.10 *Infiltrative Prostate Cancer.* Sagittal image shows an ill-defined hypoechoic mass (*arrows*) involving both the peripheral zone and the inner gland in the region of the prostate apex. Biopsy revealed poorly differentiated adenocarcinoma.

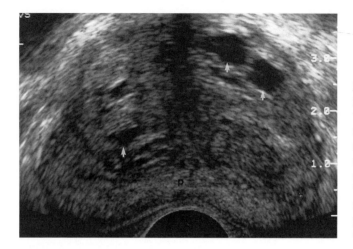

Figure 15.11 *Benign Prostatic Hypertrophy—Cystic Changes.* Transverse image through the mid-prostate shows enlargement, inhomogeneity, and cystic changes (*arrows*) characteristic of benign prostatic hypertrophy. The peripheral zone (p) is normal and slightly echogenic compared with the hypertrophied central gland.

INFLAMMATION

ACUTE PROSTATITIS/ABSCESS

Acute bacterial infection of the prostate is a clinical diagnosis with no indication for imaging. However, if symptoms fail to abate with antibiotic therapy, then abscess is suspected. TRUS is indicated to diagnose abscess and provide guidance for aspiration and drainage [13]. Prostate abscess is most common in diabetic and immunocompromised patients and in patients with indwelling urinary catheters. Causative bacteria are most commonly *Escherichia coli*, *Staphylococcus*, and gram-negative colon bacteria. Findings are

- Fluid collection with ill-defined borders, irregular walls, and occasionally septations (Fig. 15.13). Fluid may be homogeneous hypoechoic or inhomogeneous with debris. Abscesses are found primarily in the inner gland, although the PZ is commonly involved in the inflammatory process.
- Fluid collection is compressible and deforms with transducer pressure.
- Hypoechoic halo may surround the fluid collection.
- Gas in the abscess produces ring-down and comet tail artifacts.
- Color flow imaging shows periabscess hypervascularity.
- US-guided aspiration is recommended to obtain fluid for culture and for treatment by drainage. Appropriate antibiotic therapy based upon bacterial culture and sensitivity is also needed.

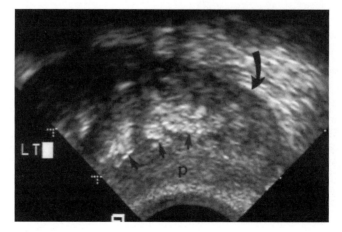

Figure 15.12 *Benign Prostatic Hypertrophy—Calcifications.* An angled transverse scan through the left base region of the prostate demonstrates calcifications, associated with benign prostatic hypertrophy, along the surgical capsule (*small arrows*). The peripheral zone (p) is normal. Note the normal sharp demarcation of the prostate (*curved arrow*) from the periprostatic fat.

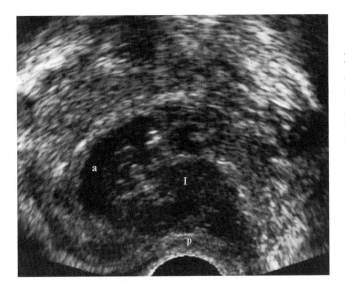

Figure 15.13 *Prostatic Abscess.* Transverse image through the mid-prostate shows heterogeneous low density in the inner gland (I) and in the peripheral zone (p) with an irregularly shaped and poorly defined fluid collection (a) that proved to be an abscess. Transrectal US-guided needle placement allowed complete aspiration with culture of the purulent material. Subsequent antibiotic therapy appropriate for the cultured *Escherichia coli* organisms resulted in complete resolution.

CHRONIC PROSTATITIS

Chronic inflammation of the prostate may be caused by incomplete treatment of bacterial prostatitis. *Chlamydia* and *Mycoplasma* may also cause chronic prostatitis. Commonly no organism is identified. Persistent symptoms include urgency, frequency, nocturia, and perineal pain.

- The prostate shows diffuse nodularity and inhomogeneous parenchyma.
- Prostatic calculi, small and in clusters or large and coarse, are common and characteristic. Calculi form in **corpora amylacea**, a proteinaceous material found in prostate glandular tissue. They are usually found near the urethra in prostatitis (Fig. 15.14), in distinction with the calcifications of BPH that form near the surgical capsule. Calculi may become infected and serve as a reservoir for relapsing bacterial infection.
- Thickening and irregularity of the prostatic capsule is common.
- Periprostatic veins may be dilated.

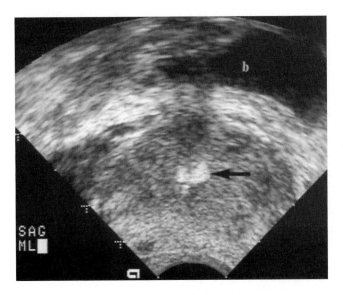

Figure 15.14 *Chronic Prostatitis.* Coarse calcification (*arrow*) in the periurethral area is characteristic of chronic prostatitis. This gland is somewhat heterogeneous but of normal size (~30 gm). Changes of chronic prostatitis are often superimposed on changes of benign hypertrophy. b, bladder.

CYSTIC LESIONS

RETENTION CYSTS

Obstruction of prostatic ductules results in cystic dilatation of glandular acini [14]. These cysts contain clear fluid and no sperm. Symptoms are rare.

- Smooth-walled unilocular cyst 1–2 cm in diameter.
- Anechoic fluid.
- Usually occur away from the midline.

CYSTIC DEGENERATION OF BPH NODULES

Cystic changes in hyperplastic nodules are common and may be caused by hemorrhage and necrosis.
- Cysts are small (<1cm) and within a nodule (Fig. 15.12).
- May contain calculi or echogenic fluid caused by hemorrhage or necrosis.

MÜLLERIAN DUCT CYST/UTRICLE CYST

Müllerian duct cysts arise from the müllerian remnant in the utricle. Utricle cysts are enlargements of the utricle. Many authors use these terms interchangeably while others believe they are two separate entities [14]. Both extend from the midline verumontanum. Symptoms depend upon size of the cyst. Most utricle cysts are small (<1 cm), whereas müllerian duct cysts are frequently large and extend well beyond the prostate.

- Midline cyst with thin walls and anechoic fluid.
- Utricle cysts commonly tubular and <1 cm in length.
- Utricle cysts fill with urine and may empty with voiding.
- Large müllerian and utricle cysts may extend well beyond the prostate and present as cystic pelvic masses.

EJACULATORY DUCT CYST

Obstruction of the ejaculatory ducts causes cystic dilatation of the duct and may be a cause of infertility, ejaculatory pain, and hematospermia [15].

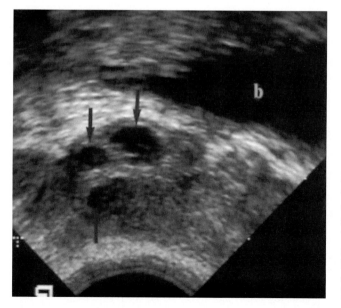

Figure 15.15 *Seminal Vesicle Cysts.* Angled transverse image of the right seminal vesicle shows three small cysts (*arrows*). This finding is strongly associated with obstruction of the seminal vesicles or ejaculatory duct, which is a cause of infertility. b, bladder.

- Cystic mass along the expected course of the ejaculatory duct.
- Small cysts are confined within the CZ.
- Large cysts may extend to the seminal vesicles [16].
- Cyst fluid contains spermatozoa.

SEMINAL VESICLE CYST

Congenital cysts of the seminal vesicles occur in association with unilateral renal agenesis, atrophic kidney, and ectopic ureter draining into the seminal vesicles [16]. Acquired cysts are found with conditions that obstruct the seminal vesicles such as infection, chronic inflammation, fibrosis, and seminal vesicle stones. Cysts also occur in association with autosomal dominant polycystic disease. Cysts of the seminal vesicles have a high association with obstruction of the vas deferens and infertility [17].

- Cystic dilatation of the seminal vesicles (Fig. 15.15).
- Dominant cyst of the seminal vesicles as large as 6–7 cm.
- Look for stones and inflammation in the seminal vesicles, obstruction of the vas deferens or ejaculatory duct, ectopic ureter, and renal anomalies.

REFERENCES

1. Melchior SW, Brawer MK. Role of transrectal ultrasound and prostate biopsy. J Clin Ultrasound 1996;24:463–471.
2. Kuligowska E, Fenlon HM. Transrectal US in male infertility: spectrum of findings and role in patient care. Radiology 1998;207:173–181.
3. Littrup PJ, Lee F, McLeary RD, et al. Transrectal US of the seminal vesicles and ejaculatory ducts: clinical correlation. Radiology 1988;168:625–628.
4. Neumaier CE, Martinoli C, Derchi LE, et al. Normal prostate gland: examination with color Doppler US. Radiology 1995;196:453–457.
5. Smith JA, Jr. Transrectal ultrasonography for the detection and staging of carcinoma of the prostate. J Clin Ultrasound 1996;24:455–461.
6. von Eschenbach A, Ho R, Murphy GP, et al. American Cancer Society guidelines for the early detection of prostate cancer: update 1997. CA Cancer J Clin 1997;47:261–264.
7. Olson MC, Posniak HV, Fisher SG, et al. Directed and random biopsies of the prostate: indications based on combined results of transrectal sonography and prostate-specific antigen density determinations. AJR Am J Roentgenol 1994;163:1407–1411.
8. Brawer MK. How to use prostate-specific antigen in the early detection or screening for prostatic carcinoma. CA Cancer J Clin 1995;45:148–164.
9. Bostwick DG. Evaluating prostate needle biopsy: therapeutic and prognostic importance. CA Cancer J Clin 1997;47:297–319.
10. Agha A, Bane BL, Culkin DJ. Cystic carcinoma of the prostate. J Ultrasound Med 1996;15:75–77.
11. Lavoipierre AM, Snow RM, Frydenberg M, et al. Prostatic cancer: role of color Doppler imaging in transrectal sonography. AJR Am J Roentgenol 1998;171:205–211.
12. Chong CL, Butler EB, Price HM, et al. Anatomy and pathology of the prostate: an overview of the prostate gland. The Radiologist 1997;4:257–276.
13. Barozzi L, Pavlica P, Menchi I, et al. Prostatic abscess: diagnosis and treatment. AJR Am J Roentgenol 1998;170:753–757.
14. Nghiem HT, Kellman GM, Sandberg SA, et al. Cystic lesions of the prostate. Radiographics 1990;10:635–650.
15. Meacham RB, Townsend RR, Drose JA. Ejaculatory duct obstruction: diagnosis and treatment with transrectal sonography. AJR Am J Roentgenol 1995;165:1463–1466.
16. King BF, Hattery RR, Lieber MM, et al. Congenital cystic disease of the seminal vesicle. Radiology 1991;178:207–211.
17. Asch MR, Toi A. Seminal vesicles—imaging and intervention using transrectal ultrasound. J Ultrasound Med 1991;10:19–23.

INDEX